INTEGRATIVE THERAPIES FOR DEPRESSION

Redefining Models for Assessment, Treatment, and Prevention

INTEGRATIVE THERAPIES FOR DEPRESSION

Redefining Models for Assessment, Treatment, and Prevention

Edited by
James M. Greenblatt, M.D.
Kelly Brogan, M.D.

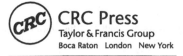

CRC Press
Taylor & Francis Group
Boca Raton London New York

CRC Press is an imprint of the
Taylor & Francis Group, an **Informa** business

CRC Press
Taylor & Francis Group
6000 Broken Sound Parkway NW, Suite 300
Boca Raton, FL 33487-2742

First issued in paperback 2021

© 2016 by Taylor & Francis Group, LLC
CRC Press is an imprint of Taylor & Francis Group, an Informa business

No claim to original U.S. Government works

Version Date: 20160406

ISBN 13: 978-1-03-224211-8 (pbk)
ISBN 13: 978-1-4987-0229-4 (hbk)

DOI: 10.1201/b19089

**Visit the Taylor & Francis Web site at
http://www.taylorandfrancis.com**

**and the CRC Press Web site at
http://www.crcpress.com**

Contents

Acknowledgments

This book was inspired by all of our patients suffering from inconsistent and ineffective treatments for depression. Our patients' desperate pleas for relief are reminders of our commitment and responsibility as treatment providers. We hope that this textbook will redefine the model for assessment, treatment, and prevention of depression.

We would like to thank all of the contributing authors for donating their time, energy, and passion in producing this textbook. We are fortunate to have collaborated with such a gifted group of dedicated clinicians and researchers in the field of integrative psychiatry to present a new model for future physicians to follow.

We also wish to thank Winnie To for her limitless administrative support and research assistance throughout this endeavor. Her organization, patience, and diligence have been instrumental in the successful completion of this project.

Finally, we would like to express our gratitude to CRC Press for giving us the opportunity and platform to help our colleagues and future physicians understand the utility of integrative approaches toward mental health care. We hope that this textbook will innervate future healthcare leaders to challenge conventional approaches and embrace the evidence-based strategies presented in this text.

James M. Greenblatt, MD and Kelly Brogan, MD, ABIHM

Acknowledgements

Foreword

Depression is one of the most serious and costly health problems facing the world today and is the leading cause of death and disability from adolescence through middle age. Approximately 15% of adults will experience severe depressed mood during their lifetimes, and approximately 15% will eventually commit suicide. Depression is the second most costly disorder in the United States, with an estimated annual cost of $80 to $130 billion.[1] Antidepressants are the third most commonly prescribed medications to Americans and the most commonly prescribed medications to Americans between the ages of 18 and 44.[2] In spite of widespread prescribing of antidepressants in developed world regions, the majority of depressed persons in North America and Western Europe do not receive adequate treatment for their symptoms with conventional prescription antidepressants.[3] This is probably the result of poor screening by mental health–care providers, underreporting by patients, and disagreement over uniform criteria for measuring response, remission, relapse, and recurrence of major depressive disorder.[4,5] There is considerable controversy over the efficacy of antidepressants in general as evidenced by the fact that among individuals who are correctly diagnosed and appropriately treated with antidepressants following American Psychiatric Association guidelines, between 40% and 70% do not respond to treatment or respond only partially,[6,7] while roughly half of patients who achieve full remission following treatment for severe depressed mood relapse within 2 years even when continuing on antidepressants.[5,8]

Individuals who do not respond or respond only partially to antidepressants have been labeled "treatment refractory." Because the average difference in drug–placebo response in randomized controlled trials of antidepressants is only 10%, a study on antidepressants in so-called "treatment-refractory" patients, which could potentially yield significant findings, would have to enroll at least 1600 patients.[9] To date neither the pharmaceutical industry nor the National Institutes of Mental Health (NIMH) has funded the large studies needed to evaluate the effectiveness of conventionally used pharmaceutical antidepressants in current widespread use to treat severe depressed mood. One side of the debate contends that the majority of drug industry–sponsored studies on antidepressants have failed to demonstrate significant response differences between antidepressants and placebos,[6,10] while the other side maintains that meta-analyses purporting to show *no benefits* of antidepressants are methodologically flawed or ideologically biased, and that rigorous analysis of findings shows that antidepressants are indeed more effective than placebos.[11] The outcome of the debate over antidepressant efficacy will probably take many more years to resolve and will ultimately rest on expert consensus over complex methodological problems involved in research designs and systematic reviews. The limitations of available conventional treatments of depression suggest that contemporary biomedical models do not adequately explain the causes of major depressive disorder and other mood disorders.

Available antidepressants are limited by adverse effects that reduce adherence, including cognitive impairment, sexual dysfunction, nausea, weight gain, and cardiovascular effects. Other unresolved issues affecting available antidepressants include unfavorable outcomes with long-term use, "paradoxical" depression-inducing effects, antidepressant-induced switching in bipolar disorder, the development of tolerance to beneficial "mood-elevating" effects, reduced efficacy when an antidepressant that was previously effective is tried for recurring depressed mood, and so-called "discontinuation syndromes" when antidepressants are abruptly stopped.

The high cost of many newer antidepressants is a serious obstacle to care for a significant percentage of depressed individuals, especially the elderly and patients on fixed incomes, who cannot afford to use a recommended antidepressant. In response to the high cost of antidepressants, it has been argued that the cost-effectiveness of many older, less expensive antidepressants and expensive recently introduced drugs is roughly equivalent.[12] In addition to general problems related to the limited efficacy of antidepressants, many depressed patients fail to improve with conventional treatment for several reasons:

- Brief medication visits covered by insurance may preclude adequate assessment and treatment planning.
- Single-drug treatments are often used at inappropriate doses resulting in poor response or high rates of adverse effects, resulting in early discontinuation before a therapeutic regimen has been tried.
- Combining two or more drugs when treating resistant depression frequently leads to a higher incidence of adverse effects, medication nonadherence, and treatment failure.
- When psychiatrists treat patients complaining of depressed mood, psychotherapy is often underutilized or not provided, resulting in diminished treatment response.
- Conventional psychiatric care stresses management of severe depressed mood with relatively less emphasis on maintenance and prevention strategies.

In the context of serious unresolved concerns about the efficacy, safety, tolerability, and affordability of conventional pharmaceutical antidepressants, select alternative treatment modalities of depressed mood are being validated by the findings of placebo-controlled studies, and in some cases systematic reviews of studies. Examples of empirically validated nonpharmaceutical treatments of depressed mood reviewed in this book include select natural products including the herbals St. John's Wort, saffron, and golden root; the vitamin folic acid; a methyl donor called SAMe; the amino acid 5-HTP; omega-3 essential fatty acids; and the pro-hormone DHEA. Select natural products including St. John's Wort, SAMe, 5-HTP, EPA (an omega-3 fatty acid), and acetyl-L-carnitine have been evaluated for their antidepressant efficacy alone or as adjuvants to prescription antidepressants. Accumulating research findings confirm that combining antidepressants with these natural products accelerates the rate of treatment response with few or no safety issues, and improved outcomes. As the authors of this unique volume point out, numerous large, well-designed studies have validated the safety and antidepressant efficacy of SAMe alone and in combination with antidepressants. Folate and vitamin B12 are required cofactors for the synthesis of SAMe, and should be taken together with SAMe for optimal results. It has been established that severely depressed persons found to have low serum folate levels are significantly less likely to respond to antidepressants; therefore, all severely depressed persons should be encouraged to take folate in a form that ensures optimal bioavailability in the brain. Depressed mood also responds to oral doses of the amino acid 5-hydroxy-tryptophan (5-HTP), the immediate precursor of serotonin, taken alone or as an adjuvant to antidepressants. 5-HTP crosses the blood-brain barrier more readily than a related molecule, L-tryptophan, and is converted to serotonin. Similar to a combined regimen of SAMe and an antidepressant, 5-HTP and antidepressants potentiate each other, resulting in a more complete and more rapid response. An important benefit of augmenting an antidepressant with a natural product is the achievement of equivalent response rates at reduced antidepressant dosages resulting in fewer adverse effects and improved medication adherence. Other nonpharmaceutical treatments of mood disorders reviewed in this book that may be safely combined with pharmaceutical antidepressants include exercise, diet, bright light exposure, and mind-body approaches. Other effective nonpharmaceutical treatments of depressed mood include exercise, mind-body therapies such as Yoga, Tai Chi, and Qigong, acupuncture, and bright-light exposure.

Dozens of expert contributing authors of *Integrative Therapies for Depression* have made an unprecedented contribution to the rapidly growing field of integrative mental health care. Through concise reviews of over 3000 published studies discussing cutting-edge research in neurobiology, nutrition, hormonal dysfunction, environmental stresses, and pharmacological and genetic factors in the pathogenesis of mood disorders, this book challenges the current limited biomedical approaches to the assessment of mood disorders. The book summarizes important emerging theories and research findings on the range of nonpharmaceutical therapies used to treat mood disorders,

including vitamins, botanicals and other natural products, exercise, bright light, mind-body practices, and spiritual approaches. Three chapters discussing rational evidence-based approaches to
integrative management of mood disorders in pregnant women, adolescents, and the elderly make
this textbook unique. This text fills an enormous gap in the conventional model of therapeutics for
mood disorders and should be required reading for psychiatrists, psychologists, family therapists,
and all clinicians who devote their days to caring for individuals afflicted with melancholia.

James Lake, MD
International Network of Integrative Mental Health

REFERENCES

1. Greden, J.F., Riba, M.B., and McInnis, M.G. 2011. *Treatment Resistant Depression: A Roadmap for Effective Care.* Washington, DC: American Psychiatric Publishing.
2. Pratt, L., Brody, D., Gu, Q. et al. 2011. Antidepressant use in persons aged 12 and over: United States, NCHS Data Brief, No 76. Hyattsville, MD: National Center for Health Statistics.
3. Demyttenaere, K., Bonnewyn, A., Bruffaerts, R. et al. 2008. Clinical factors influencing the prescription of antidepressants and benzodiazepines: Results from the European study of the epidemiology of mental disorders (ESEMeD). *J Affect Disord* 110: 84–93.
4. Simon, G., Fleck, M., Lucas, R. et al. 2004. Prevalence and predictors of depression treatment in an international primary care study. *Am J Psychiatry* 161: 1626–1634.
5. Rush, A.J., Kraemer, H.C., Sackeim, H.A. et al. 2006. Report by the ACNP Task Force on response and remission in major depressive disorder. *Neuropsychopharmacology* 31(9): 1841–1853.
6. Kirsch, I. 2008. Challenging received wisdom: Antidepressants and the placebo effect. *McGill J Med* 11: 219–222.
7. Keitner, G.I. and Mansfield, A.K. 2012. Management of treatment-resistant depression. *Psychiatr Clin North Am* 35(1): 249–265.
8. Schrader, G. 1994. Natural history of chronic depression: Predictors of change in severity over time. *J Affect Disord* 32(3): 219–222.
9. Thase, M. 2006. The failure of evidence-based medicine to guide treatment of antidepressant non-responders. *J Clin Psychiatry* 67(12): 1833–1835.
10. Kirsch, I. 2009. *The Emperor's New Drugs: Exploding the Antidepressant Myth.* London, UK: The Bodley Head.
11. Fountoulakis, K.N. and Möller, H.J. 2012. Antidepressant drugs and the response in the placebo group: The real problem lies in our understanding of the issue. *J Psychopharmacol* 26(5): 744–750.
12. Peveler, R., Kendrick, A., Thompson, C. et al. 2004. Cost-effectiveness of antidepressants in primary care Abstract 9D, Symposium 9, Recent advances in the treatment of psychiatric disorders in primary care: A U.S./U.K. perspective. APA Annual Meeting, New York, NY.

Editors

James M. Greenblatt, MD, currently serves as Chief Medical Officer and Vice President of Medical Services at Walden Behavioral Care in Waltham, Massachusetts. Walden Behavioral Care is one of the first hospitals in the country to provide a full continuum of care for patients with psychiatric disorders with programs in Massachusetts and Connecticut. Greenblatt is also an assistant clinical professor at Tufts University School of Medicine in Boston, Massachusetts. Prior to joining Walden, Greenblatt founded and served as the Medical Director of Comprehensive Psychiatric Resources, a private psychiatric practice focused on utilizing integrative medicine that has treated patients from all over the world seeking comprehensive psychiatric recommendations.

A pioneer in the field of integrative medicine, Greenblatt has treated patients with mood disorders and complex eating disorders since 1990. After receiving his medical degree and completing his psychiatry residency at George Washington University, Washington, DC, Greenblatt went on to complete a fellowship in child and adolescent psychiatry at Johns Hopkins Medical School, Baltimore, Maryland. He has lectured throughout the United States on the scientific evidence for nutritional interventions in psychiatry and mental illness.

His books, *Answers to Anorexia: A Breakthrough Nutritional Treatment that is Saving Lives* (North Branch, MN: Sunrise River Press, 2010), *The Breakthrough Depression Solution: A Personalized 9-Step Method for Beating the Physical Causes of Your Depression* (North Branch, MN: Sunrise River Press, 2011), and *Answers to Appetite Control: New Hope for Binge Eating and Weight Management* (Boston, MA: James M. Greenblatt, 2014) draw on his many years of clinical experience and expertise in integrative medicine while treating patients with eating and mood disorders. His latest book, *Preserving Memory and Optimal Brain Health*, the first of its kind, discusses the therapeutic use of low-dose lithium. *The Breakthrough Depression Solution* has been translated into Chinese and Japanese and has allowed Greenblatt to train physicians in Asia on complementary therapies for the treatment of mood disorders. Greenblatt's knowledge in the areas of biology, genetics, psychology, and nutrition as they interact in the treatment of mental illness has also led to numerous interviews by the media on television as well as in written articles for consumer audiences.

He continues to provide educational workshops and trainings for physicians across the country. He is committed to educating professionals on the limitations of the current models of treatment for mental illness, and offers practical integrative solutions based on personalized, biochemical testing.

Greenblatt is currently working on his fourth book which will discuss complementary therapies in the treatment of attention deficit-hyperactivity disorder. Greenblatt is also working on a second edition of the *Breakthrough Depression Solution* book for the consumer audience, which will feature exciting new research supporting integrative therapies for the treatment of depression.

For more information, please visit www.JamesGreenblattMD.com.

Kelly Brogan, MD, ABIHM, is a holistic women's health psychiatrist on faculty at George Washington University, Washington, DC, and in private practice in Manhattan, New York. She uses a functional medicine approach with her patients, and specializes in working with women who are pregnant or postpartum, or preconception. Brogan has been a clinical instructor at New York University School of Medicine, where she did her fellowship and a residency in reproductive psychiatry. She graduated from Cornell University Medical College, New York, and has an MA and BS from the Massachusetts Institute of Technology, Cambridge, in brain and cognitive science/systems neuroscience. She is board certified in psychiatry, psychosomatic medicine, and integrative holistic medicine, and has published widely. Her academic areas of interest include toxicology/environmental medicine, nutrition, inflammatory models of mental illness, autoimmunity, and epigenetics. She has published in the fields of psycho-oncology, women's health, perinatal mental health, alternative medicine, and infectious disease. She is on the board of Green Med Info, Pathways to Family Wellness, NYS Perinatal Association, and Fisher Wallace, and is medical director for Fearless Parent. She is a mother of two, a proud advocate of women's rights to a physiologic birth. For more information, please visit www.kellybroganmd.com.

Contributors

Myrto A. Ashe, MD, MPH
Unconventional Medicine
San Rafael, California

Bettina Bernstein, DO
Department of Psychiatry
Philadelphia College of Osteopathic Medicine
and
Department of Child and Adolescent
    Psychiatry and Behavioral Sciences
Children's Hospital of Philadelphia
Philadelphia, Pennsylvania

Peter Bongiorno, ND, LAc
Inner Source Health
New York, New York

Kelly Brogan, MD, ABHIM
George Washington University
Washington, DC
and
Private Practice
New York, New York

Richard M. Carlton, MD
New York, New York

Ralph E. Carson, LD, RD, PhD
FitRx
Brentwood, Tennessee

Emily Deans, MD
Harvard Medical School
Boston, Massachusetts
and
Wellcare Physicians Group
Norwood, Massachusetts

Susan Evans, PhD
Department of Psychiatry
Weill Cornell Medical College
New York, New York

Cynthia Gariépy, ND
Clinique Cynthia Gariépy
Québec City, Canada

Sara Gottfried, MD
Gottfried Institute for Functional Medicine
Berkeley, California

James M. Greenblatt, MD
Walden Behavioral Care
Waltham, Massachusetts
and
Department of Psychiatry
Tufts University School of Medicine
Boston, Massachusetts

Kayla Grossmann, RN
Wellness Link LLC
Boston, Massachusetts

Ann Hathaway, MD
Integrative Functional Medicine and
    Bioidentical Hormones
San Rafael, California

Natalie L. Hill, M.Div., LICSW
Smith College School for Social Work
Northampton, Massachusetts
and
Walden Behavioral Care
Waltham, Massachusetts

Bonnie J. Kaplan, PhD
Cumming School of Medicine
University of Calgary
Alberta, Canada

Jay Lombard, DO
Genomind, Inc.
King of Prussia, Pennsylvania

Barbara Mainguy, MA
Coyote Institute
Orono, Maine

Chandler Marrs, MS, MA, PhD
Lucine Health Sciences, Inc.
Henderson, Nevada

Robin May-Davis, MD
Robin May-Davis Psychiatry
Austin, Texas

Lewis Mehl-Madrona, MD, PhD
Coyote Institute
Orono, Maine
and
Departments of Family Medicine and Psychiatry
Eastern Maine Medical Center
and
Department of Psychiatry
Acadia Hospital
Bangor, Maine

Priyank Patel
Walden Center for Education and Research
Waltham, Massachusetts

Judith E. Pentz, MD
Green Lotus Healing Center
Albuquerque, New Mexico

Vesna Pirec, MD, PhD
Insight Behavioral Health Centers
Rush University Medical School
University of Illinois at Chicago
Chicago, Illinois

Lara Pizzorno, MAR, MA, LMT
SaluGenecists, Inc.
Seattle, Washington

Basant Pradhan, MD
Cooper University Hospital
Cooper Medical School of Rowan University
Camden, New Jersey

Dean Raffelock, DC, Dipl. Ac., DAAIM
Raffelock and Associates Consulting
Ashland, Oregon

Noshene Ranjbar, MD
Child and Adolescent Psychiatry Division
University of Arizona
Tucson, Arizona

Julia J. Rucklidge, PhD
Department of Psychology
University of Canterbury
Christchurch, New Zealand

Asha Shah, MD
Maine-Dartmouth Family Medicine Residency
Augusta, Maine
and
Coyote Institute
Orono, Maine

William Shaw, PhD
The Great Plains Laboratory, Inc.
Lenexa, Kansas

Healy Smith, MD, ABIHM
New York Presbyterian Hospital
Weill Cornell Medical College
New York, New York

Martha Stark, MD
Department of Psychiatry
Beth Israel Deaconess Medical Center
Harvard Medical School
Boston, Massachusetts

Gregory Thorkelson, MD
Department of Psychiatry
and
Department of Gastroenterology, Hepatology,
    and Nutrition Center for Integrative
    Medicine
University of Pittsburgh Medical Center
Pittsburgh, Pennsylvania

Kat Toups, MD, DFAPA
Bay Area Wellness
Walnut Creek, California

Antolin C. Trinidad, MD, PhD
Department of Psychiatry
Norwalk Hospital
Norwalk, Connecticut
School of Medicine
Yale University
New Haven, Connecticut

Amelia Villagomez, MD
Department of Psychiatry
Child and Adolescent Psychiatry Division
University of Arizona
Tucson, Arizona

Court Vreeland, MS, DC, DACNB
The Vreeland Clinic
White River Junction, Vermont

Barbara Wingate, MD
Rittenhouse Healing Collaborative
Philadelphia, Pennsylvania

1 Shifting the Paradigm
Redefining the Treatment of Mood Disorders

Emily Deans, MD

CONTENTS

THE ECONOMIC BURDEN OF DEPRESSION

Major depressive disorder is one of the most common mental disorders in the United States and the world. The cardinal criteria involve a period of time in which there is significantly depressed mood or loss of interest or pleasure in addition to problematic changes in functioning in at least four other areas including appetite, sleep, energy, concentration, self-esteem, and suicidal thoughts. In the United States 6.9% of adults (or 16 million people) have experienced at least one episode in the previous 12 months.[1] The World Health Organization estimates 350 million people are affected worldwide, and that in a survey of 17 countries, one in 20 people reported having a depressive episode that past year.[2]

Depressive disorders and other mental illnesses are the leading cause of disability worldwide, accounting for 37% of the healthy years of life lost from noncommunicable diseases, with depression alone accounting for one-third of this burden.[3] The societal costs of loss of mental health and productivity due to depression are also profound, though harder to pin down in a dollar amount. Still, a report from the World Economic Forum estimates the total cost of mental illness globally to be $2.5 trillion in 2010.[4] Depression is sometimes a fatal disease, particularly in combination with the frequently comorbid substance abuse.

Historically, humans have viewed depression and mental illness as caused by anything from possession by supernatural forces to imbalances of humors, with more recent viewpoints postulating that depression symptoms are caused by defects in character, resilience, or poor upbringing. Since the advent of a more biological view of psychiatry, the use of antidepressant medications resulted in a now mostly discredited theory that major depressive disorder was caused by imbalances of neurotransmitters known as the monoamines, including serotonin, norepinephrine, and dopamine.

Our pathologic understanding of the brain, mental illness, and depression in particular has increased exponentially in the past 25 years. New techniques such as functional magnetic resonance imaging (fMRI) and positron emission tomography (PET) scans give us insights into the metabolism of a living brain, while producing neuronal cells from human fibroblasts can help us understand individual genetics and the activity of neurons.

The latest biological explanation of depression, derived from a much better understanding of immunity and the body's stress response system, is the inflammatory model of depression. It is now known that depression is accompanied by chronic, low-grade inflammation, which helps explain its comorbidity with auto-immune disease, obesity, cardiovascular disease, diabetes, and other inflammatory conditions. In this model, genetic vulnerability, stressful life events, and other modulators including exposure to illnesses in life or in utero, diet, sleep, and exercise all mediate a person's level of resiliency to stress.[5] As perturbations of the system continue to add up, one can develop increasing signs of inflammation along with the symptoms of depression.

LIMITATIONS OF CURRENT TREATMENT MODELS

Despite our advances in knowledge, the recommended treatments for depression have not changed substantially over the previous two decades. The gold standard remains medications (first-line being the selective serotonin reuptake inhibitors or bupropion) in combination with psychotherapy. In general, psychiatric medications despite varying mechanisms will result in a treatment response about 50%–60% of the time, and remission about 30% of the time, with these response numbers plummeting as patients fail the first round of treatments.[6] To compare, placebo response in antidepressant clinical trials hovers around 30%–40%.[7] Some of these numbers are controversial, as it became clear that pharmaceutical companies withheld publication of negative and weak trials of blockbuster antidepressants.[8] Given that antidepressant medications can have serious side effects including agitation, hyponatremia, and severe symptoms upon discontinuation, among others, clinicians must be assured that the treatments they prescribe have more benefit than risk.

Psychotherapy has its own limitations, and the research its own set of problems, including a reluctance to admit that psychotherapy, particularly when poorly chosen or implemented, can also cause side effects.[9] In addition, while the U.S. Food and Drug Administration (FDA) keeps records of unpublished and/or failed trials of antidepressants, there is no such repository of failed psychotherapy trials. Cognitive behavioral therapy has the most data, but in general, comparison of various forms of active therapies (usually psychodynamic, mindfulness-based, or cognitive-behavioral) have shown effectiveness similar to those of antidepressant medications, generally a 50%–60% response rate, with lower total remission of symptoms, and lower rates for those who have already tried treatment before. For more severe cases, however, medication treatments are preferred, and the effectiveness of psychotherapy lessens. With knowledge of industry bias, newer reviews have continued to uphold the slight advantage of combination treatment over either medication or therapy alone.[10,11]

Clinicians and patients are left with a great deal of questions and not a small amount of frustration. Our therapeutic recommendations are based on old data and tainted by publication bias. Even the gold standard fails us nearly half of the time. Each new medication approved for major depressive disorder seems to be a "me-too" pharmaceutical, based on the old monoamine hypothesis. Stigma against mental illness continues to affect research dollars. Despite the massive global burden of depression, the National Insitutes of Health (NIH) put only $415 million into depression research in 2013, compared to $5.3 billion for cancer.[12] With no psychotherapy outperforming any other, and little industry money going to new antidepressant pharmaceuticals given the new (appropriate) scrutiny and perceived saturation of the market, it seems unlikely there will be some sort of fantastic new breakthrough treatment on the horizon.

There is some progress with the approval of some different types of therapeutics for very serious depression, such as transcranial magnetic stimulation and more research into the interesting antidepressant effects of N-methyl-D-aspartate (NMDA)-antagonists such as ketamine, but for those of us looking for low-risk, low-cost, outpatient-integrative, not requiring a fancy magnet or an anesthesiologist to work with ketamine infusions, the traditional treatment landscape remains barren. Indeed, the future seems to lie in adequate delivery of treatments and new data helping us with a more personalized and effective approach to treatment.

BRIDGING THE GAP BETWEEN THEORY AND PRACTICE

This book steps in to try to fill in some of those gaps, looking at the evidence base and science behind integrative therapies and personalized medicine for depression and how they might work.

The chapters will explain in far more detail the inflammatory model of depression, and how we can modulate both our immune system and our genetic expression itself with complementary medicine and lifestyle interventions. While some of the risk for major depressive disorder is inherited, or based on factors we cannot control (such as environment in utero), there is much we can still do to decrease the symptoms and improve quality of life beyond the psychotherapy and prescription antidepressant paradigm.

Obviously we cannot alter our genes, but the way in which our genome is expressed (also known as the "epigenome") is another matter entirely. Genes are stored within chromosomes, which are bound on proteins called histones. Various biochemical mechanisms, including methylation, acetylation, and other histone protein modifications will change how, when, and how much a certain protein is made from the genetic code within individual cells and tissues. In general, increasing methylation of histones will "silence" genes, though there are exceptions, and the complete epigenetic modulation of promotor regions, genes, and gene expression is exceedingly complex and poorly understood.

Medications can alter epigenetic expression. Monoamine oxidase inhibitors are potent inhibitors of histone demethylase LSD1, and valproate, used as a mood stabilizer, is an inhibitor of histone deacetylases. Monozygotic twins have a large accumulation of epigenetic differences as they age, giving evidence that different environmental experiences alter the expression of genes and explain how psychotherapeutic, lifestyle, and medication interventions can impact the biologic expression of depression symptoms.[13]

With our growing knowledge of inflammation, epigenetics, and personalized medicine, it is possible to help our patients in a scientific and evidence-based manner despite the limitations of the standard treatment paradigm. This textbook is an exploration of clinically relevant lifestyle and integrative medicine techniques that may be used in a meaningful way by clinicians seeking to better serve their patient with depressive disorders.

REFERENCES

1. National Institute of Mental Health, *12-Month Prevalence of Major Depressive Episode Among U.S. Adults 2012.* http://www.nimh.nih.gov/health/statistics/prevalence/major-depression-among-adults. shtml. Accessed December 28, 2014.
2. Marcus, M., Yasamy, T., Ommeren, M.V. et al. 2012. *Depression: A Global Public Health Concern.* World Health Organization, Department of Mental Health and Substance Abuse.
3. World Health Organization. 2008. *The Global Burden of Disease*, 2004 Update.
4. Bloom, D.E., Cafiero, E.T., Jané-Llopis, E. et al. 2011. *The Global Economic Burden of Noncommunicable Diseases.* Geneva: World Economic Forum.
5. Berk, M., Williams, L.J., Jacka, F.N. et al. 2013. So depression is an inflammatory disease, but where does the inflammation come from? *BMC Med* 11: 200.
6. Trivedi, M.H., Rush, J.A., Wisniewski, S.R. et al. 2006. Evaluation of outcomes with citalopram for depression using measurement-based care in STAR*D: Implications for clinical practice. *Am J Psychiatry* 163(1): 28–40.
7. Sonawella, S.B. and Rosenbauam, J.F. 2002. Placebo response in depression. *Dialogues Clin Neurosci* 4(1): 105–113.
8. Turner, E.H., Matthews, A.M., Lindardatos, E. et al. 2008. Selective publication of antidepressant trials and its influence on apparent efficacy. *N Engl J Med* 358: 252–260.
9. Barlow, D.H. 2010. Negative effects from psychological treatments. *Am Psychol* 65: 13–19.
10. DeRuebis, R.J., Siegle, G.J., and Hollon, S.D. 2008. Cognitive therapy vs. medications for depression: Treatment outcomes and neural mechanisms. *Nat Rev Neurosci* 9(10): 788–796.
11. Cuijpers, P., Turner, E.H., Mohr, D.C. et al. 2014. Comparison of psychotherapies for adult depression to pill placebo control groups: A meta-analysis. *Psychol Med* 44(4): 685–695.
12. Ledford, H. 2014. If depression were cancer. *Nature* 515: 182–184.
13. Sun, H., Kennedy, P.J., and Nestler, E.J. 2013. Epigenetics of the depressed brain: Role of histone acetylation and methylation. *Neuropsychopharmacol Rev* 38(1): 124–137.

2 The Role of Inflammation in Depression

Antolin C. Trinidad, MD, PhD

CONTENTS

INTRODUCTION

One of the most enduring core concepts in understanding clinical depression or major depressive disorder (MDD) and how it differs from other types of depression are the so-called concepts of vegetative signs and symptoms as comprising the essential features of MDD: lethargy, sleep disturbances, concentration problems, and somatic preoccupations that are not associated with observable or detectable physical abnormalities. Aches, pains, and "flu-like" symptoms are common complaints among depressed people, as is the admission: "I just do not feel that I am myself anymore." These same signs and symptoms are reproducible in situations where patients receive interferon therapy such as when they are in treatment for hepatitis C and certain forms of cancer.[1] Other symptoms in interferon therapies for these disorders can rapidly develop, such as pain, sleep disorders, and appetite problems, along with suicidal thinking. These adverse effects are considered major side effects of these treatments. Psychiatric involvement is often required or highly recommended. Interferon is a glycoprotein, in a class of compounds termed *cytokines*. It has functions in the human immune system that range from antiviral to the activation of natural killer cells and macrophages.[2] Disorders characterized by heightened activity of the immune system such as systemic lupus erythematosus, other connective tissue disorders, and coronary artery disease are associated with a high prevalence of depression.

In part because of the ability of interferon to induce MDD-like manifestations, investigators then questioned whether MDD itself is associated with, if not caused by, inflammation. Several layers of evidence now strongly implicate inflammatory mechanisms in depression. Inflammatory cytokines are elevated in the peripheral blood and cerebrospinal fluid (CSF) of people with major depression who are physically healthy.[3] Cytokines interact with many central nervous system (CNS) functions including neurotransmitter metabolism, neuroendocrine regulation, and neural plasticity. Cytokines affect the synthesis and usage of neurotransmitters that modulate mood such as the monoamines serotonin, norepinephrine, and dopamine. Some effects of increased cytokines associated with major depressive disorders (MDDs) include

- Influences the release and reuptake of monoamines
- Influences the hypothalamic-pituitary-adrenal (HPA) axis and the secretion of corticotropin-releasing hormones (CRHs)
- Decreases neurogenesis and increases apoptosis
- Impairs neuronal branching
- Decreases neuronal plasticity
- Diverges kynurenine pathway of tryptophan metabolism into a neurotoxic path

When administered to humans, cytokines stimulate the release of CRHs that then stimulate the release of adrenocorticotropic hormone (ACTH); both CRH and ACTH are known to be elevated in MDD. Although a certain level of cytokines may have trophic effects to neurons and may promote neurogenesis, an excessive level or activity of cytokines can do the opposite—it can increase apoptosis and reduce neurogenesis in some areas such as the hippocampus.[4]

HYPERAROUSAL OF THE HYPOTHALAMIC-PITUITARY-ADRENAL AXIS

In patients who have a clear-cut physical reason for inflammatory processes like autoimmune disease or even exogenous cytokine/interferon administration for therapeutic purposes, the cluster of signs and symptoms of depression may be explainable through these physiological processes. However, in patients with only MDD as the disorder without an identifiable physical abnormality, mere stress can trigger the cascade of inflammatory processes.[5]

Both the sympathetic nervous system and the hypothalamic-pituitary-adrenal (HPA) axis mediate these responses through the pulsatile release of catecholamines that can activate inflammatory signaling pathways. Although cortisol is an anti-inflammatory hormone, chronic stress can make the organism cortisol resistant. In a chronically stressed organism, high levels of cortisol are an index of both the chronic activation of the HPA axis and that organism's relative resistance to cortisol effects. Translating these findings to clinically relevant observations, hyperarousal, irritability, anxiety, and sleep disturbances are frequently seen in depression. These symptoms can be explained by a hyperarousal of the HPA axis. Depression also comes often with cognitive decline, which can be the result of cytokine-induced CNS apoptosis. Clinical and preclinical studies show that stress and depression are associated with neuronal loss in the hippocampus and limbic structures.[6,7]

While hyperarousal and associated symptoms such as anxiety and decreased sleep may promote behaviors associated with a fight-or-flight response potentially crucial for survival, they come with a price. The evidence suggests that certain structures of the central nervous system may be "worn down" through time, and that depression is a syndrome that may be a downstream effect of this process that starts much earlier. Inflammation may be the mechanism by which these processes work their way in the organism. In depression, the chronic inflammatory mechanisms themselves can induce structural changes in the brain such as hippocampal apoptosis. In turn, such structural changes can perpetuate organismal inability to cope with the stress, because the organism is less able to solve problems effectively (an example of which are the cognitive deficits that happen in major depression), thus perpetuating the cycle. This process is schematized in Figure 2.1.

However, this mechanism underlies situations wherein chronic stress happens such as in inescapable, threatening situations occurring over a period of time. Depression happens even in situations where such a dynamic is not present. In those cases, the likely mechanism is an inherently dysfunctioning inflammatory process, or an exogenously induced depression such as the administration of interferon-α in patients undergoing hepatitis C treatment.

Depression is of course heterogeneous in causation and too complex to be understood solely on the basis of one mechanism. Sex is a factor that affects the depression and inflammation relationship. It has been pointed out that the association of inflammatory markers with depression is more robust among men than it is among women.[8,9] The association of inflammation with metabolic syndrome

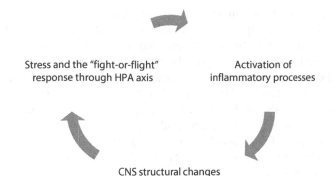

Stress and the "fight-or-flight"
response through HPA axis

Activation of
inflammatory processes

CNS structural changes

FIGURE 2.1 How stress produces CNS structural changes.

and the amount of visceral fat has been speculated as one possible mechanism—it is known that visceral fat cells release cytokines and that metabolic syndrome has been associated with increased inflammatory markers. Indeed, adipose tissues, long thought to be relatively passive storage sites of fat, are now known to function as glands, secreting various hormones and metabolically regulating substances. Because men tend to have higher quantities of visceral fat, this may explain the association with inflammation and depression as attaining a higher rate in men than in women. Other pro-inflammatory lifestyle factors such as cigarette smoking and alcohol use may be important factors as well in scrutinizing the intersection between gender, depression, and inflammation.

ACUTE AND CHRONIC INFLAMMATION

It is useful to distinguish between acute and chronic inflammation and the corresponding cascades of inflammatory changes in each category. One model of acute inflammation is experimental sepsis. In the latter state, the cytokine cascade includes tumor necrosis factor α (TNF-α), interleukin 1β (IL-1β), IL-6, IL-1ra, soluble TNF-R, IL-10, and C-reactive protein. TNF-α and IL-1 stimulate the production of IL-6, which has both pro-inflammatory and anti-inflammatory functions. In chronic, low-grade inflammation, the origin of TNF is thought to be adipose tissue. The levels of these inflammatory markers may increase several-fold, then decrease as the infection subsides. Chronic, low-grade inflammation is a state hypothesized to occur when there is a two- to threefold increase in these levels (lower amplitude than in sepsis models) over a period of time. Chronic, low-grade inflammation occurs with chronic medical disorders like diabetes, obesity, cardiac disease, and aging. In a study of elderly, depressed subjects, it has been hypothesized that the chronic inflammatory profile co-occurs with the activity of two enzymatic pathways, the indoleamine-2,3-dioxygenase (IDO) and the guanosine-triphosphate-cyclohydrolase-1 (GTP-CH1) pathways, both of which are involved in the biosynthesis of monoamines. This finding is related to increased tryptophan catabolism in turn associated with the depressive symptoms of lassitude, reduced motivation, anorexia, and pessimism. In contrast, variations in markers of GTP-CH1 activity correlated more with neurovegetative symptoms, including sleep disturbance, digestive symptoms, fatigue, sickness, and motor symptoms.[10]

Because there are high levels of circulating cytokines in obesity, it can be considered a state of chronic inflammation with or without depression. But what exactly is the relationship between obesity, depression, and inflammation? In an attempt to answer this question, a structural equation model, which makes it possible to examine the validity of competing models specifying different patterns of relations among variables, examined the relations among depression, adiposity, leptin levels, and inflammation. Using this method, there is support for a model that points to depressive symptoms promoting weight accumulation, which in turn activates an inflammatory response—in other words, the depression seems to come first, then the weight gain.[11] Indeed, depression has been associated with significant reduction in physical activity among those who are depressed.[12,13] There is also evidence that the relationship may be bidirectional: depression increases the risk for obesity, but obesity also increases the risk for depression.[14] But, other studies do not support such linear relationships—some studies question whether there is a relationship between obesity and depression at all. Despite these questions, there is a strong association in the literature between significant or extreme obesity and depression. There is also family correlation. Multivariate logistic regression analyses in a sample of 482 nuclear families segregating extreme obesity and normal weight indicated that body mass index (BMI), race, marital status, chronic medical conditions, and family history were the predicators of depression for both the genders. Thus, those with family histories of depression seem to have higher risks of obesity as well.[15] The summative idea seems to be that whatever the basic pathophysiologic mechanism is, there are intimate correlations between lowered physical activity, obesity, depression, and measures of chronic inflammation.

RESTORING HOMEOSTATIC MECHANISMS: THE ROLES OF ANTIDEPRESSANTS, EXERCISE, AND MEDITATION

The monoamine theory of depression has been the prevailing and dominant theory that explained a possible biochemical basis for major depression during the latter parts of the twentieth century. The theory posits that there lies a disorder in monoaminergic neurotransmission in the pathophysiology of major depression. The monoamine theory is at best simplistic and underplays what is involved in complex central nervous system processes that modulate stress effects. It also inadequately addresses the attendant restorative mechanisms to attain homeostasis. Inflammatory mechanisms are a sign that there exists a lack of or failing homeostasis underlying depression. To restore homeostasis thus becomes of paramount importance when considering a road to recovery. Three factors that potentially complement each other in restoring homeostatic mechanisms to counteract the adverse effects of inflammation are antidepressants, physical exercise, and meditation.

In the monoamine theory of depression, the role of antidepressants in MDD treatment has originally been conceptualized as primarily occurring through their actions on synaptic transmissions in serotonergic, noradrenergic, and dopaminergic systems in the central nervous system. Though intracellular mechanisms are also thought to be important factors in the mechanisms of antidepressant action—for example, in the case of lithium as an adjunctive/adjuvant element in certain types of depression whose actions are primarily in the cytoplasm—the specific site that has gathered the most interest is transmission at the synaptic junction. But with the recognition of inflammation as a potential factor in depression, antidepressant mechanisms beyond the synapse have been re-evaluated. In an attempt to directly attenuate inflammation in some selective serotonin reuptake inhibitor (SSRI) treatment nonresponders, the addition of celecoxib, an anti-inflammatory drug, produced greater antidepressant response, although further replication studies of this paradigm with a larger number of subjects remain lacking.[16] Again, beyond their specific actions at the synapse, preclinical and clinical studies implicate SSRI effects on various steps in the inflammatory response including the reduction of levels of TNF-α, an acute-phase cytokine produced by macrophages, and various interleukins. In one study, a group of subjects with major depression has a higher level of pretreatment TNF-α compared to controls; in post-treatment with sertraline, there was a lowering of these levels compared to those who were not treated.[17] Moreover, administration of the TNF-α antagonist etanercept to patients with moderate to severe psoriasis and ankylosing spondylitis resulted in improved symptoms of depression measured by the Beck Depression Inventory. This improvement was independent of the effect of etanercept on joint pain.[18] Although there are studies that conflict with the finding of SSRIs lowering interleukin levels, meta-analysis of the role of antidepressants generally suggests a positive correlation. The SSRIs as an antidepressant class have been shown to be particularly able to lower levels of IL-1β and IL-6. There is clinical correlation in this relationship in that the lowered levels of these interleukins also significantly lower the severity of depression in the studies that were analyzed.[19]

NEUROINFLAMMATION

Another area where the intersection of stress, depression, immunity, and antidepressant action lies is on hippocampal neurogenesis. First, neurogenesis, or the formation of new neurons, is blocked by inflammation alone. Clinical states involving CNS inflammation reduce neurogenesis, and in some cases, this effect can be diminished by anti-inflammatory drugs alone. This finding was reported in rats that underwent a bacterial lipopolysaccharide injection to induce inflammation. Neuroinflammation was blocked by indomethacin.[20] It is known that apoptosis in the hippocampus accelerates during chronic stress. Such chronicity contributes to atrophy of hippocampal structures, mediated by the HPA axis which in turn is influenced by inflammatory mechanisms. In major depression, this factor is hypothesized to underlie the cognitive decline that can accompany it as a symptom. It seems that in contrast to the effects of stress on the hippocampus, the chronic administration of antidepressants (both serotonergic and noradrenergic) increases neurogenesis or the development of new neurons. A crucial factor is chronic administration—this agrees with the well-known observation that it takes time for antidepressants to effectuate clinically observable symptomatic benefits. The subgranular zone (SGZ) of the hippocampus is one of two major neurogenic zones. Neural progenitors in the adult brain give rise to new neurons; these progenitors are particularly plentiful in the SGZ. Atypical antipsychotics, often used for antidepressant purposes, promote proliferation of neural progenitors in the SGZ and the survival of these progenitors into mature neurons. Older antipsychotics do not have these effects.[21]

PHYSICAL EXERCISE

It has been shown by several studies that physical exercise alone may have robust antidepressant properties. Exercise also promotes neurogenesis. The practical benefits of enhanced neurogenesis are most visible in aging subjects where physical exercise enhances learning and memory and executive function, and counteracts age-related brain atrophy in certain areas.[22] In the hippocampus where enhanced neurogenesis contributes to positive cognitive change, there are at least two growth factors mediating synaptic plasticity: brain-derived neurotrophic factor (BDNF) and insulin-like growth factor-1 (IGF-1). In animal studies, exercise increases BDNF in several brain regions. IGF-1 gene expression in turn is increased in hippocampal neurons as a result of exercise. There are also some suggestions that both BDNF and IGF-1 mediate the antidepressant and anxiolytic effects of exercise. While CNS IGF-1 is a growth factor, it also affects peripheral insulin functioning, in that exercise increases peripheral IGF-1, which then leads to improved insulin sensitivity. Pro-inflammatory cytokines from whatever etiology impair IGF-1 functioning; regular exercise reduces circulating pro-inflammatory cytokines, thereby restoring impaired IGF-1 functioning.[23]

There is also a relationship between exercise and the body's reaction to infection. A novel experiment to investigate this relationship is the immune activation induced by experimental infection, the infusion of low-dose *Escherichia coli*. There is a two- to threefold increase in TNF-α. If these same subjects were then subjected to 3 hours of ergonomic cycling, this burst is blunted, suggesting that exercise suppresses endotoxin-induced rise of TNF-α. The cytokine IL-6 has a unique function in that it induces anti-inflammatory cytokines such as IL-1-ra and IL-10. IL-6 also suppresses TNF-α production in in vitro studies. During rapid bursts of exercise, there is a rise of IL-6. Thus, even short bursts of exercise have shown to cause changes that can be deemed anti-inflammatory.[24]

It is, however, the customary recommendation for exercise to be regular and sustained and not just activities to be done in random fits and starts. How does long-term, regular exercise change the immunologic picture? Studies on elite swimmers in training showed lowered immunoglobulin measures.[25] These finding have been confirmed by earlier studies on athletes and intense exercise; there seems to be a lowering of lymphocytes, suppressed natural immunity, and high levels of pro-inflammatory cytokines likely associated with muscle damage. Such a dynamic brings to question the ability of intense exercise to allow subjects to resist infection. But it is likely that in sustained moderate exercise, there is greater recruitment of the HPA axis to respond and be a greater factor in the modulation of the totality of immunity. Chronic exposure to increased cytokines blunts the cortisol response. In addition to it, sustained, moderate exercise mediates the anti-inflammatory dynamic by the reduction of visceral fat mass and the reduction of circulating adipokines.[26] At this point in the discussion, the interlocking factors of physical exercise, adiposity/obesity, immune functions, and depression can be adequately appreciated: an increase in physical activity over a period of time reduces adiposity which then decreases the risk of depression, a state that is reflected in the changing homeostasis of immune measures.

MEDITATION

In terms of mental homeostasis, or keeping the mind at a steady, nonstressed condition despite the unpredictable vicissitudes of daily life, the ancient practice of meditation, traditionally associated with Asian culture and philosophy, has been known to contribute to mental well-being among its practitioners. Its role in contemporary treatments of mental illness, especially depression and anxiety, effloresced not only because of migration and a more rapid transmission of cultural practices, but also because Western-derived medical modes of healing such as pharmacological interventions have borne imperfect results in many instances; they have also induced side effects that can be intolerable to some. Many of those who suffer from mental illnesses turn to methods or interventions that deviate from the strictly biomedical models. Meditation for depression has been shown effective either as an adjunct or by itself. In discussing this intervention, it is important to start from a more basic point, which is defining what meditation is. Such a definition is crucial to discussing its effects on inflammation. Meditation is often confused with the generic phrase "relaxation exercises." However, meditation is most associated with therapeutic benefits that stem from physiologic mechanisms involving the nexus of the cortex, the HPA axis, and the immune system. For these purposes, the definition offered by Jonathan Nash and Andrew Newberg is especially cogent. They define meditation as contemplative practices that relate to "either a family of mental training techniques (the 'method definition'), or in relation to the particular altered states of consciousness that arise from the implementation of the technique (the 'state definition')".[27] They propose the inclusion of both method and state as parts of the same dynamic process that unfolds over time. The "method" thus attains the "state," which is an enhanced mental state (EMS) akin to an alteration in consciousness associated with feelings of enhanced well-being, knowledge, bliss, focus, and detachment. Such a definition relates meditation as methods and states that address levels of consciousness, alertness, and awareness. These levels in turn can be thought of as variations of cortical function. As such, the neurobiological correlates of meditation have been amply documented by functional magnetic resonance imaging (MRI) and electroencephalogram (EEG). Cortical and subcortical areas of the brain implicated in meditative states are summarized by Tobias Esch.[28]

One of the pathways by which the contemplative state attained through meditation or the EMS is by downregulation of the HPA axis. Evidence for this can be gleaned from lowered cortisol in subjects who undergo meditation.[29,30] Because meditation is a heightened function of focus and attention at least in one of its stages, this process activates the prefrontal area, particularly the right side, and the cingulate cortex. It also activates the limbic system which has rich interconnections with the hypothalamus, which then connects with the parasympathetic system to affect heart rate and respiration rate and to facilitate a sense of quiescence achieved during meditation. The locus ceruleus (LC) connects with the hypothalamus as well; activation of the LC increases the release of CRH.[31] Inhibition of the release of CRH then effectuates a corresponding change in the immunologic environment. A pool of studies show benefits of various methods of meditation on depression, anxiety, and other forms of psychological or psychiatric states.[32]

Measures of inflammatory function and the immune system have recently been included in studies of meditation as an intervention for stress, distress, and depression in an effort to study these effects at the cellular level. In a subject pool of dementia caregivers, a brief daily yogic meditation intervention reversed the pattern of increased NF (nuclear factor)-κB-related transcription of pro-inflammatory cytokines and decreased IRF1 (interferon response factor 1)-related transcription of innate antiviral response genes previously observed in healthy individuals.[33] Another study also focused on a sample of dementia caregivers; the study group, whose average age is 60 years old, underwent yogic meditation while the controls underwent relaxation training. Results showed not only significant differences in the Hamilton Depression Rating Scale (Ham-D) scores but also differences in telomerase activity, with the study group showing significantly improved telomerase activity. Telomere length has been used as a "psychobiomarker" linking chronic psychological stress and diseases in aging. A telomere is a region of repetitive DNA sequences at the end of a chromosome, which protects the end of the chromosome from deterioration. Shortened telomere length and reduced telomerase are risk factors for shortened mortality and also predict several other health and stress issues, in turn, indicative of psychological stress.[34] These findings speak to other findings in the literature suggesting that the association between inflammatory markers and depression attain a stronger relationship in aging populations, and that interventions to diminish depression and/or inflammation connote compelling results in this population.

CONCLUSION

The mental health professions have been used to conceptualizing MDD as a categorical clinical state with a set of signs and symptoms uniquely characterizing it. Whatever the physiological correlates were associated with MDD that have been observed in previous investigations, there was an implicit idea that they were epiphenomena, meaning they occur because of an independent disorder operating to produce these physiological correlates. The monoamine hypothesis was thought to be a crucial mechanism underlying MDD—it is now suspect whether it is even correct as a sole explanation. Since the discovery that measures of inflammatory states are altered in depression along with the discovery that signs and symptoms of MDD can be reproduced by the infusion of cytokines, the reverse idea has gained traction. It is now entirely possible that what we call MDD is the epiphenomenon—a constellation of signs and symptoms of an underlying bigger disorder whose clinical manifestations subsume obesity, cardiac diseases, and other chronic inflammatory conditions. The physiological nexus that entangles these conditions is a chronic dysfunction of the HPA axis and its attendant stoking of inflammatory function aberrancies. What is clear is that in terms of therapies, antidepressant medications, especially SSRIs, are a complementary (see Figure 2.2), not contradictory, intervention to attenuate the chronic inflammatory malfunction along with physical exercise and meditation.

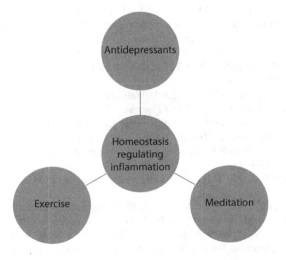

FIGURE 2.2 Complementary functions of antidepressants, exercise, and meditation.

REFERENCES

1. Koh, C., Heller, T., Haynes-Williams, V. et al. 2013. Long-term outcome of chronic hepatitis C after sustained virological response to interferon-based therapy. *Aliment Pharmacol Ther* 37(9): 887–894.
2. Gonzales-Navajas, J., Lee, J., David, M. et al. 2012. Immunomodulatory functions of type 1 interferons. *Nature Rev Immunol* 12: 125–135.
3. Raison, C.L. and Miller, A.H. 2011. Is depression an inflammatory disorder? *Curr Psychiatry Rep* 13: 467–475.
4. Kubera, M., Obuchowicz, E., Goehler, L. et al. 2010. In animal models, psychosocial stress-induced (neuro) inflammation, apoptosis and reduced neurogenesis are associated to the onset of depression. *Prog Neuropsychopharmacol Biol Psychiatry* 35(3): 744–759.
5. Zunszain, P.A., Anacker, C., Cattaneo, A. et al. 2011. Glucocorticoids, cytokines, and brain abnormalities in depression. *Prog Neuropsychopharmacol Biol Psychiatry* 35(3): 722–729.
6. Duman, R.S. 2004. Depression: A case of neuronal life and death? *Biol Psychiatry* 56(3): 140–145.
7. Lucassen, P., Meerlo, P., Naylor, A.S. et al. 2010. Regulation of adult neurogenesis by stress, sleep disruption, exercise and inflammation: Implications for depression and antidepressant action. *Eur Neuropsychopharmacol* 20: 1–17.
8. Vogelzangs, N., Duivis, H.E., Beekman, A.T.F. et al. 2012. Association of depressive disorders, depression characteristics and antidepressant medication with inflammation. *Transl Psychiatry* 2: 1–9.
9. Vogelzangs, N., Kritchevsky, S.B., Beekman, A.T.F. et al. 2008. Depressive symptoms and change in abdominal obesity in older persons. *Arch Gen Psychiatry* 65: 1386–1393.
10. Capuron, L., Schroecksnadel, S., Feart, C. et al. 2011. Chronic low-grade inflammation in elderly persons is associated with altered tryptophan and tyrosine metabolism: Role in neuropsychiatric symptoms. *Biol Psychiatry* 70(2): 175–182.
11. Miller, G.E., Freedland, K.E., Carney, R.M. et al. 2003. Pathways linking depression, adiposity, and inflammatory markers in healthy young adults. *Brain Behav Immun* 17(4): 276–285.
12. Simon, G.S., Ludman, E.J., and Linde, J.A. 2008. Association between obesity and depression in middle-aged women. *Gen Hosp Psychiatry* 30(1): 32–39.
13. Dixon, J.B., Dixon, M.E., and O'Brien, P.E. 2003. Depression in association with severe obesity changes with weight loss. *Arch Intern Med* 163(17): 2058–2065.
14. Luppino, F.S., de Wit, L.M., Bouvy, P. et al. 2010. Overweight, obesity, and depression a systematic review and meta-analysis of longitudinal studies. *Arch Gen Psychiatry* 67(3): 220–229.
15. Dong, C., Sanchez, L.E., and Price, R.A. 2004. Relationship of obesity to depression: A family-based study. *Int J Obesity* 28: 790–795.
16. Abbasia, S., Hosseinia, F., Modabberniac, A. et al. 2012. Effect of celecoxib add-on treatment on symptoms and serum IL-6 concentrations in patients with major depressive disorder: Randomized double-blind placebo-controlled study. *J Affect Disord* 141(2–3): 308–314.
17. Sutcigil, L., Oktenli, C., Musabak, U. et al. 2007. Pro- and anti-inflammatory cytokine balance in major depression: Effect of sertraline therapy. *Clin Dev Immunol* 2007: 76396.
18. Arisoy, O., Beş, C., Çifci, C. et al. 2011. FC09-05—The effect of TNFα blockers on psychometric measures in treatment resistant ankylosing spondylitis patients: A pilot study. *Eur Psychiatry* 26(1): 1862.
19. Hannestad, J., DellaGioia, N., and Bloch, M. 2011. The effect of antidepressant medication treatment on serum levels of inflammatory cytokines: A meta-analysis. *Neuropsychopharmacology* 36: 2452–2459.
20. Monje, M.L., Toda, H., and Palme, T.D. 2003. Inflammatory blockade restores adult hippocampal neurogenesis. *Science* 302: 1760–1764.
21. Manev, H., Uz, T., Smalheiser, N.R. et al. 2001. Antidepressants alter cell proliferation in the adult brain in vivo and in neural cultures in vitro. *Eur J Pharmacol* 411(1–2): 67–70.
22. Cotman, C.W., Berchtold, N.C., and Christie, L. 2007. Exercise builds brain health: Key roles of growth factor cascades and inflammation. *Trends Neurosci* 30(9): 464–475.
23. Duman, R.S. 2005. Neurotrophic factors and regulation of mood: Role of exercise, diet and metabolism. *Neurobiol Aging* 26(1): 88–93.
24. Petersen, A.M.W. and Pedersen, B.K. 2005. The anti-inflammatory effect of exercise. *J Appl Physiol* 98: 1154–1162.
25. Gleeson, M., McDonald, W.A., Pyne, D.B. et al. 2000. Immune status and respiratory illness for elite swimmers during a 12-week training cycle. *Int J Sports Med* 21(4): 302–307.
26. Gleeson, M., Bishop, N.C., Stensel, D.J. et al. 2011. The anti-inflammatory effects of exercise: Mechanisms and implications for the prevention and treatment of disease. *Nature Rev Immunol* 11: 607–615.

27. Nash, J.D. and Newberg, A. 2013. Toward a unifying taxonomy and definition for meditation. *Frontiers Psychol* 4: 1–17.
28. Esch, T. 2014. The neurobiology of meditation and mindfulness. *Studies Neurosci Consciousness Spirituality* 2: 153–173.
29. Walton, K.G., Fields, J.Z., and Levitsky, D.K. 2004. Lowering cortisol and CVD risk in postmenopausal women: A pilot study using the transcendental meditation program. *Ann NY Acad Sci* 1032: 211–215.
30. Matouseka, R.H., Dobkina, P.L., and Pruessnerb, J. 2010. Cortisol as a marker for improvement in mindfulness-based stress reduction. *Complement Ther Clin Pract* 16(1): 13–19.
31. Newberg, A. and Iversen, J. 2003. The neural basis of the complex mental task of meditation: Neurotransmitter and neurochemical considerations. *Med Hypotheses* 61(2): 282–291.
32. Hofmann, S.G., Sawyer, A.T., Witt, A.A. et al. 2010. The effect of mindfulness-based therapy on anxiety and depression: A meta-analytic review. *J Consult Clin Psychol* 78(2): 169–183.
33. Black, D.S., Cole, S.W., and Irwin, M.R. 2013. Yogic meditation reverses NF-κB and IRF-related transcriptome dynamics in leukocytes of family dementia caregivers in a randomized controlled trial. *Psychoneuroendocrinology* 38(3): 348–355.
34. Lavretsky, H., Epel, E.S., Siddarth, P. et al. 2013. A pilot study of yogic meditation for family dementia caregivers with depressive symptoms: Effects on mental health, cognition, and telomerase activity. *Int J Geriatr Psychiatry* 28(1): 57–65.

3 The Gut-Brain Axis
The Role of the Gut in Brain Health

Court Vreeland, MS, DC, DACNB and
Kelly Brogan, MD, ABIHM

CONTENTS

INTRODUCTION

Current psychiatric care has failed many patients with mood disturbances, and perhaps it's because the paradigm is incorrect. In many ways, modern psychiatry has served as a repository for the diagnostic and therapeutic limitations of conventional medicine. When a patient's symptoms of malaise, brain fog, lethargy, inattention, insomnia, agitation, and flat mood slip through the cracks of the discrete territories of specialty medicine, patients are referred for psychiatric prescription treatment. When they are treated with nonsteroidal anti-inflammatory drugs (NSAIDs), statins, acid blockers, antibiotics, and birth control pills, the mechanistic insults of these medications are poorly appreciated by prescribers, side effects are dismissed, and patients are, again, referred for psychiatric care. What happens when psychiatric care itself is predicated on medication treatment with placebo-driven short-term effects,[1–3] and worse functional outcomes in the long term?[4–6]

Escalating incidence of mood disorders may be attributable to multiple sources. Some of these include socioeconomic changes, urbanicity, dietary changes (Western-style diet), sedentary behavior, excessive screen-based information consumption, lack of adequate sunlight, reduced offline social support, and an overall disconnect from nature.[7]

The impact of these lifestyle changes may be found in transgenerational shifts to the gut microbiome—the ecology of microbes that inhabit our gastrointestinal (GI) system. Research, both recent and from the turn of the twentieth century, indicates that proper GI function might also play a role in mood disorder. Through several factors like microbial balance, gut barrier integrity, immune stimulation, and altered systemic inflammatory load, the health of the gut is increasingly being seen as vital to mental health.

GUT-BRAIN AXIS COMPONENTS

The gut-brain axis is complex and involves the following systems: central nervous system (CNS), neuroendocrine system, neuroimmune system, sympathetic and parasympathetic nervous systems, enteric nervous system, and intestinal microbiota.[8] Alterations of the microbiota with the stresses of everyday life and the Western lifestyle are thought to play a key role. The microbiota is best viewed as a type of inner organ. It is widely known that disruptions in the function of other organs may cause changes in CNS function. The same applies to disruptions of the microbiota. It has long been held that human fetuses are sterile at birth. This medical dogma is changing as of late with some studies on neonatal meconium showing the presence of microbial DNA.[9] Even the placenta has been found to harbor its own unique microbial fingerprint.[10] These findings suggest an integral role for microbiota from fetal to infant development that set the stage for adult health. If that is not convincing of the relevance of microbial contribution, then the sheer size of the numbers of organisms present should be.

By the age of one, the microbial profile looks similar to that of an adult, although it maintains its own individuality with respect to others.[11] Total adult load is estimated at 1800 genera, 40,000 species, 1–2 kg in weight, 100 trillion in number,[12] and possesses 100 times the genes found in the human genome.[13] Established functions of microbiota on human health are known and include regulation of the mucosal immune system, regulation of GI motility, epithelial barrier regulation, digestive and metabolic support including neurotransmitter production, and the prevention of colonization by pathogens.[8] It is perhaps through disruptions of these functions, disruptions of some yet undiscovered connection, or more likely, disruptions of a combination of these factors that changes in CNS functioning may be seen.

HISTORICAL PERSPECTIVES

It was not all that long ago that most of medicine viewed GI hyperpermeability as pseudoscience. Even less credence was given to how this permeability might affect the rest of the body or the brain. However, as far back as the early twentieth century it was suggested that microbial balance, and its subsequent purposeful manipulation, could positively affect mood. It was not uncommon to see the terms *autointoxication*, *intestinal stasis*, or *intestinal toxemia* in medical journals. Respected medical journals used the terms interchangeably, although *autointoxication* held great favor among authors. Scientists connected these phenomena to many things; however, most common among them were fatigue and mood change. While terms like *autointoxication*, *intestinal stasis*, and *intestinal toxemia* fell out of favor, and their mechanisms proved to be inaccurate, the idea of a connection between GI problems and mood never completely disappeared. Although the turn of the twentieth century was rife with what proved to be the half-truths of autointoxication, some scientists were laying the groundwork for the field of study we know today.

As early as 1904 it was observed that institutionalized adults (for mania or melancholia) had an increased blood reaction to intestinally derived *Escherichia coli*, suggesting the presence of preexisting immune priming to intestinal bacteria. In 1906, a physician from New York named Fenton Turck reported that psychological stress in laboratory animals was capable of altering gut permeability. Similarly, he showed that dietary factors could also affect permeability. In an experiment in which he fried bread in cottonseed oil for 30 minutes (likely producing trans fatty acids) and fed it to laboratory animals, he found increases in intestinal permeability as compared to control animals.

Other authors focused on the role of low-grade immune response in the genesis of melancholia. The idea of immune response and melancholia was eventually linked in 1920. Even the idea of endotoxins (an accepted concept today) has its origins 100 years ago. Turck believed these endotoxins were produced by intestinal bacteria and could get out of the GI tract, inducing systemic illness. Most of the research of the day regarding endotoxins focused on their roles in GI disorders like food poisoning. In 1913, microbiologist Arcangelo Distaso stated that nervous disorders that also included constipation and/or diarrhea as components seemed to be connected to the liberation of endotoxins from gram-negative bacteria. Distaso had very little clinical evidence to support his claim; however, it may have served as a conceptual foundation for today's research on lipopolysaccharides (LPSs).

In 1922, research first discovered what modern physicians would recognize as small intestinal bacterial overgrowth (SIBO). The physician who described it, Issac Jankelson, linked it to "neurasthenia." Neurasthenia was a term in the early twentieth century used to describe a cluster of modern day comorbidities like irritable bowel syndrome, chronic fatigue, myalgic encephalomyelitis, fibromyalgia, anxiety, and depressive disorders. In the late 1920s, physician and microbiologist Lloyd Arnold found that environmental stress, pathogenic bacteria, nutritional deficiencies, or drastic changes in diet could cause SIBO and intestinal permeability. He focused heavily on dietary effects and found that dietary factors were critically important when laboratory animals were infected with pathogens. Arnold was also one of the first physicians to consider how the paleolithic diet could affect microbiota and its effect on human survival.

Continuing in the 1920s and into the 1930s, more authors began to report on the effects of altered microbiota and intestinal intolerance for carbohydrates. This was either through direct alteration of microbiota or through reduced gastric acid production. The authors reported alternating constipation and diarrhea as well as anxiety as major presenting symptoms. They also reported improvement in symptoms with supplementation with acidophilus milk. Still other authors studying patients with mental disorders found that many (54%) demonstrated alterations in gastric acid production (as compared to 20% of healthy controls). Most of the patients demonstrated hypochlorhydria. It was concluded that because of the lack of hydrochloric acid in the stomach, bacteria that might otherwise be killed were allowed access to the rest of the GI tract, creating imbalances that eventually manifested as mood change.[7]

It was also during the early twentieth century that the contributions of diet to the microbiota balance began to be examined. In 1910, it was noted that diets high in protein increased proteolytic bacteria while reducing lactobacillus and Bifidobacterium species in cats and monkeys. Conversely, the opposite was true if animals were placed on a carbohydrate diet that also included milk. The animals in these experiments were also observed to show changes in cognition and mood. While study in the area of "autointoxication" and the microbiota-brain connection was popular in the early twentieth century, further studies conducted in the 1940s and 1950s were largely ignored and dismissed. Autointoxication fell out of favor, possibly because of the term itself. It was connected to just about every acute and chronic medical disorder of the day creating a high degree of skepticism in the medical community. Studies began to arise that contradicted the findings of the early twentieth century. This, combined with a healthy dose of skepticism and concern about newly marketed and unregulated treatments for autointoxication, doomed the brain-gut connection—at least for most of the rest of the century. There was a spark of interest in the 1960s when it was noted that antibiotics and *Lactobacillis acidophilus* could reduce cognitive symptoms associated with hepatic encephalopathy, but the interest was fleeting. With autointoxication "debunked," other theories rose to explain the connections between GI disturbance and cognitive change. Freud's theories were popular as were many other top-down explanations. The era of the somaticizing patient was upon medicine.[7]

Ultimately, poor explanation, a concept of panacea, charlatanism, and a greater interest in cognitive theories ended the autointoxication theory. Promising lines of research that could explain true gut-brain connectivity (intestinal permeability, LPS endotoxemia, probiotic strain investigation, cytokine changes) were impeded.[7] It would take another 70 years before the research would start to explore the gut-brain connection again.

"LEAKY" GUT

Given the historical perspective, it is easy to see why medicine has not received the concept of GI hyperpermeability with open arms. From a research standpoint, the concept was specifically avoided for the better part of the twentieth century. However, new lines of research support the idea of hyperpermeability and effects it might have on brain function. In order to grasp the concept of the gut affecting the brain, one must first understand the concept of "leaky gut."

According to Groschwitz and Hogan, "The intestinal epithelium is a single-cell layer that constitutes the largest and most important barrier against the external environment."[14] This barrier is *selectively* permeable. It is important that it remains selectively permeable so nutrients are properly absorbed but toxins, enteric flora, and antigens are not.[14] The absorption of antigenic substances stimulates a potent immune response that may disrupt host inflammatory balance, ultimately leading to changes in cytokines, immunity, neurotransmitters, and synaptic plasticity. Before proceeding, it is important the reader understands what cytokines are. "Cytokines are nonantibody proteins released by cells on contact with antigens and that act as intercellular mediators."[15] They may be inflammatory, anti-inflammatory, or modulatory. When the immune system is stimulated, cytokines are released and communicate with the brain. In this way, the immune system acts as a sensory organ,[14] which may influence mood.

Permeability through the GI epithelial barrier is regulated through two routes: transcellular and paracellular. The transcellular route involves selective transporters for amino acids, electrolytes, short-chain fatty acids, and sugars for passage directly through epithelial cells. The paracellular pathway is associated with transport between cells. Tight junctions, desmosomes, and adherens junctions located at the apical and lateral borders of the cells regulate paracellular flow. In an ideal scenario both paracellular and transcellular permeability remain selective and appropriate. However, there are factors that alter permeability. In vitro and in vivo animal studies have shown exogenous factors (alcohol, NSAIDs, and physical and psychological stress), cytokine production (IFN-γ, IL-4, IL-13, and TNF-α), and immune cells (T cells, mast cells, and eosinophils) change intestinal permeability. Still other studies have shown microbial dysbiosis, high fructose diet, and certain nutrient deficiencies like vitamins A and D, magnesium, zinc, and calcium also result in increased intestinal permeability.[16] This change in GI permeability is currently postulated to be a predisposing and aggravating factor in many established autoimmune and inflammatory conditions including inflammatory bowel disease, food allergy, celiac disease, and diabetes.[14]

Of particular interest with respect to intestinal permeability and its effect on host mood is the concept of lipopolysaccharide (LPS) stimulation of the immune system. LPS translocation through the gut barrier (and subsequent elevations in serum) is commonly referred to as endotoxemia. LPSs are found on the surface of gram-negative bacteria and function to stabilize membrane integrity. They elicit a very strong immune response. By far the largest potential source of LPS in the human body is the gut. Under normal circumstances, exceptionally small amounts of LPS are found circulating in the blood. This would indicate that in a healthy person, the gut barrier does a reasonably good job keeping LPS in the gut lumen. In people with disorders known to be associated with inflammation like obesity and diabetes, the levels of circulating LPS are higher, suggesting a breakdown of the intestinal barrier.[17] Immune response to gut bacteria has also been demonstrated in patients with major depression. This suggests intestinal hyperpermeability. LPS translocated through an overly permeable intestinal barrier are capable of modifying the biochemistry of the CNS. This is through its ability to stimulate a strong immune response and, therefore, shift inflammatory load. The effects of LPS stimulation on the CNS are not entirely unknown. Fever is a very good example. Exposure to LPS induces an inflammatory cytokine response via IL-1β, IL-6, and TNF-α. In turn, this stimulates cyclooxygenase 2 (COX-2) to synthesize prostaglandin E2 (PGE2) in the CNS, resulting in fever.[18]

Qin showed that peripheral LPS stimulation in animals was associated with a significant increase in neuroinflammation. In this study, LPS or tumor necrosis factor alpha were injected into adult wild-type mice. LPS injection caused a rapid spike in brain TNF-α that persisted for an astounding 10 months. Conversely, TNF-α injection caused serum and liver levels to rise for only 9 hours and 1 week, respectively. In the end, both systemic administration of LPS and TNF-α caused microglia to activate brain pro-inflammatory mediators; however, LPS was far more powerful and long lasting.

Additionally, LPS stimulation caused progressive loss of dopamine neurons in the substantia nigra. The activation of glial cells is particularly concerning as research has demonstrated activation may become continuous and uncontrolled. The resulting neurotoxicity cannot be "turned off" even if the instigating stimulus is removed.[19] Although glial activation is a necessary and protective step in the brain, chronic activation is associated with increased brain inflammation. This glial activation, perhaps driven by LPS stimulation from a highly permeable gut, leads to a pro-inflammatory state in the brain. In a susceptible person, this may cause mood disturbance. In fact, LPS stimulation and consequential systemic inflammatory response are tied to major depression. A systemic inflammatory response causes pro-inflammatory cytokine production (such as IL-6, IL-1β, and TNF-α), increased markers of T-lymphocyte activation, decreased serum zinc levels, and an increased induction of indoleamine 2,3 dioxygenase.[18] This culminates in increased brain inflammation, reduced availability of tryptophan for serotonin production, blood-brain barrier breakdown, and further degradation of gut barrier integrity.

Major depression shares significant comorbidity with inflammatory disease. Confounding factors make it difficult to determine if the patient is depressed because of an inflammatory comorbidity, or if the depression and their systemic illness are both rooted in high inflammatory load. Evidence is growing that both are likely of inflammatory origin. It has been reported by some that increased serum levels of IgM and IgA against LPS correlate to symptoms of MDD like fatigue, GI disturbance, autonomic disturbance, and subjective feelings of infection.[20] High antibody titers to LPS indicate gut barrier breakdown. With this information the picture of depression as an inflammatory disorder rooted in poor gut barrier function becomes clearer.

In a landmark study published in 2001 it was shown that, indeed, it is possible to induce mood changes in human beings with endotoxins (LPS). Reichenberg et al. showed in a double blind, crossover study, an injection with *Salmonella abortus-equi* endotoxin was associated with transient increases in anxiety and depressed mood in otherwise healthy subjects. Additionally, it was found memory was adversely affected with both verbal and nonverbal memory scores significantly reduced. The cytokine changes that were noted included increases in TNF-α, IL-6, and IL-1 receptor antagonist. The changes in mood and memory were highly correlated with levels of cytokines. Interestingly, other than a mild increase in rectal temperature, there were no other physical symptoms associated with endotoxin injection.[21] The lack of changes in physical symptoms supports the concept of persistent, low-grade inflammation disrupting mood without overt physical illness. This is what has been referred to as "sickness behavior" or behavioral adaptations to systemic inflammation that may have been evolutionarily adaptive as a means to conserve energetic resources for recovery. This concept is supported by studies demonstrating continuous, low-dose endotoxin infusion (rather than bolus) as more likely representative of human low-grade inflammation because of a sustained inflammatory response.[22] This makes sense in the context of a leaky gut as the source of endotoxin. It is likely to be a slow, steady flow of LPS into systemic circulation causing increased inflammatory load over months or perhaps years.

A hyperpermeable intestinal barrier is not selective for LPS but may also permit transit of antigenic proteins and environmental toxins. Polychlorinated biphenyls are particularly offensive chemicals and are linked to risk for depressive symptoms. In addition, they themselves can break down the gut and blood-brain barrier.[17]

CAUSES OF LEAKY GUT

So the question is, how does one develop "leaky gut?" Factors like alcohol, NSAIDs, physical and psychological stress, cytokine production, and immune cells increase intestinal permeability. Still other studies have shown microbial dysbiosis, high fructose diet, the Western diet, and certain nutrient deficiencies like vitamins A and D, magnesium, zinc, and calcium also result in increased intestinal permeability. Additionally, unnatural foods such as those treated with herbicides and pesticides and genetically modified organisms (GMOs) have been shown to alter the GI environment.

Stress is a major factor in many peoples' lives. It also breaks down the gut barrier and results in a reduced ability to control gut inflammation. Stress is a potent activator of the sympathetic nervous system (SNS) and though the SNS seems to display mild anti-inflammatory properties in the gut, the parasympathetic system has very powerful anti-inflammatory effects. As an example, stimulation of the vagus nerve in laboratory animals has been shown to prevent endotoxin-induced shock by reducing pro-inflammatory cytokine production.[23] The natural push-pull of the autonomic system means that powerful SNS activation causes decreased PNS activation resulting in a net loss of inflammatory control in the gut leading to barrier breakdown. Chronic stress also downregulates production of secretory IgA. Secretory IgA (SIgA) is an antibody produced in mucosal linings and plays a major role in host immunity. SIgA helps prevent antigens in the gut from being able to stick to the walls of the intestines. If these antigens are not excreted, they are able to produce an inflammatory response that may break down the gut barrier. Together with the intestinal microbiota, SIgA contributes to maintaining intestinal inflammatory response within physiological limits. Downregulation of SIgA, associated with stress, can have negative repercussions on intestinal function and integrity. This can take the form of increased adhesion of pathogenic agents to the intestinal epithelium and/or an altered balance of inflammation leading to greater intestinal permeability.[24]

Another mechanism that may increase permeability is the Western diet. This diet is often high in fructose and unhealthy fats. Fructose has been implicated in insulin resistance, fatty liver, and metabolic syndrome. Some studies have shown that fructose may induce fatty liver directly through increasing bacterial toxin (LPS) translocation from the gut and increased endotoxemia.[25] The fatty liver induced by fructose can be ameliorated when combined with antibiotics, suggesting that fructose may alter intestinal permeability through dysbiosis and activation of the immune system.[16] Further supporting this is the information showing that in mice who have been genetically modified not to have a specific receptor for endotoxins (and therefore cannot generate an inflammatory response), called a toll-like receptor, fructose exposure does not cause fatty liver or insulin resistance.[26] Additionally, Western diets are often high in calories. High-calorie diets are associated with higher levels of plasma LPS.[16] Excessive carbohydrate and fat intake have both been shown to increase translocation of LPS out of the gut and into the bloodstream.[27] Still more studies have shown the Western diet is able to shift microbial balance to one less favorable and more likely to produce obesity and a greater inflammatory load.[16] This all culminates in breakdown of the gut barrier in a self-perpetuating cycle of inflammation.

Vitamin and mineral deficiencies may also lead to increased gut permeability. It is through these nutrients' ability to change cytoskeletal structure or expression of tight junction proteins that they may be involved in changes in gut barrier function. Retinoic acid plays a major role in the expression of genes related to epithelial barrier and tight junctions. Vitamin A status regulates the cellular availability of retinoic acid. It has been shown that a reduction in vitamin A adversely affects barrier function and tight junction expression.[28] Similarly, magnesium deficiencies have been shown to reduce tight junction expression and reduce *Bifidobacterium* content in the gut.[29] In animal models, zinc deficiency has been shown to directly break down tight junctions and/or sensitize barrier cells to external stressors capable of increasing gut permeability like alcohol. Eventually, this leads to the breakdown of the gut barrier through zinc dyshomeostasis.[30] Finally, the vitamin D receptor (VDR) is hugely important in mucosal barrier function. It preserves junctional complexes, stimulates epithelial cell renewal, and modulates the immune function associated with mucosal barriers.[16] Further, administration of vitamin D to experimental animals increases colonic epithelial cell resistance to injury.[31]

Dysbiosis is also a cause of leaky gut. Dysbiosis is a term that is used to describe an imbalance that may develop between the "good" bacteria in the gut and the "bad" bacteria.[32] From the moment the gut is colonized, the microbiota serve an important protective function as they drive the functional interactions of all the elements of the adaptive immune system. This must be done by altering function not only within mucosal associated lymphoid tissue such as Peyer's patches, but also through structures outside of the gut like extraintestinal lymphoid tissue. This would obviously imply that the microbiota must at the very least be able to communicate with structures outside of the gut, or possibly even have access through the GI barrier. Any subsequent disruption of the balance of said microbiota may alter the permeability of the barrier.[33] As with all things in the body, homeostasis and balance are key. Microbial balance is determined by many factors, which can be separated into two categories: host genetic factors and environmental factors.[34]

At this time, genetic factors are not modifiable; however, changes in the environment occur frequently. The things that may alter microbial balance include diet, antibiotic use, psychological and physical stress, radiation, altered GI peristalsis,[35] and lifestyle factors like exercise, alcohol, and smoking. The environmental factors are capable of creating dysbiosis known to generate inflammation and are seen in inflammatory bowel disease.[34] A hallmark of inflammatory bowel disease is breakdown of intestinal barrier function, which is driven, in part, by microbiota changes. Although more study is necessary to understand the complex relationship between gut microbiota changes and gut permeability,[16] current knowledge of pathogens suggests a strong link. Common mechanisms of disruption of GI permeability include the aforementioned inflammation, altered fluid and electrolyte transport, and tight junction interference. Enteric pathogens may also create toxins and proteases, which damage cells, initiate apoptosis of epithelial cells, or disrupt cytoskeletal structure. *Vibrio cholerae* is known to disrupt barrier function by disrupting tight junctions, intestinal ion and fluid transport, and inflammatory response. Enteropathogenic *E. coli* (EPEC) is also capable of breaking down tight junctions and altering intestinal ion secretion. Finally, *Clostridium perfringens*, a common cause of food poisoning, also destabilizes tight junctions through a number of mechanisms.[14]

In the past year, there has been an exploration of the impact of herbicides such as Monsanto's RoundUp (glyphosate) on our gut microbiome. As it turns out, this chemical is very active in the disruption of beneficial bacteria via its impact on the "shikimate pathway" previously assumed not to exist in humans.

By imbalancing this flora, pesticides/herbicides also disrupt the production of essential amino acids such as tryptophan, a serotonin precursor, and promote production of p-cresol, a compound that interferes with metabolism of other "xenobiotics" or environmental chemicals, making the individual more vulnerable to their toxic effects. Even vitamin D3 activation in the liver may be negatively impacted by glyphosate's effect on liver enzymes, potentially explaining epidemic levels of deficiency.

There is also evidence that insecticidal toxins such as "Bt" are transferred into the blood of pregnant women and their fetuses, and that glyphosate herbicide transfers to breast milk.[36] Genetic modification of foods, in addition to guaranteeing exposure to pesticides and herbicides, confers risks of gene transference to human gut bacteria, even after a singular exposure.[37]

Most people think of ibuprofen as an innocuous, over-the-counter comfort for aches and pains. Some are so lulled into a sense of safety and efficacy, that they keep these pills in their purses and nightstands for even daily use. In addition to other known risks, its effects on the small and large intestine may be best summarized by Mäkivuokko et al., who state[38]: "The initial biochemical local sub-cellular damage is due to the entrance of the usually acidic NSAID into the cell via damage of the brush border cell membrane and disruption of the mitochondrial process of oxidative phosphorylation, with consequent ATP deficiency."

Resulting increases in permeability allow for luminal factors to access the immune system and to set off autoimmune and inflammatory processes. More recent evidence suggests that unbalanced gut bacteria set the stage for NSAID-induced permeability through neutrophil stimulation.[39] Damage from NSAID use is visible within 12–24 weeks of use[39]; however, more sensitive chemical testing reveals damage may develop as quickly as 2 weeks after beginning use with inflammation starting after just 3 days.[40] Recommending enteric-coated NSAIDs is not beneficial. It only shifts damage from the proximal GI tract to the distal areas.[40]

CYTOKINES AND BRAIN CHEMISTRY

With the knowledge that factors like stress, diet, microbiota changes, and other environmental factors may increase intestinal permeability leading to immune activation through LPS stimulation and subsequent inflammatory cytokine production, the behavioral effects may be best explained through the communication between body and brain.

Cytokines may act on central sites where the blood-brain barrier is weak or may actually cause breakdown of the blood-brain barrier (BBB). They may be transported in by selective transporters, therefore bypassing the BBB. Cytokines may act on peripheral nerves that send information into the CNS causing changes in feedback to the brain. Cytokines can affect the secretion of molecules that are not limited by the BBB but can themselves affect neurochemistry. Finally, immune cells that have infiltrated the CNS through an already compromised BBB can synthesize them.[40]

It has been shown that IL-1 has the capability of altering catecholamines. In experiments in rats, the injection of IL-1 increased the catabolites of norepinephrine (NE). This, of course, suggests there was an increased release of NE in response to IL-1. This response was seen globally in the brain; however, the greatest response was seen in the hypothalamus. Others have reported changes in dopamine metabolism in response to IL-1 injection; however, the data here are less consistent. Injection of IL-1β into rats in the first few days of life actually results in a permanent decrease in dopamine in the hypothalamus and supercervical ganglion. This occurs at surprisingly low doses. The mechanism by which IL-1 can create neurochemical changes appears to be through the cyclooxygenase (COX) enzymes. COX inhibitors prevent increases in 3-methoxy-4-hydroxyphenyl(ethylene)glycol (MHPG), which is a major metabolite of NE. In an interesting connection with the gut, abdominal vagotomy reduces increases in hypothalamic NE stimulated by IL-1β. This suggests the vagus may be important for proper modulation of immune response and proper neurochemical response.[41]

IL-1 may also affect serotonin and tryptophan metabolism. Interestingly, several experiments have shown that IL-1 administration increases brain tryptophan and 5-hydroxyindoleacetic acid (5-HIAA), the major catabolite of serotonin. This was not region specific. In the case of serotonin metabolism, COX inhibitors did not change the increase in tryptophan or 5-HIAA seen in the brain. Additionally, subdiaphragmatic vagotomy did not alter the serotonergic response to IL-1. According to some authors, increases in brain tryptophan and 5-HIAA are mediated by the sympathetic system because these changes can be prevented with ganglionic blockers. Therefore, they conclude that the increases in brain tryptophan reflect sympathetic activity.[41] The idea of IL-1 *increasing* brain tryptophan and 5-HIAA seems contradictory to current knowledge about depression and the serotonin hypothesis, so the question becomes, do the increased levels of 5-HIAA reflect increased turnover of serotonin? This makes sense in the context of depression, as increased serotonin turnover and mood disorder are associated.[42] Additionally, those who are depressed have demonstrated in studies higher levels of pro-inflammatory cytokines. These include IL-1, IL-6, and tumor necrosis factor.[43,44] In addition to affecting catecholamine and serotonin metabolism, IL-1 affects other neurotransmitters. Reductions in acetylcholine, glutamate, and gamma-aminobutyric acid (GABA) have been demonstrated as well as increases in histamine turnover.[41]

Interleukin-6 (IL-6) has been studied with respect to NE metabolism with no effects noted. However, changes in the HPA axis are noted in animal models as measured by plasma ACTH and corticosterone. Some authors have demonstrated IL-6 to increase 3,4-dihydroxyphenylacetic acid (DOPAC), a major metabolite of dopamine. This was particularly prevalent in the prefrontal cortex. These same authors also noted an increase in 5-HIAA in the hippocampus and prefrontal cortex.[41] Again, this may represent increased turnover of serotonin. Interestingly, IL-6 has also been demonstrated to increase serotonin itself in the hippocampus.[41] Perhaps this is related to the endocrine response to IL-6 and may not be relevant in mood disorder. More study is necessary.

Tumor necrosis factor-α (TNF-α) also activates the HPA axis, although IL-1 seems to be the most potent. TNF-α has been reported to increase brain MHPG and tryptophan, but only at very high doses. However, sensitization to TNF-α appears to be a phenomenon worth considering. Successive exposures to TNF-α produced marked enhancement in MHPG accompanied by changes in behavior such as decreases in activity and social exploration.[41]

Interferon-γ (IFNγ) has considerable effects on the metabolism of tryptophan and therefore can affect levels of serotonin in the brain. IFNγ has the capability to activate an enzyme called indoleamine-2,3-dioxygenase (IDO). IDO is found throughout the body and in human immune cells including macrophages and microglia. The vast majority of circulating tryptophan is metabolized by an enzyme called tryptophan-2,3-dioxygenase (TDO), where it is converted into kynurenine and other metabolites with the pathway eventually ending in niacin synthesis. This pathway is effective with less than 1% of circulating tryptophan being available for conversion to serotonin in the brain.[45] Under normal conditions, TDO is the dominant enzyme, however, with immune stimulation IDO can be activated. This has the effect of reducing serum tryptophan by as much as 25%–50%. This is important because the rate-limiting enzyme in serotonin production is tryptophan hydroxylase. It is only 50% saturated under normal circumstances, and therefore, serotonin synthesis varies with tryptophan availability.[45]

One can see how any reduction in serum tryptophan might present a problem. Although IFNγ is probably the most potent activator of IDO, other cytokines may activate it as well. TNF-α in combination with IL-6 or IL-1 can induce IDO, perhaps creating an additive effect of reducing tryptophan concentrations even further.[45] A human model of this phenomenon is seen in patients with hepatitis C (HCV). Patients with chronic HCV are often treated with long-term interferon therapy. Interferons also have the potential to activate IDO, albeit at a lower level.[41] Patients with HCV are treated with interferons for periods of 6–12 months. During the treatment period, up to a third of patients will report symptoms of depression (via standardized depression scales but self-reporting of depression results in even higher rates). The interferons administered increases inflammatory cytokine profiles, similar to those seen in depression. Although interferons are administered peripherally, central levels of inflammatory cytokines have been observed to rise. This is evidence of central communication. Also noted in HCV patients treated with interferons is an increase in the kynurenine:tryptophan ratio in the blood and cerebrospinal fluid (CSF). This suggests more tryptophan is being converted into kynurenine, making less available for conversion into serotonin. It also demonstrates increased activity of IDO in response to pro-inflammatory cytokine exposure.

Now that it is clear that cytokines can change neurochemistry, what about neurochemical responses to endotoxins? As it turns out, there is evidence of that as well. Administration of LPS decreases brain levels of NE; however, serotonin is not affected. Other evidence has shown small changes in dopamine metabolism to LPS stimulation. Levels of tryptophan and 5-HIAA have been shown to increase in response to LPS, perhaps more evidence of increased serotonin turnover. An experiment in rats demonstrated increases in extracellular DOPAC, NE, MHPG, and 5-HIAA after LPS injection.[41] Clearly, whether the mechanism affecting brain chemistry is through cytokine stimulation, direct LPS stimulation, or both, an effect is observed, and addressing this in the depressed patient might prove therapeutically valuable.

GUT-BRAIN COMMUNICATION

It is becoming quite clear that a bidirectional relationship exists between the human GI tract and the rest of the body, including the central nervous system. As with all bidirectional relationships, functional integrity of each system is required for optimal performance. A major part of this bidirectional system is the microbiota.

MICROBIAL EFFECTS ON THE CNS

The effects of microbial balance on CNS function begin early in life. The HPA axis is a neuroendocrine system. It may be thought of as a system that is highly subject to changes in the environment and is highly programmable. It has been shown that HPA response is different in animals that are handled and cared for as neonates versus animals who experience maternal deprivation. Maternal deprivation causes exaggerated HPA response to stress, and this response exists throughout the life of the animal. This altered HPA response is associated with the incidence of age-related neuropathology. It has been speculated that because of the bidirectional relationship early in life between neural and immune systems at a time when the CNS is particularly susceptible to environmental influences, microbial colonization and subsequent effects on the immune system might alter the development of HPA responsiveness. This has been demonstrated in animals, with genetically engineered germ-free mice displaying exaggerated HPA response to mild stress. This response can be corrected by colonization from pathogen-free controls in the experiment. Additionally, it was shown that colonizing the germ-free mice with enteropathogenic *E. coli* could actually increase the stress response. This suggests that not only is the presence of commensal bacteria critical, but the absence of pathogens may be as well. Another important finding from the study was a reduction of brain-derived neurotrophic factor (BDNF) and reduced protein levels in the cortex and hippocampus of germ-free mice compared to pathogen-free mice. This is an important factor because BDNF is involved in many regulatory processes in the brain, including mood and cognition.[46] In addition, levels of norepinephrine and serotonin have been shown to be reduced in germ-free animals. This was noted in both the hippocampus and cortex.[47] Conclusions can be made that postnatal colonization may play a significant role in early development and can have long-lasting impacts on sensory and neural processing of information as it relates to endocrine response to stress.[46] This information is quite suggestive, and most authors are showing that there is a critical window for colonization of the gut. After this window, the addition of bacteria from pathogen-free mice is not effective in reducing the stress response. If nothing else, this has implications on the high rate of cesarean births in the United States.

Changes in HPA axis function are well documented in depression. The connection is so strong that some authors consider it to be a causal factor. Elevated serum cortisol and CSF corticotropin-releasing hormone is well documented in the depressed patient. Stress is also linked to changes in the HPA axis. As reviewed previously, stress also affects gut immunity and gut barrier integrity. Stress has another effect. It has been shown to alter the microbiome. It can promote the growth of pathogenic *E. coli* O157:H7.[47] The brain itself has been shown to be responsive to the introduction of bacteria into the GI tract. This connection is thought to be from an immune response communicated to the brain via the vagus nerve. In one experiment, *Salmonella* Typhimurium (STM) was introduced into the stomach of mice to mimic an infection. STM also infects humans. STM-induced activation of the paraventricular nucleus and the supraoptic nucleus was seen,[48] and the introduction of bacteria to mice has been shown to produce anxiety-like behavior.[49] The question remains, does the stress alter the bacterial profile significantly enough to change CNS signaling, or does microbial overgrowth increase perceived stress? A combination of both is likely.

Still other evidence has shown gut microbiota can influence not only visceral pain perception (an easy connection to make) but also somatic pain. This information is further support for a connection between the microbiome and the CNS.[47]

Animal studies support the theory that microbiota can affect behavior. In mice, subclinical oral administration of *Campylobacter jejuni* produced anxiety. Perhaps more interesting is that the brainstem was also shown to be active in these animals. The communication line is likely the vagus. The information sent to the CNS from a stimulus like *Campylobacter jejuni* ultimately leads to autonomic, neuroendocrine, and behavioral change. Other studies have shown that dietary-induced changes designed to increase the diversity of the microbiome had a positive effect on memory and reduced anxiety-like behavior.[47]

The next logical step then is to understand just how microbial changes may be able to directly affect the CNS. It is well accepted that the commensal organisms present in the gut produce serotonin, melatonin, GABA, catecholamines, histamine, and acetylcholine. Although these neurotransmitters do not cross the blood-brain barrier in any appreciable amount, they may alter visceral reflexes which may affect CNS function. One interesting theory is that these neurotransmitters are produced so that bacteria may communicate with the host—so called "inter-kingdom signaling." Further, *Lactobacilli* have been shown to increase the activity of IDO, further altering tryptophan metabolism.[47]

The mechanism of communication may be through short-chain fatty acids (SCFAs). SCFAs "are the end products of anaerobic bacterial fermentation in the GI tract. Under physiological conditions, their production is entirely dependent on commensal microbes" (p. 13).[47] A major SCFA is butyric acid. Bacteria such as *Clostridium* species produce it. Studies have shown that injection of butyrate produces changes in the hippocampus and frontal cortex and displays antidepressant effects. One factor noted was an increase in BDNF in the frontal cortex of the mice in the experiment. Butyrate also has large effects locally in the GI tract, so this may be the mechanism through which it affects the host's mood and behavior. Other SCFAs may also have effects. Propionic acid has also been shown in experiments to create behavioral change.[47]

Evidence linking omega-3s with reduced clinical presentation in various psychiatric disorders abounds. While this link remains controversial, the mechanism may actually be through commensal bacteria. Mice fed a diet containing fish oil had a threefold increase in bifidobacteria and reduced quantities of *Bacteroides*. The connection may be through the ability of omega-3s to alter SCFA production.[47]

BENEFICIAL EFFECTS OF PROBIOTICS

Probiotics have long been known to have beneficial effects as noted by the historical perspectives section of this chapter. The exact mechanisms by which they may affect mood are less clear, but are likely to be mechanistically related to cytokine production and immune/inflammatory activation. The term *probiotic* has been defined as a live organism that, when ingested in adequate amounts, exerts a health benefit. Many bacteria are purported to be probiotic; however, few have actually been studied. Recently, a new term has been introduced in the literature—*psychobiotic*. The authors defined this as a live organism that, when ingested in adequate amounts, produces a health benefit in patients suffering from psychiatric illness. Clinical studies have been performed with promising results. Irritable bowel syndrome (IBS) is a common disorder that is known to include disturbances of the gut-brain axis. Depression and anxiety are not uncommon in patients with IBS. Placebo-controlled trials comparing *B. infantis* and *L. Salivarius* show that the former significantly improves all symptoms. Still other placebo-controlled trials have shown the combination of *L. helveticus* R0052 and *B. longum* reduced psychological stress as measured by the Hopkins Symptom Checklist, the Hospital Anxiety and Depression Scale, and the Coping Checklist. This study also showed a reduction in urinary free cortisol levels. Elevated cortisol is frequently seen in depression.[50] Probiotic-containing yogurt has even shown to be beneficial when compared to placebo after 3 weeks in a self-reported experiment. Finally, in patients with chronic fatigue syndrome who were given a yogurt drink containing *Lactobacillus casei* or a placebo, those receiving the probiotic had significant improvements in anxiety.[50]

BUILDING A HEALTHY MICROBIOME

Building and maintaining a healthy microbiome is essential to optimizing brain function. Building a healthy microbiome begins before one even has control of it. With the knowledge that microbes likely inhabit the placenta, umbilical cord and fetal membranes, and amniotic fluid,[51,52] it becomes clear that the overuse of antibiotics is of major concern. Cesarean section rates in the United States might also be of concern.

According to the Centers for Disease Control and Prevention (CDC), one-third of all births in the United States are done by cesarean section. This is a sterile birth. During vaginal delivery, the contact with maternal vaginal and intestinal flora is an important source for the start of the infant's colonization. During cesarean delivery, this direct contact is absent, and nonmaternally derived environmental bacteria play an important role for infants' intestinal colonization.[52] Evidence has shown mode of delivery to affect colonization in infants. Babies born vaginally were colonized predominantly by *Lactobacillus*, whereas cesarean delivery (CD) babies were colonized by a mixture of potentially pathogenic bacteria typically found on the skin and in hospitals, such as *Staphylococcus* and *Acinetobacter,* suggesting babies born by CD were colonized with skin flora in lieu of traditionally vaginal types of bacterium.[52]

Differences in the microbiome between babies born vaginally and via cesarean section have been demonstrated to be present anywhere from 6 months postpartum to 7 years. Clinical relevance to these differences is scant. However, there are epidemiological studies showing possible changes in physiology as it relates to mode of delivery. It is well established that intestinal bacteria play an important role in the developing immune system. Atopic diseases appear more often in infants after cesarean delivery than after vaginal delivery.

Additionally, diseases like allergic rhinitis, asthma, celiac disease, diabetes mellitus type 1, and gastroenteritis are also more likely with cesarean delivery. Interestingly, the risks for allergic rhinitis and asthma go up with repeat cesarean.[52] Given this evidence and experimental animal evidence of changes to HPA axis function and stress response, these changes likely have longer-lasting influences on mood stability as well. Another critically important window for building a healthy microbiome is breastfeeding. In addition to direct maternal contact, breast milk itself acts as a stimulator for proper microbiome development. As some studies have shown delayed lactation in cesarean births, both the sterility of cesarean birth and delayed lactation might have long-lasting adverse effects on fetal microbiome development.[52] Breast milk is the perfect microbiome-starter. It is much more than protein, carbohydrate, and fat. It contains immune factors, bacteria (termed *entero-mammary transfer*[53]), and over 200 unique oligosaccharides designed to help build and maintain the microbiome. Patients and doctors should strive for low intervention births with breastfeeding being encouraged immediately after birth.

Given this information, the use of antibiotics during pregnancy also requires examination. In particular, treatment for group B *Streptococcus* needs a closer look. A review from the *Cochrane Database of Systematic Reviews* stated, "This review finds that giving antibiotics is not supported by conclusive evidence. The review identified four trials involving 852 GBS positive women. Very few of the women in labor who are GBS positive give birth to babies who are infected with GBS and antibiotics can have harmful effects such as severe maternal allergic reactions, increase in drug-resistant organisms and exposure of newborn infants to resistant bacteria, and postnatal maternal and neonatal yeast infections" (p. 2).[54] Given the effects of a mother's microbiota on a baby's, a reexamination of this practice is necessary.

After the earliest years, other factors play a significant role in keeping the microbiome healthy. Exercise is a critical factor. Increased exercise levels are associated with an increased diversity of the microbiome.[55] A study in rats found similar results, concluding that "Exercise was shown to enhance the relative abundance of three genera, with Lactobacillus being the most abundant, while another three genera were shown to be more abundant before exercise training (*Streptococcus, Aggregatibacter* and *Sutterella*)."[56] Similarly, another study in rodents showed *Lactobacillus* and *Bifidobacterium* (among others) were increased in an exercise group as compared to controls. The researchers concluded that exercise was an important factor in determining diversity of the microbiome. Additionally, *Lactobacillus* and *Bifidobacterium* have the capacity to produce the organic acid lactate, which is converted into butyrate, an important regulatory short-chain fatty acid in the gut.[57]

Since diet is perhaps the most modifiable aspect of human health, it requires consideration in maintaining a healthy microbiome. Prebiotic compounds are a logical place to start. Prebiotics can be defined as food ingredients that "selectively stimulate the growth and/or activity of those bacteria that contribute to colonic and host health" (p. 1418).[58] Prebiotics, or nondigestible oligosaccharides, are of very little caloric value but enhance mineral absorption, lower the risk of infection and diarrhea, modulate the immune system, and favorably impact microbiota. The major dietary source of prebiotics is fructans, including chicory root extract, inulin, oligofructose, and short-chain fructooligosaccharides. Prebiotics work mostly by stimulating growth of beneficial bacteria in the gut. The consumption of prebiotics has been demonstrated to increase bifidobacteria and lactobacilli as well as butyrate producers like *Eubacterium, Faecalibacterium*, and *Roseburia*. Prebiotics have also been shown to increase total short-chain fatty acid content. However, more study is necessary in this area.[59]

In addition to prebiotic consumption, our food choices matter a great deal. The high-fat/high-sugar Western diet alters the genetic composition and metabolic activity of the microbiome. We must also consider these diets are generally also very low in fiber. These changes are now being recognized as contributing to the ever-increasing chronic disease burden. Evidence in mice has shown that changes in macronutrient content can change gut microbiota in just one day.

In humans, this process has been demonstrated to occur over weeks to months in some experimental models. A more recent experiment has shown that, yes indeed, human gut microbiota responds within days as well.[60] What does the change in microbial content look like? High-carbohydrate diets, regardless of the glycemic index of that diet increase saccharolytic bacteria. High-fat diets reduce bacterial numbers while increasing the excretion of short-chain fatty acids.[61]

Perhaps more important than the macronutrient distribution of the diet is the fiber intake. A study comparing fecal microbiota of European children and that of children from a rural African village of Burkina Faso is an interesting comparison. Diets in this African village are high in fiber content, similar to that of early human settlements at the time of the birth of agriculture. The differences were striking. The African children showed enrichment in *Bacteroidetes* and depletion in *Firmicutes*. Also, bacteria from the genera *Prevotella* and *Xylanibacter* were present in much greater quantity compared to in European children. In fact, these were completely lacking in European children. This is important because *Prevotella* and *Xylanibacter* are important for breaking down plant starches. Short-chain fatty acids were also significantly more prevalent in African children. The study authors "hypothesize that gut microbiota coevolved with the polysaccharide-rich diet of BF individuals, allowing them to maximize energy intake from fibers while also protecting them from inflammation and noninfectious colonic diseases."[62]

Another characterization of the ancestral microbiome has been attempted by Schnorr et al.[63] who assessed the fecal microbiota of 27 Hazda hunter-gatherers, among the last remaining traditional cultures who rely exclusively on foraged plants, berries, and tubers as well as hunted game. They compared the phylogenetic diversity, taxonomic relative abundance, and short-chain fatty acid profile of these samples to those of 16 urban Italians eating a classical Mediterranean diet. The researchers found significant variation between the two community samples, most notably that the Hazda microbiome was dominated by *Firmicutes*, that 22% of the bacteria were as of yet unclassified, and that *Bifidobacteria* was notably absent. There were also significant gender differences including female Hazda samples notable for *Treponema* strains, considered to be opportunistic or pathogenic, suspected to aid in degradation of the relatively higher tuber intake. The fatty acids produced by Hazda microbiota were primarily propionate (rather than butyrate), which travels to the liver for gluconeogenesis (sugar formation). The Hazda samples also bore more resemblance to other catalogued African rural samples than to Western samples.

Authors of this study stress the need for thorough understanding of the presence of important confounding variables regarding one's diet such as the growth location, method of harvesting, and manufacturing processes. The role of soil appears paramount. Soil within the United States lacks many vital nutrients,[64] due in part to harmful industrialization of agriculture practices that interfere with natural ecosystems, supporting plants rich in nutrients. Similarly, fungicides and biocides have decimated the microbial ecology of the soil[65] in ways that fundamentally derail plant-based communication about the botanical environment. Plants are a dynamic reflection of their own microbiomes,[66] passing vital information about shared environments onto human consumers.

The Western diet, which is generally too rich in all macronutrients and too low in indigestible fibers, significantly contributes to an unfavorable microbiome and is associated with the rapid increase in noninfectious intestinal disease.[60] All of these diseases demonstrate a high degree of inflammation making it possible that this is partly the mechanism through which the Western diet contributes to chronic disease, including mood disorder. Diets rich in fiber and calorically calibrated appear to be most beneficial for building and maintaining a healthy microbiome. In practice, recommending a paleolithic-inspired diet rich in vegetables and protein and low in high glycemic fruits and grain is a practical approach.

CONCLUSION

The interconnectedness of the gut, brain, immune, and hormonal systems is exceedingly difficult to unwind. Until we begin to appreciate this complex relationship, we will not be able to prevent or intervene effectively in depression, slated to become the second-leading cause of disability in this country, within the decade. For true healing and meaningful prevention, it is advisable for patients to take steps every day toward sending their body the message that it is not being attacked, it is not in danger, and it is well nourished, well supported, and calm.

As a society, we can begin to think about protecting the microbiome by demedicalizing birth and infant nutrition, and as individuals, by avoiding antibiotics, NSAIDs, gluten-containing grains, and genetically modified and nonorganic food. Promising interventions for depression from a gut-brain perspective include probiotics, fermented foods as part of a high natural fat diet, and relaxation response for optimal digestion, anti-inflammatory, and insulin sensitizing effects. This is termed *psychoneuroimmunology*, and likely represents the future of mental health care, compelling clinicians and researchers alike to appreciate the connectedness of different bodily systems, as well as our connectedness as a species to the environmental ecosystem in and around us.

REFERENCES

1. Kirsch, I. and Sapirstein, G. 1998. Listening to Prozac but hearing placebo: A meta-analysis of antidepressant medication. *Am Psychol Assoc* 1(2): 1–16.
2. Moncrieff, J. and Kirsch, I. 2005. Efficacy of antidepressants in adults. *BMJ* 331(7509): 155–157. doi:10.1136/bmj.331.7509.155.
3. Kirsch, I., Deacon, B.J., Huedo-Medina, T.B. et al. 2008. Initial severity and antidepressant benefits: A meta-analysis of data submitted to the Food and Drug Administration. *PLoS Med* 5(2): e45. doi:10.1371/journal.pmed.0050045.
4. Littrell, J.L. and Lacasse, J.R. 2012. The controversy over antidepressant drugs in an era of evidence-based practice. *Soc Work Ment Health* 10(6): 445–463. doi:10.1080/15332985.2012.699444.
5. Goldberg, D., Privett, M., Ustun, B. et al. 1998. The effects of detection and treatment on the outcome of major depression in primary care: A naturalistic study in 15 cities. *Br J Gen Pract* 48(437): 1840–1844.
6. Van Weel-Baumgarten, E.M., van den Bosch, W.J., Hekster, Y.A. et al. 2000. Treatment of depression related to recurrence: 10-year follow-up in general practice. *J Clin Pharm Ther* 25(1): 61–66.
7. Bested, A.C., Logan, A.C., and Selhub, E.M. 2013. Intestinal microbiota, probiotics and mental health: From Metchnikoff to modern advances: Part I—Autointoxication revisited. *Gut Pathogen* 5(1): 5.
8. Grenham, S., Clarke, G., Cryan, J.F. et al. 2011. Brain-gut-microbe communication in health and disease. *Front Physiol* 2: 94.
9. Mshvildadze, M., Neu, J., Shuster, J. et al. 2010. Intestinal microbial ecology in premature infants assessed with non-culture-based techniques. *J Pediatr* 156(1): 20–25.
10. Aagaard, K., Ma, J., Antony, K.M. et al. 2014. The placenta harbors a unique microbiome. *Sci Transl Med* 6(237): 237ra65.
11. Palmer, C., Bik, E.M., DiGiulio, D.B. et al. 2007. Development of the human infant intestinal microbiota. *PLoS Biol* 5(7): e177.
12. Frank, D.N., and Pace, N.R. 2008. Gastrointestinal microbiology enters the metagenomics era. *Curr Opin Gastroenterol* 24(1): 4–10.
13. Kurokawa, K., Itoh, T., Kuwahara, T. et al. 2007. Comparative metagenomics revealed commonly enriched gene sets in human gut microbiomes. *DNA Res* 14(4): 169–181.
14. Groschwitz, K.R. and Hogan, S.P. 2009. Intestinal barrier function: Molecular regulation and disease pathogenesis. *J Allergy Clin Immunol* 124(1): 3–20.
15. Yirmiya, R. 2000. Depression in medical illness: The role of the immune system. *West J Med* 173(5): 333–336.
16. Teixeira, T.F., Collado, M.C., Ferreira, C.L. et al. 2012. Potential mechanisms for the emerging link between obesity and increased intestinal permeability. *Nutr Res* 32(9): 637–647.

17. Bested, A.C., Logan, A.C., and Selhub, E.M. 2013. Intestinal microbiota, probiotics and mental health: From Metchnikoff to modern advances: Part II—Contemporary contextual research. *Gut Pathogen* 5(1): 3.

18. Vojdani, A. and Lambert, J. 2011. Functional neurology and immunology: VI. Crossing Barriers—Gut-to-brain lessons from interdisciplinary collaboration. *Funct Neurol Rehabil Ergon* 1(4): 631–644.

19. Qin, L., Wu, X., Block, M.L. et al. 2007. Systemic LPS causes chronic neuroinflammation and progressive neurodegeneration. *Glia* 55(5): 453–462.

20. Maes, M., Kubera, M., and Leunis, J.C. 2008. The gut-brain barrier in major depression: Intestinal mucosal dysfunction with an increased translocation of LPS from gram negative enterobacteria (leaky gut) plays a role in the inflammatory pathophysiology of depression. *Neuro Endocrinol Lett* 29(1): 117–124.

21. Reichenberg, A., Yirmiya, R., Schuld, A. et al. 2001. Cytokine-associated emotional and cognitive disturbances in humans. *Arch Gen Psychiatry* 58(5): 445–452.

22. Taudorf, S., Krabbe, K.S., Berg, R.M. et al. 2007. Human models of low-grade inflammation: Bolus versus continuous infusion of endotoxin. *Clin Vaccine Immunol* 14(3): 250–255.

23. Vida, G., Peña, G., Deitch, E.A. et al. 2011. α7-cholinergic receptor mediates vagal induction of splenic norepinephrine. *J Immunol* 186(7): 4340–4346.

24. Campos-Rodríguez, R., Godínez-Victoria, M., Abarca-Rojano, E. et al. 2013. Stress modulates intestinal secretory immunoglobulin A. *Front Integr Neurosci* 7: 86.

25. Bergheim, I., Weber, S., Vos, M. et al. 2008. Antibiotics protect against fructose-induced hepatic lipid accumulation in mice: Role of endotoxin. *J Hepatol* 48(6): 983–992.

26. Spruss, A., Kanuri, G., Wagnerberger, S. et al. 2009. Haub S, Bischoff SC, Bergheim I. Toll-like receptor 4 is involved in the development of fructose-induced hepatic steatosis in mice. *Hepatology* 50(4): 1094–1104.

27. Amar, J., Burcelin, R., Ruidavets, J.B. et al. 2008. Energy intake is associated with endotoxemia in apparently healthy men. *Am J Clin Nutr* 87(5): 1219–1223.

28. Osanai, M., Nishikiori, N., Murata, M. et al. 2007. Cellular retinoic acid bioavailability determines epithelial integrity: Role of retinoic acid receptor alpha agonists in colitis. *Mol Pharmacol* 71(1): 250–258.

29. Pachikian, B.D., Neyrinck, A.M., Deldicque, L. et al. 2010. Changes in intestinal bifidobacteria levels are associated with the inflammatory response in magnesium-deficient mice. *J Nutr* 140(3): 509–514.

30. Zhong, W., McClain, C.J., Cave, M. et al. 2010. The role of zinc deficiency in alcohol-induced intestinal barrier dysfunction. *Am J Physiol Gastrointest Liver Physiol* 298(5): G625–G633.

31. Kong, J., Zhang, Z., Musch, M.W. et al. 2008. Novel role of the vitamin D receptor in maintaining the integrity of the intestinal mucosal barrier. *Am J Physiol Gastrointest Liver Physiol* 294(1): G208–G216.

32. Tamboli, C.P., Neut, C., Desreumaux, P. et al. 2004. Dysbiosis in inflammatory bowel disease. *Gut* 53(1): 1–4.

33. Anders, H.J., Andersen, K., and Stecher, B. 2013. The intestinal microbiota, a leaky gut, and abnormal immunity in kidney disease. *Kidney Int* 83(6): 1010–1016.

34. Doré, J., Simrén, M., Buttle, L. et al. 2013. Hot topics in gut microbiota. *United European Gastroenterol J* 1(5): 311–318.

35. Hawrelak, J.A. and Myers, S.P. 2004. The causes of intestinal dysbiosis: A review. *Altern Med Rev* 9(2): 180–197.

36. Aris, A. and Leblanc, S. 2011. Maternal and fetal exposure to pesticides associated to genetically modified foods in Eastern Townships of Quebec, Canada. *Reprod Toxicol* 31(4): 528–533.

37. Samsel, A. and Seneff, S. 2013. Glyphosate's suppression of cytochrome P450 enzymes and amino acid biosynthesis by the gut microbiome: Pathways to modern diseases. *Entropy* 15: 1416–1463.

38. Mäkivuokko, H., Tiihonen, K., Tynkkynen, S. et al. 2010. The effect of age and non-steroidal anti-inflammatory drugs on human intestinal microbiota composition. *Br J Nutr* 103(2): 227–234.

39. Sigthorsson, G., Tibble, J., Hayllar, J. et al. 1998. Intestinal permeability and inflammation in patients on NSAIDs. *Gut* 43(4): 506–511.

40. Tacheci, I., Kopacova, M., Rejchrt, S. et al. 2010. Non-steroidal anti-inflammatory drug induced injury to the small intestine. *Acta Medica (Hradec Kralove)* 53(1): 3–11.

41. Dunn, A.J. 2006. Effects of cytokines and infections on brain neurochemistry. *Clin Neurosci Res* 6(1–2): 52–68.

42. Barton, D.A., Esler, M.D., Dawood, T. et al. 2008. Elevated brain serotonin turnover in patients with depression: Effect of genotype and therapy. *Arch Gen Psychiatry* 65(1): 38–46.

43. Owen, B.M., Eccleston, D., Ferrier, I.N., and Young, A.H. 2001. Raised levels of plasma interleukin-1β in major and postviral depression. *Acta Psychiatr Scand* 103(3): 226–228.

44. Levine, J., Barak, Y., Chengappa, K.N. et al. 1999. Cerebrospinal cytokine levels in patients with acute depression. *Neuropsychobiology* 40(4): 171–176.

45. Christmas, D.M., Potokar, J., and Davies, S.J. 2011. A biological pathway linking inflammation and depression: Activation of indoleamine 2,3-dioxygenase. *Neuropsychiatr Dis Treat* 7: 431–439.

46. Sudo, N., Chida, Y., Aiba, Y. et al. 2004. Postnatal microbial colonization programs the hypothalamic-pituitary-adrenal system for stress response in mice. *J Physiol* 558(1): 263–275.

47. Forsythe, P., Sudo, N., Dinan, T. et al. 2010. Mood and gut feelings. *Brain Behav Immun* 24(1): 9–16.

48. Wang, X., Wang, B.R., Zhang, X.J. et al. 2002. Evidences for vagus nerve in maintenance of immune balance and transmission of immune information from gut to brain in STM-infected rats. *World J Gastroenterol* 8(3): 540–545.

49. Collins, S.M., and Bercik, P. 2009. The relationship between intestinal microbiota and the central nervous system in normal gastrointestinal function and disease. *Gastroenterology* 136(6): 2003–2014.

50. Dinan, T.G., Stanton, C., and Cryan, J.F. 2013. Psychobiotics: A novel class of psychotropic. *Biol Psychiatry* 74(10): 720–726.

51. Funkhouser, L.J. and Bordenstein, S.R. 2013. Mom knows best: The universality of maternal microbial transmission. *PLoS Biol* 11(8): e1001631.

52. Neu, J. and Rushing, J. 2011. Cesarean versus vaginal delivery: Long-term infant outcomes and the hygiene hypothesis. *Clin Perinatol* 38(2): 321–331.

53. Jost, T., Lacroix, C., Braegger, CP. et al. 2014. Vertical mother-neonate transfer of maternal gut bacteria via breastfeeding. *Environ Microbiol* 16(9): 2891–2904.

54. Ohlsson, A. and Shah, V.S. 2014. Intrapartum antibiotics for known maternal Group B streptococcal colonization. *Cochrane Database Syst Rev* 2014(6): 1–43.

55. Ray, K. 2014. Gut microbiota. Tackling the effects of diet and exercise on the gut microbiota. *Nat Rev Gastroenterol Hepatol* 11(8): 456.

56. Petriz, B.A., Castro, A.P., Almeida, J.A. et al. 2014. Exercise induction of gut microbiota modifications in obese, non-obese and hypertensive rats. *BMC Genomics* 15: 511.

57. Queipo-Ortuño, M.I., Seoane, L.M., Murri, M. et al. 2013. Gut microbiota composition in male rat models under different nutritional status and physical activity and its association with serum leptin and ghrelin levels. *PLoS One* 8(5): e65465.

58. Slavin, J. 2013. Fiber and prebiotics: Mechanisms and health benefits. *Nutrients* 5(4): 1417–1435, doi:10.3390/nu5041417.

59. Institute of Medicine (US) Food Forum. 2013. *The Human Microbiome, Diet, and Health: Workshop Summary*. Washington, DC: National Academies Press; 5, Influence of Diet and Dietary Components on the Microbiome. Available from: http://www.ncbi.nlm.nih.gov/books/NBK154087/

60. David, L.A., Maurice, C.F., Carmody, R.N. et al. 2014. Diet rapidly and reproducibly alters the human gut microbiome. *Nature* 505(7484): 559–563.

61. Fava, F., Gitau, R., Griffin, B.A. et al. 2013. The type and quantity of dietary fat and carbohydrate alter faecal microbiome and short-chain fatty acid excretion in a metabolic syndrome "at-risk" population. *Int J Obes (Lond)* 37(2): 216–223.

62. De Filippo, C., Cavalieri, D., Di Paola, M. et al. 2010. Impact of diet in shaping gut microbiota revealed by a comparative study in children from Europe and rural Africa. *Proc Natl Acad Sci USA* 107(33): 14691–14696.

63. Schnorr, S.L., Candela, M., Rampelli, S. et al. 2014. Gut microbiome of the Hadza hunter-gatherers. *Nat Commun* 5: 3654. doi:10.1038/ncomms4654.

64. Fan, M.S., Zhao, F.J., Fairweather-Tait, S.J., Poulton, P.R., Dunham, S.J., and McGrath, S.P. 2008. Evidence of decreasing mineral density in wheat grain over the last 160 years. *J Trace Elem Med Biol* 22(4): 315–324, doi: 10.1016/j.jtemb.2008.07.002.

65. East, R. 2013. Microbiome: Soil science comes to life. *Nature* 501(7468): S18–S19. doi:10.1038/501S18a.

66. Hill, P.W., Marsden, K.A., and Jones, D.L. 2013. How significant to plant N nutrition is the direct consumption of soil microbes by roots? *New Phytol* 199(4): 948–955. doi:10.1111/nph.12320.

4 Clostridia Bacteria in the GI Tract Affecting Dopamine and Norepinephrine Metabolism

William Shaw, PhD

CONTENTS

INTRODUCTION

Ilya Ilyich Mechnikov, the Nobel Prize–winning biologist, was one of the first scientists to promote the idea that the microorganisms in the intestinal tract could affect health and was the first to recommend the use of beneficial lactobacilli to promote long life, essentially starting the probiotics (beneficial microorganisms) industry about a century ago. A Google search of the term *probiotics* yields 11,900,000 references. The term *dysbiosis* most commonly refers to an imbalance of microorganisms in the intestinal tract. A PubMed search indicates that the first appearance of this term in its database was in 1959 and that there are now 1005 uses of the term in articles in its database. However, the acceptance of this term took many years to gain general acceptance. Fifteen years ago, a bureaucrat from one of the laboratory regulatory agencies declared that this term was not permitted to be used by the laboratory of the author and that all such references would have to be deleted. For many years, it was thought by many in the medical community that the intestinal flora was an inert passenger and of little interest to health. Even a longer time passed until the role of intestinal microorganisms in brain function and psychiatric illness began to be studied in earnest. A PubMed search of the terms "gut microbiota and psychiatric illness" retrieved 50 articles with the earliest published in 2008, while a search of "bacteria and psychiatric illness" retrieved 9244 articles dating back to 1947. Thus, infection was widely accepted as a potential cause of psychiatric disease and a worthy research subject, but the role of the intestinal flora in psychiatric disease was not readily accepted as a worthwhile research endeavor until recently.

DISCOVERY OF CLOSTRIDIA METABOLITES

At the children's hospital where the author was the laboratory director, he was given the project of setting up urine organic acids testing. At this time, urine organic acids testing was almost exclusively performed for diagnosis of inborn errors of metabolism. One of the first steps he took was to set up to test as many chemicals in urine as possible, not just those associated with genetic diseases. He tested for food additives, vitamins, minerals, a variety of drug metabolites, and other substances. He then approached the director of a children's psychiatric hospital to begin screening for metabolic causes of psychiatric diseases. The hospital director, a psychiatrist, indicated that he had the perfect patient for the project, a teenage boy with a variety of severe behavior disorders including depression, attention deficit disorder, and oppositional defiant disorder. He then said he was certain this boy had a biological cause of his illnesses, not bad parenting, and that he would send a urine sample. An analysis of his sample indicated that his patient had an increase of the chemical later identified as 3-(3-hydroxyphenyl)-3-hydroxypropionic acid (HPHPA) in the urine. The child's urine was tested while he was in outpatient treatment for attention deficit, oppositional defiant disorder, and depression, and it revealed high concentrations of the HPHPA compound (Figure 4.1). At a later date, the condition of the boy deteriorated, he was hospitalized, and another urine sample was submitted. This time the concentration of the HPHPA was massive, so massive that it obliterated nearly all of the other peaks in the chromatogram and could not be quantitated. The amount, however, was likely 1000 times or more than amounts found in normal individuals.

Studying metabolism in patients with mental illness is very challenging because many of the patients are on a variety of drugs, with each drug having multiple metabolites. Many researchers have wasted years identifying a new compound found in urine, only to discover that they had merely found a new drug metabolite. In a study by this author and Dr. Walter Gattaz, a research psychiatrist at the Central Mental Health Institute of Germany in Mannheim, drug-free samples from patients with schizophrenia diagnoses were evaluated. Five of the 12 samples (41.7%) contained a very high concentration of a compound identified by gas chromatography/mass spectrometry (GC/MS) as a derivative of the amino acid phenylalanine, which has since been identified as HPHPA.

Despite the seeming novelty of this compound's identification, it had been referenced 50 years prior.[1] This research indicated that HPHPA, which they called (-)-beta-meta-hydroxyphenylhydracrylic

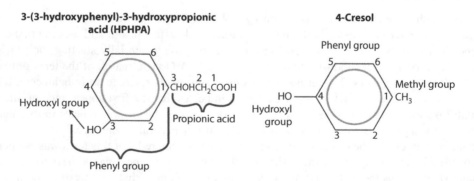

FIGURE 4.1 Biochemical structures of phenolic metabolites derived from clostridia bacteria.

acid, had been identified as one of the major phenolic acids present in elevated amounts in urine samples of patients with a large variety of mental illnesses. This association of elevated HPHPA in mental illness has been confirmed by the author. Remarkably, there was no follow-up of this important discovery by the earlier research team or any other research groups until the author's rediscovery. A similar discovery of genetic factors in peas (eventually recognized as the chromosomes) by the monk Mendel in 1865 was mostly overlooked for 35 years until rediscovered in 1900 by Hugo de Vries, Carl Correns, and Erich von Tschermak.[2]

Later, Shaw et al. found that HPHPA was elevated in many children with autism[3] and initially suspected that this compound might be an intestinal yeast metabolite. However, the author found that in a clinical research project on the effects of antifungal drugs on autism, there was not a significant decrease in HPHPA in the urine after antifungal drug therapy.[4] The mean value for the HPHPA actually increased some after antifungal therapy. This increase indicated to the author that this compound could not be due to the yeast but was probably due to a different microorganism. Since several children and adults with *Clostridium difficile* infection of the intestinal tract had high values of HPHPA in their urine, and the production of a similar compound, monohydroxyphenylpropionic acid is characteristic of different species of clostridia[5,6] but not other bacteria, I suspected that one or more species of the bacteria genus *Clostridium* were producing this compound.

KNOWN DISEASE-CAUSING CLOSTRIDIA BACTERIA

Some of the common species of *Clostridium* are *Clostridium tetani* that causes tetanus, *C. botulinum* that causes the food poisoning botulism, and *C. perfringens* and *C. difficile* that cause diarrhea.[7] *C. perfringens*, *C. novyi*, *C. bifermentans*, *C. histolyticum*, *C. septicum*, and *C. fallax* may all cause gangrene.[7] Many other species of *Clostridium* are normal inhabitants of the intestinal tract and may not be scientifically described or even named as a species. It is estimated that there are perhaps 100 different species of clostridia bacteria in the human intestine, but most are not considered pathogenic. The major reason for a lack of knowledge about these organisms is that they are strict anaerobes that cannot tolerate oxygen. Since they must be processed in an oxygen-free environment, most hospital laboratories do not have the capability to identify these organisms by culture methods.

The exception is *C. difficile*, which is most commonly identified by the toxins it produces in the stool rather than by the isolation of the organism. *C. difficile* overgrowth of the intestinal tract causes a severe and potentially fatal disorder called *pseudomembranous colitis*.[8] This overgrowth is frequently associated with the use of oral antibiotics, indicating that this organism is resistant to many of the common antibiotics such as penicillin, ampicillin, tetracyclines, cephalosporins, chloramphenicol, and others.[9] This organism is usually treated with either metronidazole (Flagyl®) or vancomycin followed by a replenishment of the intestine with *Lactobacillus acidophilus*.[8] Since many bacteria can genetically transfer drug resistance to other similar species and even unrelated species, it is my opinion that multiple species of clostridia may now be resistant to the most common antibiotic drugs.

4-CRESOL AS AN ADDITIONAL URINARY MARKER FOR *CLOSTRIDIUM DIFFICILE*

In addition to the discovery of HPHPA as a marker for gastrointestinal (GI) clostridial overgrowth, 4-cresol (para-cresol) (Figure 4.1) has been used as a specific marker for *C. difficile*.[10] 4-Cresol, a phenolic compound, is classified as a type-B toxic agent and can cause rapid circulatory collapse and death in humans.[11] Yokoyama et al.[12] recently proposed that intestinal production of 4-cresol may be responsible for a growth-depressing effect on weanling pigs. Signs of acute 4-cresol toxicity in animals typically include hypoactivity, salivation, tremors, and convulsions. Clinical signs of toxicity[13] following inhalation include irritation of mucous membranes, excitation and convulsions, hematuria at high 4-cresol concentrations, and death. High amounts of 4-cresol have been found in autism,[13] and the amount of 4-cresol in the urine has been found elevated in initial samples and in replica samples of autistic children below 8 years of age. Increased levels of this compound in autism are correlated with the degree of severity of symptoms. 4-Cresol is apparently produced by *C. difficile* as an antimicrobial compound that kills other species of bacteria in the GI tract, allowing the *C. difficile* to proliferate.

MECHANISM BY WHICH CLOSTRIDIA METABOLITES ALTER HUMAN NEUROTRANSMITTER METABOLISM AND CAUSE PSYCHIATRIC DISORDERS AND GI DISEASE

The probable biochemical mechanism by which the phenolic compounds affect behavior was discovered by Goodhart et al.[14] who found that 4-cresol and similar phenols are potent inhibitors of dopamine-beta-hydroxylase, a key enzyme in catecholamine metabolism, which is responsible for converting dopamine to norepinephrine. 4-Cresol and related phenols are postulated to covalently modify dopamine-beta-hydroxylase by a direct insertion of an aberrant 4-cresol radical into an active site tyrosine residue at position 216 of the protein, leading to irreversible inactivation of the enzyme. It is interesting that the *inactivation* of the enzyme requires vitamin C (ascorbic acid), so vitamin C *deficiency* might actually offer protection against the negative effects of this enzyme inhibitor. This fact could be very clinically important, and vitamin C supplementation should probably be avoided until clostridia treatment has been completed. Although HPHPA has not yet been verified to be an inhibitor of dopamine-beta-hydroxylase, its structure is similar to 4-cresol (Figure 4.1), and many similar phenols have been proved to be strong inhibitors of this enzyme.[14] In addition, a number of observations of organic acid test results provide indirect evidence for dopamine-beta-hydroxylase inhibition by HPHPA.

The author observed that urine samples of many individuals with severe clinical symptoms of neuropsychiatric diseases had elevated levels of the dopamine metabolite homovanillic acid (HVA), while the epinephrine and norepinephrine metabolite vanillylmandelic acid (VMA) was not elevated or was low. At the same time, the ratio of the two metabolites or the HVA/VMA ratio was extremely elevated. The same urine samples for these individuals commonly had elevated amounts of the phenolic substances 4-cresol or HPHPA. Elevated HPHPA and/or 4-cresol have now been detected in a wide variety of disorders (Table 4.1).

TABLE 4.1

Disorders Associated with Elevated Amounts of Urinary Metabolites HPHPA and/or 4-Cresol from Clostridia Bacteria

Autism and Pervasive Developmental Disorder	Obsessive Compulsive Disorder
Attention deficit	Tic disorders
Arthritis	Tourette's syndrome
Depression	Parkinson's syndrome
Bipolar depression	Alzheimer's disease
Ulcerative colitis	Psychosis
Anorexia	Schizophrenia
Anxiety	Seizure disorder
Chronic fatigue syndrome	

METABOLIC PATHWAY FOR PRODUCTION OF HUMAN NEUROTRANSMITTERS INHIBITED BY CLOSTRIDIA METABOLITES

The combined metabolic pathway for production of human neurotransmitters in the brain, adrenal glands, and sympathetic nervous system is outlined in Figure 4.2 along with the production of clostridia bacterial substances that alter this pathway. The key starting material for both human and clostridia pathways is the amino acid phenylalanine. The human pathway requires the L-isomer. The specificity for the amino acid optical isomer required for the clostridia pathway is unknown.

In humans, phenylalanine and/or tyrosine from dietary proteins or amino acid supplements are absorbed from the intestinal tract where these amino acids cross the blood-brain barrier and enter the brain. Phenylalanine in the brain is converted to tyrosine by phenylalanine hydroxylase. The ring of tyrosine is then hydroxylated to dihydroxyphenylalanine (DOPA) by tyrosine hydroxylase. DOPA is then converted to dopamine by DOPA decarboxylase which requires a vitamin B_6 cofactor. The fate of further dopamine metabolism depends on the neuron type. In dopamine-containing neurons, dopamine is the final product. In the absence of clostridia metabolites, dopamine is converted primarily to homovanillic acid which can be measured in the urine organic acid test. In norepinephrine-containing brain neurons, neurons of the peripheral central nervous system, and

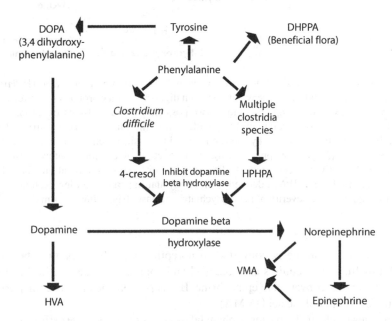

FIGURE 4.2 Integration of human and microbial metabolism involving neurotransmitters as cause of neuropsychiatric disorders. In the absence of 4-cresol and HPHPA from clostridia bacteria, phenylalanine in the central and peripheral nervous systems is converted in sequence to tyrosine, 3,4-dihydroxyphenylalanine (DOPA), dopamine, and norepinephrine. Norepinephrine may be converted to epinephrine in the adrenal gland. Dopamine is metabolized to homovanillic acid (HVA) while norepinephrine and epinephrine are converted to vanillylmandelic acid (VMA). When certain clostridia bacteria are present in the gastrointestinal tract, phenylalanine is increasingly converted to 4-cresol or 3-(3-hydroxyphenyl)-3-hydroxypropionic acid (HPHPA). This conversion depletes the supply of phenylalanine to produce neurotransmitters. In addition, 4-cresol and HPHPA inhibit the conversion of dopamine to norepinephrine by the irreversible inhibition of the key enzyme dopamine beta-hydroxylase. The inhibition of dopamine beta-hydroxylase leads to an imbalance of neurotransmitters in which dopamine is elevated and norepinephrine is depressed. Elevated dopamine can cause depletion of glutathione and increased oxidative species, leading to brain damage.

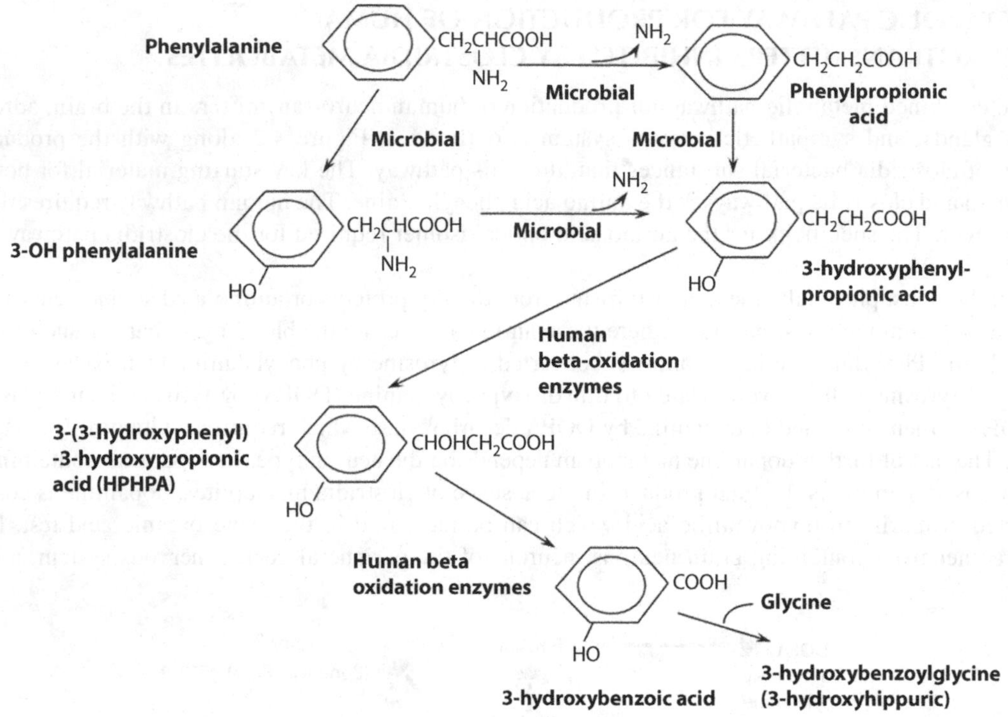

FIGURE 4.3 Biochemical synthesis of 3-(3-hydroxyphenyl)-3-hydroxypropionic acid (HPHPA) from phenylalanine in the gastrointestinal tract. Phenylalanine from digested dietary proteins is converted by clostridia enzymes to form 3-hydroxyphenylpropionic acid by two possible pathways. 3-Hydroxypropionic acid is then converted to HPHPA by fatty acid oxidation (beta-oxidation) in the mitochondria of various human tissues. HPHPA may be further metabolized to 3-hydroxybenzoic acid, which is then conjugated with glycine to form 3-hydroxybenzoylglycine (3-hydroxyhippuric acid). (In the actual biochemical pathway, the organic acids would be present as derivatives of coenzyme A. This step is omitted for simplification.) The clinical significance of this pathway is that HPHPA is derived from phenylalanine so that a high protein meal containing phenylalanine may increase the severity of neuropsychiatric disease, triggering abnormal behavior, anorexia, or seizures.

in the adrenal gland, dopamine is converted to norepinephrine by dopamine-beta-hydroxylase. Dopamine-beta-hydroxylase requires ascorbic acid and copper as cofactors. In the adrenal gland, norepinephrine is further converted to epinephrine. Both epinephrine and norepinephrine may then be converted to vanillylmandelic acid (VMA).

In certain species of clostridia bacteria, phenylalanine is converted to HPHPA by a pathway that requires both human and bacterial enzymes (Figure 4.3). If *C. difficile* is present, it is largely converted to 4-cresol. These by-products are then absorbed into the body through the intestinal tract where they have the ability to inhibit dopamine-beta-hydroxylase. These by-products covalently bind to the enzyme active site, irreversibly inhibiting the active site ability to convert dopamine to norepinephrine.

WHY ELEVATED DOPAMINE CAUSED BY CLOSTRIDIA METABOLITE INHIBITION OF DOPAMINE-BETA-HYDROXYLASE IS NEUROTOXIC

Dopamine in the cytosol at pH 7.4 is unstable[15] because the protons of the hydroxyl groups are dissociated and much more rapidly converted to unstable quinones that generate severe oxidative stress (Figure 4.4). Each molecule of unstable quinone generates about 1000 molecules of oxygen

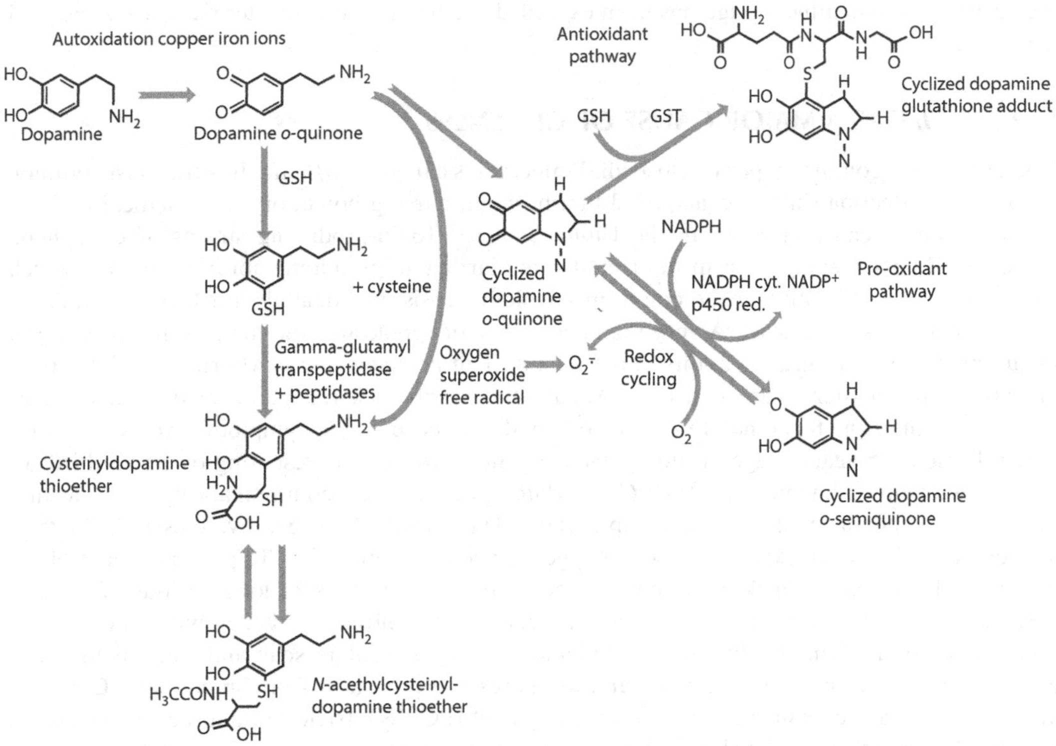

FIGURE 4.4 Toxic effects of excess dopamine. Inhibition of dopamine beta-hydroxylase by clostridia metabolites 4-cresol and HPHPA result in excess accumulation of dopamine in the synaptic vesicles, causing dopamine to leak into the cytoplasm. The pH in the synaptic vesicles is approximately 2 pH units less than the pH of the cytoplasm, 7.4. The low pH in the synaptic vesicles prevents the conversion of dopamine to its more unstable form, dopamine o-quinone. However, as dopamine accumulates, it leaks into the cytoplasm where it is increasingly converted to dopamine o-quinone especially in the presence of high concentrations of copper or iron ions. The dopamine o-quinone may then react with glutathione or cysteine. The glutathione dopamine adduct is then converted to cysteinyldopamine thioether and then to N-acetylcysteinyl-dopamine thioether. This adduct is toxic and leads to apoptosis of brain cells in the presence of high concentrations of dopamine. Thus, detoxification reactions may sometimes lead to greater toxicity to the tissues. Dopamine o-quinone that does not react with cysteine or glutathione is converted to cyclized dopamine o-quinone which can enter a pro-oxidant pathway or an antioxidant pathway. If cyclized dopamine o-quinone is converted by a P450 enzyme to cyclized dopamine o-semiquinone, the semiquinone reacts with molecular oxygen to form oxygen superoxide free radical, simultaneously regenerating cyclized dopamine o-quinone which then repeats the same cycle. It is estimated that each molecule of cyclized dopamine o-quinone formed produces 1000 molecules of oxygen superoxide free radicals. The excess dopamine commonly found in both schizophrenia and autism eventually leads to severe brain damage due to the massive production of oxygen superoxide free radicals and the over-production of toxic N-acetylcysteinyl-dopamine thioether.

superoxide radicals. In addition, cysteine and glutathione adducts are converted to metabolites that cause apoptosis of neurons.[16] Therefore, dopamine uptake into monoaminergic vesicles prevents both the accumulation of free dopamine in the cytosol and the oxidation of dopamine to o-quinones and amino acid adducts because the pH inside monoaminergic synaptic vesicles is 2.0–2.4 pH units lower than the pH in the cytosol. At this low pH, the protons of dopamine hydroxyl groups are strongly bound to the oxygen of hydroxyl groups. Low pH of monoaminergic vesicles results because a specific ATPase hydrolyzes ATP to ADP, inorganic phosphate and one proton (H+), creating a proton gradient.[15] When dopamine-beta-hydroxylase is inhibited by the phenols from clostridia, the amount of dopamine in the cytosol is likely much greater because the capacity of the vesicles for dopamine storage has been exceeded, leading to much greater oxidative stress and neuron death.

C. DIFFICILE AS A MAJOR CAUSE OF GI ILLNESS

One of the most common types of clostridial infection is called *C. difficile*. It is the most common nosocomial infection (infection acquired in a hospital, nursing home, or other medical facility) and nosocomial cause of death in the United States.[17] Toxin-producing strains of *C. difficile* can cause illness ranging from mild or moderate diarrhea to pseudomembranous colitis, which can lead to toxic dilatation of the colon (megacolon), sepsis, and death.[17] It affects hospitalized patients as well as outpatients. A very high percentage of people are colonized with this bacteria, including 5%–15% of healthy adults, more than 80% of neonates and newborns, and 50%–60% of patients in long-term care facilities. Apparently infants lack receptors on the mucosa surfaces of the intestine that bind clostridia, so they do not have severe symptoms even when colonized. Persons 65 years of age or older have been most affected, representing over two-thirds of patients with clostridia infection.[17] All *Clostridium* species share a common ability, spore formation, which is characteristic of the group (genus). The growing or vegetative clostridia bacteria are readily killed when exposed to heat, oxygen, or certain antibiotics. To preserve themselves, the clostridia develop a thick wall and become spores that can live for long periods of time on surfaces like bathroom fixtures, sinks, and toilets. Hand sanitizers or wipes with alcohol have no effect on eliminating *C. difficile*, while hand washing with plain soap and water is the most effective method to kill this organism and its spores and prevent it from spreading.[18] Common antibacterial soaps containing parachlorometaxylenol (PCMX), triclosan, and hexachlorophene may be absorbed through the skin and cause severe toxicity including neurological damage[19] and are not recommended.

C. DIFFICILE DOCUMENTED AS A MAJOR CAUSE OF DEPRESSION

Several types of medications are thought to increase risk of *C. difficile* infection (CDI), including antidepressants, and given that depression is the third most common medical condition worldwide, a team from the University of Michigan[20] investigated the exact nature of this risk. First, the team studied CDI in people with and without depression and found that people with major depression had a much higher chance of CDI (a 36% increase) than people without depression. The population-based rate of CDI in older Americans was 282.9/100,000 person-years (95% confidence interval [CI] 226.3–339.5) for individuals with depression and 197.1/100,000 person-years for those without depression (95% CI 168.0–226.1). The odds of CDI were 36% greater in persons with major depression based on evaluation of 4047 hospitalized patients tested for *C. difficile*. This association held for a variety of depressive disorders and nervous or psychiatric problems. Dr. Mary Rogers who led this study explained:

> Depression is common worldwide. We have long known that depression is associated with changes in the gastrointestinal system. The interaction between the brain and the gut, called the "brain-gut axis" is fascinating and deserves more study. Our finding of a link between depression and *Clostridium difficile* should help us better identify those at risk of infection and perhaps, encourage exploration of the underlying brain-gut mechanisms involved.

Based on the data obtained from The Great Plains Laboratory, the likely mechanism by which *C. difficile* causes depression is now known to be likely caused by 4-cresol secretion. Since HPHPA elevations in the urine are even more common than 4-cresol elevations, it is possible that an even higher percentage of depression is due to overgrowth with non-*difficile* species of clostridia bacteria. The author has consulted with psychiatrist clients whose patients with depression have had HPHPA and/or cresol elevated in their urine samples.

STOOL TESTING AS A METHOD FOR ASSESSING GI CLOSTRIDIA INFECTIONS

As mentioned earlier, *C. difficile* is the only species out of 100 species of clostridia from the GI tract to be commonly tested in hospital laboratories throughout the world. However, this species is not commonly cultured but is detected by its toxin formation. An overview of clostridia testing is presented in Table 4.2. The GI damage caused by *C. difficile* is thought to be due to exposure to two toxins produced by *C. difficile*, toxin A and toxin B, with toxin B considered to be more toxic.[17] The toxins can be tested by immunoassay of stool samples which is a fairly rapid test. Toxigenic stool culture, which requires growing the bacteria in a culture and detecting the presence of the toxins, is the most sensitive test for *C. difficile*, and it is still considered to be the gold standard.[17] However, toxigenic stool culture can take 2–3 days for results. Polymerase chain reaction (PCR) evaluation for the *C. difficile* toxins is also becoming more available. Virtually all of the research on *C. difficile* is related to the effects of this species of bacteria on the intestinal tract. Toxin-negative *C. difficile* strains are considered nonpathogenic for the infection of the intestine,[17] but cresol producing strains

TABLE 4.2

Comparison of Testing Methods for the Detection of Clostridia Bacteria

Species Tested	Method	Advantages	Disadvantages
C. difficile	Stool toxin A by immunoassay or PCR	Detects strains causing gastrointestinal disease and diarrhea; relatively fast, specific, and cheap	Does not detect strains producing high amounts of 4-cresol or HPHPA causing neuropsychiatric disorders
C. difficile	Stool toxin B by immunoassay or PCR	Detects strains causing gastrointestinal disease and diarrhea; relatively fast, specific, and cheap	Does not detect strains producing high amounts of 4-cresol or HPHPA causing neuropsychiatric disorders
C. difficile	Toxigenic stool culture	Gold standard for the detection of *C. difficile* causing gastrointestinal disease; more sensitive than toxins A and B tests	Time consuming, relatively expensive; may not detect strains producing high amounts of cresol or HPHPA causing neuropsychiatric disorders
C. difficile producing 4-cresol	GC/MS of urine as part of organic acids	Detects the compound 4-cresol which is a powerful inhibitor of dopamine-beta-hydroxylase which causes neuropsychiatric diseases; specific for *C. difficile*	May not be as sensitive as toxin assays for detecting strains of *C. difficile* causing gastrointestinal disease
Clostridia bacteria causing neuropsychiatric disorders producing HPHPA	GC/MS of urine as part of organic acid test	Detects the compound HPHPA which is a powerful inhibitor of dopamine-beta-hydroxylase which causes neuropsychiatric diseases; not specific for any specific species of clostridia but lack of specificity may not be clinically important since HPHPA is a major cause of a variety of neuropsychiatric disorders	Does not test all species of clostridia, but this may actually be advantageous since the test only measures the clostridia bacteria producing HPHPA; if the other clostridia species don't produce HPHPA, there may be no clinical significance in their measurement
Stool culture of all clostridia or PCR of total clostridia	Culture of stool or PCR of stool	Academic value of knowing total number of clostridia in stool	Does not distinguish between beneficial and pathogenic species of clostridia; clinically irrelevant; does not indicate the presence of *C. difficile* unless done as separate test

that don't produce toxins A and B may be pathogenic due to their effects on brain metabolism and for the inherent toxicity of 4-cresol itself.

In addition, urinary 4-cresol elevations associated with *C. difficile* overgrowth are much less common than urinary HPHPA elevations associated with other clostridia species. A survey of 1000 consecutive samples submitted for urine organic acids at The Great Plains Laboratory found that 15.2% were abnormally elevated for HPHPA, 6.8% were abnormally elevated for 4-cresol, and 1.6% were abnormally elevated for both HPHPA and 4-cresol, with a total positive percentage of 23.6%. Therefore, if only stool testing for *C. difficile* is performed on a patient, at least 15.2/23.6 or 64.4%, nearly two-thirds, of patients with clinically significant infections with other clostridia infections may be missed.

People sometimes assume that a test using DNA is more accurate than other types of testing. However, DNA testing is fraught with complexities. The nucleic acids of clostridia are extremely diverse. The content of the nucleic acid bases guanosine and cytosine (G+C) is used to classify bacteria species. The G+C content of DNA of clostridia species ranges from 21% to 54%.[21] The majority of intestinal species have G+C contents in the lower half of this range. Ribosomal RNA cataloging confirms that clostridia occupy six independent sublines with multiple branches including non-*Clostridium* species. The failure to offer documentation on which species are being detected and how validation was performed should lead to caution by the user of such testing, especially when such tests are labeled "experimental." Similar complexities exist with culturing clostridia, since results are commonly reported from 0 to 4+. Since many clostridia species are not pathogenic, what does a high clostridia level of 4+ indicate since beneficial, neutral, and harmful species are lumped together in one category? In reality, the results of current stool tests for total clostridia are virtually meaningless and may lead to inappropriate patient treatment.

Scientists at the Department of Microbiology IIT Research Institute, Chicago, Illinois, and the Department of Pathology Loyola University Medical Center, Maywood, Illinois, decided to evaluate one commercial laboratory offering stool methods based on a proprietary DNA method to identify gut microbiota including anaerobes[22]:

> A total of 34 stool samples were sent for Stool Testing. The stool pool was tested extensively, using conventional methodologies, on two separate days and found to be free of entero pathogenic bacteria, yeast and parasites. Thirty-one specimens were spiked with bacterial pathogens at clinically significant levels that are within the sensitivity of culture based methods, and at higher levels well above the Subject Laboratory's reported lower limit for detection of pathogens. Three "control" specimens were unaltered and contained no bacterial, fungal or parasitic pathogens. All 31 stool specimens containing bacterial pathogens were reported negative for the indicated pathogens by the Subject Laboratory. Seventeen samples of the parasite-free samples were reported as "Parasite present, taxonomy unavailable."

In addition to difficulties with stool testing, there are some commercial laboratories that offer markers for clostridia bacteria in organic acid profiles when in fact these markers are predominantly for other bacterial species.[3] One of these compounds, 3,4-dihydroxyphenylpropionic acid (DHPPA), a compound found at very low amounts in the urine, is a by-product of chlorogenic acid, a common substance found in beverages and in many fruits and vegetables including apples, pears, tea, coffee, sunflower seeds, carrots, blueberries, cherries, potatoes, tomatoes, eggplant, sweet potatoes, and peaches. Because of the chemical similarities, similar retention times in many chromatographic systems, and the similar mass spectra of 3-(3-hydroxyphenyl)-3-hydroxypropionic acid (HPHPA) and DHPPA, it is important to differentiate the sources of these compounds. The breakdown of chlorogenic acid to form DHPPA is mediated mainly by harmless or beneficial bacteria such as lactobacilli, bifidobacteria, and *E. coli,* and not by clostridia bacteria.

It is estimated that there are about 10 billion cells of clostridia per gram of stool. *C. ramosum* is the most common (53% of all subjects tested) with a mean count of about one billion per gram of stool.[23] The prevalence of some *Clostridium* species is highly dependent on diet. Stool samples of vegetarians did not contain *C. perfringens*, whereas meat and fish eaters had high amounts.[23]

Since HPHPA is associated with multiple species of clostridia but not *C. difficile*, there is really no available confirmation test for determining the specific species of *Clostridium* producing HPHPA. However, the precursors of HPHPA are produced by *C. sporogenes, C. botulinum, C. caloritolerans, C. mangenoti, C. ghoni, C. bifermentans, C. caproicum,* and *C. sordellii* with the first three producing the largest amounts.[3]

As mentioned above, stool testing for total clostridia is suboptimal since it cannot currently differentiate harmful or beneficial species. Since HPHPA resolves after treatment with vancomycin or metronidazole, I always recommend treatment based on the HPHPA value, with a follow-up test 30 days after completion of treatment. Confirmation testing of *Clostridium difficile* could be performed when 4-cresol is elevated. However, the prevalent testing for *Clostridium difficile* toxins A and B is only focused on strains that cause GI damage. Strains that produce 4-cresol but not toxins A or B may still cause significant psychiatric disease, so performing these toxin tests may muddy the interpretation of the clinical situation if these tests are negative.

ORIGIN OF HPHPA AND CLINICAL SIGNIFICANCE

The biochemical pathway for the production of HPHPA involves enzymes from both clostridia bacteria and humans (Figure 4.3). Phenylalanine derived from dietary proteins is the starting material. Phenylalanine is then converted by GI clostridia to phenylpropionic acid and 3-hydroxyphenylpropionic acid. The fact that clostridia are the *only* species that produce phenylpropionic acid is the fact that allows the metabolite of this compound HPHPA to be used as a marker for clostridia bacteria.[3] The same human enzymes that break down fatty acids by the beta-oxidation pathway to produce energy in the mitochondria convert 3-hydroxyphenylpropionic acid to HPHPA. Further metabolism of HPHPA produces 3-hydroxy-benzoic acid, which is then conjugated with glycine to form 3-hydroxybenzoylglycine (also called 3-hydroxyhippuric acid). The ability to detoxify HPHPA will likely determine the severity of clinical symptoms caused by dopamine-beta-hydroxylase inhibition. Administration of the amino acid glycine may be useful to accelerate HPHPA detoxification. On the other hand, because of its biochemical similarity to tyrosine (4-hydroxyphenylalanine), 3-hydroxyphenylalanine, one of the precursors to HPHPA, might interfere in the production of L-DOPA from tyrosine or possibly produce analogs of L-DOPA, dopamine, and norepinephrine (not shown in Figure 4.3) which would also cause severe disruption of dopamine metabolism.[3]

Since phenylalanine from protein is the starting material for HPHPA production, it is likely that some psychiatric patients may avoid protein foods to minimize production of this compound. Some of the organic acid test results from a patient with severe anorexia are shown in Figure 4.5. In this profile, the clostridia HPHPA marker in urine is five times the upper limit of normal, the dopamine metabolite HVA is 3.6 times the upper limit of normal, and the HVA/VMA ratio is a remarkable 14.4 times the upper limit of normal. Anorexia could be an adaptive response to prevent the further accumulation of toxic HPHPA from phenylalanine in dietary proteins. Similar protein food shunning is common in patients with genetic urea cycle disorders who cannot effectively detoxify ammonia from the breakdown of amino acids in protein. Many of the people with this disorder develop a vegetarian food preference before they receive a diagnosis.

TREATMENT OF CLOSTRIDIA INFECTIONS

Clostridia species are highly infectious due to spore formation, and other family members or pets should also be tested. When the person affected defecates and the toilet is flushed, the clostridia spores can aerosolize and spread to other areas of the bathroom. Clostridia spores have been found on the toothbrushes of individuals with *C. difficile* infection who used their home toilets. Therefore, all bathroom surfaces should be cleaned with dilute (1:10) household bleach to kill spores to prevent reinfection of the infected person or infection of other family members or pets.

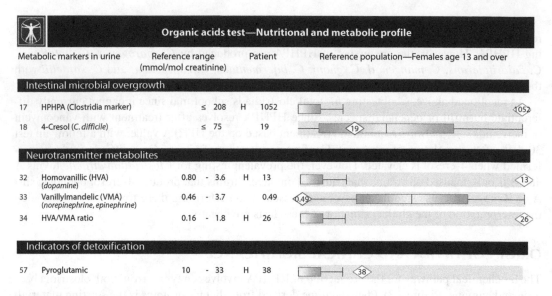

Metabolic markers in urine	Reference range (mmol/mol creatinine)	Patient		Reference population—Females age 13 and over
Organic acids test—Nutritional and metabolic profile				
Intestinal microbial overgrowth				
17 HPHPA (Clostridia marker)	≤ 208	H	1052	1052
18 4-Cresol (*C. difficile*)	≤ 75		19	19
Neurotransmitter metabolites				
32 Homovanillic (HVA) (*dopamine*)	0.80 - 3.6	H	13	13
33 Vanillylmandelic (VMA) (*norepinephrine, epinephrine*)	0.46 - 3.7		0.49	0.49
34 HVA/VMA ratio	0.16 - 1.8	H	26	26
Indicators of detoxification				
57 Pyroglutamic	10 - 33	H	38	38

FIGURE 4.5   Partial results of an organic acid profile on urine of adult female with severe anorexia. The clostridia HPHPA marker in the urine organic acid test is five times the upper limit of normal, the dopamine metabolite HVA is 3.6 times the upper limit of normal, and the HVA/VMA ratio is 14.4 times the upper limit of normal. Furthermore, VMA which is derived from epinephrine and norepinephrine is extremely low so that epinephrine production from the adrenal gland is diminished and the patient will likely have reduced tolerance to stress. The function of the sympathetic nervous system may also be adversely affected since these neurons employ norepinephrine as the major neurotransmitter. The high dopamine metabolite likely used up glutathione so that there is a high amount of pyroglutamic acid. Pyroglutamic acid is an inverse marker of glutathione deficiency, so a high amount of pyroglutamic acid indicates glutathione deficiency. In the graphs above, if the metabolite is in the normal range, the entire normal range is graphed. If the metabolite is elevated, only the upper part of the normal range is graphed. The letter H indicates high, meaning the value exceeds the upper limit of normal. The patient's value is indicated in a diamond on each graph and is also printed to the right side of the reference range.

Despite the common treatment practice of a 7–10 day course of oral vancomycin or metronidazole, this does not appear to be the most clinically effective method for treatment (Figure 4.6). Figure 4.6 shows that HPHPA disappears after about 3 weeks of metronidazole treatment but that high values of HPHPA are present again after metronidazole ceases due to spore formation. The antibiotics metronidazole and vancomycin are very effective when given orally in treating the growing vegetative cells of clostridia but are ineffective against spores.[24] Therefore, intermittent treatment protocols have evolved such that there is a waiting period without antibiotic treatment to allow antibiotic resistant spores to revert to their antibiotic susceptible vegetative forms. Use of these protocols markedly reduces the recurrence rate for clostridia.[24] The pulsing protocol in Figure 4.7 is based on treatment for 1 day followed by 2 days without treatment. This cycle of 1 day on and 2 days off is then repeated for a month. The scientific study[24] for the improved efficacy of this pulsing protocol is based on the use of oral vancomycin. However, there is no reason to think that a similar protocol using metronidazole would not also be effective.

The use of probiotics to treat clostridia has been evaluated alone and in conjunction with vancomycin or metronidazole.[24] A significant decrease in recurrences of *C. difficile* (16.7%) was observed in patients treated with high-dose vancomycin (2 g per day) and *Saccharomyces boulardii* compared with patients who received high-dose vancomycin and placebo (50%). However, *S. boulardii* treatment had no impact on recurrence rates of patients treated with low-dose vancomycin or metronidazole. Several strains of lactobacilli have also been tested as treatments for *C. difficile* infections.

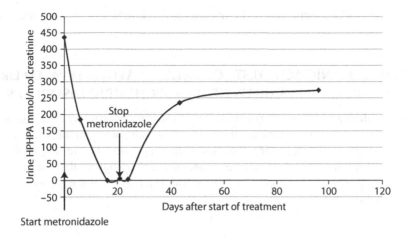

FIGURE 4.6   After obtaining a baseline urine sample (day 0), a child with autism was treated with metronidazole for 21 days. Urine samples were collected subsequently which indicate regrowth of clostridia after presumed germination of spores. (Data from Shaw, W., *Nutr Neurosci* 13(3): 135–143, 2010.)

In three case series,[24] a total of 41 patients with recurrent *C. difficile* infections were treated with *L. rhamnosus GG* (the main probiotic bacteria in Culturelle®). As a result, 50%–84% of the patients had no further recurrences.

The use of stool transplants is a new experimental treatment modality[25] that is gaining increasing interest as a treatment for those patients in which three courses of vancomycin or metronidazole have failed. However, the U.S. Food and Drug Administration considers this treatment experimental and requires a considerable amount of documentation to use this method. The author has also received reports of children vomiting up feces after administration of stool from a suitable donor. This treatment modality, however, is not only difficult to obtain, but is very expensive. The pulsing method of antibiotic administration together with several months of follow-up with probiotics likely

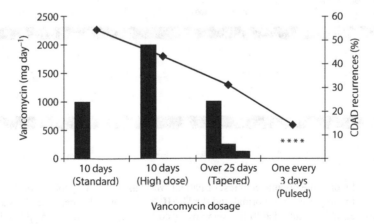

FIGURE 4.7   Effectiveness of different treatment strategies for recurrent *Clostridium difficile* associated disease (CDAD). Different vancomycin regimes (bars) compared to the frequency of recurrences (r) in 200 patients followed for at least 2 months post-treatment. Asterisks indicate one dose every 3 days. The standard dose was 1000 mg per day, the high dose 2000 mg per day, the tapered dose starting at 1000 mg per day and then decreasing to 125 mg per day, and the pulsed dose administered at a dose from 125–500 mg every 3 days over a mean of 27 days. (Data from McFarland, L.V., *J Med Microbiol* 54: 101–111, 2005.)

represents the best available approach, and clinician feedback indicates that this method is highly successful.

EXAMPLES OF ORGANIC ACID TESTS OF PATIENTS WITH ELEVATED URINE CLOSTRIDIA MARKERS IN VARIOUS NEUROPSYCHIATRIC DISORDERS

The final figures indicate examples of organic acid profiles of individuals with gastrointestinal clostridia overgrowth and severe long-term colitis (Figure 4.8), schizoid symptoms (Figure 4.9), early Parkinson's disease (Figure 4.10), and irritable bowel with depression before (Figure 4.11) and after (Figure 4.12) treatment. It is evident from an examination of these figures that the same underlying mechanism involving inhibition of dopamine metabolism is a major factor in many different neuropsychiatric disorders (Table 4.2).

CONCLUSION

The finding of Armstrong and Shaw that a unique phenolic biochemical, now termed HPHPA, was found to be elevated in a wide variety of mental illnesses has been confirmed by the author to be a product of the combined metabolism of human and clostridia bacteria species, with three species of clostridia being the highest producers. Of course, it is possible that additional nonspeciated types of clostridia may also be producers. In addition, a similar phenolic biochemical 4-cresol is produced mainly by the clostridia species *C. difficile*, one of the most common hospital infections.

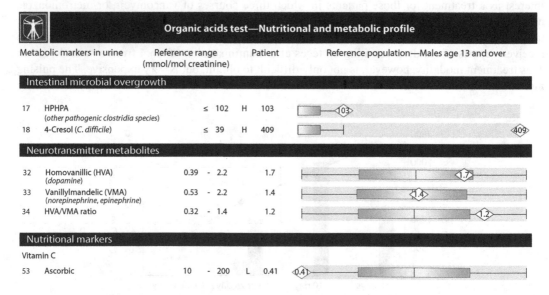

FIGURE 4.8 Results of urine organic acid test of patient who has had severe colitis for 25 years. Although 4-cresol is 10 times the upper limit of normal and the HPHPA is slightly elevated, the HVA and HVA/VMA ratios are not elevated presumably due to the very low ascorbic acid (vitamin C). Apparently the very low vitamin C reduced the inactivation of dopamine-beta-hydroxylase by 4-cresol so that the HVA and HVA/VMA ratios were not affected. The 4-cresol is so high that many of the patient's symptoms may be due to the toxicity of 4-cresol itself. In the graphs above, if the metabolite is in the normal range, the entire normal range is graphed. If a metabolite is elevated, only the upper part of the normal range is graphed. The letter H indicates high, meaning the value exceeds the upper limit of normal. The patient's value is indicated in a diamond on each graph.

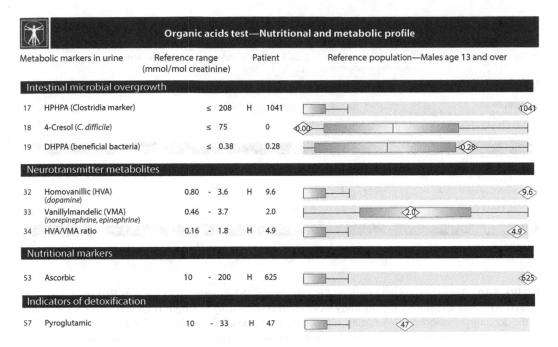

Organic acids test—Nutritional and metabolic profile			
Metabolic markers in urine	Reference range (mmol/mol creatinine)	Patient	Reference population—Males age 13 and over
Intestinal microbial overgrowth			
17 HPHPA (Clostridia marker)	≤ 208	H 1041	1041
18 4-Cresol (*C. difficile*)	≤ 75	0	0.00
19 DHPPA (beneficial bacteria)	≤ 0.38	0.28	0.28
Neurotransmitter metabolites			
32 Homovanillic (HVA) (*dopamine*)	0.80 - 3.6	H 9.6	9.6
33 Vanillylmandelic (VMA) (*norepinephrine, epinephrine*)	0.46 - 3.7	2.0	2.0
34 HVA/VMA ratio	0.16 - 1.8	H 4.9	4.9
Nutritional markers			
53 Ascorbic	10 - 200	H 625	625
Indicators of detoxification			
57 Pyroglutamic	10 - 33	H 47	47

FIGURE 4.9   Urine organic acid profile of a vegetarian patient with schizoid symptoms. Note that ascorbic acid (vitamin C) is elevated which likely accelerates the deactivation of dopamine-beta-hydroxylase by HPHPA. Elevated pyroglutamic acid is an indicator of glutathione deficiency. The elevated pyroglutamic acid marker may indicate brain toxicity due to formation of dopamine amino acid adducts and dopamine quinones that deplete glutathione. The patient may have adopted a vegetarian diet to reduce the amount of protein containing phenylalanine that increases HPHPA, increasing the degree of mental illness. In the graphs above, if the metabolite is in the normal range, the entire normal range is graphed. If a metabolite is elevated, only the upper part of the normal range is graphed. The letter H indicates high, meaning the value exceeds the upper limit of normal. The patient's value is indicated in a diamond on each graph.

These bacteria have been implicated as a common infection in a major study of depression and other mental illnesses. The major biochemical mechanism by which the clostridia metabolites affect both the brain and the sympathetic nervous system is the irreversible inhibition of dopamine beta-hydroxylase, resulting in elevated dopamine in the brain and sympathetic nervous system. The elevated dopamine forms quinones that induce toxic levels of free radicals, causing brain dysfunction and apoptosis of neurons. It appears that this complex metabolic interaction is the first example of how abnormal intestinal flora can have profound effects on brain function. Many other such interactions will likely be forthcoming.

Future challenges will be to discover how abnormally elevated phenols cause such a variety of neuropsychiatric disorders. Undoubtedly many of these modulating factors will be genetic differences in the metabolism of phenolic compounds, such as phenol sulfotransferase and detoxification reactions involving glutathione and formation of glucuronides, as well as genetic differences in the human biochemical pathways for the conversion of bacterial phenylpropionic acid to HPHPA and as polymorphisms in dopamine-beta-hydroxylase.

ACKNOWLEDGMENTS

The author thanks Lori Knowles-Jimenez and Heather Getz for their assistance in editing the content of this chapter.

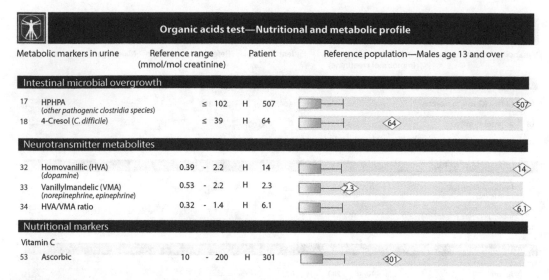

FIGURE 4.10   Urine organic acid profile of elderly man with beginning symptoms of Parkinson's disease. Both HPHPA and 4-cresol are significantly elevated. It is interesting that both HVA and VMA are elevated, but the dopamine metabolite HVA is markedly elevated as is the HVA/VMA ratio. Vitamin C is also elevated which is a cofactor in the inactivation of dopamine-beta-hydroxylase. Parkinson's disease is associated with decreased amounts of dopamine in the brain, but in the early stages of the disease clostridia metabolites HPHPA and 4-cresol may paradoxically cause elevated dopamine which at high concentrations leaks from the synaptic vesicles and is converted to quinones and amino acid adducts which damage dopamine containing neurons. If a metabolite is elevated, only the upper part of the normal range is graphed. The letter H indicates high, meaning the value exceeds the upper limit of normal. The patient's value is indicated in a diamond on each graph.

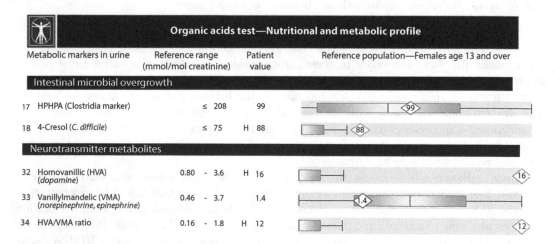

FIGURE 4.11   Organic acid profile of a 65-year-old woman with irritable bowel and severe depression prior to treatment.

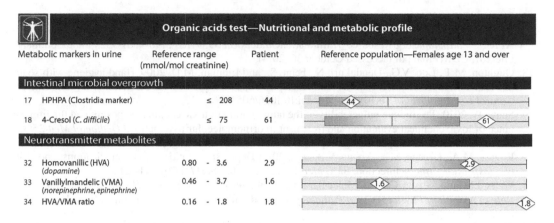

Metabolic markers in urine	Reference range (mmol/mol creatinine)		Patient	Reference population—Females age 13 and over
Intestinal microbial overgrowth				
17 HPHPA (Clostridia marker)	≤ 208		44	
18 4-Cresol (*C. difficile*)	≤ 75		61	
Neurotransmitter metabolites				
32 Homovanillic (HVA) (*dopamine*)	0.80	- 3.6	2.9	
33 Vanillylmandelic (VMA) (*norepinephrine, epinephrine*)	0.46	- 3.7	1.6	
34 HVA/VMA ratio	0.16	- 1.8	1.8	

FIGURE 4.12   Organic acid profile of same woman in Figure 4.11 after antimicrobial treatment resolved both depression and irritable bowel. Note that 4-cresol and neurotransmitters are in normal range.

REFERENCES

1. Armstrong, M.J. and Shaw, K.N.F. 1957. The occurrence of (-)-β-m-hydroxyphenylhydracrylic acid in human urine. *J Biol Chem* 225: 269–278.
2. Simunek, M., Hoßfeld, U., and Wissemann, V. 2011. "Rediscovery" revised—The cooperation of Erich and Armin von Tschermak-Seysenegg in the context of the "rediscovery" of Mendel's laws in 1899–19011. *Plant Biol* 13(6): 835–841. doi:10.1111/j.1438-8677.2011.00491.
3. Shaw, W. 2010. Increased urinary excretion of a 3-(3-hydroxyphenyl)-3-hydroxypropionic acid (HPHPA), an abnormal phenylalanine metabolite of *Clostridia* spp. in the gastrointestinal tract, in urine samples from patients with autism and schizophrenia. *Nutr Neurosci* 13(3): 135–143.
4. Shaw, W., Kassen, E., and Chaves, E. 2000. Assessment of antifungal drug therapy in autism by measurement of suspected microbial metabolites in urine with gas chromatography-mass spectrometry. *Clin Pract Altern Med* 1: 15–26. Available at: http://www.greatplainslaboratory.com/camarticle/index.html
5. Elsden, S.R., Hilton, M.G., and Waller, J.M. 1976. The end products of the metabolism of aromatic amino acids by Clostridia. *Arch Microbiol* 107: 283–288.
6. Bhala, A., Bennett, M., McGowan, K., and Hale, D. 1993. Limitations of 3-phenylpropionylglycine in early screening for medium chain acyl dehydrogenase deficiency. *J Pediatr* 122: 100–103.
7. Sande, M. and Hook, E. 1983. Other clostridial infections. In *Principles of Internal Medicine*, 10th ed. Ed. R. Petersdorf et al. New York, NY: McGraw-Hill, pp. 1009–1013.
8. Afghani, B. and Stutman, H. 1994. Toxin related diarrheas. *Pediatr Ann* 23: 549–555.
9. Finegold, S. 1986. Anaerobic infections and *Clostridium difficile* colitis emerging during antibacterial therapy. *Scand J Infect Dis* 49: 160–164.
10. Sivsammye, G. and Sims, H.V. 1990. Presumptive identification of *Clostridium difficile* by detection of p-cresol (4-cresol) in prepared peptone yeast glucose broth supplemented with *p*-hydroxyphenylacetic acid. *J Clin Microbiol* 28(8): 1851–1853.
11. Phua, T.J., Rogers, T.R., and Pallett, A.P. 1984. Prospective study of *Clostridium difficile* colonization and paracresol detection in the stools of babies on a special care unit. *J Hyg (Cambridge)* 93: 17–25.
12. Yokoyama, M.T., Tabori, C., Miller, E.R., and Hogberg, M.G. 1982. The effects of antibiotics in the weanling pig diet on growth and the excretion of volatile phenolic and aromatic bacterial metabolites. *Am J Clin Nutr* 35: 1417–1424.
13. Persico, A.M. and Napolioni, V. 2012. Urinary p-cresol (4-cresol) in autism spectrum disorder. *Neurotoxicol Teratol* 36: 82–90.
14. Goodhart, P.J., DeWolf, Jr., W.E., and Kruse, L.I. 1987. Mechanism-based inactivation of dopamine β-hydroxylase by p-cresol and related alkylphenols. *Biochemistry* 26: 2516–2583.
15. Munoz, P., Huenchuguala, S., Paris, I., and Segura-Aguilar, J. 2012. Dopamine oxidation and autophagy. *Parkinson's Dis* 2012: Article ID 920953. doi:10.1155/2012/920953.
16. Zhang, J., Kravtsov, V., Amarnath, V. et al. 2000. Enhancement of dopaminergic neurotoxicity by the mercapturate of dopamine: Relevance to Parkinson's disease. *J Neurochem* 74: 970–978.

17. Carrico, R.M. 2013. Association for Professionals in Infection Control and Epidemiology (APIC) Implementation Guide: Guide to preventing *Clostridium difficile* infections. Washington, DC: APIC. http://apic.org/Resource_/EliminationGuideForm/59397fc6-3f90-43d1-9325-e8be75d86888/File/2013CDiffFinal.pdf (accessed October 30, 2014).

18. Oughton, M.T., Loo, V.G., Dendukuri, N., Fenn, S., and Libman, M.D. 2009. Hand hygiene with soap and water is superior to alcohol rub and antiseptic wipes for removal of *Clostridium difficile. Infect Control Hosp Epidemiol* 30(10): 939–44. doi:10.1086/605322.

19. Shaw, W. 2010. The unique vulnerability of the human brain to toxic chemical exposure and the importance of toxic chemical evaluation and treatment in orthomolecular psychiatry. *J Orthomol Med* 25(3): 125–134. Available at http://www.greatplainslaboratory.com/home/eng/articles/hand_soap_article.pdf

20. Rogers, M.A., Greene, M.T., Young, V.B. et al. 2013. Depression, antidepressant medications, and risk of *Clostridium difficile* infection. *BMC Med* 11: 121. doi:10.1186/1741-7015-11-121.

21. Wells, J.M. and Allison, C. 1995. Molecular genetics of intestinal anaerobes. In *Human Colonic Bacteria: Role in Nutrition, Physiology, and Pathology*, Ed. G.R. Gibson and G.T. MacFarlane, Boca Raton, FL: CRC Press, p. 28.

22. Gingras, B.A., Duncan, S.B., Schueller, N.J., and Schreckenberger, P.C. 2014. Assessment of the diagnostic accuracy of recently introduced DNA stool screening test. *Int J Hum Nutr Funct Med* 2: 3–8.

23. Conway, P. 1995. Microbial ecology of the human large intestine. In *Human Colonic Bacteria: Role in Nutrition, Physiology, and Pathology*, Ed. G.R. Gibson and G.T. MacFarlane, Boca Raton, FL: CRC Press, pp. 1–24.

24. McFarland, L.V. 2005. Alternative treatments for *Clostridium difficile* disease: What really works? *J Med Microbiol* 54: 101–111.

25. van Nood, E., Vrieze, A., Nieuwdorp, M. et al. 2013. Duodenal infusion of donor feces for recurrent *Clostridium difficile. N Engl J Med* 368: 407–415.

5 Stress, Fear, Trauma, and Distress
Underlying Factors in Depression

Peter Bongiorno, ND, LAc

CONTENTS

INTRODUCTION

Depressive illness is a complex syndrome that has an array of possible etiologies and treatment interventions. An understanding of stress, trauma, fear, and distress are essential to adequately understand the underlying drivers of depression and to guide best care.

This chapter is going to define these terms, review the concepts of Hans Selye's model of General Adaptation, and Bruce McEwen's allostatic load as they relate to depression. It will review stress-response mechanisms in light of the hypothalamic-pituitary-adrenal axis. Additionally, treatment options related to stress and allostatic load will be reviewed. The chapter will conclude with a discussion of the prenatal environment's culpability in the future offspring's stress response in an effort to prevent depressive illness in the next generation.

DEFINITIONS OF STRESS, FEAR, TRAUMA, AND DISTRESS

Stress, fear, trauma, and distress are somewhat hard to define. These are clearly related to each other, and to the pathophysiology that can culminate in depression. For the health community to be able to effectively treat any illness, it is key to ascribe among all practitioners adequate and universally accepted definitions to the label, factors, and conditions of a disease. Using a simple analogy, if a physician does not know the definition of hyperglycemia, she would be challenged to treat diabetes properly, and she would not understand the tools available to help. Given that there is no single biological marker for depression, it is important to acknowledge, and hopefully agree on, the definitions regarding the major factors in depression: stress, trauma, fear, and distress. These are not single entities, but they exist as a continuum.

STRESS

The clinical presentation of depression shares many features with the stress response. Changes in cognition, affective responses, arousal, and dysregulation of both autonomic function and the neuroendocrine system are found in both depression and the stress response.

While stress is universally recognized as highly significant in depression, the definition of stress varies among physicians. Along with this, there is little agreement on the best ways to handle stress. Hungarian endocrinologist Hans Selye first used the term *stress* after completing his medical training at the University of Montreal in the 1920s. He defined it as a "non-specific strain on the body caused by irregularities in normal body functions. This stress resulted in the release of hormones."[1] Stressors can take many different forms: changes in environmental milieu, weather, social structure, and interpersonal interaction. The stress response can also be initiated by perceived danger, from the onset of new illness, from exposure to toxins, and even by food sensitivity.

While typically thought of as negative in connotation, stress is not exclusively considered pathologic. Interestingly, Selye's "strain on the body" can also be experienced even in environments where there is no apparent stress or unpleasant experience. Accordingly, Hans Selye defined the "eustress" state as a situation where the organism seeks out a particular situation that can also affect the release of glucocorticoids and increase in sympathetic activity.[2] For example, the desire to exercise or engage in sexual activity may fit under this definition.

For the purposes of this chapter, "stress" will refer to a dissonant and subjectively challenging experience. This is the type of stress that leads to the activation of the limbic system and hypothalamic-pituitary-adrenal (HPA) axis to protect the body against adversity. This type of stress will also lead to the secretion of stress hormones like corticotropin-releasing hormone (CRH), adrenocorticotropic hormone (ACTH), and cortisol.

It is widely accepted that difficult life challenges (such as loss of a loved one, accidents, illness, work stresses, and interpersonal problems) can cause stress. There exist a host of physiologic assaults that can generate a "silent" stress response. For example, persistent organic pollutants create a negative effect on insulin sensitivity in the body.[3] This can raise inflammation, and create a greater likelihood for depressive illness to occur.

FEAR

Fear may be considered a more specific type of stress or strain on the body. According to Shin and Liberzon, fear is "an unpleasant emotion caused by the belief that someone or something is dangerous, likely to cause pain, or a threat" and is the "underlying cause of many of our actions and anxiety."[4] Fear causes human physiology to also gird for challenging times. Fear will drive Selye's stress response of hormone and glucocorticoid release.

Critical for survival, a fear-driven response to danger will drive behavioral changes, causing the organism to take a defensive or offensive posture. It will also unleash a series of physiological changes such as increased breathing rate, heart rate, blood pressure, and diminution of nonessential physiology for that moment (e.g., digestive secretions, sexual interest). According to Phil Gold, director of the Clinical Branch of Neuroendocrinology at the National Institute of Mental Health, "an extensive circuitry has thus been developed for generating and modulating fear and response, to both simulate appropriate behavior characterized by speed and simplicity and inhibit more complex, novel, and untested response."[5]

TRAUMA

According to the American Psychological Association, trauma is an "emotional response to a terrible event like an accident, rape or natural disaster." While stress and fear are a normal part of the human experience, the psychiatric definition of "trauma" places it as "an event outside normal human experience."[6] Shock and denial are protective and common reactions that occur acutely after a traumatic event. However, in the longer term, the response may also include unpredictable emotions, flashbacks, strained relationships, and somatic presentation, such as digestive distress, headaches, or other common complaints.[7]

Prolonged chronic stress or fear can lead to someone becoming traumatized. Stress and fear bring discomfort, and hopefully the impetus to create changes that are healthful in the long term and to avoid trauma. Trauma, on the other hand, can leave the person feeling helpless and unable. Traumatic stress can cause durable changes in brain areas such as the amygdala, hippocampus, and prefrontal cortex.[8]

Stress and fear will elicit a response to enable survival and hopefully bring resolution so the person can return to his or her original state and homeostasis. Homeostasis is defined as the stability of the physiologic systems that maintain life.[9] However, trauma can have enduring psychological effects, becoming a deeply distressing or disturbing experience[10] that results in preoccupation, avoidance, and vigilance.

DISTRESS

Chronic stress and fear, and/or trauma can lead to distress. Most definitions of distress suggest an "aversive, negative state in which coping and adaptation processes fail to return an organism to physiological and/or psychological homeostasis."[11] Distress suggests a maladaptive state where the organism's biological systems are altered and the ability to cope is significantly compromised.[12] In 1999, Moberg published the paper entitled, "When Does Stress Become Distress?" In this paper, he proposed that the organism's "use of reserve resources to cope with prolonged or severe stress has a negative impact on other bodily functions (including behavior) and leads to distress."[13]

Great strides in understanding stress and distress have come from animal models. Animal studies have shown that long-term immobilization restraint testing will produce distress, while shorter-term restraint does not. For example, in one study, immobilization stress on rats produced ulcers only after 6 hours of exposure, but not before this time point.[14]

Any animal or person's likelihood of moving into distress will be affected not only by duration, but also by that organism's constitution, nature of the stress, predictability of the stress, intensity of the stressors, and whether there is a sense of control in the situation. There is little in the way of a cause-and-effect relationship among these factors, resultant behaviors, and the onset of distress. For each animal or person, distress does not always present itself with the same maladaptive behaviors, such as fits of anger or reclusion. Sometimes the clinical changes are more internal, like blood pressure volatility, or immunosuppression.[15]

Sense of control and choice can avoid stress and fear moving into distress. When an animal or human finds it has options and can exercise control over its environment, then it displays more adaptive behaviors, versus the maladaptive type seen when in a state of distress.[16] Animal study suggests that animals who cannot escape restraint but can control their exposure to a shock experience showed fewer signs of distress versus those who are not able to stop the shock.[17]

THE STRESS RESPONSE, ADAPTATION AND ALLOSTASIS

When experiencing stress, the body naturally deploys a number of behavioral and physiologic responses designed to weather the current challenge in an effort to return to homeostasis. According to McEwen, during a stressful event (known as a stressor) the central nervous system and the body communicate in a bidirectional fashion via the endocrine, immune, and autonomic systems.[18] The interconnectedness of these systems supports a mind-body response, initiating changes in behavior, autonomic nervous system, activation in immune and cytokine cascades, as well as secretion of the hormones of stress (such as glucocorticoids and catecholamines).

In the short run, these responses are beneficial, for they serve to promote physiological and psychological survival. These physiological and behavioral responses are both stressor and person specific. Some individuals handle stressors better and more effectively than others. As a result, individuals will have different methodologies to attempt to achieve homeostasis. In the middle term, regulatory processes, behaviors, and physiology are challenged but functioning relatively normally. In the long term, consistent bombardment of stress, fear, and/or trauma and the knee-jerk attempts at homeostasis will contribute to the enduring negative effects of chronic stress and behavioral changes that could encourage unhealthy lifestyle and illness, engendering further stress in the process.

SELYE'S GENERAL ADAPTATION SYNDROME

Austrian-Canadian endocrinologist Hans Selye is credited with bringing the classical theory of stress to modern medicine. Connecting stress to the sympathetic nervous and HPA axis reaction to stress,[19] Selye outlined current perception of the flight-or-flight response. As mentioned briefly above, he went on to recognize the short, middle, and long-term consequences of stress, and recognized the continuum of the stress response as the general adaptation syndrome (GAS).

Simply put, the first stage of the GAS is the alarm reaction. In this phase, the adrenal cortex releases glucocorticoids, while the medullary part of the adrenal glands sends out the catecholamines. These function to help create a physiologic and behavioral response that brings the organism back to homeostasis.

If homeostasis is achieved but some level of stressor is still present, then it is understood that the organism has begun to adapt to a new normal or setpoint—this adaptation is the second stage of the GAS. For example, to keep up with the new stressor, higher levels of catecholamines and glucocorticoids are now needed.

If the stress remains constant and persists, the organism might then experience the third stage, which is exhaustion. In this situation the adaptive response is no longer physiologically viable. This means the organism will need to battle the stressor without its physiologic protectors (such as cortisol and catecholamines) working at levels sufficient to produce a homeostatic balance. This is typically where overt pathology may present itself, and this is the likely stage of chronic depression. The GAS occurs in three stages:

1. Alarm stage
2. Resistance stage
3. Exhaustion stage

ALLOSTASIS

Selye's classic model is still as applicable today as it was revolutionary when first proposed. However, for the purposes of understanding the relationship of the GAS to depression, it is equally as important to share additional concepts that have been worked out to further elucidate his model. Since Selye's seminal work, it has been established that the molecules of stress, such as glucocorticoids, cytokines, and catecholamines, can have both salutatory and deleterious results on physiology. It is possible that the "exhaustion" phase may not be so much a true depletion of these molecules, but instead could be the resultant effect of these being at too high a level for too long a time, whereby they are not recognized (as is the case of glucocorticoid resistance) or contribute to a chronic assault and damage of their own (as can be the case with chronic inflammation).[20]

Bruce McEwen's research team created a new term: *allostasis*, or *allostatic overload*, to recognize the paralleled healthful and noxious results of the stress response. The molecules of the stress response, including cortisol, epinephrine, and cytokine cascades, can clearly help the organism with the adaptive changes that allow for survival. For example, cortisol creates a gluconeogenic response in the liver that releases blood sugar more freely into the bloodstream. This allows glucose to remain much more available to the brain and muscle tissue. Available glucose is a key in the fight-or-flight response. Epinephrine readies the body for "fight or flight." Unfortunately, the mediators of the stress response will also contribute to allostatic overload, whereby the chemicals will contribute to wear and tear on the body, and cause longer-term damage if unremitting.

ALLOSTASIS VERSUS HOMEOSTASIS

In his 2005 article "Stressed or Stressed Out?" McEwen also clarifies the inherent ambiguity of these terms. He defines *homeostasis* as encompassing the more basic systems that are essential for life, while *allostasis* includes those that maintain these systems in balance.[9] This clarification underscores how the body does not remain constant, but instead equilibrates in a dynamic flux of sorts. This dynamic equilibrium is what is considered as stable.

While the allostatic load works to dynamically rebalance, it can, at the same time, damage tissues, deplete reserves, and encourage depressive illness, as well as other diagnosable diseases. The hippocampus has a high concentration of cortisol receptors. Neuronal apoptosis is increased by hypercortisolemic stress in the hippocampus. In patients with major depression, hippocampal volume is negatively correlated with symptom severity. In Vietnam veterans with posttraumatic stress disorder (PTSD), smaller hippocampal volumes correlate with longer combat exposure.[21]

In 2002, McEwen and his team also acknowledged that altered and chronic allostatic load will contribute to physical illness. His team drew up 10 markers of allostatic function to measure healthful aging and analyzed data from a 7 year longitudinal study of a community-based cohort, whose age at baseline was between 70 and 79 years. They found that the level of allostatic load can independently predict functional decline in elderly men and women. The markers they measured were

1. 12 hour overnight urinary cortisol excretion
2. 12 hour overnight urinary excretion of norepinephrine
3. 12 hour overnight urinary excretion of epinephrine
4. Serum dehydroepiandrosterone sulfate (DHEA-S)
5. Average systolic blood pressure
6. Average diastolic blood pressure
7. Ratio of waist-to-hip circumference
8. Serum high-density lipoprotein (HDL) cholesterol
9. Ratio of total-to-HDL cholesterol in the serum
10. Blood glycosylated hemoglobin

While the research did not consider depression as an endpoint, almost all of these factors chosen for this study are considered altered in and related to depression in some way. Catecholamine levels are altered in depression.[22] Glucocorticoids are often high or dysregulated in depression.[23] Elevated levels of serum DHEA may be associated with the biological pathophysiology of depression.[24] Lower serum HDL-C levels are a marker for major depression and suicidal behavior in depressed men.[25,26] There is also a relationship between higher blood glucose, elevated blood glycosylated hemoglobin, and elevated risk of depressive symptoms.[27] Higher blood pressure by itself does not seem to be strongly correlated with depression,[28] and may even be lowered in depressive illness[29] (maybe suggestive of the exhaustive stage of the GAS). Visceral adipose tissue plays a role in the relationship between obesity, depression, and cardiovascular disease.[30]

This list is not a complete representation of the neuroendocrine and immunologic players that make up allostatic load, but the results revealed that allostatic load significantly correlates with functional decline, illustrated by increased rates of cardiovascular disease and metabolic disturbance, as well as declines in physical and cognitive function, and mortality. This correlation was substantially larger than had been previously found in other research. The authors concluded that measure of allostatic load is indeed an independent predictor of functional decline in elderly men and women. Interestingly, the individual components of allostatic load were only modestly different from normal, and had only mild and generally statistically insignificant associations with outcomes. In depression, this may also be the case. In the authors' discussion, they suggested that "a multisystem measure of physiologic dysregulation is better at predicting future health than individual physiologic markers or risk factors, especially when dysregulation in individual systems are small."[31]

ANATOMY AND PHYSIOLOGY OF THE STRESS RESPONSE

Maintaining homeostatic balance in the face of threats that are real or perceived requires initiation of endocrine, nervous, and immunologic reactions, collectively known as the *stress response*.[32] The stress response can be both helpful and protective, and can also elicit maladaptive and destructive responses in certain individuals. These pernicious responses are more commonly associated with the behaviors of depressive illness. For example, animals exposed to long-term social subordination will present with altered HPA set points, ineffective hippocampal and dentate gyrus cell survival, glucocorticoid resistance, cognitive changes, withdrawal of behavior, and lowered immune status in the effort to produce coping mechanisms to the stressor.[33,34] The stress response interacts with many body systems and will play a role in the pathogenesis of depression. Below, we briefly summarize its effect on the HPA, allostatic load, thyroid function, hormonal balance, and inflammation.

Stress, fear, trauma, and distress lead to initial and ongoing cortical signal input to the hypothalamus (Figure 5.1). This signaling will lead to HPA alterations resulting in CRH production in the medial parvocellular subdivision of the paraventricular nucleus.[35] Raised levels of CRH are known to have neurotoxic effects.[36] As the final common pathway in the stress response, CRH is released to the hypothalamus and feeds directly to the anterior pituitary. There, binding initiates ACTH release. ACTH travels through the bloodstream and initiates adrenal cortex release of cortisol.[37] The action of CRH on ACTH release is also strongly potentiated by arginine vasopressin (also known as antidiuretic hormone). CRH and ACTH production is augmented when the hypothalamic paraventricular neurons are chronically activated. Oxytocin counters this effect. Normally, cortisol will negatively feedback through the action of mineralocorticoid and glucocorticoid receptors, to exert negative feedback on the hippocampus, the pituitary, and the hypothalamus.[38]

In chronic stress as well as disease states, the glucocorticoid feedback system can fail, allowing for greater levels of cortisol.[34] Higher levels of cortisol initially increase serotonin levels by both increasing tryptophan hydroxylase activity (which helps convert tryptophan to serotonin) and by increasing the availability of tryptophan itself.[39] However in a dose-dependent manner, chronically high allostatic loads of cortisol and the other molecules of stress will, over the long term, have the opposite effect and decrease serotonin levels.[40]

The 5-HT (serotonin) receptor is also affected. The 5-HT receptor 1A responds initially with great receptivity in acute cortisol increase,[41] but with decreased sensitivity with chronically higher levels.[42] Paradoxically, the 5-HT_2 receptor seems to upregulate with higher chronic cortisol in animal studies, although human studies are not conclusive.[43] Genetic susceptibility due to 5-HT receptor polymorphisms may also enhance the stress effect.

Low thyroid levels are a factor in depression, and can be an early or even first symptom of oncoming depression.[44] Regarding the hypothalamic-pituitary-thyroid (HPT) axis, high stress states and allostatic load will also alter the thyroid axis, whereby high levels of ACTH will affect levels of thyroid releasing factor and thyroid stimulating hormone (TSH). Repeated and chronic stress can

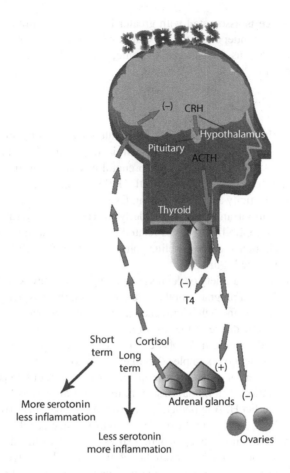

FIGURE 5.1 Stress response and the hypothalamic, pituitary, adrenal, thyroid, and ovarian axes.

lower serum levels of tetraiodothyronine (T4).[45] Glucocorticoids will also influence the de-iodinase enzyme responsible for peripheral conversion of T4 to active triiodothyronine (T3).[46]

The stress effect on the hypothalamic-pituitary-ovarian (HPO) axis also may play a role in serotonin alterations, as high and chronic stress will diminish reproductive organ capacity and activity. Estrogen is the predominant female hormone known for its ability to affect the levels of serotonin in the brain by changing the ability of nerve cells to recognize this important mood transmitter, as well as by lowering levels of an enzyme called monoamine oxidase, which breaks down serotonin.[47]

The stress response also upregulates inflammation in the body. High levels of glucocorticoids initially will tamp down the immune system, and lower inflammatory response. Neuropsychiatric disorders such as major depression have been associated with eventual decreased responsiveness to glucocorticoids (called glucocorticoid resistance), which is believed to be related in part to impaired functioning of the glucocorticoid receptor. Glucocorticoid resistance, in turn, can encourage greater levels of inflammation as well as hyperactivity of CRH and the sympathetic nervous system pathways, and will contribute to a variety of disease processes as well as behavioral alterations.[20] While most work surrounding cortisol focuses on the glucocorticoid receptor (GR), the mineralocorticoid receptor (MR) is beginning to be recognized for its importance in the stress response. Considered a low-capacity, but high-affinity cortisol receptor, the MR activity seems to determine the initial appraisal of a stressor and may prevent or reverse symptoms of stress-related depression,[48] while the GR controls, normalizes, and coordinates the activated stress responses.[49]

Glucocorticoid resistance is associated with greater levels of inflammation. Even for relatively healthy subjects, stressors are independently associated with greater inflammation, as evidenced by hypercoagulability and thrombus formation.[50] Chronic, low-grade inflammation in the body and brain contribute to depression.[51]

PRENATAL STRESS

Impaired functioning of the HPA axis has been associated with several physical and psychiatric disorders, such as the metabolic syndrome,[52] fibromyalgia, depression,[53] and PTSD.[54,55] While daily life stressors modulate present HPA activity, the prenatal environment and childhood experience may be far more impacting on the overall tone of the HPA. Gestational stress is a likely powerful player for offspring brain plasticity and development. Exposure to maternal stress in utero and early childhood adversity is an important factor for underlying HPA axis alterations that may mediate the effects on individual susceptibility to stress-related disorders. In simpler terms, like the volume setting on a stereo, events in utero set the baseline volume levels of the HPA and decide how overall "loud or soft" it will "play" (see Figure 5.2).

Studies have linked maternal anxiety or depression during pregnancy with HPA axis reactivity in infants and children.[56,57] When a pregnant mother is under stress, the offspring will be more likely to sustain altered brain physiology and behavioral changes with life-long consequences, including predisposition to depression. As evidence of the role of allostatic load in this early life process, several animal studies have reported specific links between prenatal stress exposure manifesting as glucocorticoid resistance in offspring. For example, Zucchi et al. showed in animal research how maternal stress will alter microRNA control of fetal transcriptomes which upregulate pathologic processes in the brain, such as inflammation.[58] In human research, maternal anxiety or depression during pregnancy has been shown to predict HPA hyperactivity, as well as changes in cortisol, in infants and preadolescent children.[56,57] Stressful maternal experiences will modify genetic expression in the brain in an epigenetic fashion. Stress impacts epigenetic expression, activating the genes that will make the offspring more prone to mood disorder, even though the genes themselves have not changed.[59]

The first evidence in humans of an association between prenatal psychosocial stress exposure and subsequent alterations in the regulation of the HPA axis was found in a study of 31 healthy young adults, whose mothers experienced major negative life events during their pregnancy. These offspring revealed much higher cortisol levels, when exposed to a stressor, relative to controls.

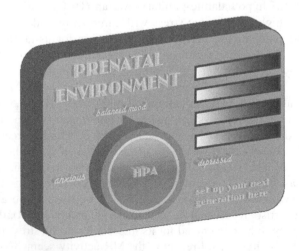

FIGURE 5.2 *In utero* events affect life long HPA activity. (Reprinted with permission from Bongiorno, P. 2015. *Holistic Solutions for Anxiety and Depression*. New York: WW Norton, p. 109.)

These results may reflect higher CRH neuronal activity and increased pituitary reactivity to stimulation in prenatally stressed subjects when exposed to psychosocial stress.[60]

From an integrative standpoint, it should also be noted that dietary imbalances, such as poor nourishment and low birth weight, maternal overeating, and processed fat diets will also contribute to HPA and mood disorder in the next generation. Increases in anxiety and decreases in learning capacity are found in offspring whose pregnant moms had higher intakes of unhealthy foods. These effects did not vastly change if the newborn pups were given a normal diet, suggesting that dietary imbalances before birth may not be fully reversible if the offspring eats more balanced after being born.[61] Emerging science supportive of the epigenetic impact of nutrition on the fetus underscores the importance of educating women about the importance of a healthy diet before and during pregnancy.

Factors after birth and in childhood will continue to affect HPA function. Studies on rat pups reveal that overfeeding of neonates will show increased HPA hyperresponsiveness and predisposition to mood disorder.[62] Victims of child abuse, those who experienced maternal separation as evidenced through parental loss in the 9/11 terrorist attacks,[63] as well as children exposed to the 1995 Oklahoma City bombing all displayed significant HPA dysregulation and predisposition to anxiety and depression.[64] Patients with PTSD who were exposed to childhood sexual abuse or other trauma reveal manifestations of allostatic load in the form of neuroanatomical changes such as smaller hippocampal volumes.[65,66]

LABORATORY TESTING IN THE STRESS-RESPONSE CONTEXT

While there is no formal testing available for the assessment of allostatic load, future markers will likely more consistently use an adrenal stress panel, which tests saliva levels of cortisol and DHEA. This is useful, for it more accurately describes cortisol function in the body and is typically easier to administer than a blood test.

Among the number of useful tests, allostatic load testing, as outlined in McEwen's work, may prove especially valuable in understanding and creating individualized treatment options for the patient with depression.

PREVENTING STRESS RESPONSE IN THE NEXT GENERATION

Along with proper nutrition, mind-body modalities in the prenatal and childhood period may hold the greatest promise in balancing HPA axis function and preventing depression in the next generation. There is evidence that pregnant women enjoy health benefits from mind-body therapies when used in conjunction with conventional prenatal care. In a meta-analysis, progressive muscle relaxation was the most common intervention used in pregnant women. Other studies used a multimodal psychoeducation approach or a yoga and meditation intervention and showed there was modest evidence for the efficacy of mind-body modalities during pregnancy. Treatment group outcomes included higher birth weight, shorter length of labor, fewer instrument-assisted births, and reduced perceived stress and anxiety.[67]

CONCLUSION

Depression is a multifactorial condition in terms of presentation and cause. Stress responses may be set up in the prenatal environment or can be initiated or augmented in childhood and adulthood from stressful experiences. Stressors, fears, and traumas can lead to distress and culminate in a chronic allostatic load that is responsible for the signs and symptoms of depression, and can contribute to other diseases including metabolic disease, autoimmunity, and cancer. A strong understanding of this process can help the integrative practitioner choose treatment options specific to the needs of each patient.

REFERENCES

1. Centre for Human Studies on Stress. What Is Stress? http://www.humanstress.ca/stress/what-is-stress/history-of-stress.html (accessed March 9, 2014).
2. Selye, H. 1975. *Stress without Distress*. New York, NY: New American Library.
3. Ruzzin, J., Petersen, R., Meugnier, E. et al. 2010. Persistent organic pollutant exposure leads to insulin resistance syndrome. *Environ Health Perspect* 118(4): 465–471.
4. Shin, L.M. and Liberzon, I. 2010. The neurocircuitry of fear, stress, and anxiety disorders. *Neuropsychopharmacology* 35(1): 169–191.
5. Gold, P.W. 2005. Stress system dysregulation in depression: From molecular biology to new treatment opportunities. In *Biology of Depression*, Licinio J. and Wong, M-L. (eds.). Weinheim, Germany: Wiley.
6. No author. Trauma. Washington, DC: American Psychological Association. http://www.apa.org/topics/trauma/ (accessed January 10, 2014).
7. Lewis, S. 1999. *An Adult's Guide to Childhood Grief and Trauma*. London, UK: Routledge.
8. Bremner, J.D. 2006. Traumatic stress: Effects on the brain. *Dialogues Clin Neurosci* 8: 445–461.
9. McEwen, B. 2005. Stressed or stressed out: What is the difference? *J Psychiatry Neurosci* 30: 315–318.
10. Cox, F. 2013. Trauma. *Br J Pain* 7: 265.
11. Carstens, E. and Moberg, G.P. 2000. Recognizing pain and distress in laboratory animals. *ILAR J* 41(2): 62–71.
12. Moberg, G.P. 2000. Biological response to stress: Implications for animal welfare. In *The Biology of Animal Stress*, Ed. G.P., Moberg and J.A. Mench. Wallingford, UK: CAB International, pp. 1–21.
13. Moberg, G.P. 1999. When does stress become distress? *Lab Anim* 28(4): 422–426.
14. Ushijima, I., Mizuki, Y., and Yamada, M. 1985. Development of stress-induced gastric lesions involves central adenosine A1-receptor stimulation. *Brain Res* 339: 351–355.
15. National Research Council (US) Committee on Recognition and Alleviation of Distress in Laboratory Animals. *Recognition and Alleviation of Distress in Laboratory Animals*. Washington, DC: National Academies Press. http://www.ncbi.nlm.nih.gov/books/NBK4027/ (accessed September 9, 2014).
16. Mench, J.A. 1998. Why it is important to understand animal behavior. *ILAR J* 39: 20–26.
17. Maier, S.F. and Watkins, L.R. 2005. Stressor controllability and learned helplessness: The roles of the dorsal raphe nucleus, serotonin, and corticotropin releasing hormone. *Neurosci Biobehav R.* 29(4–5): 829–841.
18. McEwen, B.S. 1998. Protective and damaging effects of stress mediators. *N Engl J Med* 338: 171–179.
19. Selye, H. 1936. A syndrome produced by diverse nocuous agents. *Nature* 138: 32.
20. Pace, T.W., Hu, F., and Miller, A.H. 2007. Cytokine-effects on glucocorticoid receptor function: Relevance to glucocorticoid resistance and the pathophysiology and treatment of major depression. *Brain Behav Immun* 21: 9–19.
21. Vasterling, J.J., Duke, L.M., Brailey, K. et al. 2002. Attention, learning, and memory performances and intellectual resources in Vietnam veterans: PTSD and no disorder comparisons. *Neuropsychology* 16: 5–14.
22. Potter, W.Z. and Manji, H.K. 1994. Catecholamines in depression: An update. *Clin Chem* 40: 279–287.
23. Steckler, T., Holsboer, F., and Reul, J.M. 1999. Glucocorticoids and depression. *Baillieres Best Pract Res Clin Endocrinol Metab* 13: 597–614.
24. Kurita, H., Maeshima, H., Kida, S. et al. 2013. Serum dehydroepiandrosterone (DHEA) and DHEA-sulfate (S) levels in medicated patients with major depressive disorder compared with controls. *J Affect Disord* 146: 205–212.
25. Maes, M., Smith, R., Christophe, A. et al. 1997. Lower serum high-density lipoprotein cholesterol (HDL-C) in major depression and in depressed men with serious suicidal attempts: Relationship with immune-inflammatory markers. *Acta Psychiatr Scand* 95: 212–221.
26. Teofilo, M.M., Farias, D.R., Pinto, T. et al. 2014. HDL-cholesterol concentrations are inversely associated with Edinburgh Postnatal Depression Scale scores during pregnancy: Results from a Brazilian cohort study. *J Psychiatr Res* 58: 181–188.
27. Hamer, M., Batty, G.D., and Kivimaki, M. 2011. Haemoglobin A1c, fasting glucose and future risk of elevated depressive symptoms over 2 years of follow-up in the English Longitudinal Study of Ageing. *Psychol Med* 41: 1889–1896.
28. Shinn, E.H., Poston, W.S., Kimball, K.T. et al. 2001. Blood pressure and symptoms of depression and anxiety: A prospective study. *Am J Hypertens* 14: 660–664.

29. Hildrum, B., Mykletun, A., Stordal, E. et al. 2007. Association of low blood pressure with anxiety and depression: The Nord-Trøndelag Health Study. *J Epidemiol Community Health* 61: 53–58.
30. Wiltink, J., Michal, M., Wild, P.S. et al. 2013. Associations between depression and different measures of obesity. *BMC Psychiatry.* 13: 223.
31. Karlamangla, A.S., Singer, B.H., McEwen, B.S. et al. 2002. Allostatic load as a predictor of functional decline. MacArthur studies of successful aging. *J Clin Epidemiol* 55: 696–710.
32. Smith, S.M. and Vale, W.W. 2006. The role of the hypothalamic-pituitary-adrenal axis in neuroendocrine responses to stress. *Dialogues Clin Neurosci* 8: 383–395.
33. Blanchard, R.J., McKittrick, C.R., and Blanchard, D.C. 2001. Animal models of social stress: Effects on behavior and brain neurochemical systems. *Physiol Behav* 73: 261–271.
34. Carroll, B.J., Curtis, G.C., and Mendels, J. 1976. Neuroendocrine regulation in depression, I: Limbic system-adrenocortical dysfunction. *Arch Gen Psychiat* 33: 1039–1044.
35. Vale, W., Spiess, J., Rivier, C. et al. 1981. Characterization of a 41-residue ovine hypothalamic peptide that stimulates secretion of corticotropin and beta-endorphin. *Science* 213: 1394–1397.
36. Wong, M.L., Loddick, S.A., Bongiorno, P.B. et al. 1995. Focal cerebral ischemia induces CRH mRNA in rat cerebral cortex and amygdala. *Neuroreport* 6: 1785–1788.
37. van Praag, H.M. 2004. Can stress cause depression? *Prog Neuropsychopharmacol Biol Psychiatry* 28: 891–907.
38. Swaab, D.F., Bao, A.M., and Lucassen, P.J. 2005. The stress system in the human brain in depression and neurodegeneration. *Ageing Res Rev* 4: 141–194.
39. Davis, S., Heal, D.J., and Stanfort, S.C. 1995. Long-lasting effects of acute stress on the neurochemistry and function of 5-hydroxytryptaminergic neurones in the mouse brain. *Psychopharmacology* 118: 267–272.
40. Weiss, J.M., Goodman, P.A., Losito, B.G. et al. 1981. Behavioral depression produced by an uncontrollable stressor: Relationship to norepinephrine, dopamine, and serotonin levels in various regions of rat brain. *Brains Res. Rev* 3: 167–205.
41. Young, A.H., Goodwin, G.M., Dick, H. et al. 1994. Effects of glucocorticoids on 5-HT1a presynaptic function in the mouse. *Psychopharmacology* 114: 360–364.
42. Crayton, J.W., Joshi, I., Gulati, A. et al. 1996. Effect of corticosterone on serotonin and catecholamine receptors and uptake sites in rat frontal cortex. *Brain Res* 728: 260–262.
43. Firk, C. and Markus, C.R. 2007. Review: Serotonin by stress interaction: A susceptibility factor for the development of depression? *Psychopharmacology* 21: 538–544.
44. Davis, J.D. and Tremont, G. 2007. Neuropsychiatric Aspects of Hypothyroidism and Treatment Reversibility. *Minerva Endocrinol* 32: 953–959.
45. Helmreich, D.L., Parfitt, D.B., Lu, X.Y. et al. 2005. Relation between the hypothalamic-pituitary-thyroid (HPT) axis and the hypothalamic-pituitary-adrenal (HPA) axis during repeated stress. *Neuroendocrinology* 81: 183–192.
46. Bianco, A.C., Nunes, M.T., Hell, N.S., and Maciel, R.M. 1987. The role of glucocorticoids in the stress-induced reduction of extrathyroidal 3,5,3′-triiodothyronine generation in rats. *Endocrinology* 120: 1033–1038.
47. Carrasco, G.A., Barker, S.A., Zhang, Y. et al. 2004. Estrogen treatment increases the levels of regulator of G protein signaling-Z1 in the hypothalamic paraventricular nucleus: Possible role in desensitization of 5-hydroxytryptamine(1A) receptors. *Neuroscience* 127: 261–267.
48. Ter Heegde, F., De Rijk, R.H., and Vinkers, C.H. 2015. The brain mineralocorticoid receptor and stress resilience. *Psychoneuroendocrinology* 52: 92–110.
49. DeRijk, R.H. Personal communication.
50. von Känel, R., Hamer, M., Malan, N.T. et al. 2013. Procoagulant reactivity to laboratory acute mental stress in Africans and Caucasians, and its relation to depressive symptoms: The SABPA study. *Thromb Haemost* 110: 977–986.
51. Berk, M., Williams, L.J., Jacka, F.N. et al. 2013. So depression is an inflammatory disease, but where does the inflammation come from? *BMC Med* 11: 200.
52. Bjorntorp, P. and Rosmond, R. 2000. The metabolic syndrome—A neuroendocrine disorder? *Br J Nutr* 83: S49–S57.
53. Holsboer, F. 2000. The corticosteroid receptor hypothesis of depression. *Neuropsychopharmacology* 23: 477–501.
54. Parker, G. 1990. The parental bonding instrument. A decade of research. *Soc Psychiatry Psychiatr Epidemiol* 25: 281–282.

55. Yehuda, A. 1997. Sensitization of the hypothalamic–pituitary–adrenal axis in posttraumatic stress disorder. *Ann NY Acad Sci* 821: 57–75.
56. Field, T. 2004. Prenatal depression effects on the fetus and the newborn. *Infant Behav Dev* 27: 216–229.
57. O'Connor, T.G. 2005. Prenatal anxiety predicts individual differences in cortisol in pre-adolescent children. *Biol Psychiatry* 58: 211–217.
58. Weinstock, M. 2005. The potential influence of maternal stress hormones on development and mental health of the offspring, *Brain Behav Immun* 19: 296–308.
59. Zucchi, F.C., Yao, Y., Ward, I.D. et al. 2013. Maternal stress induces epigenetic signatures of psychiatric and neurological diseases in the offspring. *PLoS ONE* 8(2): e56967.
60. Entringer, S., Kumsta, R., Hellhammer, D.H. et al. 2009. Prenatal exposure to maternal psychosocial stress and HPA axis regulation in young adults. *Horm Behav* 55: 292–298.
61. Bilbo, S.D. and Tsang, V. 2010. Enduring consequences of maternal obesity for brain inflammation and behavior of offspring. *FASEB J* 24: 2104–2115.
62. Spencer, S.J. and Tilbrook, A. 2009. Neonatal overfeeding alters adult anxiety and stress responsiveness. *Psychoneuroendocrinology* 34: 1133–1143.
63. Pfeffer, C.R., Altemus, M., Heo, M., and Jiang, H. 2007. Salivary cortisol and psychopathology in children bereaved by the September 11, 2001 terror attacks. *Biol Psychiatry* 61: 957–965.
64. Pfefferbaum, B., Tucker, P., North, C.S. et al. 2012. Autonomic reactivity and hypothalamic pituitary adrenal axis dysregulation in spouses of Oklahoma City bombing survivors 7 years after the attack. *Compr Psychiatry* 53: 901–906.
65. Stein, M.B., Koverola, C., Hanna, C. et al. 1997. Hippocampal volume in women victimized by childhood sexual abuse. *Psychol Med* 27: 951–959.
66. Villarreal, G., Hamilton, D.A., Petropoulos, H. et al. 2002. Reduced hippocampal volume and total white matter volume in posttraumatic stress disorder. *Biol Psychiat.* 52: 119–125.
67. Beddoe, A.E. and Lee, K.A. 2008. Mind-body interventions during pregnancy. *J Obstet Gynecol Neonatal Nurs* 32: 165–175.
68. Bongiorno, P. 2015. *Holistic Solutions for Anxiety and Depression*. New York: WW Norton, p. 109.

6 Mitochondrial Dysfunction and Physiological Depression

Dean Raffelock, DC, Dipl. Ac., DAAIM

CONTENTS

INTRODUCTION

The word *integrative*, when used in reference to the practice of psychiatry, can denote the understanding of the intricate interconnectedness of the mind-body interface: that physiologic disease can cause psychological symptoms and that psychological distress can cause physical disease.

Integrative psychiatry focuses on finding and treating the root cause(s) of mood disease. It implies treating the source of the symptoms, not solely being satisfied with providing symptomatic relief. Here is an analogy to illustrate this important distinction: Imagine you are seeking help from your own physician and during your consultation in his or her examining room, the fire alarm sounds. The alarm is excessively loud, piercing, and disruptive, so your physician rises to quickly turn off the red fire alarm switch located on the office wall, then calmly sits down again and continues conversing with you. Are you satisfied with that response? On the one hand you would be quite relieved that the loud, disruptive noise is now silenced. Yet, most likely, you would soon become quite uncomfortable with the lack of thoroughness and curiosity demonstrated by your doctor. You would probably request that he or she speedily inquire if there is an actual fire burning that might require calling the fire department and/or evacuating the building. Similarly, prescribing psychoactive medication (or prolonged psychoanalysis) when a patient's depression is caused by any of the physiologic conditions discussed in this book could also be seen as treating the symptoms but failing to look for and treat the actual cause. It is necessary and compassionate to turn off a loud distress signal (symptom), but the *cause* of the alarm sounding should also be investigated and resolved whenever possible.

This chapter focuses on one of the frequently misdiagnosed physiologic causes of depression, mitochondrial dysfunction.[1–9] So much has been researched and written about mitochondria, the organelles essential for producing the physiologic energy to power most cellular activities, that this chapter will necessarily be limited to a brief overview of aerobic metabolism and then predominantly focus on the nutrients required for optimal mitochondrial function.[10–20]

MITOCHONDRIA: A FUNCTIONAL OVERVIEW

Our mitochondria are the energy powerhouses of the cell. They could accurately be compared to armored nuclear power plants because they activate and safely contain (when healthy) the intense explosions required to cleave the high-energy bond between two oxygen atoms. These oxygen-cleaving explosions would cause devastating, widespread oxidative damage (akin to a nuclear melt-down) if they occurred anywhere else in the body. This catabolic oxygen combustion helps break down food (carbohydrates, proteins, and fats) and converts it into energy units called ATP (adenosine triphosphate), plus water, heat, and carbon dioxide.

Mitochondria are the only organelles that have their own individual DNA. This mitochondrial DNA primarily codes for ATP production. When healthy, our mitochondria prevent close to 99% of the oxygen they process from becoming corrosive oxygen free radicals. Damaged, toxic, or inefficient mitochondria can cause a great deal of oxidative stress. Mitochondrial DNA is particularly susceptible to damage because of its proximity to oxygen combustion in the inner membrane and because of the lack of protective histones. A mutation in mitochondrial DNA can cause aberrant replication and a reduction in the manufacturing and recharging of ATP. This drop in ATP production particularly affects the functions of the most energy-demanding, bioactive tissues in the body like the brain and nerves, endocrine glands, organs (liver, kidneys, lungs, heart, etc.), and muscles.

Within a unit of ATP is a high-energy phosphate bond that stores the energy required to power most of the body's physiological functions. These functions include those that affect all organ systems including the brain.[3] Stored energy is released when ATP is converted to ADP (adenosine diphosphate) and P (phosphate). This is somewhat like the charging and recharging of a battery except that an ATP molecule needs to be recharged close to 1000 times per day. When ATP (the battery) runs down into ADP and P, the recharger (mitochondrion) reattaches the phosphate, thus recharging ADP back into ATP (oxidative phosphorylation) so it can provide physiologic energy to meet the cell's requirements once again. ATP supplies the energy for a cell to perform its function, including energy to keep up the cell membrane's voltage (electrical charge) via mineral ion pumps.

The average human cell (except erythrocytes) contains about 2500 mitochondria, so there are over one quadrillion energy-producing mitochondria within the human body. One quadrillion is three times the amount of human cells (including erythrocytes) in the body, and twice the number of microbes found in the human intestinal biome. The importance of optimal mitochondrial health cannot be overestimated.

ANAEROBIC VERSUS AEROBIC METABOLISM

Our cells produce ATP through either anaerobic or aerobic metabolism. Anaerobic energy production does not require the presence of oxygen like aerobic metabolism does. Anaerobic metabolism, which takes place within the cellular cytosol, separates a molecule of glucose into two molecules of pyruvate in a process called *glycolysis*. The pyruvate is then fermented into lactate and ethanol (or gets converted into acetyl coenzyme A). The energy produced from the breakdown of pyruvate forms ATP from ADP and P. Anaerobic energy metabolism is inefficient compared to aerobic metabolism because it produces only two units of ATP per molecule of glucose. If our cells lacked mitochondria, they would be dependent on glycolysis for energy with tragic health consequences as evidenced by the varied symptoms of mitochondrial genetic diseases. Depending solely on glycolysis for energy would be like trying to keep a fire going by continuously feeding it tiny twigs. Thanks to our mitochondria, approximately 90% of the body's energy is aerobically produced.

When these quadrillion mitochondria are functioning properly, they continually help transform two molecules of acetyl coenzyme A (acetyl co-A) into 36 units of ATP (adenosine triphosphate). This is an exponential improvement in energy production over glycolysis. The first phase of this aerobic energy transformation is known as the citric acid cycle (or Krebs cycle or tricarboxylic acid cycle) and takes place in the outer compartment of the mitochondria. Here a series of four

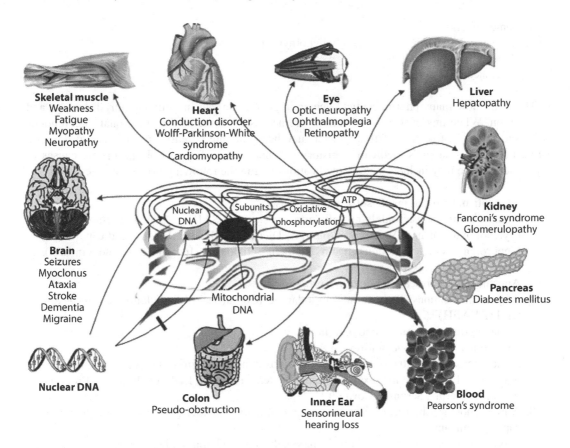

FIGURE 6.1 Mitochondrion.

dehydrogenase enzymes remove four pairs of electrons, which are then used to form NADH (from niacin) and FADH (from riboflavin). From there, NAD+/NADH and FAD/FADH help transport the electrons through the electron transport chain (ETC) where they undergo oxidative phosphorylation within the inner membrane of the mitochondrion.

Oxidative phosphorylation produces ATP utilizing energy manufactured from redox reactions within the electron transport chain. The second step of this process is performed by an electrochemical proton gradient that activates ATP synthase. ATP synthase uses the energy from the flow of protons to combine ADP and P. ATP is produced by oxidative phosphorylation utilizing electrons generated by the oxidation of organic acids within the citric acid cycle.

The key point here is that mitochondria are exponentially better at producing ATP than is glycolysis, and any physiological process that causes mitochondrial dysfunction can cause widespread cellular energy deficits and fatigue, adversely affecting virtually all organ systems including the brain (Figure 6.1).[1–9]

CAUSES OF MITOCHONDRIAL DYSFUNCTION

An increasing number of factors are now associated with causing mitochondrial damage and dysfunction. Among these are

1. Oxidative stress
2. Radiation exposure
3. Environmental toxins

4. Some infections
5. Hormone deficiencies (most notably hypothyroidism)
6. Genetic mitochondrial diseases
7. Pharmaceutical agents

There are now many pharmaceutical agents implicated in causing mitochondrial damage and dysfunction. When any of these medications are necessary, some of the nutritional interventions discussed in the last section of this chapter may help mitigate potential mitochondrial damage. Being aware of a patient's medication history can help screen for possible iatrogenic causes of depression. These may include specific medications within the following drug categories:

1. Alcoholism medications: Disulfiram (Antabuse)[21]
2. Analgesics and nonsteroidal anti-inflammatory drugs (NSAIDs): Aspirin; acetaminophen (Tylenol®); diclofenac (Voltaren®, Voltarol®, Diclon®, Dicloflex®, Difen®, and Cataflam®); fenoprofen (Naflon®); indomethacin (Indocin®, Indocid®, Incron ER®, Indocin-SR®), naproxen (Aleve®, Naprosyn®)[21]
3. Anesthetics: Bupivacaine, lidocaine, propofol[21]
4. Angina medications: Perhexaline, amiodarone (Cordarone®), diethylaminoethoxyhexesterol (DEAEH)[21]
5. Antiarrhythmics: Amiodarone (Cordarone)[21]
6. Antibiotics: Tetracycline, antimycin A[21]
7. Antidepressants: Amitriptyline (Lentizol), amoxapine (Asendin®), citalopram (Cipramil®), fluoxetine (Prozac®, Symbyax®, Sarafem®, Fontex®, Foxetin®, Ladose®, Fluctin®, Prodep®, Fludac®, Oxetin®, Seronil®, Lovan®)[21]
8. Antipsychotics: Chlorpromazine, fluphenazine, haloperidol, risperidone, quetiapine, clozapine, olanzapine[21]
9. Anxiety medications: Alprazolam (Xanax®), diazepam (Valium®, Diastat®)[21]
10. Barbiturates: Amobarbital (Amytal®), aprobarbital, butabarbital, butalbital (Fiorinal®), hexobarbital (Sombulex®), methylphenobarbital (Mebaral®), pentobarbital (Nembutal®), phenobarbital (Luminal®), primidone, propofol, secobarbital (Seconal®, Talbutal®), thiobarbital[21]
11. Cholesterol medications: Statins—atorvastatin (Lipitor®, Torvast®), fluvastatin (Lescol®), lovastatin (Mevacor®, Altocor®), pitavastatin (Livalo®, Pitava®), pravastatin (Pravachol®, Selektine®, Lipostat®), rosuvastatin (Crestor®), simvastatin (Zocor®, Lipex®), bile acids—cholestyramine (Questran®), clofibrate (Atromid-S®), ciprofibrate (Modalim®), colestipol (Colestid®), colesevelam (Welchol®)[21]
12. Chemotherapy medications: Mitomycin C, porfiromycin, Adriamycin (also called doxorubicin and hydroxydaunorubicin and included in the following chemotherapeutic regimens—ABVD, CHOP, and FAC)[21]
13. Dementia medications: Tacrine (Cognex®), Galantamine (Reminyl®)[21]
14. Diabetes medications: Metformin (Fortamet®, Glucophage®, Glucophage XR, Riomet), troglitazone, rosiglitazone, buformin[21]
15. HIV/AIDS medications: Atripla®, Combivir®, Emtriva®, Epivir® (abacavir sulfate), Epzicom®, Hivid® (ddC, zalcitabine), Retrovir® (AZT, ZDV, zidovudine), Trizivir®, Truvada®, Videx® (ddI, didanosine), Videx® EC, Viread®, Zerit® (d4T, stavudine), Ziagen®, Racivir®[21]
16. Epilepsy/seizure medications: Valproic acid (Depacon®, Depakene®, Depakene syrup, Depakote®, Depakote ER, Depakote sprinkle, divalproex sodium)[21]
17. Mood stabilizers: Lithium[21]
18. Parkinson's disease medications: Tolcapone (Tasmar®), Entacapone (COMTan®, also in the combination drug Stalevo®)[21]

Of particular note for the psychiatrist are the antidepressant, antipsychotic, antianxiety, and mood stabilizer medications listed and presently known to cause mitochondrial damage and dysfunction. Many more references and potential mechanisms of action are included within the article[21] by John Neustadt and Steve R. Pieczenik (2008). Since this article was published, no doubt more pharmaceutical agents have and will be researched and shown to cause mitochondrial damage. This further emphasizes caution when prescribing psychoactive medication and makes a stronger case for diagnosing and treating the root cause(s) of the symptoms of depression whenever possible.

MITOCHONDRIAL COUPLING AND UNCOUPLING

The electron transport chain directs the flow of electrons and helps to recycle NAD+ and FADH. This high-energy process also produces water, and when operating efficiently, minimal amounts of harmful reactive oxygen species. It is estimated that, when healthy, only 1% of the oxygen we breathe is converted into the high-energy, corrosive, reactive oxygen species (ROS): superoxide, hydroxyl radical, and hydrogen peroxide. Because of this ROS production, antioxidants (including superoxide dismutase, catalase, and glutathione peroxidase/reductase) are located within the mitochondria in order to prevent massive free radical damage. The process of combining oxidative phosphorylation and the electron transport chain is often referred to as mitochondrial *coupling*. There are numerous factors that can interfere with this coupling process and cause *uncoupling*. Mitochondrial uncoupling can significantly increase oxidative stress and mitochondrial DNA mutations, reduce aerobic energy (ATP) production, and affect virtually all organ systems.[3]

IMPORTANT MITOCHONDRIAL NUTRITIONAL COFACTORS

Most physicians learn about mitochondrial function by memorizing a chart similar to Figure 6.2. Most likely the exchange of electrons and protons involved in the citric acid cycle, oxidative phosphorylation, and the electron transport chain were emphasized (see Figure 6.2), but for most the nutritional cofactors and key mitochondrial antioxidants were not required learning. This information is essential for improving mitochondrial function and helping to mitigate potential damage and symptoms of depression cause by specific medications (and other causes of uncoupling). As always, the physician must decide if the benefits of prescribing a drug outweigh the risks, especially if evidence-based alternative options are available. Figure 6.3 depicts many of the nutritional cofactors necessary for a mitochondrion to function efficiently.

KEY MITOCHONDRIAL NUTRITIONAL COFACTORS

Fatty acids, amino acids, and sugars must all be converted to acetyl co-A in order to be processed within the mitochondrion for aerobic energy production. The process that breaks down fatty acid, glycerol, and cholesterol molecules to generate acetyl-coA in the mitochondria is called beta-oxidation. The L-carnitine (in its acyl-carnitine form) is necessary to transport fatty acids across the inner mitochondrial membrane and into the mitochondrial matrix so they can be converted into acetyl co-A and enter the citric acid cycle.[9] Carnitine is synthesized from the amino acids lysine and methionine. This conversion requires three methyl groups (requiring cofactors B-6, B-12, folate, trimethylglycine, methionine, serine), plus vitamin C, B-3, biotin, and iron. The process that breaks down amino acids into acetyl co-A is called *deamination*. Vitamins B-6 (pyridoxyl-5-phosphate), B-12 (methylcobalamin), folate (5-MTHF), and biotin are required for deamination. Sugar is broken down via glycolysis and requires vitamins B-1, B-3, B-5, and biotin.

Once food fuel is transported into the mitochondrial matrix, it enters the citric acid cycle (CAC) and travels through eight enzymatic steps that require 10 vitamins and minerals (B-1 [thiamin pyrophosphate], B-2 [riboflavin occurring as flavin-adenine-dinucleotide], B-3 [niacin occurring

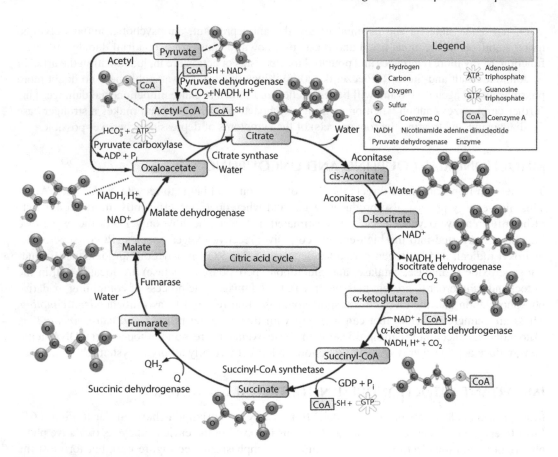

FIGURE 6.2 Citric acid cycle.

as nicotinamide dinucleotide and NADH], B-5, B-6 [occurring as pyridoxal-5-phosphate], alpha lipoic acid, magnesium, sulfur, iron, and phosphorus), as well as 12 amino acids (aspartate, arginine, cysteine, glutamic acid, glutamine, histidine, isoleucine, methionine, phenylalanine, proline, tyrosine, and valine) to complete each cycle. The eight organic acids formed during the citric acid cycle (CAC) are oxaloacetate, citrate, cis-aconitate, isocitrate, alpha-ketoglutarate, succinate, fumarate, and malate. These organic acids are then oxidized to provide the electrons for oxidative phosphorylation (OP) and the electron transport chain (ETC). The organic acids formed during the CAC can be measured using organic acid testing (see Chapter 4) where a specific build-up of any organic acid can point to the nutritional cofactors that may be necessary to provide in supplement form in order to better facilitate its transformation into the next organic acid in the CAC.

Oxidative phosphorylation and the ETC require the presence of coenzyme Q10, magnesium, zinc, and vitamins C, K, B-2, and B-3 in order to produce and recycle ATP. Table 6.1 depicts many of the nutritional cofactors required to modulate oxidative phosphorylation.

As oxidative stress increases, the amount of high-energy intermediates decreases, and the amounts of oxidized intermediates increase. This causes a significant diminishment in aerobic energy production and lower overall energy reserves. Oxidative stress lowers the ratio of reduced to oxidized intermediates. Glutathione is considered the most important mitochondrial antioxidant. Under conditions of oxidative stress, oxidized glutathione disulfide increases, while reduced glutathione decreases. Under normal, healthy conditions, the ratio between reduced glutathione and glutathione disulfide should be 100:1 (Table 6.1).

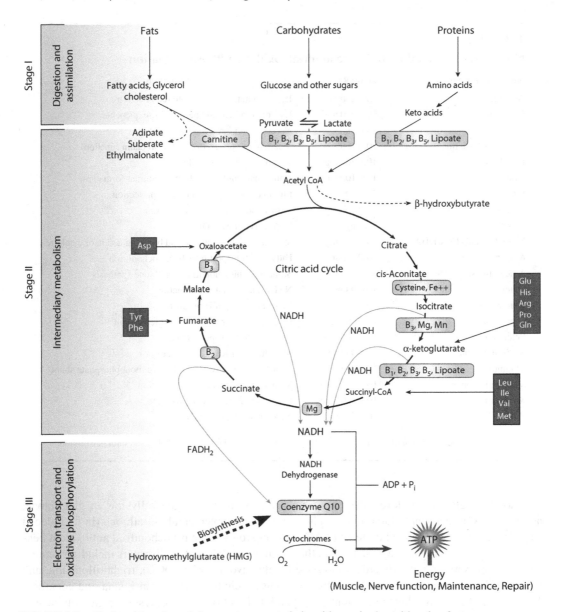

FIGURE 6.3 Citric acid cycle and electron transport chain with required nutritional cofactors.

MITOCHONDRIAL ANTIOXIDANTS

Mitochondria contain three important antioxidant molecules to protect themselves from oxidative damage. These are (1) glutathione, (2) coenzyme Q10, and (3) lipoic acid. Glutathione (GSH) is the major free radical scavenger in the brain. It is the universal cellular reduction-oxidation balancing molecule. Diminished GSH levels elevate cellular vulnerability toward oxidative stress and accumulating ROS. Oxidative stress has been associated with major depressive disorder, bipolar disorder, and schizophrenia.[1–9] GSH is a tripeptide (glutamyl-cysteinyl-glycine) that regulates oxidizing cell processes that shift with the flow of NAD^+ and NADH. Selenium and vitamin C are important cofactors. The enzyme glutathione reductase requires FAD from riboflavin (B2) and copper. Glutathione is profoundly important for mitochondrial function and the antioxidant cascade.

TABLE 6.1

Nutritional Modulators of Mitochondrial Oxidative Phosphorylation

Nutritional Agent	Daily Range	Influence
Ascorbate	500–6000 mg	Part of glutathione—lipoate redox activity
Catechin	50–1000 mg	Hydroxyl radical and peroxynitrite quencher
Copper	1–3 mg	Necessary for Zn-CuSOD
CoQ 10 (ubiquinone)	20–1000 mg	Maintenance of electron transport chain function
Ferulic acid	100–300 mg	Hydroxyl radical quencher
Glutathione	100–1000 mg	Antioxidant and Phase II mercapturate formation
Lipoic add	50–1000 mg	Multiple roles in mitochondrial protection
Magnesium	50–1000 mg	Mitochondrial Krebs cycle activator
Manganese	2–5 mg	Necessary for MnSOD
N-3 fatty acid (EPA/DHA)	500–300 mg	Mitochondrial membrane and blocking action of cytokine
N-acetyl-carnitine	50–1000 mg	Fatty acid transport into the mitochondrion
N-acetyl-cysteine (NAC)	50–1500 mg	Stimulates mitochondrial glutathione synthesis
Niacin	10–50 mg	NADH and NADPH production
Niacinamide	200–2000 mg	NADH and NADPH production
Riboflavin	10–200 mg	$FADH_2$ activator and Krebs cycle nutrient
Selenium	100–500 mcg	Activator of GSH peroxidase
Sodium succinate	100–4000 mg	Mitochondrial Krebs cycle activator
Thiamin	10–200 mg	Transketolase activator for hexose monophosphate shunt
Vitamin E-(tocopherols)	100–1000 mg	Mitochondrial membrane protection
Vitamin K	100–1000 mcg	Electron transport chain protector
Zinc	10–50 mg	Necessary for Zn-CuSOD

Source: Lukaczer, D. *Clinical Nutrition: A Functional Approach.* 2nd ed., IFM, 2004. Used with permission.

Mitochondrial glutathione levels decrease with age.[15] Neurons are generally low in glutathione, and aging lowers neuronal glutathione levels even more. Supplemental glutathione (in its reduced form) or its precursor N-acetyl cysteine (NAC) can help to increase mitochondrial antioxidant benefits.[15] NAC is emerging as a useful agent in the treatment of psychiatric disorders including depression, schizophrenia, bipolar disorder, obsessive-compulsive disorder (OCD), trichotillomania, and grooming disorder and are helpful in substance abuse including that of marijuana and cocaine.[16] The benefits of NAC for these conditions go beyond its function as a precursor for glutathione and are linked to its effects on neurotransmitters and inflammatory cytokines.[16]

Coenzyme Q10 is a steroid-like structure and belongs to the family of oxidoreductases. It is formed through the same acetylation pathway as cholesterol (HMG CoA reductase), and its production can be similarly downregulated by statin drugs. This enzyme participates in oxidative phosphorylation. It controls the rate of citric acid cycle processing via the oxidation of succinate to fumarate. Reduced CoQ10 accepts hydrogen atoms from reduced FADH2. Without adequate CoQ10, cells do not make adequate ATP. CoQ10 is available as a supplement in ubiquinone and ubiquinol forms. These are the oxidized and reduced forms with ubiquinol said to be better assimilated, particularly in older individuals who may lack hepatic conversion capacity.[17]

Lipoic acid is a cellular antioxidant and plays an essential role in mitochondrial dehydrogenase reactions. It is necessary for glycolysis and the citric acid cycle. It is the "B-vitamin" most commonly omitted from multivitamin formulas because of its expense. It interacts with glutathione and vitamin C to aid in the recycling of vitamin E and is helpful in protecting cell membranes.

KEY NUTRIENTS HELPFUL IN ASSISTING MITOCHONDRIAL FUNCTIONING

The list of necessary nutritional requirements for optimal functioning of mitochondria is rather long. As is apparent, B-vitamins (including B-1, B-2, B-3, B-5, B-6, biotin, and lipoic acid), coQ10, mineral chelates using CAC organic acid salts (succinate, fumarate, malate, citrate, and alpha keto-glutarate), glutathione/N-acetyl cysteine, acetyl L-carnitine, vitamin C, essential fatty acids and amino acids, and vitamin K are all essential for optimal mitochondrial functioning. In addition, medium-chain triglycerides (i.e., MCT oil) may be helpful because of more efficient entry into the mitochondria.

Pyrroloquinoline quinone (PQQ) is a redox agent capable of both reducing and oxidizing, so while not a pure antioxidant, PQQ is linked to providing powerful antioxidant support to mitochondria.[17] PQQ also stimulates spontaneous growth of new mitochondria (mitochondrial biogenesis) within aging cells, and protects the brain's cells and neurotransmitter systems against neurotoxicity and amyloid-beta protein.[18–20,22–24] As mitochondrial research continues, other nutraceuticals, and perhaps pharmaceutical supports, are being discovered. Showing promise, at the writing of this chapter, are nicotinamide adenine dinucleotide (NAD), NADH, and nicotinamide riboside for promoting sirtuin (SIRT1 and SIRT3) gene activation.[25–27] Undoubtedly, more nutraceutical mitochondrial enhancers will be forthcoming as research continues.

MITOCHONDRIAL DYSFUNCTION, OXIDATIVE STRESS, AND DEPRESSION: CONNECTING THE DOTS

Research is now suggesting a strong associative relationship between mitochondrial dysfunction, oxidative stress, and depression. New research is now attempting to uncover the neurobiological mechanisms that cause oxidative stress to trigger depression in susceptible people. Some of the proposed mechanisms have to do with a combination of neuro-inflammation, neurovascular unit dysfunction, and blood-brain barrier hyperpermeability causing alterations in endothelial nitric oxide levels and endothelial nitric oxide synthase uncoupling.[22] In their study Souhel Najjar, Daniel M. Pearlman, Orrin Devinsky, and colleagues[27] theorize a number of neurobiological mechanisms that may directly cause or, in combination, contribute to depression. They state that the combination of oxidative stress and neuro-inflammation are implicated in the neurobiology of major depressive disorder, and they propose a number of neurobiological mechanisms, that when triggered by the combination of oxidative stress and neuro-inflammation, that may cause or contribute to depression.[23–30] These include

- Decreased serotonergic and increased glutamatergic tone with increased glutamatergic tone continuing to increase oxidative stress and neuro-inflammation.[31]
- Upregulated ratios of T helper 1 (Th1) cells and proinflammatory cytokines: (a) microglial activation, (b) astroglial loss and activation, and (c) decreased $CD4^+CD25^+FOXP3^+$ regulatory T (T_{Reg}) cell counts.[32–40]
- Experimental evidence suggesting that increased ROS synthesis (oxidative stress) and neuro-inflammation exhibit a bidirectional relationship, and that ROS can activate microglia and increase proinflammatory cytokine synthesis—for example, by stimulating transcription factor nuclear factor κB (NFκB)—and activated microglia and proinflammatory cytokines can, in turn, perpetuate oxidative stress.[41–45]

Now that oxidative stress and neuro-inflammation have been associated with depression,[46–49] more research looking to uncover the neurobiological connections between the three will be forthcoming.

CONCLUSION

Mitochondrial dysfunction is an important example of a physiologic process that can mimic and masquerade as psychological depression. It is beneficial for the busy integrative physician to maintain this awareness. Oxidative stress is now being seen as one of the fundamental causes of mood disorders. Recent research supports this premise.[1-9] Mitochondrial dysfunction is the most important cause of endogenous oxidative stress because of the corrosive ROS generated when high-energy oxygen cleavage is inefficiently contained.

There are many factors that may have a disabling (uncoupling) effect on mitochondrial function. These include oxidative stress, radiation exposure, environmental toxins, infection, hormone deficiencies (most notably hypothyroidism), genetic mitochondrial diseases, and ingestion of numerous pharmaceutical agents. A careful medication history may reveal potential causes of mitochondrial damage and dysfunction leading to symptoms of low energy, fatigue, and physiological depression.

An adequate supply of the nutrients required for the citric acid cycle and oxidative phosphorylation to take place efficiently is essential to maintain and improve mitochondrial function. These nutrients are not recycled indefinitely and need to be replenished through nutrient-dense diets and, in compromised health, specific nutraceutical supplementation. A strong case can be made for supplementing mitochondrial nutritional cofactors for preventative reasons, especially in the aging population. The medical detractor statement "Taking vitamins will just give you expensive urine" repeated to many patients over too many decades does not hold up to the scrutiny of modern, research-based, nutrition science. Individual humans use up specific vitamins, minerals, amino acids, fatty acids, and antioxidants at unique rates (biochemical individuality) based on genetics, epigenetics, dietary choices, stress levels, and other lifestyle factors. Deficiency or insufficiency of one or more of the required nutrients necessary for optimal mitochondrial functioning may be an underlying cause or complicating factor in patients presenting with depression.

REFERENCES

1. Tobe, E.H. 2013. Mitochondrial dysfunction, oxidative stress, and major depressive disorder. *Neuropsychiatr Dis Treat* 9: 567–573.
2. Konradi, C., Eaton, M., MacDonald, M.L. et al. 2004. Molecular evidence for mitochondrial dysfunction in bipolar disorder. *Arch Gen Psychiatry* 61(3): 300–308.
3. Johns, D.R. 1995. Mitochondrial DNA and disease. *N Engl J Med* 333(10): 638–644.
4. Streck, E.L., Goncalves, C.L., Furlanetto, C.B. et al. 2014. Mitochondria and the central nervous system: Searching for a pathophysiological basis of psychiatric disorders. *Rev Bras Psiquiatr* 36(2): 156–167.
5. Fattal, O., Budur, K., Vaughan, A.J. et al. 2006. Review of the literature on major mental disorders in adult patients with mitochondrial diseases. *Psychosomatics* 47: 1–7.
6. Shao, L., Martin, M.V., Watson, S.J. et al. 2008. Mitochondrial involvement in psychiatric disorders. *Ann Med* 40(4): 281–295.
7. Jou, S.H., Chiu, N.Y., and Liu, C.S. 2009. Mitochondrial dysfunction and psychiatric disorders. *Chang Gung Med J* 32(4): 370–379.
8. Anglin, R.E., Garside, S.L., Tarnopolsky, M.A. et al. 2012. The psychiatric manifestations of mitochondrial disorders: A case and review of the literature. *J Clin Psychiatry* 73(4): 506–512.
9. Clay, H.B., Sillivan, S., and Konradi, C. 2011. Mitochondrial dysfunction and pathology in bipolar disorder and schizophrenia. *Int J Dev Neurosci* 29(3): 311–324.
10. Foster, D.W. 2004. The role of the carnitine system in human metabolism. *Ann NY Acad Sci* 1033: 1–16.
11. Almeida, O.P., Ford, A.H., Hirani, V. et al. 2014. B vitamins to enhance treatment response to antidepressants in middle-aged and older adults: Results from the B-VITAGE randomised, double-blind, placebo-controlled trial. *Br J Psychiatry* 205(6): 450–457.
12. Young A.J., Johnson, S., Steffens, D.C. et al. 2007. Coenzyme Q10: A review of its promise as a neuroprotectant. *CNS Spectrums* 12(1): 62–68.
13. Bhagavan, H.N. and Chopra, R.K. 2006. Coenzyme Q10: Absorption, tissue uptake, metabolism and pharmacokinetics. *Free Radic Res* 40: 445–453.

14. Ernster, L. 1977. *Facts and Ideas about the Function of Coenzyme Q10 in the Mitochondria*. Amsterdam: Elsevier, pp. 15–18.

15. Benzi, G. and Moretti, A. 1995. Age and peroxidative stress-related modifications of the cerebral enzymatic activities linked to mitochondria and the glutathione system. *Free Rad Biol Med* 19: 77–101.

16. Dean, O., Giorlando, F., and Berk, M. 2011. *N*-acetylcysteine in psychiatry: Current therapeutic evidence and potential mechanisms of action. *J Psychiatry Neurosci* 36(2): 78–86.

17. Failla, M.L., Chitchumroonchokchai, C., and Aoki, F. 2014. Increased bioavailability of ubiquinol compared to that of ubiquinone is due to more efficient micellarization during digestion and greater GSH-dependent uptake and basolateral secretion by Caco-2 cells. *J Agric Food Chem* 62(29): 7174–7182.

18. Rucker, R., Chowanadisai, W., and Nakano, M. 2014. Potential physiological importance of pyrroloquinoline quinone. *J Biol Chem* 285: 142–152, *EMBO Mol Med* 6(6): 721–731.

19. Chowanadisai, W., Bauerly, K.A. Tchaparian, E. et al. 2010. Pyrroloquinoline quinone stimulates mitochondrial biogenesis through cAMP response element-binding protein phosphorylation and increased PGC-1alpha expression. *J Biol Chem* 285(1): 142–152.

20. Zhang, P., Xu, Y., Sun, J. et al. 2009. Protection of pyrroloquinoline quinone against methylmercury-induced neurotoxicity via reducing oxidative stress. *Free Radic Res* 43(3): 224–233.

21. Neustadt, J. and Pieczenik, S.R. 2008. Medication-induced mitochondrial damage and disease. *Mol Nutr Food Res* 52(7): 780–788.

22. Scanlon, J.M., Aizenman, E., and Reynolds, I.J. 1997. Effects of pyrroloquinoline quinone on glutamate-induced production of reactive oxygen species in neurons. *Eur J Pharmacol* 326(1): 67–74.

23. Hara, H., Hiramatsu, H., and Adachi, T. 2007. Pyrroloquinoline quinone is a potent neuroprotective nutrient against 6-hydroxydopamine-induced neurotoxicity. *Neurochem Res* 32(3): 489–495.

24. Zhang, J.J., Zhang, R.F., and Meng, X.K. 2009. Protective effect of pyrroloquinoline quinone against Abeta-induced neurotoxicity in human neuroblastoma SH-SY5Y cells. *Neurosci Lett* 464(3): 165–169.

25. Sasaki, Y., Araki, T., and Milbrandt, J. 2006. Stimulation of nicotinamide adenine dinucleotide biosynthetic pathways delays axonal degeneration after axotomy. *J Neurosci* 26(33): 8484–8491.

26. Belenky, P., Racette, F.G., Bogan, K.L. et al. 2007. Nicotinamide riboside promotes Sir2 silencing and extends lifespan via Nrk and Urh1/Pnp1/Meu1 pathways to NAD+. *Cell* 129(3): 473–484.

27. Najjar, S., Pearlman, D.M., Devinsky, O. et al. 2013. Neurovascular unit dysfunction with blood-brain barrier hyperpermeability contributes to major depressive disorder: A review of clinical and experimental evidence. *J Neuroinflammation* 10: 142.

28. Chi, Y. and Sauve, A.A. 2013. Nicotinamide riboside, a trace nutrient in foods, is a vitamin B3 with effects on energy metabolism and neuroprotection. *Curr Opin Clin Nutr Metab Care* 16(6): 657–661.

29. Ozcan, M.E., Gulec, M., Ozerol, E. et al. 2004. Antioxidant enzyme activities and oxidative stress in affective disorders. *Int Clin Psychopharmacol* 19: 89–95.

30. Ng, F., Berk, M., Dean, O., and Bush, A.I. Oxidative stress in psychiatric disorders: Evidence base and therapeutic implications. *Int J Neuropsychopharmacol* 11: 851–876.

31. Berk, M., Copolov, D.L., Dean, O. et al. 2008. N-acetyl cysteine for depressive symptoms in bipolar disorder—A double-blind randomized placebo-controlled trial. *Biol Psychiatry* 64: 468–475.

32. Maes, M., Ruckoanich, P., Chang, Y.S. et al. 2011. Multiple aberrations in shared inflammatory and oxidative & nitrosative stress (IO&NS) pathways explain the co-association of depression and cardiovascular disorder (CVD), and the increased risk for CVD and due mortality in depressed patients. *Prog Neuropsychopharmacol Biol Psychiatry* 35: 769–783.

33. Scapagnini, G., Davinelli, S., Drago, F. et al. 2012. Antioxidants as antidepressants: Fact or fiction? *CNS Drugs* 26: 477–490.

34. Maes, M., Mihaylova, I., Kubera, M. et al. 2011. IgM-mediated autoimmune responses directed against multiple neoepitopes in depression: New pathways that underpin the inflammatory and neuroprogressive pathophysiology. *J Affec Disord* 135: 414–418.

35. Galecki, P., Szemraj, J., Bienkiewicz, M. et al. 2009. Lipid peroxidation and antioxidant protection in patients during acute depressive episodes and in remission after fluoxetine treatment. *Pharmacol Rep* 61: 436–447.

36. Gibson, S.A., Korade, Z., and Shelton, R.C. 2012. Oxidative stress and glutathione response in tissue cultures from persons with major depression. *J Psychiatr Res* 46: 1326–1332.

37. Najjar, S., Pearlman, D.M., Alper, K. et al. 2013. Neuroinflammation and psychiatric illness. *J Neuroinflammation* 10: 43.

38. Steiner, J., Bogerts, B., Sarnyai, Z. et al. 2012. Bridging the gap between the immune and glutamate hypotheses of schizophrenia and major depression: Potential role of glial NMDA receptor modulators and impaired blood-brain barrier integrity. *World J Biol Psychiatry* 7: 482–492.

39. Steiner, J., Bielau, H., Brisch, R. et al. 2008. Immunological aspects in the neurobiology of suicide: Elevated microglial density in schizophrenia and depression is associated with suicide. *J Psychiatr Res* 42: 151–157.
40. Frick, L.R., Williams, K., and Pittenger, C. 2013. Microglial dysregulation in psychiatric disease. *Clin Dev Immunol* 2013: 608654.
41. Gosselin, R.D., Gibney, S., O'Malley, D. et al. 2009. Region specific decrease in glial fibrillary acidic protein immunoreactivity in the brain of a rat model of depression. *Neuroscience* 159: 915–925.
42. Banasr, M. and Duman, R.S. 2008. Glial loss in the prefrontal cortex is sufficient to induce depressive-like behaviors. *Biol Psychiatry* 64: 863–870.
43. Haroon, E., Raison, C.L., and Miller, A.H. 2012. Psychoneuroimmunology meets neuropsychopharmacology: Translational implications of the impact of inflammation on behavior. *Neuropsychopharmacology* 37: 137–162.
44. Liu, Y., Ho, R.C., and Mak, A. 2012. Interleukin (IL)-6, tumour necrosis factor alpha (TNF-alpha) and soluble interleukin-2 receptors (sIL-2R) are elevated in patients with major depressive disorder: A meta-analysis and meta-regression. *J Affect Disord* 139: 230–239.
45. Raison, C.L., Lowry, C.A., and Rook, G.A. 2010. Inflammation, sanitation, and consternation: Loss of contact with coevolved, tolerogenic microorganisms and the pathophysiology and treatment of major depression. *Arch Gen Psychiatry* 67: 1211–1224.
46. Hong, M., Zheng, J., Ding, Z.Y. et al. 2013. Imbalance between Th17 and T_{reg} cells may play an important role in the development of chronic unpredictable mild stress-induced depression in mice. *Neuroimmunomodulation* 20: 39–50.
47. Anderson, G., Berk, M., Dodd, S. et al. 2013. Immuno-inflammatory, oxidative and nitrosative stress, and neuroprogressive pathways in the etiology, course and treatment of schizophrenia. *Prog Neuropsychopharmacol Biol Psychiatry* 42: 1–4.
48. Salim, S., Chugh, G., and Asghar, M. 2012. Inflammation in anxiety. *Adv Protein Chem Struct Biol* 88: 1–25.
49. Block, M.L., Zecca, L., and Hong, J.S. 2007. Microglia-mediated neurotoxicity: Uncovering the molecular mechanisms. *Nat Rev Neurosci* 8: 57–69.

7 Micronutrient Deficiencies and Mitochondrial Dysfunction

Chandler Marrs, MS, MA, PhD

CONTENTS

INTRODUCTION

Mitochondria provide 90% of the adenosine triphosphate (ATP) required to maintain cellular function and viability via the interconnected processes of the Krebs/tricarboxylic acid cycle (TCA) and the electron transport chain (ETC).[1] Impediments to ATP production imperil cell function and viability, eventually leading to cell death. Organ systems requiring the most ATP are especially susceptible to slight permutations in mitochondrial efficiencies (e.g., the brain, heart, muscles, and gastrointestinal system). Nutrient insufficiency is a key contributor to mitochondrial structural and functional derangement, capable of initiating and maintaining a variety of disease processes from diabetes and cardiovascular disease to the neurodegeneration observed in Alzheimer's and Parkinson's.[2] Nutrient insufficiency has become increasingly prevalent where Western dietary practices predominate and may underlie many of the diseases plaguing modern cultures. A growing body of evidence suggests that there is a connection between nutrient availability, mitochondrial health, and human health.

MITOCHONDRIAL DISEASE BASICS

PRIMARY MITOCHONDRIAL DISORDERS ARE COMMON

Mitochondrial disorders can be characterized as primary or secondary, where primary represents clear heritability and secondary denotes functional or acquired diseases generally attributable to lifestyle variables. This chapter will focus primarily on secondary disorders. By way of background, however, brief descriptions of both are included.

The prevalence of primary mitochondrial disease, heritable mtDNA mutations passed matrilineally, is estimated at rates as high as 1 in 500 individuals,[3] making the potential for mitochondrial-based dysfunction in any population quite high. The more severe, primary mitochondrial diseases are generally identified in infancy and early childhood. However, not all carriers of mtDNA mutations become recognizably ill during childhood. Sometimes symptoms do not emerge until much later in life, if at all. There appears to be a threshold ratio of mutated to normal mtDNA that must be reached before symptoms arise.[4] When they do arise, even individuals with the same mitochondrial genotype express symptoms differentially. In other words, genotype and phenotype are not closely associated.

It is possible, therefore, for primary mitochondrial disease to remain latent until adulthood. Individuals with mitochondrial mutations present with extended histories of psychiatric disorders, migraines, GI disturbances, and other ailments, not commonly attributable to mitochondria in primary care.[5] Sometimes it is not until a child is born into the family with frank mitochondrial illness that the family history is reviewed, and latent mitochondrial diseases in the adult relatives are discovered.

SECONDARY MITOCHONDRIAL DAMAGE IS WIDESPREAD

Mitochondria are particularly susceptible to epigenetic influence[6] and environmentally induced damage. Physiological stressors, lifestyle variables, environmental, and pharmaceutical exposures can trigger symptoms in formerly asymptomatic or silent carriers of mtDNA mutations and/or evoke entirely new disease processes where primary disease had not been previously recognized. These secondary insults to mitochondria induce structural or functional changes in the organelle, that if left untreated, produce mtDNA mutations, ultimately, blurring the lines between primary and secondary disease process altogether, especially transgenerationally.[7] Given the sheer number of toxicants and other variables capable of inducing mitochondrial damage, it is safe to say that most individuals will face mitochondrial insult as a matter of modern life.

PSYCHIATRIC COMORBIDITIES

Depression has been observed in up to 70% of individuals with primary mitochondrial disease including 50% of children,[8] while bipolar disorder and panic disorder are noted in 17% and 11%,[9] respectively. In one study, the estimated lifetime prevalence of psychiatric diagnosis in individuals with primary mitochondrial disease was 47%, including the 42% lifetime prevalence of personality disorder.[10] Psychosis is a prominent symptom of both primary and secondary mitochondrial disease but is frequently misdiagnosed as schizophrenia or bipolar disorder.[11] Similarly, mitochondrial abnormalities have been identified in patients with depression, bipolar disorder, and schizophrenia.[12]

The data are not clear as to what degree psychiatric symptoms are present in secondary or acquired mitochondrial dysfunction, because those connections are not often assessed. Given the number of mechanisms by which toxicants and/or nutrient deficiencies can impact mitochondrial functioning, it is likely that psychiatric sequelae are common. Unfortunately, the period between onset of psychiatric symptoms and diagnosis of mitochondrial disease spans an average of 13 years,[5] during which time medications that directly damage mitochondria and are capable of inducing mitochondrial disorders, independent of the original disease process, are administered,[13] while treatments supporting mitochondrial function are withheld.

It is important to recognize that in mitochondrial medicine, disease boundaries no longer apply. Inasmuch as mitochondria affect cellular functioning globally, mitochondrial damage and disease will present broadly. These disorders will vary between patients, even those with the same mutations[14] and/or same nutrient deficit-based liabilities. The individual's heritable, environmental, and nutritional dispositions contribute significantly to disease presentation. It is with those caveats that one must interpret the data regarding linkages proposed among mitochondrial dysfunction and specific disease processes that manifest through individual organ, system, or tissue pathologies or within discrete diagnostic categories such as those ascribed to by psychiatry or any other discipline. These linkages, while present, are artifactual boundaries of the study design and may not exist in mitochondrial medicine.

LET FOOD BE MEDICINE

One of the more interesting aspects of mitochondrial therapeutics for both primary and secondary disorders, is that successful treatment protocols involve nutrition—supplying the mitochondria with nutrients that facilitate TCA and ETC efficiency. That is, mitochondrial medicine involves dietary and other lifestyle changes, combined with the appropriate nutrient supplements to normalize mitochondrial functioning and reduce disease burden.[15] And so, with all the advances in modern medicine, it appears that we are back to nutrients, back to Hippocrates and "let food be medicine," and back to the mitochondria as key regulators of health and disease. How is it possible that nutrition, not pharmaceuticals, might solve some the most vexing medical issues of modernity? The answer is basic biochemistry. An examination of how secondary mitochondrial dysfunction develops clarifies the relationship between diet and mitochondrial functioning.

MITOCHONDRIA NEED NUTRIENTS

Dietary nutrients provide the building blocks for cell functioning and survival in every tissue of the body. Without those nutrients a myriad of health problems arise. What we eat plays a huge role in human health. Cellular respiration, specifically, depends upon the transformation of dietary energy, derived from carbohydrates, fats, and proteins, into cellular energy or ATP.[16] Dietary vitamins and minerals are essential components for hundreds of metabolic reactions in the body and act as catalysts and coenzymes for enzymatic reactions participating in mitochondrial respiration and energetics. Vitamins provide structural components for enzymes and mitochondrial cyto-chromes,[17] act as electron and proton carriers in the ATP[18]–generating electron transport chain, and scavenge for free radicals,[19] the by-product of ATP production and key initiator of mito-chondrial damage.[20] Mitochondrial functioning, therefore, can be compromised significantly by nutrient deficiency.[21]

Specifically, from pyruvate to acetyl CoA, the enzymes of the pyruvate dehydrogenase complex (PDC) are heavily dependent on thiamine, but also require riboflavin, pantothenic (B5) acid, and lipoic acid in addition to iron, sulfur, niacin (B3), cysteine, magnesium, and manganese. Beta oxi-dation, which breaks down fatty acids, requires L-carnitine.[22] Both use the energy released from these processes to reduce the electron carriers nicotinamide adenine dinucleotide (NAD[+]), yielding NADH, and flavin adenine dinucleotide (FAD), yielding FADH2. NAD and FAD require niacin and riboflavin, respectively.

From there, energy from the electrons is used to pump hydrogen ions (protons) into the mito-chondrial intermembrane space. The five complexes of the ETC require additional nutrients includ-ing ubiquinone, riboflavin, iron, sulfur, and copper.[19] Ubiquinone or coenzymeQ (CoQ) transports electrons from complexes I and II to complex III.[23] CoQ synthesis requires vitamins B2, B6, B12, folate, pantothenic acid, niacin, and vitamin C. Heme synthesis, required for complex IV to pro-ceed, requires seven nutrients: pyridoxine, pantothenate, zinc, riboflavin, iron, copper, and biotin.[24] Biotin deficiency leads to loss of complex IV functionality directly via a reduction in heme synthe-sis.[25] Nutrient deficits in complex IV "result in oxidant leakage, DNA damage, accelerated mito-chondrial decay, and cellular aging".[26] ATP synthesis occurs in complex V.

As a by-product of ATP production both during physiological and abnormal electron transport, the mitochondria release reactive oxygen species (ROS). During normal function 1%–5% of all oxygen consumed by the cell is converted to ROS.[11] CoQ and vitamins C, E, niacin, and folate are free radical scavengers.[27] Damaged or nutrient-deficient mitochondria increase ROS production, as does nutrient overload. Without the proper balance of nutrients to maintain mitochondrial efficien-cies and buffer ROS production, the feed-forward cascade of oxidative damage, cellular aging, and disease ensues.

MITOCHONDRIAL ENERGETICS AND CELLULAR HOMEOSTASIS

Since mitochondria are fundamental to cellular energetics and homeostasis, interference with nor-mal mitochondrial function via insufficient nutrients impairs carbohydrate and lipid metabolism[28] and, thus, cellular energetics. As one might imagine, impaired cellular energetics leads to pathology in regions where cellular energy demands are highest, the central nervous system (why we see so many psychiatric and cognitive symptoms linked to mitochondrial functioning), the gastrointestinal and cardiovascular systems, and muscles. Symptoms as diverse as cyclic vomiting,[29] gastroparesis and pseudo bowel obstructions,[30] myalgias[31] and myopathies,[32] neuropathies,[33] migraines,[34] seizures or syncope,[35] ataxia and tremors,[17] hormone disorders,[36] depression,[37] bipolar, anxiety, psychosis, fatigue,[38] exercise intolerance,[39] cognitive impairment[5] (in previously high-functioning individuals), diabetes,[40] and metabolic disturbances[41] have been attributed to mitochondrial distress amenable to nutrient therapies. Autonomic instability,[42] affecting everything from mood stability[43] to car-diac functioning,[44] wakefulness, and sodium and potassium balance,[45] can be expected as well. According to Dr. Richard Boles, former director of the Metabolic and Mitochondrial Disorders Clinic at Children's Hospital Los Angeles: "Mitochondrial dysfunction doesn't really cause any-thing, what it does is predisposes towards seemingly everything."[46]

In addition to the disease processes evoked by insufficient energy metabolism, the mitochon-dria also regulate inflammatory cascades,[47] steroidogenesis,[48] neurotransmission,[49] neurodegenera-tion,[1] ion homeostasis,[50] heme synthesis,[20] ROS production and detoxification, and, ultimately, cell death.[51] For women, in particular, hormone dysregulation, ovarian, thyroid,[52] and adrenal, and the menstrual and reproductive disorders that ensue, represent some of the least recognized signs of mitochondrial dysfunction.[53]

DISRUPT MITOCHONDRIA INDUCE DISEASE

Where there are deteriorating mitochondria, cell damage, cell death, and organ damage will follow. Affected systems depend upon the individual's unique combination of heritable predispositions and environmental exposures. This makes mitochondrial disorders simultaneously some of the most complex disease processes known to man, but also, the easiest to recognize. That is, when a patient presents with a complex and endless array of seemingly unrelated symptoms, there is a good chance the mitochondria are involved and a likelihood that nutrient deficiency is present.[16] Nutrient deficiency, imbalance, and in some cases, nutrient dependency are remediable if identified and treated.[11] The problem, however, is that most of modern medicine is under the false impression that malnutrition was resolved generations ago. It was not. Malnutrition is alive and well in modern culture. Indeed, the 2014 Global Report on Nutrition found that all 193 countries assessed, including all first-world Westernized countries, struggle with multiple interleaving forms of malnutrition ranging from child and adult micronutrient insufficiency to obesity.[54]

ENVIRONMENTAL FACTORS AFFECTING MITOCHONDRIAL HEALTH

NUTRIENT DEFICIENCIES IN THE LAND OF PLENTY

It may be surprising that nutrient deficiencies would exist in the postindustrial age, where food is abundant, obesity endemic, and nutrient fortification common; but they do. Though the estimates of nutrient deficiency vary from study to study, by nutrient, and by population sampled, consistently, the data show both a high prevalence of both frank and marginal vitamin and mineral deficits where Western diets that are rich in empty calories predominate.[55] Nutrient deficiencies exist across all economic and social strata and are not solely limited to states of starvation or undernourishment, as is commonly assumed. Malnutrition is evident in overweight[56] and sedentary individuals and in presentably fit and highly active individuals,[57] including athletes.[58,59]

Nutrient deficiency in modern culture is not strictly about food scarcity or caloric intake, but nutrient availability itself; nutrient availability can be hampered by a number of variables, many of which have coalesced over recent decades. For example, modern agricultural practices have depleted crop nutrients, and thus, dietary nutrient availability in harvested food has declined significantly. Simultaneously, increased pharmaceutical dependence and environmental pollutant exposures have deranged nutrient absorption and metabolism via a number of physiological mechanisms, many of which involve the mitochondria. As a consequence, all but the most conscientious among us are at risk for one or more vitamin or mineral deficiencies. Just how bad is it? The breadth and depth of environmental factors affecting mitochondria nutrient status and, by association, human health, are staggering.

CONVENTIONAL AGRICULTURE AND FOOD NUTRIENT AVAILABILITY

In our efforts to produce the largest and most attractive fruits and vegetables, we've cultivated out 95% of the genetic variation from food crops; reducing to almost nothing the ~200,000 plant metabolites that provide nutrition.[60] When fruits, vegetables, and grains are selected for high yield, approximately 80%–90% of the dry weight yield comes from carbohydrates and not the dozens of other nutrients and thousands of phytochemicals that would normally be present.[61]

To make matters worse, we have substituted nutritionally rich and diverse crops with ones that originate from engineered plant seeds laced with glyphosate, adjuvants, and other chemical toxicants, grown in topsoil that has been almost fully depleted of minerals.[62] In Canada and the United

States, 85% of the mineral content in top soil has been depleted over the last 100 years (through 1992). Similarly, Europe and South America have seen 72% and 76% reductions, respectively.[63] This has led to a 6%–38% reduction in the vitamin and mineral content of many fruits and vegetables between 1950 and 1999.[64] Surprisingly, no data are available for the last 15 years, but one might surmise that the trends identified over the last half century have continued.

The heavy use of agrochemicals is believed to be at the center of many of the observed nutrient deficiencies in harvested foods. RoundUp®, with glyphosate (by far the most prominent among those chemicals, with 527 million pounds of product used worldwide in 2011),[65] serves as an example of how agrochemicals have invaded commercial food production to disrupt nutrient availability in the crops and nutrient absorption in the organisms that eat those crops. Glyphosate does the following:

- *Destroys gut bacteria.* Research shows that glyphosate destroys beneficial gut bacteria, leaving the more pathogenic species intact.[61] The disruption of gut bacteria significantly influences the synthesis and absorption of nutrients.
- *Chelates minerals.* Because glyphosate also binds to the minerals that do absorb, it acts as a chelator, effectively inactivating remaining minerals.[66] The chelated metals (iron, zinc, manganese, cobalt) contribute to mineral deficiencies but also vitamin deficiencies inasmuch as minerals are required for the enzyme activity that regulates vitamin synthesis.
- *Accumulates.* Glyphosate is present in significantly higher concentrations in individuals who eat genetically modified (GM)-based foods compared to those who eat predominantly organic foods and also in chronically ill versus healthy individuals.[67]
- *Damages mitochondria.* RoundUp damages complexes I and III of the electron transport cycles, reducing ATP production by some 40%.[68] Early evidence of this was demonstrated over 30 years ago.[69]

Crop nutrient depletion is an unrecognized problem in health care. Food no longer has the nutrient availability it once did, and worse yet, carries with it a cocktail of chemicals that damage microbiotic balance, mitochondrial functioning, and a myriad of other processes fundamental to basic organismal health.[70] With this in mind, nutrient insufficiency should not be considered a problem of economically driven, calorie insufficiency, as it has been historically, but rather, a fundamental loss of nutrients in the available food sources. For the practitioner, this means that patients eating a largely conventional diet, even if replete with healthy fruits and vegetables, may be nutrient insufficient, particularly in the face of stressors like illness and toxicant exposures.[71] Identifying and remedying nutrient deficiencies may reduce the burden of illness.

PHARMACEUTICAL AND ENVIRONMENTAL EXPOSURES DEPLETE MITOCHONDRIAL NUTRIENTS

Extending this discussion further, it should be evident that nutrient-depleted food sources are not the only insults to mitochondrial health. From a mechanistic standpoint, anything that limits mitochondrial functioning, risks evoking illness. Medications, vaccines, and environmental toxicants induce mitochondrial damage via numerous pathways that ultimately reduce nutrient availability and increase ROS-mediated damage.[1,72]

Pharmaceuticals alter gut microbiota. The balance of gut microbiota, covered in Chapter 3, is critical for vitamin synthesis, absorption, and metabolism. Disturbed gut microbiota and nutrient imbalance are quick to follow. Nutrient imbalance directly impairs mitochondrial functioning inasmuch as vitamins, minerals, and other dietary nutrients are required for ATP synthesis and to temper oxidative stress.

In addition to disturbing gut microbiota, many pharmaceuticals deplete nutrient availability within the mitochondria itself.[73] For example, thiamine is necessary for both carbohydrate[74] and fatty acid metabolism,[23] making thiamine availability indispensable for cellular energetics. Even subtle thiamine deficiency evokes serious health conditions, particularly in the central nervous system where ATP demands and thiamine turnover[75] are highest. A number of medications deplete thiamine, including antibiotics, metformin, the loop diuretics, thiazide and thiazide derivatives, estrogens in hormone replacement therapies, and oral contraceptives.[76] Vaccines should be included on this list, as case reports and therapeutic evidence link thiamine deficiency to many post-vaccine reactions.[43] Thiamine deficiency, once considered a risk limited to chronic alcoholics and patients requiring extended parenteral feeding, has re-emerged across multiple populations, bringing with it corresponding symptoms of the long forgotten beriberi and Wernicke's encephalopathy.[77]

Statins, on the other hand, deplete CoQ.[78] CoQ is a naturally occurring, fat-soluble compound responsible for electron transport. Reduced CoQ leads to impaired mitochondrial energy production. CoQ can be synthesized de novo, but is largely derived from diet. CoQ synthesis depends on sufficient concentrations of vitamins B2, B6, B12, folate, pantothenic acids, niacin, and vitamin C. Insufficient dietary intake or availability of the B vitamins leads to reduced CoQ. That means CoQ can be depleted pharmaceutically, via insufficient intake of dietary CoQ and/or via insufficient B vitamins. Combine all three factors, and the risk for mitochondropathies increases. In addition to vitamin depletion, all classes of psychotropic drugs directly induce mitochondrial damage, as do antibiotics, NSAIDs, and many other popular medications.[74]

These are but a few examples of pharmaceutically induced nutrient depletion and effects on the mitochondria. Additional information on medication-induced nutrient depletion can be found on the websites of Linus Pauling Institute,[79] the University of Maryland,[80] and the Natural Medicine's Comprehensive Database: Drug Influences on Nutrient Levels and Depletion.

MITOCHONDRIAL RISK NOT A PREREQUISITE FOR FDA APPROVAL

The impact of pharmaceuticals on mitochondrial functioning has only recently, and still not fully, become an endpoint in pharmaceutical research. It is not required by the U.S. Food and Drug Administration (FDA)[81] and how those medications dually impact nutrients and the mitochondria is not clear. An in vivo analysis of some 550 pharmaceuticals revealed 34% induced mitochondrial damage by disrupting reactions within the ETC.[82] Each drug was investigated independently and in culture. We can only anticipate how real-life applications of polypharmacy, coupled with environmental exposures, poor diet, and heritable predispositions might increase those liabilities, at least additively, if not synergistically. Moreover, most pharmacological research assesses only acute toxicities on healthy drug naïve animals. In the real world, healthy and drug naïve can no longer be said to exist, suggesting that acquired mitochondrial damage is far more likely than represented by the current research.[83]

ENVIRONMENTAL POLLUTANTS

The final factors in what is already a damaging collection of mitochondrial toxicants include the environmental pollutants. However, aside from the research delineating the toxic effects of RoundUp and glyphosate, there are far fewer studies evaluating the effects of environmental pollutants on mitochondrial integrity[84] and none on nutrient depletion. Perhaps one of the clearest and most extreme examples of environmentally induced damage to mitochondrial function comes from the Gulf War. With the widespread exposures to environmental and pharmaceutical toxicants, fully one-third of Gulf War Vets subsequently developed complex, multisystem illnesses that have been clearly linked to mitochondrial damage[85] and nutrient depletion.[83]

CHRONIC ILLNESS AND POOR NUTRITION

Within this context, it should be evident how the modern environment is, in many ways, detrimental to health. We consume nutritionally depleted foods, laden with chemicals, rely on pharmaceuticals to solve what may be symptoms originating from poor nutrition, all the while being exposed to regular and complex mixtures of environmental toxicants. Alone, any one of these factors can contribute to the onset and maintenance of disease; together no one really knows how these exposures are affecting health.

If the epidemiological data are any indication, the impact of the modern environment on health is negative and rapidly worsening.[86] The incidence of psychiatric illness and psychotropic medication use is growing, particularly in regions where Western diets predominate. According to the most recent data, psychiatric disorders plague one in four Americans (26%) compared to non-Western countries where the rate of psychiatric illness hovers around 4%.[87] Concurrently, chronic health issues directly associated with diet and lifestyle like obesity, heart disease, and diabetes continue to increase,[88] year in and year out, as do those not traditionally associated with diet and lifestyle like autoimmune disease.[89] If we view mitochondria as a final common pathway between diet, environment, and health, then these trends represent a single disease process, expressed differentially. To the extent that a growing body of research finds nutrient therapies successful in mitochondrial medicine,[90] there is hope that increased awareness, research, and diagnostic capabilities will improve patient outcomes and reverse these trends.

MITOCHONDRIA AND BRAIN FUNCTION

MITOCHONDRIA AND THE BRAIN

Despite the historically poor clinical recognition of ailing mitochondria in psychiatry and primary care, every presentation of mitochondrial disease, whether primary or acquired, affects brain function in some manner or another. The brain has the highest concentration of mitochondria and uses more energy per unit mass than any other organ.[15] The tightly regulated systems of neural communication require ATP-controlled functions like ion channels, receptors, vesicle release, and neurotransmitter recycling[91] to function properly. Abnormalities in mitochondrial structure or function derail neural communication and homeostasis and can become both the cause and consequence of a broad array of neuropsychiatric conditions, including those that lead to irreversible neurodegeneration like Alzheimer's, Parkinson's, and amyotrophic lateral sclerosis (ALS).[92] In addition to a fundamental need for ATP, healthy mitochondria are required to regulate the inflammatory cascades, manage and buffer ROS exposure and damage, and temper the effects of Ca^{2+} influx.[93] As in the body, cerebral mitochondria represent a common pathway for a variety of disease processes.

COMPENSATORY REACTIONS OF CEREBRAL MITOCHONDRIAL DYSFUNCTION

Slight to increasingly prominent derivations in brain bioenergetics will set off compensatory reactions to offset unmet energy demands in mitochondria. Three key changes include the reallocation of resources by the orexin/hypocretin neurons, increased brain lactate, and inflammation. Understanding the mechanisms by which these reactions occur allows the practitioner to identify symptoms and rationalize treatment approaches more effectively.

OREXIN/HYPOCRETIN NEURONS

Modulation of the orexin/hypocretin (same neurons, different names) system appears to be an early compensatory reaction to reduced ATP. The orexin/hypocretin neurons require as much as five to six times the amount of intracellular ATP to maintain firing,[94] allowing them to sense and monitor brain energy resources early, before ATP levels become critical. The orexin/hypocretin neurons cease firing when ATP stores become low, thereby allowing the reallocation of energy. At the most basic level, release of the orexin/hypocretin induces wakefulness. When orexin/hypocretin neurons are turned on and firing appropriately, arousal and feeding are maintained. When orexin neurons are turned off, diminished, or dysfunctional, melatonin, the sleep-promoting hormone, is turned on. The two work in concert to manage wakefulness and sleep.

Originating in the lateral hypothalamus, orexin/hypocretin neurons project across the entire brain[95] with its two receptors (OXA and OXB) differentially distributed throughout the central nervous system and into the periphery. Within the brain, orexin/hypocretin neurons project to the thalamus, the locus coeruleus, dorsal raphe nucleus (DRN), ventral tegmental area (VTA) with particularly dense projections to monoaminergic and cholinergic nuclei in the brainstem and hypothalamic regions.[96] Peripherally, orexin/hypocretin innervation reaches the adrenals,[97] testes, and ovaries[98] suggesting a role in hormone regulation. Orexin/hypocretin receptors have also been identified in the kidney and small intestines.[99]

With illness and/or depleted energy stores, these neurons induce sleep and reduce feeding. The sleepiness, fatigue, malaise, and anorexia common in most pathogenic illnesses and also mitochondrial distress are the result of a reallocation of resources mediated by the orexin/hypocretin system. These neurons also modify pain (dynorphin receptors co-located on orexin/hypocretin neurons), digestion (via the neuropeptide galanin),[99] and cortical spreading depression in migraines and epileptogenesis,[99] among other functions. Perhaps most relevant to this discussion, low cerebrospinal fluid (CSF) concentrations of orexin have been implicated in major depression and suicidality.[100]

From this system of neurons, we can see that wakefulness and feeding are key components of healthy mitochondria. When energy resources are low, sleep and loss of appetite would be common. Consider new-onset sleep disorders, whether hypersomnia or narcolepsy, related to the orexin/hypocretin system. Similarly, consider the connection between excessive sleep, low motivation, loss of pleasure, and depressed mood as linking back to orexin/hypocretin through modulation of the serotonin (DRN) and dopamine (VTA) systems—again, compensatory reactions in the face of impaired mitochondria.

The role of these neurons in generating migraine and seizures should also be recognized. A mechanism suggested for migraine and seizures is a compensatory destabilization of brain ion homeostasis. Barring physiological changes in ion concentrations, ATP-mediated ion channel instability together with compensatory signals from orexin/hypocretin neurons could account for these events. Whether arrived at clinically or mechanistically, one should suspect depleted mitochondria underlying this constellation of symptoms. With new-onset disturbances in particular, consider the possibility of a medication or vaccine-induced reaction.

LACTATE AS A MARKER FOR MITOCHONDRIAL FUNCTIONING

Just as lactate buildup and tolerance thresholds in the muscles represent overall fitness in the face of increased metabolic demands, so too does brain lactate. Lactate is a fuel used readily in the body in response to changing metabolic needs (exertion and stressors[101]) and efficiencies (oxygen usage, nutrient cofactor availability). Exercise physiologists have been measuring lactate and other indicators of metabolic functioning (aerobic versus anaerobic) for decades using a variety of respirometry tools, from breathing apparatus to blood tests and tissue biopsies. In a grossly oversimplified manner, the extent to which one produces and utilizes lactate during training indicates one's overall fitness. Those same aerobic/anaerobic processes that occur in our body occur in the brain. Even though the brain is a huge consumer of glucose as its preferred fuel, recent evidence suggests that it also produces and consumes lactate in parallel to the body during exercise and other stressors.[102]

Brain lactate, therefore, represents a compensatory shift in mitochondrial bioenergetics from aerobic metabolism to anaerobic metabolism. The connection between lactate and mitochondrial functioning was only recently discovered and remains hotly debated.[103] It was believed that lactate remained outside the mitochondrion. Now, evidence suggests that mitochondria can convert lactate to ATP, and that lactate is shuttled in and out of mitochondria to be used when needed.[104]

Beyond just the production of lactate in brain trauma,[105] where oxygen and glucose[106] are depleted rapidly, brain lactate levels appear to correspond with shifts in aerobic/anaerobic metabolism.[107] The shift toward anaerobic metabolism and excess lactate, especially during rest and low exertion, indicates mitochondrial distress. While measuring lactate as a marker of mitochondrial dysfunction is common in sports physiology, it has only recently become more prominent with suspected mitochondrial abnormalities like myalgic encephalomyelitis/chronic fatigue syndrome,[108] multiple sclerosis,[109] or other disorders.

Most recently, magnetic resonance spectroscopy (MRS) has been used to identify lactate doublets in diseased cerebral mitochondria. The lactate molecule has two, weakly coupled, signals or resonances. When viewed on the MRS the lactate doublet presents as a double peak in the signal algorithm.[110] Evidence of lactate doublets from MRS, even when magnetic resonance imaging (MRI) shows no irregularities, can point to cerebral mitochondrial dysfunction. In patients with primary mitochondrial disease, the regional,[111] differences in brain lactate[112] correspond to the neurological and clinical symptomatology associated with each disease process. Lactate doublets have been recognized in acquired mitochondrial dysfunction like autism[113] and aging[102] (although mechanisms remain contested[114]), bipolar disorder,[115] and other mitochondrial disease processes.[116] Thus, the extent to which mitochondrial energetics shift from aerobic to anaerobic metabolism can be measured via lactate response, peripherally or centrally.

Absent testing however, clinical indications in the musculature would be reported as fatigue, muscle pain, and weakness. The sensation would be akin to "hitting the wall," a threshold of exertion with which many athletes are familiar. With mitochondrial damage or distress, however, those sensations and symptoms develop in the presence of minimal or no exertion and generally take longer to dissipate.[117] In the brain, excess lactate acutely would be indication of injury or trauma. More chronically and more conservatively, one could anticipate decrements in a variety of functions aligned with the regional distribution of lactate or a more global presentation indicating systemic illness.

With bipolar disorder, where much research has been focused, the dominant hypothesis suggests disrupted mitochondrial bioenergetics leading to neurochemical imbalance. Specifically, the evidence is pointing to impaired oxidative phosphorylation leading to a shift toward anaerobic metabolism with consequent diminished energy production, substrate availability (nutrients) and altered phospholipid metabolism.[118]

In addition to the direct effects of lactate on specific cell populations, lactate can initiate and maintain inflammatory cascades, a function that elicits, and results in, mitochondrial distress. Neuroinflammation is associated with psychiatric illness.[119]

VITAMINS AND BRAIN INFLAMMATION

Among the myriad of mechanisms capable of initiating inflammation, mitochondria figure prominently. Remarkably, many of the same nutrient deficiencies that evoke problems within the mitochondria (the B vitamins) and force them to initiate inflammatory cascades, also activate neurotoxic chemical cascades, stressing the nervous system and the mitochondria even further. Vitamin B6, for example, is a necessary cofactor in over 100 enzymes, including those involved in heme synthesis (complex IV) and CoQ synthesis.[79] It is also critical for the catabolism of the essential amino acid tryptophan. Tryptophan is required for serotonin and melatonin synthesis. Disturbances in tryptophan catabolism not only lead to disturbances in neurotransmitter activity, but also can lead to cell death or apoptosis in vital brain regions like the hippocampus, basal ganglia, and cerebellum.

In the setting of optimal physiology, tryptophan serves as a substrate for serotonin and melatonin. Excess tryptophan is degraded resulting in the by-products nicotinic acid (niacin) and nicotinamide adenine dinucleotide (NAD^+). Loss of niacin metabolism from this pathway can lead to significant disease, including pellagra, which is characterized by scaly skin lesions, delusions, and confusion. In addition to a loss of niacin synthesis, when vitamin B6 is deficient and the tryptophan pathway is disturbed, the incomplete degradation of tryptophan produces several metabolites that are neurotoxic, including quinolinic acid.[120]

Quinolinic acid is a potent and self-perpetuating neurotoxin when unopposed in the brain.[118] It generates ROS and overactivates N-methyl-D-aspartate (NMDA) glutamate receptors to the point of apoptosis, all the while inhibiting brain astrocytes' ability to clean up the excess glutamate. Once that cycle becomes initiated, quinolinic acid potentiates its own release and that of other neurotoxins, ensuring continued brain inflammation and damage.

With the appropriate vitamin B6 concentrations, quinolinic acid is not the final product of tryptophan catabolism, NAD^+ is, and any damage initiated by quinolinic acid as a natural by-product within this pathway is offset by two neuroprotective factors, kynurenine and picolinic acid. Vitamin B6 is critical for the kynurenine aminotransferase and kynurinase enzymes; enzymes that lead to neuroprotective compounds, kynurenine or picolinic acid. Kynurenine blocks the cytotoxic effects of quinolinic acid by blocking the NMDA receptor, making it unavailable to quinolinic acid, while picolinic acid is the primary metal chelator in the brain. In other words, vitamin B6 controls the balance between inflammation and anti-inflammation within the brain and the body.[121]

Defects in vitamin B6 metabolism are linked to seizure disorders[122] resistant to traditional anticonvulsants but remediable with vitamin B6. Vitamin B6 reduces brain atrophy in Alzheimer's patients,[123] tardive dyskensia in schizophrenics,[124] and diabetes in patients with depression.[125] Low vitamin B6 is believed to play a key role in the oxidative stress associated with Huntington's disease.[126] One of the more interesting studies involves preventing the hippocampal apoptosis associated with bacterial meningitis using vitamin B6.[127] In an experimental version of bacterial meningitis, vitamin B6 supplementation reduced brain inflammation and hippocampal apoptosis by upregulating the neuroprotective factors controlled by the tryptophan–kynurenine pathway.

MITOCHONDRIAL MENTAL HEALTH: A CASE FOR THIAMINE

Vitamin B1, thiamine (thiamin), is arguably one of the most important vitamins to mitochondria and mental health, and simultaneously, one of the least recognized culprits in mitochondrial impairment. Discovered over a century ago and synthesized in the late 1930s, thiamine deficiency and associated disorders gained prominence in 1950s–1960s before its gradual relegation to the list of vitamin deficiencies solved by modern medicine and foodstuff fortification.[75] With the exception of thiamine's role in alcoholism-induced Wernicke's encephalopathy and Korsakoff's syndrome and periodic dietary-driven outbreaks in Japan[128] or, more recently, Israel,[129] thiamine deficiency syndromes have all but disappeared from clinical conversations. Unfortunately, thiamine deficiency has not.

One study found that 75% and 76% of type 1 and type 2 diabetics, respectively, were thiamine deficient.[130] Obesity confers a high risk for thiamine deficiency (29%),[131] as does bariatric surgery used to correct the weight problem.[132] Post-bariatric thiamine deficiencies have been reported in as many as 49% of patients.[133] Interestingly, and concurrently, bariatric surgery increases folate concentrations. A random sampling of 500 patients admitted to the emergency room over a 3-day period in the United Kingdom found that 20% of the patients were thiamine deficient.[134] Females seem to be more deficient than males,[135] especially during pregnancy with hyperemesis gravidarum[136] and/ or thyrotoxicosis.[137] In one study of anorexia, thiamine deficiency was found in 38% of the patients tested.[138] Thiamine deficiency has been observed in schizophrenics along with a 50% decrease in the number of mammillary body neurons, important relays for limbic and extra limbic connections and memory formation,[139] and at least one case study of Wernicke's encephalopathy in bipolar disorder has been published.[81]

The use of yeasts in vaccines (HPV and HBV[140]), and/or the regular consumption of foods high in thiaminase (coffee, tea, and other foods),[141] will deactivate thiamine,[142] and render an individual thiamine deficient. A number of medications directly and indirectly deplete thiamine including all classes of antibiotics and the proton pump inhibitors used by millions of individuals worldwide.[81] Dietary insufficiency in pyridoxine and pantothenic acid or problems with GI nutrient absorption or metabolism (from disturbed gut microbiota) can initiate and/or hasten thiamine decline. When thiamine-depleting agents combine, full-blown Wernicke's can emerge in the most unlikely individuals (e.g., in non-alcoholics). Indeed, there is a growing awareness among emergency room doctors that Wernicke's and the constellation of symptoms that precede, have increased in prevalence and complexity.[143]

Thiamine's Role in Brain Health

Without thiamine, the whole mitochondrial engine slows to a halt. Thiamine, once converted to its biologically active form thiamin pyrophosphate (TPP), is a cofactor in key enzymes responsible for ATP production, including transketolase, pyruvate dehydrogenase, and alpha-ketoglutarate dehydrogenase. More recently, the role of thiamine in fatty acid metabolism has been elucidated with the recognition that 2-hydroxyacyl-CoA lyse (HACL1) is TPP dependent, linking thiamine to myelination and other critical lipid-dependent processes.[23] Thiamine deficiency, thus, can derail central and peripheral metabolism, induce tissue injury in regions with high metabolic demands, initiate a buildup of toxic intermediates like lactate, and impair myelination. White matter abnormalities are common with mitochondrial disorders,[144] and in psychiatric illness, perhaps an unrecognized link to thiamine deficiency.

Combining current dietary and environmental trends with the biochemistry of mitochondrial thiamine dependence suggests chronic and lower-level insufficiencies are present in broad swaths of the population. Arguably, this then predisposes individuals to more serious thiamine deficiency syndromes in the face of secondary or tertiary mitochondrial insults, such as the addition of a pharmaceutical product or an illness that precipitates further dietary decline. With appropriate nutrition prior to the insult, and total removal of thiamine from the diet, thiamine depletion occurs within approximately 18 days.[145] Poor diet prior to the insult would expedite that process.

From experimental evidence in rodents, we know that cerebral thiamine concentrations diminish by 80% of normal before overt neurological symptoms are observed. Conversely, recovery of function begins when thiamine concentrations increase by just 6%–26% of normal.[146] Prior to the onset of neurological symptoms, the researchers observed weight loss, progressive anorexia, hair loss, and drowsiness (orexin/hypocretin compensation). This suggests that somewhere between normal thiamine concentrations and the 80% decline is an opportunity to recognize the trajectory of thiamine deficiency and treat it. This also points to a probable nonlinear, waxing and waning of symptoms in modern thiamine-related syndromes, where dietary thiamine is periodically available and offsets, at least temporarily, the full progression of symptoms.

Long Latency Thiamine Deficiency

If thiamine deficiency is observed through the lens of mitochondrial functioning, it is possible to anticipate a much broader context of symptoms, particularly when multiple nutrients are deficient simultaneously. Using the three functional responses described previously (orexin/hypocretin deactivation, lactate, and inflammation) as an example, the parameters of a temporal and dose-response trajectory are recognizable. Specifically, early or mild mitochondrial insults would be met with orexin/hypocretin mediated slowing. Behaviorally, sleeping, fatigue, anorexia, depressed mood, reduced activity, and apathy are cardinal symptoms. Paresthesias, muscle pain, dizziness, and cognitive fuzziness might also be present.[147]

With more moderate or longer-duration thiamine deficits, where compensatory reactions in mitochondrial functioning have begun (lactate and inflammation), system instability becomes a cardinal feature. Here, the mitochondria are increasingly incapable of meeting energy demands, and minor stressors initiate symptoms. From the mental health standpoint, mood lability, irritability, fearfulness progressing to agitation, cognitive impairment,[148] and difficulty finding words, comprehending text, and memory issues become more prominent. Depending upon the patient, GI dysmotility symptoms such as gastroparesis, excessive vomiting, diarrhea, and/or bowel irritability might emerge,[24] along with neuropathic pain and ataxias, tremors, and syncope.[149]

In a small study of 20 patients, poor dietary habits were associated with functional disturbances in thiamine metabolism leading to moderate thiamine deficiency. Symptomatically, the patients presented with a variety of what might have been considered psychosomatic features, including abdominal and/or chest pain, sleep disturbances (sleep walking/talking, insomnia, terrors, panic), chronic and unremitting fatigue, recurrent fever of unknown origins, personality changes, alternating and intermittent diarrhea and constipation, nausea and vomiting, night sweats, anorexia, and other symptoms. The researchers also noted labile blood pressure, tic-like movements, and absent patellar reflexes. Thiamine supplementation resolved completely and/or improved the symptoms significantly in all 20 patients.[150]

As the thiamine deficiency progresses, symptoms include heart palpitations, hypotension, bradycardia at rest, and tachycardia with sinus arrhythmia (postural orthostatic tachycardia syndrome).[148] Ataxia and balance issues become more prominent. Nystagmus (usually horizontal) and ocular abnormalities are recognizable. Finally, mental status changes, including hallucinations, delusions, and disorientation would become prominent,[151] followed by coma and death if not identified.[152] Thiamine deficiency symptoms respond favorably to thiamine supplementation.

CLINICAL PRESENTATION AND THERAPEUTIC OPTIONS

CLINICAL PRESENTATION OF ADULT MITOCHONDRIAL DYSFUNCTION

Symptoms of secondary and nutrient-dependent mitochondrial dysfunction present broadly across multiple organ systems, and the symptoms change over time. Early symptoms may not be recognizable or concordant with those that develop as the damage progresses and secondary inflammatory cascades escalate, initiating additional disease processes.[5] Since a number of medications and vaccines induce direct mitochondrial damage but also deplete nutrients, the time course for onset is variable, dependent both upon individual predispositions and reserves and nutrient-specific threshold concentrations, above or below which symptoms appear. Finally, the prevalence of medically unexplained symptoms ranges from 25% to 75% in outpatient care.[153] Most will be referred for psychiatric evaluation, and many will receive comorbid psychiatric diagnoses that may or may not be appropriate. Given the diversity of seemingly unexplainable and unrelated symptoms attributed to mitochondrial dysfunction, including those with prominent psychiatric manifestations, the possibility for mitochondrial disease with nutrient remediable elements should be considered with all psychiatric evaluations. Listed below are common and not so common symptoms of mitochondrial illness. A complete listing of symptoms is beyond the scope of this chapter; however, a multitude of publications are available online.

FATIGUE AND DEPRESSION

Loss of energy, loss of motivation, chronic, unremitting fatigue, with or without muscle weakness and excessive sleeping or hypersomnia are cardinal symptoms of mitochondrial distress. Fatigue and related symptoms are often misdiagnosed as depression. Major depression may be the clinical expression for reduced mitochondrial respiration and impaired mitochondria-regulated immune response.[30] In some cases, the fatigue and depressive symptoms will be attributable to an untreated or undertreated thyroid condition. This should be considered. Diminished thyroid function, however, is also a marker of mitochondrial distress, and so, recognizing and supporting mitochondrial function should also improve thyroid health.

AUTONOMIC DYSREGULATION

The autonomic system is particularly sensitive to respiratory chain disorders.[147] Dysautonomias are marked by a dysregulation of autonomic input with quick sympathetic input paired with much slower parasympathetic re-regulation. Estimates suggest 70 million people worldwide and 500,000 to 3 million Americans are affected by dysautonomias.[154] The onset is common in the teenage years, frequently coincident with an illness or toxic exposure such as a vaccine. Girls seem to be more affected than boys.

The more common symptoms include temperature dysregulation, significant increase or decrease in heart rate relative to postural position (postural orthostatic tachycardia syndrome—POTS, or postural hypotension), blood pooling in the legs, syncope, dizziness, seizures, blurred or disrupted vision (ranging from intermittent loss of visual acuity to complete blindness during attack), significant noise and light sensitivity, intense salt and water cravings, nausea and vomiting (cyclic vomiting syndrome), GI dysmotility (IBS is common), mood lability, fatigue and inertia, and severe anxiety attacks. Symptoms are triggered by periods of physiologic and psychological stress, and can either be primary or occur secondary to another medical condition.

The array of possible symptoms affecting different organ systems, the variability and intermittent nature of the episodes, and the sudden emergence in previously healthy teenagers, leads many practitioners to suspect psychosocial origins and treat accordingly. Dysautonomias are not psychosocial constructs, even though psychiatric symptoms may be present, but rather indicators of mitochondrial distress and sometimes primary, though previously latent, disease processes. From a mechanistic perspective, consider the episodes triggered by stressors that place a greater demand upon ATP resources than are available. Support the mitochondrial deficiency and symptoms generally improve dramatically without the need for psychotropics.

CEREBELLAR DYSREGULATION AND ATAXIA

Cerebellar ataxia is a common symptom of mitochondrial disease and damage. Clinical presentation ranges from subtle and barely noticeable to gross gait and balance disturbances where the individual can barely stand or walk. When combined with autonomic dysregulation, patients may collapse to the floor, losing muscle strength intermittently. Ataxias, along with tremors, severe muscle weakness, and seizures have been observed post medication[155] and vaccine reactions.[148] Ataxia along with persistent fatigue and memory difficulties are noted in untreated or undertreated hypothyroidism, as well. The relationship between thyroid and mitochondrial function is close and reciprocal, and symptoms may present concordantly. Imaging tests may or may not detect evidence of cerebellar injury, and comprehensive lab testing for thyroid disease remains a problem in clinical care. When ataxia is mild and not readily observable and/or when imaging or standard lab tests are negative, depression may be diagnosed incorrectly. The presence of observable ataxia should point the practitioner toward mitochondrial distress, and a further assessment of mitochondrial symptoms and liabilities should be conducted. Thiamine[156] and CoQ deficiencies[157] have been noted with mitochondrial ataxias.

PSYCHIATRIC AND COGNITIVE DISTURBANCES

Psychiatric and cognitive manifestations of mitochondrial distress are common. In the early stages and with mild deficiencies, these symptoms may present nonspecifically as a loss of energy and loss of motivation. With more moderate and/or longer-duration mitochondrial deficiencies, mood lability, anxiety, personality changes, and psychosis may present. Cognitive deficits are common complaints among patients with secondary mitochondrial derangements relative to a medication/vaccine adverse reaction, but they are not often recognized or tested. Some of the symptoms include difficulty finding words (naming and fluency), understanding written text, decreased attention span, visual and verbal memory deficits, and an overall decline in cognitive ability.[150] In the case of recent onset psychiatric symptoms and cognitive complaints, medication history should be reviewed and changed accordingly.

MYOPATHY AND MYALGIAS

Muscles are highly metabolically active and susceptible to drug or nutrient depletion–induced muscle pain and weakness.[158] Along with generalized fatigue, symptoms of muscle weakness, pain, inflammation, cramping, and tendinopathies should not be discounted. Low CoQ, the electron transport enzyme, is a common culprit. Statins, fibrates, and nicotinic acid reduce CoQ concentrations and impair mitochondrial energy production. Zidovudine inhibits mitochondrial DNA polymerase. Antibiotics, especially the fluoroquinolones, increase mitochondrial ROS in addition to depleting Mg and thiamine. CoQ synthesis requires B vitamins, and so reduced B vitamins by any mechanism will reduce CoQ concentrations and impair electron transport in the mitochondria. Trials with CoQ10, lipoic acid, and creatine reduce muscle pain and weakness.[159] Thiamine, because of its central role in ATP metabolism, would be expected to alleviate symptoms as well, but research is lacking for these particular indications.

GASTROINTESTINAL DYSMOTILITY

Gastrointestinal dysmotility is common with mitochondrial disease and dysfunction, affecting upwards of 15% of patients with primary mitochondrial disease. The data on secondary mitochondrial disease are lacking but likely parallel the rates observed in primary disease processes. The published comorbidity between GI disturbances and psychiatric disorders is quite high ranging from 20%[160] to 80%[161] depending on the GI syndrome in question. Depression, migraine, and dysmotility may be clustered together.[33]

Symptoms may include everything from unexplained abdominal pain and chronic constipation to cyclic vomiting and diarrhea. Anorexia (remember the orexin/hypocretin neurons), gastroparesis (incomplete emptying of the stomach), and pseudo-bowel obstructions[162] are also common. Profound weight loss is possible, especially with anorexia, gastroparesis, and cyclic vomiting. These symptoms are not psychogenic, but rather appear to be a result of irregular and diminished energy resources supplying the nerves and/or the contractile cells responsible for motility. Inflammation is a core component of the disease process that can either initiate or trigger episodes; once triggered, managing the inflammation taxes mitochondrial energies even further, setting forth a chronically self-perpetuating cycle that is difficult to curtail. CoQ10 and L-carnitine have been used to successfully treat cyclic vomiting syndrome,[163] and CoQ10 has been effective with pseudo–bowel obstruction.[164]

SKIN AND HAIR

In addressing the total health of the patient, dermatological manifestations of mitochondrial distress are some of the most obvious to detect but least likely to be recognized, especially in the context of a psychiatric evaluation. The clinical presentations are varied and a full discussion is beyond the scope of this chapter (see the work by Feichtinger et al.[167]).[165] Briefly, however, hair loss (via thyroid intermediaries[166]) and hirsutism (via adrenal disruption), and various manifestations of atopic dermatitis are indicators of mitochondrial mutations or distress in complex IV.

MITOCHONDRIAL SUPPORT

Across the literature, references to the "mitochondrial cocktail"[167] are prominent. Generally speaking, the mitochondrial cocktail is based upon supporting mitochondrial functioning with vitamins, minerals, and other nutrients. While the exact ingredients and dosing varies from group to group and will be customized to the specific needs of each patient, common among these therapies are key nutrients including thiamine (B1), niacin (B3), riboflavin, pantothenic (B5), folate (B9—in some but not all, pay attention to MTHFR mutations), cobalamin (B12), vitamins C, E, and D, magnesium, lipoic acid, L-carnitine, CoQ10, zinc, iron, glutathione, essential fatty acids, and other minerals may also be used. In most cases, long-term, high-dose vitamin therapies[15] are required to recover, stabilize mitochondrial functioning, and overcome genetic enzyme polymorphisms.[168,169]

CONCLUSION

The role of vitamins and minerals in psychiatry has grown in prominence over recent decades. Increasing evidence suggests micronutrient deficiencies are not only common in patient populations but in many cases underlie many seemingly intractable disease processes. Concurrently, nutrient supplementation is linked to improved outcomes. Despite promising research, however, there remains a stigma associated with the use of micronutrients in psychiatric and primary care populations. Considered alternative, if considered at all, the treatment of vitamin or mineral deficiency is often the last resort, when it should instead be considered first line.[170]

Aside from the stigma associated with micronutrient therapies,[171] it can be difficult for the practicing physician to know which nutrients should be applied to what conditions and when. Many of the symptoms of individual vitamin deficiency syndromes overlap with each other, affect multiple organ systems simultaneously, and lead to an array of often contradictory diagnostic decisions. Conversely, the literature abounds with protocols promoting individual nutrients as one-size-fits-all, silver-bullet solutions for every disease known to man. In this context, the reluctance to use nutrients therapeutically is understandable. The purpose of this chapter was to allay some of those concerns, not by listing every nutrient-to-symptom relationship, but by providing a lens through which to view, and ultimately discern, the role nutrients in health and mental health. The lens chosen was mitochondrial dysfunction.

Mitochondria are central integrators and mediators of cellular and organismal health. By way of energy homeostasis and the myriad of other functions managed, mitochondria control cellular viability at the most fundamental level. Dysfunctional or distressed mitochondria induce disease, with high-energy organ systems affected most. Since mitochondria are entirely dependent on dietary nutrients to perform these critical functions, nutrition sits at the nexus of cellular and organismal health. With the near perfect storm of environmental factors that have coalesced over recent decades, nutritional insufficiency is all but guaranteed in most patient and nonpatient populations alike. The result of nutrient insufficiency has been a dizzying array of complex and seemingly unrelated but co-morbid diseases in Westernized cultures.

By using mitochondrial impairment as a mechanism to understand disease, the consideration of treatment options becomes more tenable than when we segregate diseases by organ system and consider them as separate and noninteracting entities. For example, fatigue, loss of energy, loss of motivation, symptoms traditionally attributable to depression, now become linked to loss of mitochondrial energetics and by association a downregulated orexin/hypocretin system, followed by lactate, and inflammatory cascades. The frequently co-morbid complaints of muscle pain and weakness commonly diagnosed as fibromyalgia or chronic fatigue can also be attributable to ailing mitochondria, as can the GI dysmotility syndromes. Similarly, lactate and inflammatory cascades represent compensatory mitochondrial actions, rather than discrete entities. Viewed in this light, the therapeutic goal becomes minimizing further mitochondrial damage and restoring and/or supporting mitochondrial functioning. Central to this approach is nutrition. Within this context, whether to supplement or not becomes an entirely different risk-to-benefit profile than is commonly calculated, but one that offers great potential to reduce the burden of multiple disease processes simultaneously.

REFERENCES

1. Neustadt, J. and Pieczenik, S.R. 2008. Medication-induced mitochondrial damage and disease. *Mol Nutr Food Res* 52: 780–788. doi:10.1002/mnfr.200700075.
2. McInnis, J. 2013. Insights on altered mitochondrial function and dynamics in the pathogenesis of neurodegeneration. *Transl Neurodegeneration* 2: 12. doi:10.1186/2047-9158-2-12.
3. Vandebona, H. et al. 2009. Prevalence of mitochondrial 1555A-G mutation in adults of European descent. *N Engl J Med* 360: 642–644.
4. Wallace, D.C. and Chalkia, D. 2013. Mitochondrial DNA genetics and the heteroplasmy conundrum in evolution and disease. *Cold Spring Harb Perspect Biol* 5(11): a021220. doi:10.1101/cshperspect.a021220.
5. Cohen, B.H. and Gold, D.R. 2001. Mitochondrial cytopathy in adults: What we know so far. *Cleveland Clin J Med* 68: 625–642.
6. Minocherhomji, S., Tollefsbol, T.O., and Singh, K.K. 2012. Mitochondrial regulation of epigenetics and its role in human disease. *Epigenetics* 7: 326–334.
7. Csoka, A.B. and Szyf, M. 2009. Epigenetic side-effects of common pharmaceuticals: A potential new field in medicine and pharmacology. *Med Hypotheses* 73: 770–780.
8. Anglin, R.E., Tanropolsky, M.A. Mazurek, M.F., and Rosebush, P.I. 2012. The psychiatric presentation of mitochondrial disorders in adults. *J Neuropsychiatry Clin Neurosci* 24(4): 394–409.
9. Fattal, O. et al. 2007. Psychiatric comorbidity in 36 adults with mitochondrial cytopathies. *CNS Spectrums* 12(6): 429–438.
10. Inczedy-Farkas, G., Remenyi, V., Gal, A., Varga, Z., Balla, P., Udvardy-Meszaros, A., Bereznai, B., and Molnar, M.J. 2012. Psychiatric symptoms of patients with primary mitochondrial DNA disorders. *Behav Brain Funct* 8: 9. doi:10.1186/1744-9081-8-9.
11. Clay, H., Sillivan, S., and Konradi, C. 2011. Mitochondrial dysfunction and pathology in bipolar disorder and schizophrenia. *Int J Dev Neurosci* 29: 311–324.
12. Shao, L., Martin, M.V., Watson, S.J., Schatzberg, A., Akil, H., Myers, R.M., Jones, E.G., Bunney, W.E., and Vawter, M.P. 2008. Mitochondrial involvement in psychiatric disorders. *Ann Med* 40(4): 281–295. doi:10.1080/07853890801923753.
13. Finsterer, J. 2012. Mitochondrion-toxic drugs given to patients with mitochondrial psychosis. *Behav Brain Funct* 8: 45.
14. Hudson, G., Gomez-Duran, A., Wilson, I.J., and Chinnery, P.F. 2014. Recent mitochondrial DNA mutations increase the risk of developing common late-onset human diseases. *PLoS Genetics* 10(5): e1004369. doi:10.1371/journal.pgen.1004369.
15. Kidd, P.M. 2005. Neurodegeneration from mitochondrial insufficiency: Nutrients, stem cells, growth factors, and prospects for brain rebuilding using integrative management. *Altern Med Rev* 10(4): 268–293.
16. El Bacha, T., Luz, M., and Da Poian, A. 2010. Dynamic adaptation of nutrient utilization in humans. *Nature Education* 3(9): 8.
17. Huskisson, E., Maggini, S., and Ruf, M. 2007. The role of vitamins and minerals in energy metabolism and well-being. *J Int Med Res* 35: 277–289.
18. Berg, J.M., Tymoczko, J.L., and Stryer L. 2002. Metabolic pathways contain many recurring motifs. In *Biochemistry*, 5th ed. New York, NY: Freeman. Available at: http://www.ncbi.nlm.nih.gov/books/NBK22398/
19. Pieczenick, S.R. and Neustadt, J. 2007. Mitochondrial dysfunction and molecular pathways of disease. *Exp Mol Pathol* 83: 84–92.
20. Federico, A., Cardaioli, E., Da Pozzo, P., Formichi, P., Gallus, G.N., and Radi, E. 2012. Mitochondria, oxidative stress and neurodegeneration. *J Neurol Sci* 322(1–2): 254–62. doi:10.1016/j.jns.2012.05.030.
21. Depeint, F., Bruce, W.R., Shangari, N., Mehta, R., and O'Brien, P.J. 2006. Mitochondrial function and toxicity: Role of the B vitamin family on mitochondrial energy metabolism. *Chem Biol Interact* 163: 94–112.
22. Wanders, R.J.A., Komen, J., and Kemp, S. 2011. Fatty acid omega-oxidation as a rescue pathway for fatty acid oxidation disorders in humans. *FEBS J* 278: 182–194. doi:10.1111/j.1742-4658.2010.07947.x.
23. Hroudová, J., Fišar, Z., and Raboch, J. 2013. *Mitochondrial Functions in Mood Disorders*. In *Mood Disorders*, Ed. N. Kocabasoglu, InTech, doi:10.5772/53254. Available at: http://www.intechopen.com/books/mood-disorders/mitochondrial-functions-in-mood-disorders
24. Ames, B. 2006. Low micronutrient intake may accelerate the degenerative diseases of aging through allocation of scarce micronutrients by triage. *PNAS* 103: 7589–17594, doi:10.1073/pnas.0608757103.
25. Atamna, H., Newberry, J., Erlitzki, R., Schultz, C.S., and Ames, B.N. 2006. Biotin deficiency inhibits heme synthesis and impairs mitochondria in human lung fibroblast. *J Nutr* 137: 25–30.

26. Ames, B.M., Atamna, H., and Killilea D.W. 2005. Mineral and vitamin deficiencies can accelerate the mitochondrial decay of aging. *Mol Aspects Med* 26(4–5): 363–378.

27. Kucharska, J. 2008. Vitamins in mitochondrial function. In *Mitochondrial Medicine: Mitochondrial Metabolism, Diseases, Diagnosis and Therapy*, Ed. A. Gvozdjáková. New York, NY: Springer, pp. 367–384.

28. Casteels, M., Sniekers, M., Fraccascia, P., Mannaerts, G.P., and Van Veldhoven, P.P. 2007. The role of 2-hydroxyacyl-CoA lyase, a thiamin pyrophosphate-dependent enzyme, in the peroxisomal metabolism of 3-methyl-branched fatty acids and 2-hydroxy straight-chain fatty acids. *Biochem Soc Trans* 35: 876–880. doi:10.1042/BST0350876.

29. Sunku, B. 2009. Cyclic vomiting syndrome. *Gastroenterol Hepatol* 5(7): 507–515.

30. Chapman, T.P., Hadley, G., Fratter, C., Cullen, S.N., Bax, B.E., Bain, M.D., Sapsford, R.A., Poulton, J., and Travis, S.P. 2014. Unexplained gastrointestinal symptoms: Think mitochondrial disease. *Digest Liver Dis* 46: 1–8.

31. Myhill, S., Booth, N.E., and McLaren-Howard, J. 2009. Chronic fatigue syndrome and mitochondrial dysfunction. *Int J Clin Exp Med* 2(1): 1–16.

32. Abdullah, M., Vishwanath, S., Elbalkhi, A., and Ambrus, J.L. 2012. Mitochondrial myopathy presenting as fibromyalgia: A case report. *J Med Case Rep* 6: 55. doi:10.1186/1752-1947-6-55.

33. Finsterer, J. 2005. Mitochondrial neuropathy. *Clin Neurol Neurosurg* 107(3): 181–186.

34. Sparaco, M., Feleppa, M., Lipton, R.B., Rapoport, A.M., and Bigal, M.E. 2006. Mitochondrial dysfunction and migraine: Evidence and hypotheses. *Cephalalgia* 26(4): 361–372.

35. Finsterer, J. and Mahjoub, S.Z. 2013. Presentation of adult mitochondrial epilepsy. *Seizure* 22(2): 119–123.

36. Feldt, M.M. and Kerr, D.S. United Mitochondrial Disease Foundation. Mito101—Endocrinology. Available at: http://www.umdf.org/atf/cf/%7B858ACD34-ECC3-472A-8794-39B92E103561%7D/mito101_Endocrinology_Feldt_Kerr.pdf

37. Burnett, B.B., Gardner, A., and Boles, R.G. 2005. Mitochondrial inheritance in depression, dysmotility and migraine? *J Affect Disord* 88(1): 109–116.

38. Filler, K., Lyon, D., Bennett, J., McCain, N., Elswick, R., Lukkahatai, N., and Saligan, L.N. 2014. Association of mitochondrial dysfunction and fatigue: A review of the literature. *BBA Clin* 1: 12–23. doi:10.1016/j.bbacli.2014.04.001.

39. Chowanadisai, W., Keen, C.L., Liu, J., Rucker, R.B., Sharman, E., and Shenoy, S.F. 2011. Well-functioning cell mitochondria promote good health. *Calif Agric* 65(3):136–140. doi:10.3733/ca.v065n03p136.

40. Maassen, A.J., Hart, L.M., Van Essen, E., Heine, R.J., Nijpels, G., Jahangir Tafrechi, R.S., Raap, A.K., Janssen, G.M., and Lemkes, H.H. 2004. Mitochondrial diabetes: Molecular mechanisms and clinical presentation. *Diabetes* 53 (suppl 1): S103–S109. doi:10.2337/diabetes.53.2007.S103.

41. Lee, H.K. and Shim, E.B. 2013. Extension of the mitochondria dysfunction hypothesis of metabolic syndrome to atherosclerosis with emphasis on endocrine disrupting chemicals and biophysical laws. *J Diabetes Investig* 4(1): 19–33.

42. Zelnick, N., Axelrod, F.B., Leshinsky, E., Griebel, M.L., and Kolodny, E.H. 1996. Mitochondrial encephalomyopathies presenting with features of autonomic and visceral dysfunction. *Pediatr Neurol* 14(3): 251–254.

43. Tobe, E.H. 2014. Cerebellar dysregulation and heterogeneity of mood disorders. *Neuropsychiatr Dis Treat* 10: 1381–1384.

44. Kanjwal, K., Karabin, B., Kanjwal, Y., Saeed, B., and Grubb, B.P. 2010. Autonomic dysfunction presenting as orthostatic intolerance in patients suffering from mitochondrial cytopathy. *Clin Cardiol* 33(10): 626–629.

45. Lonsdale, D. 2015. Thiamine and magnesium deficiencies: Keys to disease. *Med Hypotheses* 84(2): 129–134. doi: 10.1016/j.mehy.2014.12.004. Epub: December 15, 2014.

46. Bridge-Cook, P. 2014. Cyclic vomiting syndrome and mitochondrial dysfunction: Research and treatments. *Hormones Matter.* Available at: http://www.hormonesmatter.com/cyclic-vomiting-syndrome-mitochondrial-dysfunction/

47. Naviaux, R.K. 2014. Metabolic features of the cell danger response. *Mitochondrion* 16: 7–17. Available at: http://dx.doi.org/10.1016/j.mito.2013.08.006

48. Miller, W.L. 2013. Steroid hormone synthesis in mitochondria. *Mol Cell Endocrinol* 379: 62–73.

49. Sheng, Z.H. 2014. Mitochondrial trafficking and anchoring in neurons: New insight and implications. *J Cell Biol* 204: 1087–1098.

50. O'Rourke, B., Cortassa, S., and Aon, M.A. 2005. Mitochondrial ion channels: Gatekeepers of life and death. *Physiology* 20: 303–315. doi:10.1152/physiol.00020.2005.

51. Kroemer, G., Galluzzi, L., and Brenner, C. 2007. Mitochondrial membrane permeabilization in cell death. *Physiol Rev* 87: 99–163.

52. Cioffi, F., Senese, R., Lanni, A., and Golglia, F. 2013. Thyroid hormones and mitochondria: With a brief look at derivatives. *Mol Cell Endocrinol* 379: 51–61.

53. Velarde, M.C. 2014. Mitochondrial and sex steroid hormone crosstalk during aging. *Longevity Healthspan* 3: 2. doi:10.1186/2046-2395-3-2.

54. International Food Policy Research Institute (IFPRI). 2014. Global Nutrition Report 2014: Actions and Accountability to Accelerate the World's Progress on Nutrition. Washington, DC: IFPRI.

55. Fairfield, K.M. and Fletcher, R.H. 2002. Vitamins for chronic disease prevention in adults: Scientific review. *J Am Med Assoc* 287(23): 3116–3126. doi:10.1001/jama.287.23.3116.

56. Via, M. 2012. The malnutrition of obesity: Micronutrient deficiencies that promote diabetes. *ISRN Endocrinol* 2012: Article ID 103472. doi:org/10.5402/2012/103472.

57. Manore, M.M. 2000. Effect of physical activity of thiamine, riboflavin and vitamin B6 requirements. *Am J Clin Nutr* 72: 598s–606s.

58. Constantini, M.W. et al. 2010. High prevalence of vitamin D deficiency in athletes and dancers. *Clin J Sports Med* 20: 368–371.

59. Lovell, G. 2008. Vitamin D status in females in elite gymnastics. *Clin J Sports Med* 18: 159–161.

60. Daniel, E. and Ryan, E.P. The nutrigenome and gut microbiome: Chronic disease prevention in crop phytochemical diversity. In *The Molecular Basis of Plant Genetic Diversity*, Ed. Mahmut Caliskan. (InTech: Chapters published 2012 under CC BY 3.0 license doi:10.5772/2639), pp. 357–398.

61. Shehata, A.A., Schrödl, W., Aldin, A.A., Hafez, H.M., and Krüger, M. 2013. The effect of glyphosate on potential pathogens and beneficial members of poultry microbiota in vitro. *Curr Microbiol* 66(4): 350–8. doi:10.1007/s00284–012–0277-2. Epub 2012 Dec 9.

62. Mesnage, R., Bernay, B., and Seralini, G-E. 2012. Ethoxylated adjuvants of glyphosate-based herbicides are active principles of human cell toxicity. *Toxicology* 16: 313(2–3): 122–8. doi:10.1016/j.tox.2012.09.006.

63. Marler, J.B. and Wallin J.R. 2006. Human health, the nutritional quality of harvested food and sustainable farming systems. Nutrition Security Institute. Available at: http://www.nutritionsecurity.org/PDF/NSI_White%20Paper_Web.pdf

64. Davis, D.R., Epp, M.D., and Riordan, H.D. 2004. Changes in USDA food composition data for 43 garden crops, 1950–1999. *J Am Coll Nutr* 23(6): 669–682.

65. Benbrook, B. 2012. Impacts of genetically engineered crops on pesticide use in the U.S.—The first sixteen years. *Environ Sci Europe* 24: 24. doi:10.1186/2190-4715-24-24.

66. Sorenson, M.T., Poulsen, H.D., and Hojberg, O. 2014. Memorandum on "the feeding of genetically modified glyphosate resistant soy products to livestock." Aarhus University, Denmark: Danish Centre for Food and Agriculture.

67. Kruger, M., Schledorn, P., Schrödl, W., Hoppe, H.-W., Lutz, W., and Shehat, A.A. 2014. Detection of glyphosate residues in animals and humans. *J Environ Anal Toxicol* 4: 210. doi:10.4172/2161-0525.1000210.

68. Peixoto, F. 2005. Comparative effects of the RoundUp and glyphosate on mitochondrial oxidative phosphorylation. *Chemosphere* 61(8): 1115–1122.

69. Olufunso, O.O., Babunmi, E.A., and Bassir, O. 1979. Effect of glyphosate on rat liver mitochondria *in vivo*. *Bull Environ Contam Toxicol* 22(1): 357–364.

70. Samsel, A. and Seneff, S. 2013. Glyphosate's suppression of cytochrome P450 enzymes and amino acid biosynthesis by the gut microbiome: Pathways to modern diseases. *Entropy* 15: 1416–1463. doi:10.3390/e15041416.

71. Curl, C.L., Fenske, R.A., and Elgethun, K. 2003. Organophosphorus pesticide exposure of urban and suburban preschool children with organic and conventional diets. *Environ Health Perspect* 111(3): 377–382.

72. Kalghatgi, S., Spina, C.S., Costello, J.C., Liesa, M., Morones-Ramirez, J.R., Slomovic, S., Molina, A., Shirihai, O.S., and Collins, J.J. 2013. Bactericidal antibiotics induce mitochondrial dysfunction and oxidative damage in mammalian cells. *Sci Transl Med* 5(192): 192ra85. doi:10.1126/scitranslmed.3006055.

73. Scatena, R. 2007. The role of mitochondria in pharmacotoxicology: A reevlauation of an old, newly emerging topic. *Am J Physiol Cell Physiol* 293: C12–C21. doi:10.1152/ajpcell.00314.2006.

74. Lonsdale, D. 2003. A review of the biochemistry, metabolism and clinical benefits of thiamin(e) and its derivatives. *Evid Based Complement Altern Med* 3(1): 49–59. doi:10.1093/ecam/nek009.

75. Rindi, G., Patrini, C., Comincioli, V., and Reggiani, C. 1980. Thiamine content and turnover rates of some rat nervous regions, using labeled thiamine as a tracer. *Brain Res* 181(2): 369–380.

76. Natural Medicines Comprehensive Database: Drug Influences on Nutrient Levels and Depletion. Available at: http://naturaldatabase.therapeuticresearch.com/ce/ceCourse.aspx?pc=08-40&cec=0&pm=5

77. McCormick, M.L., Buchanan, J.R., Onwuameze, O.E., Pierson, R.K., and Paradiso, S. 2013. Beyond alcoholism: Wernicke-Korsakoff syndrome in patients with psychiatric disorders. *Cogn Behav Neurol* 24(4): 209–216. doi:10.1097/WNN.0b013e31823f90c4.

78. Golomb, B.A. and Evans, M.A. 2008. Statin adverse effects: A review of the literature and evidence for a mitochondrial mechanism. *Am J Cardiovasc Drugs* 8(6): 373–418.
79. Linus Pauling Institute: Micronutrient Information Center. Available at: http://lpi.oregonstate.edu/infocenter/
80. University of Maryland Medical Center: Vitamins. Available at: http://umm.edu/health/medical/reports/articles/vitamins
81. Dykens, J.A. and Will, Y. 2007. The significance of mitochondrial toxicity testing in drug development. *Drug Discov Today* 12: 777–785.
82. Will, Y. and Dykens, J. 2014. Mitochondrial toxicity assessment in industry—A decade of technology development and insight. *Expert Opin Drug Metabol Toxicol* 10(8): 1061–1067.
83. Golomb, B.B.A., Allison, M., Koperski, S., Koslik, H.J., Devaraj, S., and Ritchie, J.B. 2014. CoEnyzme Q10 benefits symptoms in Gulf War Veterans: Results of a double blind study. *Neural Comput* 26: 2594–2651.
84. Meyer, J.N., Leung, M.C., Rooney, J.P., Sendoel, A., Hengartner, M.O., Kisby, G.E., and Bess, A.S. 2013. Mitochondria as a target of environmental toxicants. *Toxicol Sci* 134(1): 1–17. doi: 10.1093/toxsci/kft102. Epub: April 29, 2013.
85. Koslik, H.J., Hamilton, G., and Golomb, B.A. 2014. Mitochondrial dysfunction in Gulf War Illness revealed by 31 phosphorus magnetic resonance spectroscopy: A case-control study. *PLoS ONE* 9(3): e92887. doi:10.1371/journal.pone.0092887.
86. *U.S. Health in International Perspective: Shorter Lives, Poorer Health.* 2013. Washington, DC: National Academies Press.
87. Lakhan, S.E. and Vieira, K.E. 2008. Nutritional therapies for mental disorders. *Nutr J* 7: 2. *PMC*. Web. 23 Nov. 2014.
88. Padwal, R.S. and Sharma, A.M. 2010. Prevention of cardiovascular disease: Obesity, diabetes and the metabolic syndrome. *Can J Cardiol* 26(Suppl C): 18C–20C.
89. Brady, D. 2012. Autoimmune disease: A modern epidemic? *Townsend Lett.* http://www.townsendletter.com/June2012/autoimmune0612.html
90. Parikh, S., Saneto, R., Falk, M.J., Anselm, I., Cohen, B.H., Haas, R., Medicine Society TM. 2009. A modern approach to the treatment of mitochondrial disease. *Curr Treat Options Neurol* 11: 414–430.
91. Ivannikov, M.V., Sugimori, M., and Llinas, R.R. 2013. Synaptic vesicle exocytosis in hippocampal synaptosomes correlates directly with total mitochondrial volume. *J Mol Neurosci* 49(1): 223–230.
92. Reddy, P.H. 2008. Mitochondrial medicine for aging and neurodegenerative diseases. *Neuromolecular Med* 10(4): 291–315. doi:10.1007/s12017-008-8044-z.
93. Picard, M. and McEwen, B. 2014. Mitochondria impact brain function and cognition. *PNAS* 111: 7–8.
94. Liu, Z.-W., Gan, G., Suyama, S., and Gao, X-B. Intracellular energy status regulates activity in hypocretin/orexin neurones: A link between energy and behavioural states. *J Physiol* 589(Pt 17): 4157–4166. doi:10.1113/jphysiol.2011.212514.
95. Sakuri, T. 2007. The neural circuit of orexin (hypocretin): Maintaining sleep and wakefulness. *Nature Rev Neurosci* 8: 171–181. doi:10.1038/nrn2092.
96. Tsujino, N. and Sakuri, T. 2009. Orexin/Hypocretin: A neuropeptide at the interface of sleep, energy homeostasis, and reward system. *Pharmacol Rev* 61(2): 162–176. doi:10.1124/pr.109.001321.
97. Randeva, H.S., Karteris, E., Grammatopoulos, D., and Hillhouse, E.W. 2001. Expression of orexin-A and functional orexin type 2 receptors in the human adult adrenals: Implications for adrenal function and energy homeostasis. *J Clin Endocrinol Metab* 86(10): 4808–4813.
98. Silveyra, P., Cataldi, N.I., Lux-Lantos, V., and Libertun, C. 2009. Gonadal steroids modulated hypocretin/orexin type-1 receptor expression in a brain region, sex and daytime specific manner. *Regul Pept* 27:158(1–3): 121–126. doi:10.1016/j.regpep.2009.08.002.
99. Takahashi, K., Arihara, Z., Suzuki, T., Sone, M., Kikuchi, K., Sasano, H., Murakami, O., and Totsune, K. Expression of orexin-A and orexin receptors in the kidney and the presence of orexin-A-like immunoreactivity in human urine. *Peptides* 27: 871–877.
100. Brundin, L., Bjorkqvist, M., Petersen, A., and Traskman-Bendz, L. 2007. Reduced orexin levels in the cerebrospinal fluid of suicidal patients with major depressive disorder. *Eur Neuropsychopharmacol* 17: 573–579.
101. Jacobs, R.A., Meinild A.K., Nordsborg, N.B., and Lundby, C. 2013. Lactate oxidation in human skeletal muscle mitochondria. *Am J Physiol—Endocrinol Metab* 304(7): E686–E694. doi:10.1152/ajpendo.00476.2012.
102. Ross, J.M., Öberg, J., Brené, S., Coppotelli, G., Terzioglu, M., Pernold, K., Goiny, M. et al. 2010. High brain lactate is a hallmark of aging and caused by a shift in the lactate dehydrogenase A/B ratio. *PNAS* 107(46): 20087–20092, doi:10.1073/pnas.1008189107.

103. Dienel, G.A. 2012. Brain lactate metabolism: The discoveries and the controversies. *J Cereb Blood Flow Metabol* 32(7): 1107–1138. doi:10.1038/jcbfm.2011.175.
104. Cruz, R.S.O., de Aguiar, R.A., Turnes, T., Penteado Dos Santos, R., de Oliveira, M.F., and Caputo, F. 2012. Intracellular shuttle: The lactate aerobic metabolism. *Scientific World J* 2012: 420984. doi:10.1100/2012/420984.
105. Oddo, M., Levine, J.M., Frangos, S., Maloney-Wilensky, E., Carrera, E., Daniel, R.T., Levivier, M., Magistretti, P.J., and LeRoux, P.D. 2012. Brain lactate metabolism in humans with subarachnoid hemorrhage. *Stroke* 43: 1418–1421. doi:10.1161/STROKEAHA.111.648568.
106. Maniega, M.M., Cvoro, V., Chappell, F.M., Armitage, P.A., Marshall, I., Bastin, M.E., and Wardlaw, J.M. 2008. Changes in NAA and lactate following ischemic stroke. *Neurology* 71(24): 1993–1999.
107. Overgaard, M., Rasmussen, P., Bohm, A.M., Seifert, T., Brassard, P., Zaar, M., Homann, P., Evans, K.A., Nielsen, H.B., and Secher, N.H. 2012. Hypoxia and exercise provoke both lactate release and lactate oxidation by the human brain. *FASEB J* 26(7): 3012–3020.
108. Shungu, D.C., Weiduschat, N., Murrough, J.W., Mao, X., Pillemer, S., Dyke, J.P., Medow, M.S., Natelson, B.H., Stewart, J.M., and Mathew, S.J. 2012. Increased ventricular lactate in chronic fatigue syndrome. III. Relationships to cortical glutathione and clinical symptoms implicate oxidative stress in disorder pathophysiology. *NMR Biomed* 25: 1073–1087. doi:10.1002/nbm.2772.
109. Narayana, P.A. 2005. Magnetic resonance spectroscopy in the monitoring of multiple sclerosis. *J Neuroimaging* 15(4 Suppl): 46S–57S. doi:10.1177/1051228405284200.
110. Lange, T. 2006. Pitfalls in lactate measurements at 3T. *Am J Neuroradiol* 27: 895–901.
111. Detre, J.A., Wang, Z.Y., Bogdan, A.R., Gusnard, D.A., Bay, C.A., Bingham, P.M., and Zimmerman, R.A. 1991. Regional variation in brain lactate in leigh syndrome by localized ^{1}H magnetic resonance spectroscopy. *Ann Neurol* 29: 218–221. doi:10.1002/ana.410290219.
112. Da Rocha, A.J., Túlio Braga, F., Carlos Martins Maia, A. Jr, Jorge da Silva, C., Toyama, C., Pereira Pinto Gama, H., Kok, F., and Rodrigues Gomes, H. 2008. Lactate detection by MRS in mitochondrial encephalopathy: Optimization of technical parameters. *J Neuroimaging* 18: 1–8. doi:10.1111/j.1552-6569.2007.00205.x.
113. Goh, S. et al. 2014. Mitochondrial dysfunction as a neurobiological subtype of Autism Spectrum Disorder: Evidence from brain imaging. *J Am Med Assoc* 71(6): 665–671. doi:10.1001/jamapsychiatry.2014.179.
114. Quistorff, B. and Grunnet, N. 2011. High brain lactate is not caused by a shift in the lactate dehydrogenase A/B ratio. *PNAS* 108(7): E21. doi:10.1073/pnas.1017750108.
115. Stork, C. and Renshaw, P.F. 2005. Mitochondrial dysfunction in bipolar disorder: Evidence from magnetic resonance spectroscopy research. *Mol Psychiatry* 10: 900–919.
116. ElBeheiry, A.A., Abougabal, A.M., Omar, T.I., and Etaby, A.N. 2014. Role of brain magnetic resonance spectroscopy in the evaluation of suspected mitochondrial diseases in children: Experience in 30 pediatric cases. *Egypt J Radiol Nucl Imaging* 45(2): 523–533. doi:10.1016/j.ejrnm.2013.12.012.
117. Learmonth, Y.C., Paul, L., McFadyen, A.K., Marshall-McKenna, R., Mattison, P., Miller, L., and McFarlane, N.G. 2014. Short-term effect of aerobic exercise on symptoms in multiple sclerosis and chronic fatigue syndrome: A pilot study. *Int J MS Care* 16(2): 76–82. doi:10.7224/1537-2073.2013-005.
118. Zinger, A., Barcia, C., Herrero, M.T., and Guillemin, G.J. 2011. The involvement of neuroinflammation and kynurenine pathway in Parkinson's disease. *Parkinson's Dis.* 2011(2011): 11, Article ID 716859, doi:10.4061/2011/716859.
119. Najjar, S., Pearlman, D.M., Alper, K., Najjar, A., and Devinsky, O. 2013. Neuroinflammation and psychiatric illness. *J Neuroinflammation* 10: 43 doi:10.1186/1742-2094-10-43.
120. Smith, A.J., Stone, T.W., and Smith, R.A. 2007. Neurotoxicity of tryptophan metabolites. *Biochem Soc Trans* 35: 1287–1289. doi:10.1042/BST0351287.
121. Midttun, O., Ulvik, A., Ringdal Pedersen, E., Ebbing, M., Bleie, O., Schartum-Hansen, H., Nilsen, R.M., Nygård, O., and Ueland, P.M. 2011. Low plasma vitamin B-6 status affects metabolism through the kynurenine pathway in cardiovascular patients with systemic inflammation. *J Nutr* 141(4): 611–617.
122. Tong, Y. 2014. Seizures caused by pyridoxine (vitamin B6) deficiency in adults: A case report and literature review. *Intract Rare Dis Res* 3(2): 52–56.
123. Douahd, G., Refsum, H., de Jager, C.A., Jacoby, R., Nicholsa, T.E., Smith, S.M., and Smith, A.D. 2013. Preventing Alzheimer's disease-related gray matter atrophy by B-vitamin treatment. PNAS 110: 9523–9528. doi:10.1073/pnas.1301816110.
124. Lerner, V., Miodownik, C., Kaptsan, A., Bersudsky, Y., Libov, I., Sela, B.A., and Witztum, E. 2007. Vitamin B6 treatment for tardive dyskinesia: A randomized, double-blind, placebo-controlled, crossover study. *J Clin Psychiatry* 68(11): 1648–1654.

125. Oxenkrug, G., Ratner, R., and Summergrad, P. 2013. Kynurenines and vitamin B6: Link between diabetes and depression. *J Bioinform Diabetes*. Available at: http://openaccesspub.org/journals/download.php?file=51-OAP-JBD-IssuePDF.pdf.

126. Sorolla, M.A., Rodríguez-Colman, M.J., Tamarit, J., Ortega, Z., Lucas, J.J., Ferrer, I., Ros, J., and Cabiscol, E. 2010. Protein oxidation in Huntington disease affects energy production and vitamin B6 metabolism. *Free Radical Biol Med* 49(4): 612–621. doi:10.1016/j.freeradbiomed.2010.05.016.

127. Zysset-Burri, D.C., Bellac D.L., Leib, S.L., and Wittwer, M. 2013. Vitamin B6 reduces hippocampal apoptosis in experimental pneumococcal meningitis. *BMC Infect Dis* 13: 393. doi:10.1186/1471-2334-13-393.

128. Kawai, C., Wakabayashi A., Matsumura, T., and Yui, Y. Reappearance of beriberi heart disease in Japan. A study of 23 cases. *Am J Med* 69(3): 383–386.

129. Fattal-Valevski, A., Kesler, A., Sela, B.A., Nitzan-Kaluski, D., Rotstein, M., Mesterman, R., Toledano-Alhadef, H. et al. 2005. Outbreak of life-threatening thiamine deficiency in infants in Israel caused by a defective soy-based formula. *Pediatrics* 115(2): e233–e238.

130. Thornalley, P.J., Babaei-Jadidi, R., Al Ali, H. et al. 2007. High prevalence of low plasma thiamine concentration in diabetes linked to marker of vascular disease. *Diabetologica* 50: 2164–2170.

131. Flancbaum, L. et al. 2006. Preoperative nutritional status of patients undergoing Roux-en-Y gastric bypass for morbid obesity. *J Gastrointest Surg* 10(7): 1033–1037.

132. Xanthakos, S.A. Nutritional deficiencies in obesity and after bariatric surgery. *Pediatr Clin North Am* 56(5): 1105–1121. doi:10.1016/j.pcl.2009.07.002.

133. Lakhani, S.V. et al. 2008. Small intestinal bacterial overgrowth and thiamine deficiency after Roux-en-Y gastric bypass surgery in obese patients. *Nutr Res* 28: 293–298.

134. Jamieson, C.P., Obeid, O.A., and Powell-Tuck, J. 1999. The thiamin, riboflavin and pyridoxine status of patients on emergency admission to hospital. *Clin Nutr* 18(2): 87–91.

135. Carrodeguas, L., Kaidar-Person, O., Smozstein, S. et al. 2005. Preoperative thiamine deficiency in obese population undergoing laparoscopic bariatric surgery. *Surg Obes Relat Dis* 1(6): 517–522.

136. Maurice, C.F., Haiser, H.J., and Turnbaugh, P.J. 2013. Xenobiotics shape the physiology and gene expression of the active human gut microbiome. *Cell* 152(1–2): 39–50.

137. Togay-Isikay, C., Yigit, A., and Mutleur, N. 2001. Wernicke's encephalopathy due to hyperemesis gravidarum: An under-recognised condition. *ANZ J Obstetr Gynecol* 41(4): 453–456.

138. Millson, C.E., Harding, K., and Hillson, R.M. 1995. Wernicke-Korsakoff syndrome due to hyperemesis gravidarum precipitated by thyrotoxicosis. *Postgrad Med J* 71(834): 249–250.

139. Winstpn, A.P., Jamieson, C.P., Madira, W., Gatward, N.M., and Palmer, R.L. 2000. Prevalence of thiamin deficiency in anorexia nervosa. *Int J Eating Dis* 28(4): 451–454.

140. Lurong, K.V.Q. and Nguyen, L.T.H. 2013. The role of thiamine in schizophrenia. *Am J Psychiatry Neurosci* 1(3): 38–46.

141. Oxford Vaccine Group. Vaccine Knowledge Project. Available at: http://www.ovg.ox.ac.uk/vaccine-ingredients#yeast%20proteins

142. Dumitrescu, L., Simionescu, O., Oprisan, A., Luca, D., Gitman, A., Ticmeanu, M., and Tanasescu, R. 2011. Update on Wernicke's: Considerations on epidemiology (II). *Rom J Neurol* 10(4): 172–178.

143. Liu, S., Bae, Y., Leggas, M., Daily, A., Bhatnagar, S., Miriyala, S., St Clair, D.K., and Moscow, J.A. 2012. Pharmacologic properties of polyethylene glycol-modified bacillus thiaminolyticus thiaminase I enzyme. *JPET* 341: 775–783.

144. Donnino, M.W., Vegas, J., Miller, J., and Walsh, M. 2007. Myths and misconceptions of Wernicke's encephalopathy: What emergency room physicians should know. *Ann Emerg Med* 50(6): 715–721.

145. Barragán-Campos, H.M., Vallée, J.N., Lô, D., Barrera-Ramírez, C.F., Argote-Greene, M., Sánchez-Guerrero, J., Estañol, B., Guillevin, R., and Chiras, J. 2005. Brain magnetic resonance imaging findings in patients with mitochondrial cytopathies. *Arch Neurol* 62(5): 737–742.

146. Fattal-Valevski, A. 2011. Thiamine (Vitamin B1). *J Evid Based Complement Altern Med* 16(1): 12–20.

147. McCandless, D.W., and Schenker, S. 1968. Encephalopathy of thiamine deficiency: Studies of intracerebral mechanisms. *J Clin Invest* 47(10): 2268–2280. doi:10.1172/JCI105912.

148. Grill, M.F. and Maganti, R.K. 2011. Neurotoxic effects associated with antibiotic use: Management considerations. *Br J Clin Pharmacol* 72(3): 381–393.

149. Lonsdale, D. 2009. Dysautonomia, a heuristic approach to a revised model for etiology of disease. *Evid Based Complement Altern Med* 6(1): 3–10. doi:10.1093/ecam/nem064.

150. Poloni, M., Mazzarello, P., Laforenza, U., Caramella, C., and Patrini, C. 1992. Thiamin contents of cerebrospinal fluid, plasma and erythrocytes in cerebellar ataxias. *Eur J Neurol* 32: 154–158. doi:10.1159/000116814.

151. Lonsdale, D. and Shamberger, R.J. 1980. Red cell transketolase as an indicator of nutritional deficiency. *Am J Clin Nutr* 33(2): 205–211.
152. Harper, C.J., Giles, M., and Finlay-Jones, R. 1986. Clinical signs in the Wernicke-Korsakoff complex: A retrospective analysis of 131 cases diagnosed at necropsy. *J Neurol Neurosurg Psychiatry* 49(4): 341–345.
153. Thompson, A.D., Guerinni, I., and Marshall, J.E. 2009. Wernicke's encephalopathy: Nutrition issues in practical gastroenterology, series #75. *Pract Gasteroenterol.* Available at http://www.medicine.virginia. edu/clinical/departments/medicine/divisions/digestive-health/nutrition-support-team/nutrition-articles/ ThomsonArticle.pdf
154. Karabatsiakis, A., Böck, C., Salinas-Manrique, J., Kolassa, S., Calzia, E., Dietrich, D.E., and Kolassa, I.-T. 2014. Mitochondrial respiration in peripheral blood mononuclear cells correlates with depressive subsymptoms and severity of major depression. *Transl Psychiatry* 4: e397. doi:10.1038/tp.2014.44.
155. Dysautonomia International. Available at: http://www.dysautonomiainternational.org/page.php?ID=34
156. Spinazzi, M., Angelini, C., and Patrini, C. 2010. Subacute sensory ataxia and optic neuropathy with thiamine deficiency. *Nat Rev Neurol* 6(5): 288–293. doi: 10.1038/nrneurol.2010.16. Epub: March 23, 2010.
157. Chihiro, Y., Toyoshima, M., Maegaki, Y., Kodama, Y., Hayami, H., Takahashi, Y., Kusunoki, S., Uchibori, A., Chiba, A., and Kawano, Y. 2013. Association of acute cerebellar ataxia and human papilloma virus vaccination: A case report. *Neuropediatrics* 44(05): 265–267. doi:10.1055/s-0033-1333873.
158. Artuch, R., Brea-Calvo, G., Briones, P., Aracil, A., Galván, M., Espinós, C., Corral, J. et al 2006. Cerebellar ataxia with coenzyme Q10 deficiency: Diagnosis and follow-up after coenzyme Q10 supplementation. *J Neurol Sci* 246: 153–158.
159. Mancuso, M., Calsolaro, V., Orsucci, D., Carlesi, C., Choub, A., Piazza, S., and Siciliano, G. 2009. Mitochondria, cognitive impairment, and Alzheimer's disease. *Int J Alzheimer's Dis* 2009: Article ID 951548. doi:10.4061/2009/951548.
160. Smithson, J. 2009. Drug induced muscle disorders. *Clin Pharmacist* 28(12): 1056–1062.
161. Rodriguez, M.C., MacDonald, J.R., Mahoney, D.J., Parise, G., Beal, M.F., and Tarnopolsky, M.A. 2007. Beneficial effects of creatine, CoQ10, and lipoic acid in mitochondrial disorders. *Muscle Nerve* 35(2): 235–242. doi:10.1002/mus.20688.
162. Mussell, M., Kroenke, K., Spitzer, R.L., Williams, J.B., Herzog, W., and Löwe, B. 2008. Gastrointestinal symptoms in primary care: Prevalence and association with depression and anxiety. *J Psychosomatic Res* 64: 605–612.
163. Mikocka-Walus, A.A., Turnbull, D.A., Moulding, N.T., Wilson, I.G., Andrews, J.M., and Holtmann, G.J. 2007. Controversies surrounding the comorbidity of depression and anxiety in inflammatory bowel disease patients: A literature review. *Inflamm Bowel Dis* 13: 225–234.
164. Giordano, C., Sebastiani, M., De Giorgio, R., Travaglini, C., Tancredi, A., Valentino, M.L., and Bellan, M. et al. 2008. Gastrointestinal dysmotility in mitochondrial neurogastrointestinal encephalomyopathy is caused by mitochondrial DNA depletion. *Am J Pathol* 173(4): 1120–1128. doi:10.2353/ ajpath.2008.080252.
165. Boles, R.G. 2011. High degree of efficacy in the treatment of cyclic vomiting syndrome with combined co-enzyme Q10, L-carnitine and amitriptyline, a case series *BMC Neurol* 11: 102. doi:10.1186/1471-2377-11-102.
166. Bergamin, C.S., Rolim, L.C., Dib, S.A., and Moisés, R.S. Unusual occurrence of intestinal pseudo obstruction in a patient with maternally inherited diabetes and deafness (MIDD) and favorable outcome with coenzyme Q10. *Arquivos Brasileiros Endocrinol Metabol* 52(8): 1345–1349.
167. Feichtinger, R.G., Speri, W., Bauer, J.W., and Kofler, B. 2014. Mitochondrial dysfunction: A neglected component of skin diseases. *Exp Dermatol* 23: 607–614.
168. Vidali, S., Knuever, J., Lerchner, J., Giesen, M., Bíró, T., Klinger, M., Kofler, B., Funk, W., Poeggeler, B., and Paus, R. Hypothalamic-pituitary-thyroid axis hormones stimulate mitochondrial function and biogenesis in human hair follicles. *J Investig Dermatol* 134: 33–42.
169. Ames, B.N., Elson-Schwab, I., and Silver, E.A. 2002. High dose vitamin therapy stimulates variant enzyme with decreased coenzyme binding affinity (increase K_m): Relevance to genetic disease and polymorphisms. *Am J Clin Nutr* 75: 616–658.
170. Tarnopolsky, M.A. 2008. The mitochondrial cocktail: Rationale for combined nutraceutical therapy in mitochondrial cytopathies. *Adv Drug Deliv Rev* 60(13–14): 1561–1567. doi:10.1016/j. addr.2008.05.001
171. Cornish, S. and Mehl-Madrona, L. 2008. The role of vitamins and minerals in psychiatry. *Integr Med Insights* 3: 33–42.

8 Vitamin Deficiencies and Depression
Evidence-Based Research

James M. Greenblatt, MD and Priyank Patel

CONTENTS

INTRODUCTION

Patients with psychiatric disorders often have poor food patterns, either from a reduced appetite, skipping meals, consuming fast or processed foods, or a general lack of interest in food altogether. In fact, patterns of poor dietary intake often predate the appearance of symptoms of these disorders.[1] In a Spanish study Sanchez-Villegas et al. followed 493 participants over a median time of 6.2 years, tracking their consumption of fast food and processed pastries and exploring possible correlations with incidence of depression.[2] They found an increased risk of depression in those with greater fast food intake.

Vitamins are an essential component of our diet for proper health maintenance. Initial studies around the turn of the century exploring the role of vitamins showed that rats fed a diet limited to purified proteins, fats, and carbohydrates did not survive.[3] However, when supplemented with what Hopkins termed "accessory factors," which were present in an unrefined diet, the rats flourished both mentally and physically. These factors proved absolutely essential to the survival of the animal. Later discoveries of nitrogen groups found within these micronutrients altered their name to what we now know as vitamins.

Each vitamin has a distinct chemical structure and has important roles in proper functioning of key reactions within cellular metabolism and gene expression. Vitamins are organic compounds that are only required in minute amounts in the diet. B-complex vitamins are a group of eight vitamins; B1, B3, B6, and B12 have been studied intensively because of their effects on the brain. With the exception of vitamin D, which requires sunlight for conversion into its active form, they are all found in common foods present in a well-rounded diet. A deficiency of these vitamins can lead to debilitating disease, each with its own unique set of physiologic symptoms. What is often overlooked, however, is the effect of vitamin deficiencies on perpetuating concurrent psychiatric symptoms. Also, genetic predispositions can alter physiologic pathways and further increase the risk of vitamin deficiency.

This chapter will explore the role of deficiencies in vitamin C, the B vitamins, and vitamin D in depression and other psychiatric disorders as well as the potential for supplementation as part of integrative treatment for these disorders.

FOLATE

Folate is a water-soluble B vitamin found in a wide variety of foods such as vegetables (asparagus and spinach), lentils, dry beans, fruits, and whole grain cereals.[3] Apart from its traditional name, folate is also referred to by its many physiologic forms: folic acid, folinic acid (leucovorin), or 5-methyltetrahydrofolate (5-MTHF).[4] Once absorbed through the jejunum in the small intestines, folate undergoes several activation reactions within the liver, leading to different biologically active forms. Chief among these is the formation of 5-MTHF, its circulatory form within the blood that can freely cross the blood-brain barrier and subsequently pass into the cerebrospinal fluid. This form plays a crucial role in the metabolism of vitamin B12. Each form must exist in dynamic equilibrium with its counterpart for proper functioning of folate's many roles.[4] Serving as a cofactor, folate is necessary for key reactions throughout the body that require methylation and nucleic acid synthesis.[5]

Due to the different forms of folate found within food and the varying bioavailability[5] of supplemental folic acid, the National Institutes of Health (NIH) makes use of the dietary folate equivalent (DFE) system. One DFE is defined as 1 μg of dietary folate and 0.6 μg of supplemental folic acid.[6] The recommended daily allowance by the NIH for adults over the age of 14 years is 400 μg DFE, with progressive levels for children based on age, ranging from 65 to 300 μg DFE. Women of childbearing age are advised to take 600 mcg DFE during pregnancy, starting before conception if possible, and 500 μg while breastfeeding. Children born to mothers with inadequate intake of supplemental folic acid during pregnancy suffer from devastating neural tube defects. Adults often present with symptoms of macrocytic or megaloblastic anemia and increased levels of the amino acid homocysteine, which can be potentially neurotoxic.[4] Additionally, several studies have linked folate deficiency to increased risk for developing cognitive deficits and depression.

Folate deficiency has several different causes. Most apparent among these is inadequate dietary intake of B vitamins.[4] Several drugs that can lead to folate deficiency are oral contraceptives, antibiotics, anticonvulsants, antacids, and alcohol. Also, patients with cancer often experience rapid depletion of folate stores due to overactive cellular proliferation.[4] Other prominent causes of folate deficiency include malabsorption through the jejunum due to inborn errors of metabolism, bacterial overgrowth, or intestinal inflammatory conditions (e.g., atrophic gastritis, irritable bowel disease [IBD]). Finally, people with genetic polymorphisms of the C677T and A1298C variants of 5, 10-methylenetetrahydrofolate reductase (MTHFR) gene show reduced enzyme activity and lower efficiency of folate metabolism, which consequently leads to a deficiency of folate and a surplus of homocysteine.[7]

In 2007, Gilbody et al. conducted a meta-analysis of all studies examining an association between this polymorphism and psychiatric conditions. Specific to depression, they included 10 studies (11,709 participants; 1280 cases of depression, 10,429 controls). Three of these were cross-sectional population-based studies, and seven were case-control studies. These studies demonstrated that people who express the homozygote (TT) variant over the wild-type (CC) variant of the C677T variant have a 1.36 times greater likelihood of developing depression than others without this genetic variant.[8] Additionally, the odds of having the T/T genotype was twice as great in depressed patients as in the general population. Patients with this genotype are likely to have reduced DNA production and repair.

The association between folate deficiency and depression has been reported by many studies dating back to the mid-twentieth century. In 1962, Herbert first reported that cognitive symptoms develop from inadequate folate intake.[9] After placing himself on a folate-free diet for 4.5 months, he experienced irritability, insomnia, and forgetfulness, the cardinal symptoms of depression.

He noted that all of his symptoms disappeared within 2 days after he started folate supplementation. Subsequently, in 1970, Reynolds et al. reported subnormal serum folate (less than 2.5 ng/mL) and vitamin B12 (less than 150 pg/mL) levels in 101 patients with depressive illness.[10] Folate deficiency was nearly twice as common as vitamin B12 deficiency among depressed patients in the sample. A 1980 study of 50 patients admitted with megaloblastosis reported greater prevalence of mood disturbance among patients with folate deficiency (56%) than among those with vitamin B12 deficiency (20%).[11] Similarly, within the same year Ghadirian et al. studied 48 adults divided into three groups based on their primary conditions: depressive, psychiatrically ill (not depressed), and medically ill. Serum folic acid levels were lowest in the depression group (2.23 ng/mL; $P < .05$) when measured after 1 week.[12] This level is just half the normal value for serum folic acid (~5 ng/mL) found in an average adult. In accordance with previous studies, these researchers show a significant negative correlation between depression scale scores and serum folic acid levels.

Carney et al. demonstrated that out of the 243 patients who were receiving inpatient psychiatric treatment, 31% had a red blood cell (RBC) folate level below 200 nm/mL and 12% below 150 nm/mL.[13] Also, RBC folate levels were lowest in the depressed subset of the population. A large-scale study of folate deficiency and depression was first attempted in the general population in 2004 by Tolmunen et al.[14] These investigators examined 2443 men between 42 and 60 years of age with no history of psychiatric conditions. The study participants were grouped in thirds based on their natural dietary intake of folate and assessed for depression via the Human Population Laboratory Depression Scale. The group with the lowest folate intake had a 67% greater risk of elevated depressive symptoms (score >5) compared to those in the highest third. After adjustments for smoking, alcohol, body mass index, socioeconomic status, marital status, education, and total fat consumptions were made, the risk for depression remained significantly elevated.

Reynolds and colleagues first determined a relationship between depression and the methionine-homocysteine cycle in the 1970s.[10] A subsequent study by Bottiglieri et al. showed that 52% of depressed patients had elevated plasma homocysteine levels.[15] These patients also exhibited notably lower serum and red blood cell folate levels. Cerebrospinal fluid (CSF) examinations further revealed marked reduction of folate, SAMe, and monoamine metabolites. In line with this previous work, several recent observational studies have been conducted to further establish an association between higher homocysteine levels and depression, especially in the elderly. The 2008 cross-sectional analysis by Almeida et al. of elderly men (greater than 70 years of age) showed not only a higher overall risk of incident depression but also that this risk increased 2% to 5% for every unit (micromoles per liter) increase in concentration of homocysteine.[16] A cohort of elderly adults over the age of 65 followed over a 4-year period showed women with higher homocysteine levels (≥11.9 umol/L) had a higher risk for developing depression than those with lower concentrations.[17] Additionally, an Australian study in 2013 found elevated homocysteine to mediate poor cognitive performance in older adults with depression.[18] Cognitive performance was measured via the Consortium to Establish a Registry for Alzheimer's Disease (CERAD) neuropsychological battery and the Mini Mental Status Exam (MMSE). Those with high homocysteine levels and major depressive disorder (MDD) had worse immediate verbal and delayed visual recall. Those with depressive symptoms not fully meeting DSM-IV criteria had lower MMSE immediate and delayed recall scores than those with normal homocysteine levels. Researchers have also attempted to explore a relationship between depression and homocysteine levels in younger adults under the age of 65. Nabi et al. conducted a large population-based study with 3392 men and women between 35 and 66 years of age. Among men, the prevalence of MDD was 31.5% in those with homocysteine levels greater than 15 umol/L.[19] Men with higher homocysteine levels also showed a greater propensity to meet diagnostic criteria for lifetime MDD.

The methionine-homocysteine pathway is tightly intertwined with the folate cycle. Vitamin B12 is an important cofactor in the de novo formation of methionine from homocysteine. It assists in the transfer of a methyl group from 5-MTHF to homocysteine to create methionine and tetrahydrofolate. Subsequently, homocysteine is created utilizing the intermediates S-adenosylmethionine (SAMe) and S-adenosylhomocysteine (SAH) from methionine. SAMe produces methyl groups necessary for DNA synthesis and catecholamines synthesis. The Hordaland-Homocysteine study, Norwegian research that studied 18,044 participants from 1992 to 1993, showed that the MTHFR C677T variant was expressed in 73% of those with homocysteine levels ≥40 µmol/L.[20] These individuals were also found to have had concurrent low folate and vitamin B12 levels. Likewise, in 2007, Zittan et al. reported similar findings. Of the 360 asymptomatic patients they observed, 18.6% expressed the homozygous C677T gene mutation variant with elevated homocysteine concentrations when compared to those with the heterozygote variant.[21] In fact, homozygote patients also had a 4.2 times higher probability of having vitamin B12 deficiency (<150 pmol/L) than the heterozygote group. Thus, studies have shown that folate and vitamin B12 deficiency is accompanied by elevated homocysteine levels at higher rates in this genetic subset of the population.

Another such study recounted that increasing folate levels from <2 nmol/L to >15 nmol/L can produce a significant decline in homocysteine levels.[22] Similar to folate deficiency, vitamin B12 deficiency can hinder the methionine-homeostasis pathway. Such deficiency can stem from either a genetic failure in absorption via the gut or from a deficiency in dietary intake that leads to a more modest increase in homocysteine levels (≥30–100 uM).[15]

In addition to contributing to the onset of depression, folate deficiency can also perpetuate symptoms, worsen clinical outcomes, reduce response to traditional antidepressants, and increase the risk of relapse in patients during treatment. Fava et al. treated 213 adults with MDD with 20 mg of fluoxetine daily for 8 weeks.[23] Individuals with sole folate deficiency showed 2.2 times greater likelihood of resistance to treatment than their normal counterparts. In a double-blinded randomized control trial (RCT), Papakostas et al. divided 55 fluoxetine-resistant MDD patients continuing onto next-step therapy into groups receiving either an increased dose of fluoxetine (40–60 mg/d) or augmenting fluoxetine with either lithium or desipramine.[24] Patients with lower serum folate levels (≤2.5 ng/mL) but no vitamin B12 or homocysteine deficiency had a nonresponse rate to treatment of 93% compared to 55% for those with normal levels. Thus, patients with low levels of serum folate have a weakened response to both initial and second-order treatments. Moreover, patients who actually showed minimal response to the initial fluoxetine 8-week treatment exhibited clinical improvement at a much later time. A follow-up study by Papakostas et al. estimated that this clinical improvement would happen 1.5 weeks later than in those with normal folate levels.[25] A further study by Papakostas et al. showed that after continuing fluoxetine treatment, treatment responders with low folate levels experienced significantly higher relapse rates.[26] There was no relationship between vitamin B12 levels and relapse rates. These studies show that maintaining proper folate levels is crucial in not only preventing the onset of depression but for its successful treatment.

Alternatively, folate therapy in depressive patients with normal folate levels has been studied as a clinical approach to improve outcomes. Studies have found that augmenting antidepressant therapy with folic acid can strongly improve treatment efficacy. In 2000, Coppen et al. conducted a double-blind RCT of 127 depressed adults with normal folate who received either daily combination therapy of 500 µg folic acid and 20 mg fluoxetine, or 20 mg fluoxetine with placebo.[27] After a 10-week period, women showed a lower mean Hamilton Rating scale score of 6.8 in the treatment group compared to a score of over 11.7 in the control group. Furthermore, 93.9% of women in the treatment group showed a reduction of more than 50% (equaling good clinical response) in their rating scores compared to only 61.1% of women in the control group. Men did not show the same type of response as women; however, the study suggests that men may require a higher dose of folic acid than women to sustain plasma levels. No additional adverse events were reported with the addition of folic acid.

Several relevant studies have demonstrated positive effects of utilizing 5-MTHF in the treatment of depression. Guaraldi et al. conducted an open-label trial of 16 elderly patients, of whom 14 were normofolatemic with major depressive disorder (Hamilton Depression Rating Scale-D21 [HAM-D-21] ≥18).[28] After 4 weeks of daily oral 5-MTHF (50 mg) treatment, patients showed significant improvement in depressive symptoms (>50% reduction on HAM-D) in 81% of the patients. Likewise, in a double-blinded randomized equivalence study, Passeri et al. further compared 5-MTHF to Trazodone (TRZ) in depressed patients with normal folate levels (HAM-D-21 ≥18) and/or dementia (MMSE = 12–23).[29] Ninety-six patients were randomized to receive either oral 50 mg/day 5-MTHF or oral 100 mg/day Trazodone for 8 weeks. Patients receiving 5-MTHF showed a greater reduction of symptoms at 4 weeks and at the end of the treatment period than the TZD group. Methylfolate (5-MTHF) led to a significantly greater improvement of immediate recall (Rey's Verbal Memory Test) than Trazodone; the rates were 53% versus 37%, respectively. Furthermore, another double-blinded RTC by Godfrey et al. studied 41 patients with low RBC folate levels (<200 µg/L) and either depression or schizophrenia. These patients received standard psychotropic medication (tri-cyclic antidepressant [TCA] or monoamine oxidase inhibitor [MAOI]) augmented with either 15 mg 5-MTHF or a placebo for 6 months.[30] The MTHF group reported significant clinical and social improvement at 3 and 6 months. This improvement was maintained over the course of the study in the MTHF group. In the placebo group, however, patients initially showed slight improvement at 3 months, yet symptoms recurred by 6 months.

Folic acid requires a four-step transformation process to be converted to the active form of folate, L-methylfolate. The importance of L-methylfolate is grounded in its ability, unlike that of folic acid, to directly cross the blood-brain barrier for the synthesis of neurotransmitters,[31] and thus to overcome the MTHFR C-T polymorphism present in many depressive patients. As a result, it requires a smaller bioequivalent dose per tablet (7.5 mg) than folic acid (52.5 mg).[32] In 2012, Papakostas et al. demon-strated that L-methylfolate may be efficacious as an adjunctive therapy in patients with MDD with partial or no response to traditional selective serotonin reuptake inhibitors (SSRIs).[33] In one trial, patients with continued SSRI use were randomized into three groups (7.5 mg/day L-methylfolate for 30 days followed by 15 mg/day for 30 days, placebo for 30 days followed by 7.5 mg/day L-methylfolate, or placebo for 60 days) and resulted in no statistically significant ($p = 0.01$) differ-ence between the treatment groups. However, a second trial with 75 patients with identical groups to the first study, except for treatment groups now receiving 15 mg/day of L-methylfolate for the first 30 days, yielded greater efficacy of L-methylfolate and SSRI combinations than SSRI monotherapy alone. Improvements were graded via response rate (32.3% versus 14.6%, $p = 0.04$) and degree of change (−5.58 versus −3.04, $p = 0.05$) in depression scores (HAM-D, Quick Inventory of Depressive Symptomatology-Self Report [QIDS-SR], and Clinical Global Impressions Scale [CGI]). Patients in both trials receiving adjuvant 15 mg/day L-methylfolate also reported fewer side effects than other combination groups.[34] Unlike traditional antidepressants, it does not appear to be associated with any weight gain, sexual dysfunction, sleep disturbances, or suicidal ideation.[35–37] Therefore, 15 mg/day of L-methylfolate augmentation with SSRI use is an effective and safe treatment strategy for treating partially or fully resistant MDD patients. In 2014, the group repeated a similar, double-blinded RCT on 75 outpatient adults with SSRI-resistant MDD (DSM-IV criteria), stratified via specific biomarker levels and genotype.[34] They discovered patients with baseline body mass index ≥30 kg/m^2, elevated plasma C-reactive protein or 4-hydroxy-2-nonenal concentrations, low S-adenosylmethionine/S-adenosylhomocystein ratio and genetic markers had greater pooled mean change from baseline on the Hamilton Depression Rating Scale (HDRS-28) and Clinical Global Impressions Scale (CGI).

Shelton et al. conducted a prospective trial where patients with major depressive disorder on 3 months of L-methylfolate responded via an automated telephone interview.[35] Patients reported a mean reduction of 8.5 points (58.2% decrease) in their nine-item Patient Health Questionnaire (PHQ-9), significant reductions in self-reported impairment in work/home/social life, and a higher medication satisfaction with L-methylfolate than their prior medication.

Folinic acid (leucovorin) was studied in an 8-week prospective study as adjunctive treatment among adults suffering from antidepressant-resistant (4 weeks of fluoxetine or venlafaxine) major depressive disorder (HAM-D-17 ≥12). In this 2002 Alpert et al. open-label study, 22 adults supple-mented their SSRI treatment with doses of Leucovorin at 15 mg for 2 weeks and then 30 mg for 6 weeks.[38] Of the 16 patients who completed the study, 19% had a HAM-D-17 ≤7 and 31% saw a 50% reduction in scores from baseline. Leucovorin is a well-known medication used in cancer patients receiving chemotherapy. This study shows that it can also provide moderate relief for patients with resistant MDD, serving as adjunct therapy with standard SSRI treatment. Folinic acid functions similarly to folic acid; however, it does not require the enzyme dihydrofolate reductase (DHFR) for its conversion, providing the ability to overcome drugs that may interact with this enzyme (e.g., methotrexate).

SAMe is a naturally occurring intermediary compound in all living cells, and reduced levels can lead to a decrease in crucial neurotransmitters.[39] Dubbed the "Sammy" Solution by *Newsweek* in 1999, this supplement has shown great promise in elevating mood and emotional well-being. It has been studied since its discovery in 1952 Italy by G. L. Cantoni and subsequently prescribed in Europe for the last 30 years. Within the United States, SAMe is sold as a dietary supplement under the Dietary Supplemental Health and Education Act (DSHEA) of 1994. It is available for purchase from local health and nutrition stores as an oral supplement under a variety of brand names and dosages. In efforts to compound and review relevant evidence regarding the role of SAMe in the treatment of depression, Mischoulon et al. in 2002 conducted a large meta-analysis.[40] In six of the eight placebo-controlled trials, SAMe was shown to be superior to placebo. In the other two studies its effects were equivalent to those of placebo. In another six comparison studies, SAMe showed equal efficacy to tricyclic antidepressants (TCAs) and greater effect than imipramine in one study. When SAMe was used in combination with TCAs, two studies reported an earlier onset of action than monotherapy alone. SAMe is generally well tolerated but should not be used in patients with bipolar disorder, as early studies show that some patients develop mania with SAMe supplementation.

VITAMIN B12

Vitamin B12 has long been known as the "tonic" or "feel good" vitamin. The water-soluble essential vitamin, also called cobalamin, contains the metal cobalt surrounded by a porphyrin-like ring.[41] The nutrient is important for the formation of red blood cells, development of the central nervous system, and DNA.[42] A decline of vitamin B12, even in a mild form, has been associated with an array of neurological and psychiatric disorders, including neuropathy, dementia, psychosis, fatigue, and cognitive impairment.[43] Recent studies further corroborate these findings, and suggest vitamin B12 deficiency as an important reversible comorbidity present in patients plagued with such conditions. A 1-year retrospective study in India (2015) of 259 patients with vitamin B12 deficiency found 21 patients with posterior dementia, 20 with frontotemporal dementia, 7 with schizophrenia, 12 with alcohol-dependent syndromes (ADS) and Parkinson's disease, 3 with bipolar affective disorder, 1 with Creutzfeldt-Jakob disease, and 8 with hypothyroidism.[44]

Defining a particular value for a deficiency can be problematic, as the true prevalence may be miscalculated because it is based on general population statistics. Nonetheless, according to two 2004 studies, 40% of Americans have low levels of vitamin B12, and 20% of elderly people have severe vitamin B12 deficiencies because of a decreased ability to absorb the vitamin.[45,46] In addition to the elderly, vegetarians are also at high risk for developing vitamin B12 deficiencies because natural sources of the vitamin come only from animal products such as eggs, meat, and dairy. Herrman et al. confirmed in his 2003 study that vegans and vegetarians had significantly lower vitamin B12 status than omnivores.[47]

The exact mechanism by which vitamin B12 affects mood and causes symptoms of depression has yet to be identified, although multiple theories have been explored in recent years. Vitamin B12 deficiency can lead to changes in one-carbon metabolism, causing increased levels of homocysteine.[48] These metabolites have toxic effects on neural development and are associated with increased levels of cortisol. Altering one-carbon metabolism also affects methylation. In fact, vitamin B12 is a methyl donor in many methylation reactions of the brain. According to the hypomethylation hypothesis, reducing methylation decreases synthesis of monoamine neurotransmitters, ultimately resulting in depression.[42] Low levels of vitamin B12 also cause degeneration and demyelination of nerves.[49] This may lead to abnormal chemical reactions in nerve cell junctions thought to cause depression, particularly in the brain cells of the median forebrain. Last, vitamin B12 is also a coenzyme in the formation of folate.[41] Thus, a vitamin B12 deficiency can produce a secondary deficiency of functional folate, a vitamin involved in the process and rate of synthesis of monoamine neurotransmitters involved in depression, such as dopamine, norepinephrine, and serotonin.

Vitamin B12 has been used as an augmentation therapy in patients who are resistant to antidepressant treatment. Kate et al. report two cases of depressed male patients who had not responded to three trials of antidepressants.[50] Both patients were found to have low vitamin B12 levels and, not surprisingly, were also found to be vegetarians. In case one, a 43-year-old man with a history of insomnia followed by the development of major depression had been unsuccessfully treated over the years with various combinations of imipramine, fluoxetine, clomipramine, mirtazapine, escitalopram, and milnacipran. The patient was ultimately given 1000 mg/day of vitamin B12 in addition to his antidepressant medication, and his symptoms improved within 3 weeks. A follow-up study 1.5 years later confirmed that daily doses of vitamin B12 led to lasting improvement of his depressive symptoms. In the second case, a 29-year-old man presented anxious-avoidant behavior and MDD for 5 years. He was treated with escitalopram, venlafaxine, and imipramine with no improvement. After his vitamin B12 deficiency was discovered, he was treated with 1000 mg/day of vitamin B12 in addition to his antidepressant medication. Improvement in his depression was seen within 4 weeks.

In addition to case reports, clinical studies also demonstrate strong correlations between vitamin B12 deficiencies and depression. A cross-sectional comparative study by Güzelcan and Van Loon indicated that patients with a vitamin B12 deficiency scored higher on the Beck Depression Inventory.[51] Levitt and Joffe found vitamin B12 levels inversely correlated with depression scores in 96 depressed patients taking no medication.[52] Mischoulon et al. showed that fluoxetine treatment for depression was less effective in patients with a low plasma level of vitamin B12.[53] Similarly, Hintikka et al. found that patients with high levels of vitamin B12 responded better to treatment for their depression than those with low levels.[54] Ellis and Nasser studied 28 patients complaining of fatigue who had normal levels of vitamin B12.[43] After 2 weeks of intramuscular injections of 5 mg of vitamin B12, patients improved in terms of general well-being, level of happiness, appetite, and level of fatigue.

VITAMIN B1

In 1936, the synthesis of thiamine (vitamin B1) by Williams et al. ushered an end to the horrific disease beriberi.[55] The disease was especially prevalent in countries where the population relied heavily on rice intake. Initial reports suggesting that the disease was caused by a dietary deficiency were made by Kanehiro Takaki, a surgeon general in the Japanese navy in 1884. He noted that when supplementing the diet of sailors with other food groups such as dairy, meats, and vegetables, there was a stark reduction in the occurrence of the disease. It was not until 1897 that the specific connection between beriberi and polished rice was established by Christiaan Eijkman.[56] He was able to successfully reverse beriberi-like symptoms in poultry fed with polished rice by including rice polishings in their diet. However, he failed to identify the key ingredient and incorrectly believed polished rice to contain a toxin that could be counteracted by rice polishings. Then, in 1901, Gerrit Grijns, a Dutch physician, correctly hypothesized that polished rice caused the disease because it lacked a key nutrient that remained within rice polishings.[57] Many years later, in 1926, Jansen and Donath were able to isolate the crystalized form of thiamine from rice polishings,[58] setting the stage for Robert Runnels Williams's discovery of the chemical structure of thiamine in 1934, and its subsequent synthesis.[55]

Thiamine deficiency is rare in developed nations today, as foods such as refined sugars and flour are fortified with thiamine after processing. It is, however, more prevalent in certain subsets of the population lacking a proper diet, such as alcoholics. Deficiency initially presents with nonspecific symptoms of lack of appetite, muscle weakness, headaches, irritability, and depressed mood.[59] More severe deficiency can lead to beriberi, which is further categorized into two distinct subtypes: wet and dry. Dry beriberi presents mainly with symptoms of polyneuritis characterized by distal extremity motor paralysis, decreased reflexes and/or numbness, and tingling. Wet beriberi also manifests muscular atrophy and cardiovascular symptoms of congestive heart failure, such as lower extremity edema, ascites, tachycardia, and elevated blood pressure along with neuropathy. Alcoholics can present with a more serious form of thiamine deficiency termed Wernicke-Korsakoff syndrome, which appears as confusion, ataxia, nystagmus, dementia, and psychosis.[3]

Data confirm a relationship between thiamine deficiency and mood alterations. In 1957, Joseph Brozek removed thiamine from the diet of men for 15–27 days and noticed initial symptoms of anorexia, vomiting, muscle weakness, and depression.[59] Utilizing the Minnesota Multiphasic Personality Inventory (MMPI), he demonstrated that respondents showed marked deterioration in the "psychoneurotic triad" of hypochondriasis, depression, and hysteria. When oral administration of thiamine was restarted, the men recovered completely, starting with improved appetite and mood. In addition, several subsequent double-blind placebo controlled randomized trials have further established the association between thiamine and depression. In a study by Benton et al., 129 adults were provided either a multivitamin that included thiamine or a placebo for 1 year.[60] After the first 3 months women showed improved mood with elevated thiamine levels compared to depressed mood with low thiamine levels. Moreover, 80 Irish women with marginal thiamine deficiency were randomized to receive either 10 mg thiamine supplementation or a placebo.[61] Those who received thiamine therapy experienced a significantly increased appetite, deceased fatigue, and improved sleep pattern along with better generalized well-being. In a 2013 Chinese study focusing on 1587 elderly adults with depressive symptoms (Center for Epidemiological Studies Depressive Scale ≥16) were more prevalent (11.3%) in patients with poor thiamine nutritional levels.[62] Last, in another study by Benton et al., targeted therapy with 50 mg of thiamine was employed to improve functional levels in relation to mood, memory, and reaction times after randomization of 120 young women with normal thiamine levels.[63] Women in the treatment group reported thinking more clearly and feeling more energized than the patients on placebo. Although there was no significant association with memory, reaction times were improved in the thiamine group.

Data have established a possible physiologic association between thiamine supplementation and elevated mood. Improvements in depressive symptoms are correlated with increased levels of thiamine in patients with both low and normal baseline thiamine levels.

VITAMIN B6

Vitamin B6 is composed of pyridoxal, pyridoxamine, and pyridoxine, with pyridoxal 5-phosphate (PLP) the predominant active form found in tissues.[64] PLP serves as a cofactor in over 100 metabolic pathways, including the metabolism of amino acids, glycogen, and sphingoid bases.[64] A deficiency in this vitamin can lead to a variety of disorders, such as seborrheic dermatitis, microcytic anemia, and epileptiform convulsions.[64] A deficiency in vitamin B6 may also be involved in the onset and progression of depression.[65] Moreover, the vitamin has been suggested as a safe treatment for depressive symptoms and as an adjunct therapy to antidepressant medications.[66,67] Although the exact mechanism by which vitamin B6 affects depression is not known, promising pathways have been suggested.

The active form of vitamin B6, PLP, is also a cofactor in the synthesis of monoamine neurotransmitters, including serotonin, dopamine, and γ-aminobutyrate.[64,65] Specifically, decarboxylase, a key enzyme involved in the synthesis of serotonin and other neurotransmitters, depends on PLP to function.[68] The serotonin deficiency hypothesis proposes that depression is caused by a deficiency of serotonin in the brain. According to this theory, depression may be associated with a decrease in the transportation of L-tryptophan, a precursor to serotonin, across the blood-brain barrier.[69] Dopamine deficiency has also been implicated in the onset of depression.[70] For this reason, vitamin

B6 has been suggested as an adjunct therapy to help enhance a positive response to standard antidepressant treatments.

Vitamin B6 is an essential cofactor in the metabolism of homocysteine. According to the vascular hypothesis of depression, a deficiency in vitamin B6 leads to an increase in the concentration of homocysteine in plasma. High homocysteine levels are associated with cerebrovascular disease, a significant risk factor for depression.[66,71] As folate and vitamin B12 are also involved in the metabolism of homocysteine, these members of the vitamin B complex may affect depression synergetically.

Several clinical trials indicate a significant connection between vitamin B6 deficiency and depression. Ford et al. performed a controlled trial on 299 elderly men without depression.[71] The men were randomly assigned to either placebo or treatment of 400 μg vitamin B12 + 2 mg folic acid + 25 mg vitamin B6 per day. The results of the study were not statistically significant; however, those treated with vitamins were 24% more likely not to develop depression during the experiment. Almeida et al. conducted a randomized, double-blind, placebo-controlled study on 273 stroke patients.[66] Vitamin B6, vitamin B12, and folate were given to the patients for 1–10.5 years and were ultimately associated with a decreased risk of major depression in the treatment group as compared to the placebo group.

Two large studies focus on vitamin B6 supplementation and depression. A cross-sectional study by Merete et al. analyzed 618 elderly Caribbean Hispanics and a comparison group of 251 elderly non-Hispanic whites.[72] Using the Center for Epidemiologic Studies Depression Scale and a semi-quantitative food frequency questionnaire, Merete and colleagues found depression twice as prevalent in the Hispanic group. In addition, non-Hispanic whites were more likely to be taking vitamin supplements, with an overall higher intake of vitamin B6 as compared to the Hispanic population. According to the study, a lower vitamin B6 intake was significantly correlated with higher depression scores. Skarupski et al. studied a population of 3503 elderly people also using the Center for Epidemiologic Studies Depression Scale and a semi-quantitative food frequency questionnaire.[65] Similarly, they found that higher intake of vitamin B6 and vitamin B12 correlated with a decreased likelihood of developing depression throughout a 12-year period. Together, these studies suggest that vitamin B6 may have protective properties against depression, particularly for the elderly population.

Hvas et al. analyzed 140 individuals with the Major Depression Inventory.[70] Eighteen subjects were found to be depressed, and a low plasma level of PLP was significantly associated with symptoms of depression. Stewart et al. found the same correlation between low levels of vitamin deficiency and depression in 101 depressed outpatients.[73]

Clinical studies have also highlighted vitamin B6 as a potential treatment for the symptoms of depression. Weizman et al. found that treatments of 150 mg/day of Vitamin B6 for 1 month decreased patients' symptoms of depression as shown on the Hamilton Depression Rating Scale.[74] Wyatt et al. summarized studies using vitamin B6 as a treatment for premenstrual syndrome. They found vitamin B6 beneficial for treating the mood symptoms of premenstrual syndrome.[67]

Vitamin B6 should be considered as a treatment or adjunct therapy for those suffering from depression, especially the elderly and patients not responding to traditional medications. The recommended daily allowance is 1.3 mg/day for adults.[65] The Food and Nutrition Board recommends an upper limit of 100 mg/day, as a higher intake of vitamin B6 may lead to sensory neuropathy.

INOSITOL

Inositol, a naturally occurring isomer of glucose, is a nutritional supplement that has been suggested as a treatment for a multitude of disorders. The nutrient is sometimes considered part of the vitamin B complex and can be found in a variety of foods such as whole-grain cereals, fruits, plants, and meats.[75] Inositol is not a prescription medication but is widely available as a supplement with a typical daily intake of 1 gram per day.[75] Oral intake of inositol directly increases inositol levels in the central nervous system, affecting brain neurochemistry.[75]

The mechanism by which inositol affects the brain and symptoms of depression is not fully understood; however, recent interest in the nutrient has illuminated general ideas of its role in the body. Inositol is a precursor to the formation of phosphatidylinositol (PI), a family of lipids required for creating the cytosolic component of the eukaryotic cell membrane. The inositol cycle requires cleavage of these phosphatidyl bonds to further create inositol triphosphate (IP$_3$) and diacylglycerol (DAG), which subsequently stimulate Ca$^+$ release and activate protein kinase C, respectively.[76] These second messengers allow for cell surface receptors of neurotransmitters to affect cellular processes.[75] Specifically, the phosphatidylinositol cycle is hypothesized to be involved in glutamate, muscarinic cholinergic, alpha 1 noradrenergic receptors, dopaminergic D$_1$ receptors, 5-HT$_{2A}$ and 5-HT$_{2C}$.[77] Therefore, researchers have suggested that inositol may be used for a spectrum of disorders typically treated with SSRIs, including depression, panic disorder, obsessive compulsive disorder, binge eating disorder, and bulimia.[78]

Many clinical studies have indicated that levels of inositol are lower in the CSF and brains of depressed patients. In 1978, Barkai et al. reported that unipolar and bipolar depressed patients had significantly reduced levels of inositol in their CSF compared to control subjects.[79] In 1997, findings by Shimon et al. supported these results. These researchers found reduced inositol levels in postmortem brains of patients with bipolar disorder and suicide victims as compared to normal controls.[80] Similarly, in 2005, Coupland et al. found that 13 patients with moderate to severe major depressive disorder had a significantly lower ratio of inositol to creatine in the prefrontal and anterior cingulate cortex areas of the brain.[81]

Clinical studies have found inositol beneficial in the treatment of depression. Levine et al. performed two pilot studies in 1993. The first demonstrated that six grams of inositol administered for 6 weeks improved the depressive symptoms of nine of eleven patients.[82] Furthermore, the only side effect reported was occasional mild flatulence. The second study concluded that oral inositol treatment increased CSF levels of inositol by almost 70%.[83] Two years later, Levine et al. further supported their results in a double-blind controlled study among 27 patients taking 12 g of inositol or placebo for 4 weeks.[84] Patients on inositol had an overall greater improvement of depressive symptoms. Evins et al. studied 17 patients with bipolar depression taking either inositol or placebo in addition to lithium or valproate for 6 weeks in a randomized double-blind experiment.[77] Although inositol was not more effective as an augmentation therapy than placebo on average, more patients on inositol experienced improvement in depressive symptoms as an overall trend. Chengappa et al. performed a pilot study investigating inositol as an augmentation therapy for bipolar depression.[85] Twenty-four bipolar patients were given either 12 g of inositol or a placebo for 6 weeks in addition to their antidepressants. Of the 22 subjects who completed the study, 50% of patients treated with inositol responded with a significant decrease in depressive symptoms, whereas only 30% of patients taking a placebo showed these results.

In identifying the safety profile for therapeutic inositol, Belmaker et al. reviewed seven previous studies (excluding ones with co-administration of other agents) that utilized a dose of 12 g per day of inositol for their research.[86] Of the 107 patients included, two patients showed mildly elevated glucose. Other side effects reported were two patients with flatulence, one with nausea, and two with insomnia. Two subsequent studies reported that patients on higher doses of inositol at 18 g per day exhibited mild side effects of nausea (24%), flatulence (15%), dizziness (9%), and sleepiness and headache (6%).[78,87] Of the two double-blind, controlled, crossover studies, one was conducted for 6 weeks on patients with bulimia nervosa and the other a 2-month study comparing inositol versus fluvoxamine in panic disorder patients. Patients on fluvoxamine reported more nausea and tiredness. The experimental doses for therapeutic inositol are significantly higher than the inositol acquired from dietary intake and have not shown any serious side effects. However, long-term effects are still unknown. More studies are needed, including young children and pregnant or nursing women as participants.

Inositol is a natural substance that is generally well tolerated.[85] Preliminary studies over the years have shown great promise for utilizing inositol as a viable alternative in patients struggling with a spectrum of disorders commonly responsive to selective serotonin reuptake inhibitors such as depression, panic disorder, obsessive-compulsive disorder (OCD), and bulimia. However it provides no benefit in patients suffering from schizophrenia, Alzheimer's dementia, attention deficit-hyperactivity disorder (ADHD), autism, and electroconvulsive therapy (ECT)-induced memory impairment.[88] Additionally, although inositol has shown equal efficacy to fluvoxamine, current research has demonstrated enhanced efficacy when used in combination or as adjunct to SSRIs. In conclusion, more studies need to be performed to fully understand the therapeutic potential and long-term safety of this nutrient.

VITAMIN D

Vitamin D is categorized as a hormone because of its paracrine, autocrine, and endocrine functions,[89] and it can be acquired through food or exposure to the sun.[90] Vitamin D2, or ergocalciferol, is only made by plants. Vitamin D3, or cholecalciferol, is created when ultraviolet light reaching the skin photochemically converts cholesterol to Vitamin D.[90] Serum 25-hydroxyvitamin D [25(OH)D] is a biological marker used to reliably measure the levels of both forms of vitamin D.[91,92] Among its many functions, vitamin D is important for facilitating calcium absorption; maintaining calcium homeostasis in tissues; influencing growth of bones and teeth; maintaining properly functioning neurons and glial cells; preventing rickets and osteomalacia; influencing tissues and organs; preventing psoriasis, muscle pain, weakness, elevated blood pressure, some forms of cancer, and autoimmune disease; and preserving mental health.[90,93] Vitamin D can be found in high amounts in fatty fish and also in milk, yogurt, orange juice, cereals, and dietary supplements.[93] A sufficient amount of vitamin D can also be produced from 5–15 minutes of daily exposure to sunlight.

Vitamin D receptors exist in neurons and glial cells in the brain, allowing vitamin D to affect neurochemistry.[91,93] Specifically, research suggests vitamin D may act on particular regions of the brain important in the development of depression, including the prefrontal cortex, hippocampus, cingulate gyrus, thalamus, hypothalamus, and substantia nigra.[89,93] Moreover, it has also been discovered that genetic variations of vitamin D receptors are associated with depression.[94] Research has shown that vitamin D controls the transcription of over 1000 genes involved in neurotrophic and neuroprotective effects, including the maintenance and development of neurons.[94] In addition, vitamin D may stimulate the release of neurotrophins.[89] Although the exact mechanism by which vitamin D affects mood is yet to be made entirely clear, clinical studies provide strong evidence of a direct connection.

In a recent study, Polak et al. investigated the association between vitamin D levels and depressive symptoms in 615 young adults.[91] Subjects in the lowest quartile of vitamin D levels were more likely to report having symptoms of depression than those in the highest quartile, suggesting that vitamin D deficiency is a potential predictor of depression. Similarly, in a study on previously deployed military personnel who committed suicide, Umhau et al. found that subjects in the lowest octile of vitamin D levels had the highest risk of suicide.[94] Milaneschi et al. found a comparable effect in the elderly population, with low levels of vitamin D correlating with a significantly higher risk of developing depression.[95] In a unique study on adolescence, Tolppanen et al. measured vitamin D levels and depressive symptoms in the same group of children at 9.8, 10.6, and 13.8 years old.[92] Interestingly, higher levels of vitamin D at age 9.8 predicted lower levels of depression at age 13.8, suggesting an association between low levels of vitamin D and early onset depression. Bertone-Johnson et al. performed a cross-sectional study on 81,189 older women and found an inverse association between vitamin D levels and depressive symptoms in the postmenopausal women.[96] In another study, Lee et al. found that lower vitamin D levels were associated with depression in a population of 3369 European men.[97] A study by Black et al. found similar results in a population of young adult males.[98]

In one study by Han et al., patients who suffered acute ischemic strokes were tested for depression.[99] The results showed that patients who had developed depression after their stroke had significantly lower levels of vitamin D than those patients who did not develop depression. Yue et al.

attained similar results in their study analyzing the association between vitamin D and symptoms of depression 6 months after an acute ischemic stroke.[89] Again, low levels of vitamin D were independently associated with post-stroke depression.

Vitamin D supplements have also been found to enhance positive mood. In a study by Lansdowne et al., healthy subjects were given 800 IU, 400 IU, or no vitamin D during 5 days of winter.[100] Study results showed that vitamin D was able to significantly enhance positive affect and also reduce negative affect. Possibly the most important of all of these studies is a recent meta-analysis of randomized control trials using vitamin D to treat depression.[101] In this analysis, all experiments with methodological flaws were excluded, including interventions that did not include vitamin D levels in the intervention group, did not measure baseline vitamin D levels, or included subjects without baseline deficiencies in vitamin D. Using these guidelines, seven of eight randomized control trials found that vitamin D significantly improved symptoms of depression, which is a comparable effect size to that of antidepressant medications. These diverse studies suggest a connection between vitamin D deficiency and depression across all age groups and both genders.

VITAMIN C

Vitamin C (ascorbic acid) cannot be synthesized by the human body. Therefore, the diet alone must provide this vital nutrient. Ample amounts are found in fruits and vegetables, and the vitamin is absorbed through the small intestines.[102] Once absorbed, it is an indispensable cofactor for hydroxylation of proline and lysine, which are essential building blocks of collagen formation. Human stores of vitamin C can supply need in times of deficiency for up to 29–90 days before symptoms occur.[103] Levels that reach a critical low may lead to clinical manifestations of scurvy.

Scurvy is not a modern disease. Writing on papyrus, Ebers in 1500 BC Egypt not only diagnosed the disease, but also treated it with onions, which are rich in vitamin C.[104] Hippocrates, credited as the father of medicine, continued to build upon the Egyptian writings in further describing the many symptoms of scurvy. When sea exploration became commonplace during the sixteenth–eighteenth centuries, scurvy was common among sailors away on long voyages without proper nutrition. The psychological effects of scurvy were chronicled by Richard Walter, a chaplain on a voyage across the Pacific. He recounted that the afflicted men lost the inhibition that deters excessive feeling, reporting that they experienced events "with emotions of the most voluptuous luxury."[105] The men would all fall into a state of deep despair and yearn to return home. He also noted the men's emotional unpredictability, describing them as easily startled or breaking down and crying at the slightest displeasure.

In the twenty-first century scurvy is almost extinct. It is extremely rare in developed nations where adequate health education and proper nutrition are readily available.[103] The small incidence of cases in these countries have occurred largely in people with psychiatric conditions, alcoholism,[106] or the elderly.[103] Depression, which often develops in cancer patients receiving chemotherapy, can potentially lead to scurvy due to poor nutrition.[107] In particular, smokers and individuals with low economic status exhibit significantly lower mean serum concentrations of vitamin C than their counterparts, putting them at greater risk for developing symptomatic disease.[107] Underdeveloped nations have higher incidence rates of scurvy throughout their populations, primarily due to malnourishment.

Scurvy is often ignored in a differential diagnosis due to the nature of its broad symptoms, which are often easily explained by more common causes. It causes gingivitis, loose teeth, dystrophic hair, and bleeding abnormalities such as petechial hemorrhages and large bleeding into the skin, muscles, joints, or deep organs.[103,107] Chronic abnormalities such as anemia and ischemic heart disease are also prominent features of the disease.[103] Perhaps most difficult to identify are the subtle changes in mood and affect seen in severe cases,[107] which can quickly turn to severe depression without prompt treatment.[108] Healthy young men who were subjected to a vitamin C depletion protocol frequently reported initial symptoms of fatigue and irritability in the absence of other symptoms.[107]

In a 2003–2004 National Health and Nutrition Examination Survey (NHANES), 16% of adults reported low energy levels and weakness with low vitamin C intake.[107] In a 1969 study by Hodges et al., a group of participants was given a diet lacking vitamin C.[109] The investigators noted that participants exhibited increased general malaise and fatigue as the disease progressed. Symptoms of depression and suicidal ideations developed only 30 days after the start of the diet, well before many of the physiologic symptoms were apparent. One hypothesis proposed to explain these symptoms is that ascorbic acid is necessary for proper functioning of the dopamine beta-hydroxylase enzyme, which catalyzes dopamine into norepinephrine.[108] The hormone is responsible for behavioral stimulation and excitement; therefore, decreased levels can lead to depression.

Zhang et al. conducted a 6-week double-blind RCT studying 15 hospitalized patients with vitamin C deficiency for response to supplemental vitamin C (500 mg daily).[110] Vitamin C therapy increased plasma and mononuclear leukocyte vitamin C concentrations. This was associated with a subsequent 34% decrease in mood disturbance.

CONCLUSION

Patients with depression are often unable to provide adequate self-care. One of the major concerns is their adoption of poor eating patterns and subsequent vitamin deficiencies. Therefore, inquiry into a patient's nutritional status is of paramount interest for clinicians. Nutritional counseling offers the psychiatrist a window into identifying potential modifiable risk factors with minimal risk for side effects. Those with greater risk for vitamin deficiencies are patients with comorbid conditions such as alcoholism, low socioeconomic status, or restrictive dietary patterns such as vegans and elderly patients. Information about dietary patterns can be established by asking patients about daily food intake regarding timing of meals, restrictions, favorite snacks, and habits. This initial assessment must also include examination of blood nutritional levels, especially folate, vitamin B12, and vitamin D. Investigation of nutritional deficiencies is also warranted in patients with current or history of treatment resistance.

Moreover, psychiatrists are encouraged to review evidence-based scientific literature regarding nutritional deficiencies and effects of potential supplementation. Adjunct nutritional supplementation must occur after careful consultation with the patient's primary care provider. Even rudimentary educational consultation regarding well-balanced, nutrition-dense meals including healthy grains, leafy greens, beans, and fruits and vegetables can provide profound benefit. Clinical nutritionist consultations are of further benefit for more complex patients requiring greater investigation and management.

Nutritional deficiencies can affect mental health, and vitamin deficiencies have been associated with a wide range of mood-related symptoms. Vitamins have the ability to alter molecular and cellular processes, which are integral for proper cognitive functioning. These nutrients serve as key cofactors in integral chemical reactions that are required for the formation of neurotransmitters and DNA synthesis. Small subsets of the population, with certain genetic polymorphisms, are at greater risk for deficiencies such as folate and vitamin B12. Significant research over the past few decades has demonstrated that vitamin deficiencies may not only lead to greater incidence of psychiatric disorders but also prolong their duration and perpetuate treatment resistance to standard therapy. With this knowledge, researchers have shown positive results in dietary augmentation and nutritional supplementation as ways of improving care for patients with mental health disorders. This provides an opportunity for clinicians to positively alter brain chemistry, with safe, cost-effective, and readily available interventions.

Industrialized societies have the highest rates of obesity due to their high caloric intake, which is often not well-balanced to provide nutrient-dense foods with adequate vitamins. The fact that dietary factors can have such a critical impact on brain health compels us to better understand them as a strategy for improving public health. However, practical aspects such as dietary design, frequency, and amount of nutrients required remain to be fully answered. Research is still needed to answer these questions, but current evidence supports the historical literature that vitamin deficiencies contribute to the onset of depression and likely prevent full remission and recovery.

ACKNOWLEDGMENTS

The authors of this chapter would like to thank Valentina Park, B.S., for her research and editorial support in the production of this chapter.

REFERENCES

1. Satyanarayana, Rao T.S., Asha, M.R., Ramesh, B.N. et al. 2008. Understanding nutrition, depression and mental illnesses. *Ind J Psychiatry* 50(2): 77–82.
2. Sanchez-Villegas, A., Toledo, E., de Irala, J. et al. 2011. Fast-food and commercial baked goods consumption and the risk of depression. *Public Health Nutr* 15(3): 424–432.
3. Berdanier, C.D. 1998. *Advanced Nutrition Micronutrients.* Boca Raton, FL: CRC Press/Taylor & Francis.
4. Mischoulon, D. and Franz, R.M. 2007. The role of folate in depression and dementia. *J Clin Psychiatry* 68(10): 28–33.
5. Smith, D.A., Kim, Y-I., and Refsum, H. 2008. Is folic acid good for everyone? *Am J Clin Nutr* 87(3): 517–533.
6. Institute of Medicine. Food and Nutrition Board. 1998. *Dietary Reference Intakes: Thiamin, Riboflavin, Niacin, Vitamin B6, Folate, Vitamin B12, Pantothenic Acid, Biotin, and Choline.* Washington, DC: National Academy Press.
7. Coppen, A. and Bolander-Gouaille, C. 2005. Treatment of depression: Time to consider folic acid and vitamin B12. *J Psychopharmacol* 19(1): 59–65.
8. Gilbody, S., Lewis, S., and Lightfoot, T. 2007. Methylenetetrahydrofolate reductase (MTHFR) genetic polymorphisms and psychiatric disorders: A HuGE review. *Am J Epidemiol* 165(1): 1–13.
9. Herbert, V. 1962. Experimental nutritional folate deficiency in man. *Trans Assoc Am Phys* 75: 307–320.
10. Reynolds, E.H., Preece, J.M., Bailey, J. et al. 1970. Folate deficiency in depressive Illness. *Br J Psychiatry* 117(538): 287–292.
11. Shorvon, S.D., Carney, M.W., Chanarin, I. et al. 1980. The neuropsychiatry of megaloblastic anaemia. *Br Med J* 281(6247): 1036–1038.
12. Ghadirian, M.A., Ananth, J., and Engelsmann F. 1980. Folic acid deficiency and depression. *Psychosomatics* 21(11): 926–928.
13. Carney, M.W., Chary, T.K., Laundy, M. et al. 1990. Red cell folate concentrations in psychiatric patients. *J Affect Disord* 9(3): 207–213.
14. Tolmunen, T., Voutilainen, S., Hintikka, J. et al. 2003. Dietary folate and depression symptoms are associated in middle-aged Finnish men. *Am Soc Nutr Sci* 133(10): 3323–3236.
15. Bottiglieri, T. 2005. Homocystein and folate metabolism in depression. *Neuro-Psychopharmacol Biol Psychiatry* 29(7): 1103–1112.
16. Almeida, O.P., McCaul, K., Hankey, G.J. et al. 2008. Homocysteine and depression in later life. *Arch Gen Psychiatry* 65(11): 1286–1294.
17. Forti, P., Rietti, E., Pisacane, N. et al. 2009. Blood homocystein and risk of depression in the elderly. *Arch Gerontol Geriatr* 51(1): 21–25.
18. Ford, A.H., Flicker, L., Singh, U. et al. 2013. Homocystein, depression and cognitive function in older adults. *J Affect Disord* 151(2): 646–651.
19. Nabi, H., Bochud, M., Glaus, J. et al. 2013. Association of serum homocystein with major depressive disorder: Results from a large population-based study. *Psychoneuroendocrinology* 38(10): 2309–2318.
20. Guttormsen, A.B., Ueland, P.M., Nesthus, I. et al. 1996. Determinants and vitamin responsiveness of intermediate hyperhomocysteinemia (≥40 micromol/liter). The Hordaland homocysteine study. *J Clin Invest* 98(9): 2174–2183.
21. Zittan, E., Preis, M., Asmir, I. et al. 2007. High frequency of vitamin B12 deficiency in asymptomatic individuals homozygous to MTHFR C677T mutation is associated with endothelial dysfunction and homocysteinemia. *Am J Physiol Heart Circ Physiol* 293(1): H860–H865.
22. Refsum, H., Nurk, E., Smith, D.A. et al. 2006. The Hordaland homocysteine study: A community-based study of homocysteine, its determinants, and association with disease. *Am Soc Nutr* 136(6): 17315–17404.

23. Fava, M., Borus, J.S., Alpert, J.E. et al. 1997. Folate, vitamin B12, and homocystein in major depressive disorder. *Am J Psychiatry* 154(3): 426–428.

24. Papakostas, G.I., Petersen, T., Mischoulon, D. et al. 2004. Serum folate, vitamin B12, and homocystein in major depressive disorder, Part 1: Predictors of clinical response in fluoxetine-resistant depression. *J Clin Psychiatry* 65(8): 1090–1095.

25. Papakostas, G.I., Petersen, T., Lebowitz, B.D. et al. 2005. The relationship between serum folate, vitamin B12, and homocystein levels in major depressive disorder and the timing of improvement with fluoxetine. *Int J Neuropsychopharmacol* 8(4): 523–528.

26. Papakostas, G.I., Petersen, T., Mischoulon, D. et al. 2004. Serum folate, vitamin B12, and homocystein in major depressive disorder, Part 2: Predictors of relapse during the continuation phase of pharmacotherapy. *J Clin Psychiatry* 65(8): 1096–1098.

27. Coppen, A. and Bailey, J. 2000. Enhancement of the antidepressant action of fluoxetine by folic acid: A randomized placebo controlled trial. *J Affect Disord* 60(2): 121–130.

28. Guaraldi, G.P., Fava, M., Mazzi, F. et al. 1993. An open trial of methyltetrahydrofolate in elderly depressed patients. *Ann Clin Psychiatry* 5(2): 101–105.

29. Passeri, M., Cucinotta, D., Abate, G. et al. 1993. Oral 5′-methyltetrahydrofolic acid in senile organic mental disorders with depression: Results of a double-blind multicenter study. *Aging (Milan, Italy)* 5(1): 63–71.

30. Godfrey, P.S., Toone, B.K., Carney, M.W. et al. 1990. Enhancement of recovery from psychiatric illness by methylfolate. *The Lancet* 336(8712): 392–395.

31. Wu, D. and Pardridge, W.M. 1999. Blood-brain barrier transport of reduced folic acid. *Pharm Res* 16(3): 415–419.

32. Willems, F.F., Boers, G.H., Blom, H.J. et al. 2004. Pharmacokinetic study on the utilization of 5-methyltetrahydrofolate and folic acid in patients with coronary artery disease. *Br J Pharmacol* 141(5): 825–830.

33. Papakostas, G., Shelton, R., Zajecka, J. et al. 2012. L-Methylfolate as adjunctive therapy for SSRI-resistant major depression: results of two randomized, double-blind, parallel-sequential trials. *Am J Psychiatry* 169(2): 1267–1274.

34. Papakostas, G., Shelton, R., Zajecka, J. et al. 2014. Effect of adjunctive L-methylfolate 15 mg among inadequate responders to SSRIs in depressed patients who were stratified by biomarker levels and genotype: Results from a randomized clinical trial. *J Clin Psychiatry* 75(8): 855–863.

35. Shelton, R.C., Sloan, M., Barrentine, L.W. et al. 2013. Assessing effects of L-methylfolate in depression management: Results of a real world patient experience trial. *Prim Care Companion CNS Disord* 15(4).

36. Scott, J.M. and Weir, D.G. 1981. The methyl folate trap. A physiological response in man to prevent methyl group deficiency in kwashiorkor (methionine deficiency) and an explanation for folic-acid induced exacerbation of subacute combined degeneration in pernicious anaemia. *Lancet* 28242: 337–340.

37. Lamars, Y., Prinz-Langenohl, R., Bramswig, S. et al. 2006. Red blood cell folate concentrations increase more after supplementation with [6S]-5-methyltetrahydrofolate than with folic acid in women of childbearing age. *Am J Clin Nutr* 84(1): 156–161.

38. Alpert, J.E., Mischoulon, D., Rubenstein, G.E. et al. 2002. Folinic acid (Leucovorin) as an adjunctive treatment for SSRI-refractory depression. *Ann Clin Psychiatry* 14(1): 33–38.

39. Spillmann, M. and Fava, M. 1996. S-adenosyl-methionine (ademethionine) in psychiatric disorders. *CNS Drugs* 6: 416–425.

40. Mischoulon, D. and Fava, M. 2002. Role of S-adenosyl-l-methionine in the treatment of depression: A review of the evidence. *Am Soc Clin Nutr* 76(5): 11585–11615.

41. Hutto, B.R. 1997. Folate and cobalamin in psychiatric illness. *Compr Psychiatry* 38(6): 305–314.

42. Milanlıoğlu, A. 2011. Vitamin B12 deficiency and depression. *J Clin Exp Invest* 2(4): 455–456.

43. Ellis, F.R. and Nasser, S. 1973. A pilot study of vitamin B12 in the treatment of tiredness. *Br J Nutr* 30(2): 277–283.

44. Issac, T.G., Soundarya, S., Christopher, R. et al. 2015. Vitamin B12 deficiency: An important reversible co-morbidity in neuropsychiatric manifestations. *Ind J Psychol Med* 37(1): 26–29.

45. Wolters, M., Strohle, A. and Hahn, A., 2004. Cobalamin: A critical vitamin in the elderly. *Prev Med* 39(6): 1256–1266.

46. Andres, E., Noureddine, H., Loukili, E.N. et al. 2004. Vitamin B12 (cobalamin) deficiency in elderly patients. *CMAJ* 171(3): 251–259.

47. Herrman, W., Schorr, H., Obeid, R. et al. 2003. Vitamin B-12 status, particularly holotranscobalamin II and methylmalonic acid concentrations, and hyperhomocysteinemia in vegetarians. *American Journal of Clinical Nutrition* 78(1): 131–136.

48. Kale, A., Naphade, N., Sapkale, S. et al. 2009. Reduced folic acid, vitamin B12 and docosahexaenoic acid and increased homocysteine and cortisol in never-medicated schizophrenia patients: Implications for altered one-carbon metabolism. *Psychiatry Res* 175(1–2): 47–53.

49. Kate, N., Grover, S., Agarwal, M. et al. 2010. Does B12 deficiency lead to lack of treatment response to conventional antidepressants? *Psychiatry* 7(11): 42–44.

50. Dommise, J. 1991. Subtle vitamin-B-12 deficiency and psychiatry: A largely unnoticed but devastating relationship? *Med Hypothesis* 34(2): 131–140.

51. Güzelcan, Y. and Van Loon, P. 2009. Vitamin B12 status in patients of Turkish and Dutch descent with depression: A comparative cross-sectional study. *Ann Gen Psychiatry* 8(1): 18–22.

52. Levitt, A.J. and Joffe, R.T. 1993. Folate, B12 and thyroid function in depression. *Biol Psychiatry* 33(1): 52–53.

53. Mischoulon, D. Burger, J.K., Spillmann, M.K. et al. 2000. Anemia and macrocytosis in the prediction of serum folate and vitamin B12 status, and treatment outcome in major depression. *J Psychosom Res* 49(3): 183–187.

54. Hintikka, J., Tolmunen, T., Tanskanen, A. et al. 2003. High vitamin B12 level and good treatment outcome may be associated in major depressive disorder. *BMC Psychiatry* 3(1): 17–18.

55. Williams, R.R. and Cline, J.K. 1936. Synthesis of vitamin B1. *J Am Chem Soc* 58(8): 1504–1505.

56. Eijkman, C. 1897. Eine beriberiähnliche krankheit der Hühner. *Virchows Archiv Pathol Anatomy* 148(3): 523.

57. Grijns, G. 1901. Over polyneuritis gallinarum. *I. Geneesk. Tijdscht. Ned. Ind* 43: 3–110.

58. Jansen, B.C.P. and Donath, W.F. 1926. On the isolation of antiberiberi vitamin. *Proc. Kon. Ned. Akad. Wet* 29: 1390–1400.

59. Brozek, J. 1957. Psychological effects of thiamine restriction and deprivation in normal young men. *Am J Clin Nutr* 5(2): 109–118.

60. Benton, D., Haller, J., and Fordy, J. 1995. Vitamin supplementation for one year improves mood. *Neuropsychobiology* 32: 98–105.

61. Smidt, L.J., Cremin, F.M., Grivetti, L.E. et al. 1991. Influence of thiamin supplementation on the health and general well-being of an elderly Irish population with marginal thiamin deficiency. *J Gerontol* 46(5): M16–M22.

62. Zhang, G., Ding, H., Chen, H. et al. 2013. Thiamine nutritional status and depressive symptoms are inversely associated among older chinese adults. *J Nutr* 143(1): 53–58.

63. Benton, D., Griffiths, R., and Haller, J. 1997. Thiamine supplementation mood and cognitive functioning. *Psychopharmacology* 129(1): 66–71.

64. Food and Nutrition Board, Institute of Medicine. 1998. *Dietary Reference Intakes for Thiamin, Riboflavin, Niacin, Vitamin B6, Folate, Vitamin B12, Pantothenic Acid, Biotin and Choline.* Washington, DC: National Academy Press, 196–305.

65. Skarupski, K.A., Tangney, C., Li, H. et al., 2010. Longitudinal association of vitamin B-6, folate, and vitamin B-12 with depressive symptoms among older adults over time. *Am J Clin Nutr* 92(2): 330–335.

66. Almeida, O.P., Marsh, K., Alfonso, H. et al. 2010. B-vitamins reduce the long-term risk of depression after stroke: The vitatops-dep trial. *Ann Neurol* 68(4): 503–510.

67. Wyatt, K.M., Dimmock, P.W., Jones, P.W. et al. 1999. Efficacy of vitamin B6 in the treatment of premenstrual syndrome: Systematic review. *BMJ* 3187195: 1375–1381.

68. Bender, D.A. 1998. Non-nutritional uses of vitamin B6. *British Journal of Nutrition* 81(1): 7–20.

69. Williams, A., Cotter, A., Sabina, A. et al., 2005. The role for vitamin B-6 as treatment for depression: A systematic review. *Family Practice* 22(5): 532–537.

70. Hvas, A.M., Juul, S., Bech, P. et al. 2004. Vitamin B6 level is associated with symptoms of depression. *Psychother Psychosom* 73(6): 340–343.

71. Ford, A.H., Flicker, L., Thomas, J. et al. 2008. Vitamins B12, B6, and folic acid for onset of depressive symptoms in older men: Results from a 2-year placebo-controlled randomized trial. *J Clin Psychiatry* 69(8): 1203–1209.

72. Merete, C., Falcon, L.M., and Tucker, K.L. 2008. Vitamin B6 is associated with depressive symptomatology in Massachusetts elders. *J Am College Nutr* 27(3): 421–427.

73. Stewart, J.W., Harrison, W., Quitkin, F. et al. 1984. Low B6 levels in depressed outpatients. *Biol Psychiatry* 19(4): 613–616.

74. Shiloh, R., Weizman, A., Weizer, N. et al. 2001. Antidepressive effect of pyridoxine (vitamin B6) in neuroleptic-treated schizophrenic patients with co-morbid minor depression-preliminary open-label trial. *Harefuah* 140(5): 369–373.

75. Taylor, M.J., Wilder, H., Bhagwagar, Z. et al. 2004. Inositol for depressive disorders. *Coch Database Syst Rev* 2004(1): CD004049.
76. Einat, H., Karbovski, H., Korik, J. et al. 1998. Inositol reduces depressive-like behaviors in two different animal models of depression. *Psychopharmacology* 144(2): 158–162.
77. Evins, A.E., Demopulos C., Yovel, I. et al. 2006. Inositol augmentation of lithium or valproate for bipolar depression. *Bipolar Disord* 8(2): 168–174.
78. Gelber, D., Levine, J., and Belmaker, R.H. 2001. Effect of inositol on bulimia nervosa and binge eating. *Int J Eating Disord* 29(3): 345–348.
79. Barkai I.A., Dunner D.L., Gross H.A., Mayo P. and Fieve R.R. 1978. Reduced myoinositol levels in cerebrospinal fluid from patients with affective disorder. *Biol Psychiatry* 13: 65–72.
80. Shimon, H., Agam, G., Belmaker, R.H. et al. 1997. Reduced frontal cortex inositol levels in postmortem brain of suicide victims and patients with bipolar disorder. *Am J Psychiatry* 154(8): 1148–1150.
81. Coupland, N.J., Ogilvie, C.J., Hegadoren, K.M. et al. 2005. Decreased prefrontal myo-inositol in major depressive disorder. *Biol Psychiatry* 57(12): 1526–1534.
82. Levine, G.J., Barak, Y., Gonzalves, M. et al. 1993. Inositol 6 gm daily may be effective in depression but not in schizophrenia. *Human Psychopharmacol* 8: 49–53.
83. Levine, G.J., Rapaort, A., Lev, L. et al. 1993. Inositol treatment raises CSF inositol levels. *Brain Res* 627(1): 168–169.
84. Levine, G.J., Barak, Y., Gonzalves, M. et al. 1995. Double-blind, controlled trial of inositol treatment of depression. *Am J Psychiatry* 152(5): 792–794.
85. Chengappa, K., Levine, J., Gershon, S. et al. 2002. Inositol as an add-on treatment for bipolar depression. *Bipolar Disord* 2(1): 47–55.
86. Belmaker, R.H., Bersudsky, Y., Benjamin, J. et al. 1995. Manipulation of inositol-linked second messenger systems as therapeutic strategy in psychiatry. *Adv Biochem Psychopharmacol* 49: 67–84.
87. Palatnik, A., Frolov, K., Fux, M. et al. 2001. Double-blind, controlled, crossover trial of inositol versus fluvoxamine for treatment of panic disorder. *J Clin Psychopharmacol* 21(3): 335–339.
88. Levine, G.J. 1997. Controlled trials of inositol in psychiatry. *Eur Neuropsychopharmacol* 7(2): 147–155.
89. Yue, W., Xiang, L., Zhang, Y-J. et al. 2014. Association of serum 25-hydroxyvitamin D with symptoms of depression after 6 months in stroke patients. *Neurochem Res* 39(11): 2218–2224.
90. Holick, M.F. 2009. Shining light on the vitamin D. *Dermato Endocrinol* 1(1): 4–6.
91. Polak, M.A., Houghton, L.A., Reeder, A.I. et al. 2014. Serum 25-hydroxyvitamin D concentrations and depressive symptoms among young adult men and women. *Nutrients* 6(11): 4720–4730.
92. Tolppanen, A-M., Sayers, A., and Fraser, W.D. 2012. The association of serum 25-hydroxyvitamin D3 and D2 with depressive symptoms in childhood—a prospective cohort study. *J Child Psychol Psychiatry* 53(7): 757–766.
93. Bertone-Johnsonnure, E.R. 2009. Vitamin D and the occurrence of depression: Causal association or circumstantial evidence? *Nutrition Rev* 67(8): 481–492.
94. Umhau, J.C., Heilig, M., George, D.T. et al. 2013. Low vitamin D status and suicide: A case-control study of active duty military service members. *Plos One* 8(1): e51543.
95. Milaneschi, Y., Shardell, M., Corsi A.M. et al. 2010. Serum 25-hydroxyvitamin D and depressive symptoms in older women and men. *J Clin Endocrinol Metabol* 95(7): 3225–3233.
96. Bertone-Johnson, E.R., Powers, S.I., Spangler, L. et al. 2011. Vitamin D intake from foods and supplements and depressive symptoms in a diverse population of older women. *Am J Clin Nutr* 94(4): 1104–1112.
97. Lee, D.M., Tajar, A., O'Neill, T.W. et al. 2011. Lower vitamin D levels are associated with depression among community-dwelling European men. *J Psychopharmacol* 25(10): 1320–1328.
98. Black, L.J., Jacoby, P., Allen, K.L. et al. 2014. Low vitamin D levels are associated with symptoms of depression in young adult males. *ANZ J Psychiatry* 48(5): 464–471.
99. Han, B., Lyu, Y., Sun, H. et al. 2014. Low serum levels of vitamin D are associated with post-stroke depression. *Eur J Neurol.* 22(9): 1269–1274.
100. Lansdowne, A.T.G. and Provost, S.C. 1998. Vitamin D3 enhances mood in healthy subjects during winter. *Psychopharmacology* 135(4): 319–323.
101. Spedding, S. 2014. Vitamin D and depression: A systematic review and meta-analysis comparing studies with and without biological flaws. *Nutrients* 6(4): 1501–1518.
102. Parade Publications. What Americans think about aging and health. *Par. Mag.* February 5 2006. 11.
103. Chang, C.W., Chen, M.J., Wang, T.E. et al. 2007. Scurvy in a patient with depression. *Digestive Dis Sci* 52(2): 1259–1261.

104. Mayberry, Jason Allen. 2004. Scurvy and Vitamin C. Food and Drug Law. http://dash.harvard.edu/bitstream/handle/1/8852139/Mayberry.html?sequence = 2 (accessed December 29, 2014).
105. Lamb, J. 2011. Captain Cook and the Scourge of Scurvy. Updated: February 17th, 2011. Available at: http://www.bbc.co.uk/history/british/empire_seapower/captaincook_scurvy_01.shtml.
106. Wang, A.H. and Still, C. 2007. Old world meets modern: A case report of scurvy. *Nutr Clin Pract* 22(4): 445–448.
107. Schleicher, R.L., Carroll, M.D., Ford, E.S. et al. 2009. Serum vitamin C and the prevalence of vitamin C deficiency in the United States: 2003–2004 National Health and Nutrition Examination Survey (NHANES). *Am J Clin Nutr* 90(5): 1252–1263.
108. Dixit, V.M. 1979. Cause of depression in chronic scurvy. *Lancet* 314 (8151): 1077–1078.
109. Hodges, R.E., Baker, E.M., Hood, J. et al. 1969. Experimental scurvy in man. *Am J Clin Nutr* 22(5): 535–548.
110. Zhang, M., Robitaille, L., Eintrach, S. et al. 2011. Vitamin C provision improves mood in acutely hospitalized patients. *Nutrition* 27(5): 530–533.

9 Mineral Deficiencies and Depression
Evidence-Based Research

James M. Greenblatt, MD and Kayla Grossmann, RN

CONTENTS

INTRODUCTION

Minerals are critical for the optimal function of the human body. These nutrients are responsible for many basic roles including fluid balance, enzyme activity, and protein synthesis. Their absence or inadequacy has been found to promote disease states across anatomic systems. A substantial body of research has linked mineral deficiencies to poor brain development, cognitive deficits, and a diversity of psychiatric symptoms. Specifically, it is well-established that several key minerals are necessary to support neurotransmitter systems. This chapter will focus on the influence of individual mineral deficiencies, including those of zinc, magnesium, and lithium, on the pathophysiology of depression. Consequently, trials demonstrating their efficacy as mono- and adjunctive antidepressant therapies will also be presented. From this collection of evidence it is clear that maintaining adequate levels of specific minerals is important for modulating depressive symptoms. Furthermore, the mechanisms through which each mineral act are unique and varied, making targeted assessment and supplementation crucial for successful outcomes.

MICRONUTRIENT DEFICIENCIES

According to the World Health Organization, micronutrient deficiencies affect more than 2 billion people worldwide and lead to severe health complications.[1] Adverse effects have been observed in growth and development, mental and neuromotor performance, immunocompetence, reproductive function, and overall morbidity and mortality.[2] Ongoing research is suggesting that subclinical micronutrient deficiencies may contribute to growing rates of psychiatric diseases, including depression.[3]

Micronutrient deficiencies were previously believed to occur only in areas of the world struggling with food shortages and high rates of hunger. However, in 2006 the United Nations acknowledged a "new type" of malnutrition defined not by food scarcity but instead by food quality and nutrient density.[4] This new paradigm for understanding malnutrition, termed "type B malnutrition," encourages a focus on the existence of micronutrient depletion even in the face of food surplus and the obesity epidemic. According to a recent study, the percentage of the U.S. population with a significantly deficient intake of any one micronutrient (less than 50% of the Recommended Daily Allowance [RDA]) ranges from 2% to greater than 20%, depending on the nutrient investigated.[5] Further evidence suggests that 30% of the population in industrialized nations where processed foods are readily available is plagued with clinically significant deficiencies in micronutrients.[6]

MINERAL DEFICIENCIES

Of the three most prevalent micronutrient groups, vitamins, minerals, and phytochemicals, deficiencies of minerals are of particular concern. Minerals originate below ground and enter the food supply through soil. As the human body cannot create enough of these minerals for effective metabolism, a balanced diet with ample drinking water is critical.[7] Yet, mineral levels are steadily declining in earth soils and consequently from the foods grown within. Unlike vitamins synthesized by plants, minerals must be absorbed from earth soils to be present in dietary foods. A 2004 study sponsored by the American College of Nutrition compared harvested crops today with those from 1950 and found a 40% decline in current crops' nutrition content.[8] An English study found a decrease in the mineral levels in foods ranging from 2% to 84% between the years 1940 and 2002.[9] The researchers cited growing pollution, rampant pesticide use, over-mining, and exploitive agricultural practices as culprits for leaching minerals out of the oceans, soils, and, consequently, our food supply.[7]

In addition, many chemicals and pharmaceuticals share common receptors with minerals within the body. Competitive blocking of binding sites prevents critical nutrients from reaching areas of greatest demand (e.g., the brain).[6] Polypharmacy is particularly problematic for mental health patients, where depending on practice setting, between 13% and 90% of patients take more than two psychotropic medications daily.[10] In the general population, common compounds such as sugar, caffeine, and alcohol foster excessive mineral excretion through the kidneys.[11] Increased demands on metabolic and immune reactions in response to disease processes such as depression further deplete minerals.[12] Common over-the-counter and prescription medications also deplete minerals.[13]

MINERAL INTERACTIONS AND DEPRESSION

Minerals have been found to contribute to major pathways in the pathophysiology of depression. A recent review article published in 2014 provides an excellent summary of the current research on mineral deficiencies and depression.[14] Minerals influence brain morphology, neurochemistry, and bioenergetics through several shared mechanisms.

Brain-derived neurotropic factor (BDNF) is an essential neurotropic factor, found within the human brain and periphery (e.g., human serum and plasma). Acting on neurons within the central and peripheral nervous system, it functions to regulate plasticity of existing neuronal synapses and facilitates maturation and differentiation of new neuronal cells. Minerals are crucial for the production and activation of BDNF and have been found to influence its levels in the body.

BDNF binds two separate receptors, the tyrosine kinase family receptor (Trk), found in greatest density around the synaptic junction for BDNF's effects on synaptic plasticity, and the pan75 neurotrophin receptor (p75[NTR]), which enhances neuronal apoptosis.[15] Within the brain, this protein is found in the hippocampal region, an area responsible for learning, memory, and complex thought.

Recent studies have proposed strong associations between neuronal plasticity and the onset of and recovery from major depression. Adults with depression and elevated stress levels experience a great reduction in the total volume of neurons, and most notably neuronal loss in the hippocampus.[16] These alterations are explained by new hypotheses of activity-dependent neuronal plasticity.[17] However, these hippocampal changes are only temporary and can be reversed by antidepressant therapy.[16] Several animal studies have demonstrated marked reduction in hippocampal BDNF expression of rats subjected to stressors such as forced swimming and a subsequent increase in BDNF levels with antidepressant therapy, particularly medications acting as serotonin-norepinephrine reuptake inhibitors (SNRIs).[18–20] A recent clinical trial demonstrated that patients with major depressive disorder have lower serum and plasma BDNF levels than their normal counterparts, and when treated with antidepressants, their serum BDNF levels greatly increased.[21] Therefore, serum levels of BDNF may reflect the true state of neuronal synapses within the hippocampus of patients with major depressive disorder.[19] Zinc, magnesium, and lithium have all been found to increase levels of BDNF.

Numerous studies have also concluded that the hyperactivation of N-methyl-D-aspartate (NMDA) receptors contributes to the pathophysiology of depression.[22,23] NMDA receptors respond to glutamate by increasing their permeability to calcium. The calcium flux through NMDA receptors is key to synaptic plasticity, learning, and memory, particularly in the hippocampal CA1 area where NMDA receptors act as "coïncidence detectors" in long-term potentiation.[20] Depressed patients have significantly smaller hippocampus volumes, suggesting that the hippocampus is connected to the onset of depression.[16] As NMDA receptor activation increases, there is a corresponding increase in glutamate levels accompanied by prolonged presence of calcium in the cell. This leads to overstimulation and excitotoxic damage, a cause of the neurodegeneration associated with depression.[24]

The literature suggests that zinc and magnesium work to prevent depressive symptoms by inhibiting NMDA receptors.[22–24] This response happens in two ways. First, in voltage-independent inhibition, certain minerals like zinc perform noncompetitive, allosteric inhibition, thereby reducing the channel-opening frequency of NMDA receptors. In the second type of inhibition, the mineral directly blocks the NMDA ion channel from opening through voltage-dependent inhibition. Through either pathway, minerals prevent the deleterious effects of NMDA receptor overactivation by slowing calcium reception and preserving the integrity of hippocampal nervous tissue.[25,26]

Inflammation plays a fundamental role to the pathophysiology of depression. The alteration of pro- and anti-inflammatory cytokines has been frequently observed in patents with major depressive disorder (MDD), although whether the relationship is cause or effect is still unclear.[27] Minerals are highly involved in psychoneuroimmunology and pivotal for preserving and reinforcing the antioxidant and immune pathways that counterbalance inflammation. Central to our biological response to oxidative stress is the Keap1/Nrf2/ARE pathway, which regulates the transcription of the antioxidant genes that maintain cellular homeostasis and the detoxification genes that eliminate toxins to prevent damage.[28] This pathway has been found to be highly responsive to dietary factors, including plant-derived compounds and minerals.[28] Deficiencies in key elements, such as zinc, have also been shown to allow greater production of injurious cytokines such as NF-κB[29] and IL-1β.[30] Other nutrients are involved in T- and B-cell activation, with insufficiencies potentiating immunosuppressive effects.[18,22] This chapter will review eight minerals associated with depression. The five minerals with the most evidence-based research include zinc, magnesium, chromium, iron, and lithium. Three other trace minerals—selenium, copper, and iodine—are also briefly discussed.

ZINC

Zinc is one of the most abundant trace minerals in the body.[31] It is a critical structural component of many proteins and a cofactor to enzymes directly involved with brain function.[32] Ongoing research suggests that zinc is highly implicated in the pathophysiology of depression. More recent research shows that dietary zinc deprivation disrupts homeostasis in the brain and creates behavioral disturbances including anorexia, dysphoria, impaired cognitive function, learning disabilities, and neurological disorders.[32]

The existence of a relationship between zinc and depression is based on three consistent findings. First, serum zinc levels are lower in patients with depression than in their healthy counterparts. Second, zinc supplementation has been shown to reduce depressive symptoms. Last, antidepressant treatments have been shown to increase zinc availability over time. Several research studies support an inverse relationship between the severity of depression and zinc levels.[33,34] In one study, researchers found that zinc levels in depressed subjects were 22% lower on average than those of healthy subjects.[35] Other reviews show zinc levels inversely proportional to depression symptoms.[23,36,37]

Zinc supplementation has been shown to reduce depressive symptoms. In a preliminary study conducted with 30 young women, a multivitamin given alongside 7 mg of zinc resulted in notable reductions in anger and depression scales, whereas the multivitamin alone elicited no change over the 10-week trial.[38] In addition, zinc supplements have been shown to improve the efficacy of antidepressant treatment, especially in treatment-resistant patients.[16] A meta-analysis of randomized controlled studies surveying results in over 450 subjects confirmed that zinc effectively lowered depressive symptoms when used as an adjunct to antidepressant medications.[39]

Antidepressant treatments have also been shown to increase zinc availability over time. Medications such as citalopram directly increase physiologic serum levels of zinc. Other combinations of antidepressant therapy have shown a redistribution of zinc levels within the brain, with greatest stores found in the hippocampal region controlling synaptic plasticity, learning, memory, and mood.[22,40]

Although a clear relationship between zinc and depression exists, two central questions remain unanswered: Are lower zinc levels a cause or an effect of depression? And what are the biological mechanisms behind the relationship between zinc and depression? Several studies have suggested that zinc decreases depressive symptoms by inhibiting NMDA receptors.[18,22] Zinc binds to allosteric sites on the extracellular N-terminal domains of the NR2 subunits of NMDA receptors.[22] Zinc joins with the NR2A subunit in higher affinity but only partially blocks this receptor.[22,24] In contrast, zinc maintains a lower affinity with the NR2B subunit but is able to completely inhibit this receptor.[22,24] Thus, the overall inhibitory effect of zinc is greater at the NR2B receptor subunit, where excitatory calcium is fully blocked.[24]

Another proposed mechanism for zinc's effects in mitigating depression involves the peptide BDNF.[41] Zinc supplementation has been shown to enhance BDNF gene expression in rat brains, affecting the cerebral cortex and hippocampus, in particular.[18] In contrast, zinc deficiency has been associated with low BDNF levels in humans.[22] BDNF also contributes to the downregulation of NMDA receptors, thereby decreasing the availability of zinc.[20]

The relationship between zinc and depression may be linked to immune response. Zinc serves as an essential immune constituent required for normal T-cell function.[18,22] Thus, an overactive immune system rapidly depletes physiologic zinc resources within the body.[24] In patients with depression, reduced zinc levels are often found together with elevated neopterin levels—a highly sensitive marker denoting the operation of cell-mediated immunity.[23]

While severe zinc deficiency is uncommon in developed nations, many people have chronically inadequate levels. Individuals at heightened risk for insufficient levels of zinc include those experiencing gastrointestinal disorders, long-standing chronic conditions (e.g., malignancy, anorexia nervosa), alcoholics, vegetarians, and pregnant or lactating women.[42] Such circumstances alter normal physiology, resulting in poor absorption, expedited losses, and increased zinc requirements. General dietary recommendations for adult men and women are a daily intake of 11 mg and 8 mg of zinc, respectively. Pregnant or nursing women should take in 25 mg/day to meet the increased demands on their bodies.[42] Large amounts of zinc are found in oysters, red meat, eggs, wheat germ, spinach, pumpkin and squash seeds, nuts, chocolate, chicken, beans, and mushrooms.

Average adults store 2–4 g of zinc throughout the body. Testing for accurate levels remains a challenge for clinicians. Approximately 98% of zinc is stored within the cells and controlled tightly via homeostatic mechanisms.[43] There is no widely accepted blood test to determine deficiency; thus, a combination of serum and hair levels is often used in clinical practice. Serum and RBC zinc levels are the most commonly used laboratory tests to assess zinc deficiency. A "zinc taste test" as first reported in *The Lancet* in 1984, can also be extremely helpful in determining physiological zinc levels.[44] If a strong metallic taste is detected from tasting a dilute zinc sulfate solution, this is predictive of adequate zinc levels. Two other functional tests for zinc deficiency include the zinc-dependent enzymes alkaline phosphatase and zinc-dependent white blood cell count.

MAGNESIUM

Magnesium is an essential mineral for a well-functioning and healthy human body. It is one of the most common intracellular cations, second only to potassium. It functions as a central regulator of metabolism, a cofactor for over 325 other enzymes, especially ATPase, and as a modulator of calcium and potassium transport.[45] Magnesium has a long history of treating depression; in fact, in 1921, magnesium become the first medically acknowledged substance to effectively treat depression.[46]

Experimental and epidemiological evidence suggests that magnesium deficiency affects many disease processes.[47] Disruption of magnesium metabolism has been reported in cardiovascular diseases, obstetric conditions, neurological diseases, affective disorders, and alcohol withdrawal.[30] An abundance of analyses have demonstrated a correlation between low levels of magnesium and depression.[48–51] When monitored, magnesium levels have been found to normalize after antidepressant therapy and with recovery from depression.[52,53]

Supplementation with magnesium has been shown to decrease symptoms of depression when used to augment antidepressants. Animal studies with laboratory mice have demonstrated a synergistic effect between magnesium and citalopram, imipramine, or tianeptine on stress response as measured by the forced swim test.[54,55]

When used with lithium, benzodiazepines, and neuroleptics, magnesium significantly reduced dose requirements.[47] Magnesium has reduced symptoms of MDD, as well as chronic fatigue syndrome, mania, and schizophrenia.[56–58] One randomized trial in senior citizens demonstrated that for individuals suffering from both depression and magnesium deficiency, magnesium supplements and medication have equally beneficial results. After receiving either 450 mg of elemental magnesium or 50 mg of imipramine daily for 12 weeks, participants showed similar improvement as measured by depression scales.[59]

Similar to zinc, magnesium is an inhibitor of NMDA receptors and an intracellular calcium antagonist.[60] Magnesium is also involved in dampening stress responses via the hypothalamic-pituitary-adrenal (HPA) axis. When reacting to stress, the hypothalamus emits corticotropin-releasing hormone (CRH), which stimulates the secretion of adrenocorticotropic hormone (ACTH) and in turn the release of cortisol from the adrenals. This pathway activates the parasympathetic nervous system to respond to the stressor and also triggers a negative feedback loop to suppress production of CRH back to appropriate resting levels. Magnesium aids in balancing the HPA axis by slowing the secretion of ACTH, thus reducing responsiveness to ACTH and preventing stress hormones from entering the brain.[61] The combination of magnesium deficiency and chronic stress leads to hyperactivation of the HPA axis. This produces excess cortisol levels that damage the hippocampus and has been correlated with depression.[61]

Magnesium deficiency has been increasing over the last 100 years. Seventy-five percent of Americans today consume less magnesium than the Recommended Daily Allowance; 20% are ingesting less than half of the daily requirement (420 mg/day for men and 320 mg/day for women).[62,63] This decrease in the average person's magnesium intake can be attributed to drastic changes in the modern American diet. Refining flour, a common practice since 1905, removes 16% of the magnesium that would be available in whole wheat flour. This one change accounts for an average decrease in daily magnesium intake by 150 mg.[64] Magnesium has also been filtered out of most drinking water reservoirs, and that which remains is often rendered useless by fluoride and other sanitation agents.[62] Last, modern diets contain increased amounts of calcium, a mineral that reduces magnesium retention and absorption.[62]

Frequently using over-the-counter and prescription medications can result in decreased magnesium (Table 9.1). Patients with diabetes mellitus and chronic malabsorption syndromes, such as Crohn's disease, gluten-sensitive enteropathy, and regional enteritis, are at greater risk of magnesium deficiencies.[64] Those over 55 years of age are more susceptible to magnesium deficiencies due to age-related decrease in gut absorption and increased renal excretion.[11]

Magnesium deficiency is difficult to assess in routine blood tests. One percent of the body's magnesium is found in blood, and less than half a percent is found in the serum.[65] Red blood count magnesium levels might be a more accurate reflection of magnesium deficiency. Clinical symptoms associated with magnesium deficiency include insomnia, constipation, anxiety, and muscle spasms. Magnesium may also be increased within the diet, as no upper intake level for dietary magnesium exists. Halibut, yogurt, nuts and seeds, oatmeal, potatoes, wheat bran, brown rice, avocados, and kidney beans are all good sources of magnesium.[65]

TABLE 9.1

Common Drugs that Deplete Essential Minerals

Drug Categories	Copper	Iron	Magnesium	Selenium	Zinc
Antacids					
Aluminum, calcium, and magnesium-containing preparations	✓	✓	✓		
Miscellaneous preparations			✓		
Anticonvulsant medications					
Valproic acid derivatives	✓			✓	✓
Antiretroviral medications					
Reverse transcriptase inhibitors	✓				✓
Anti-inflammatory medications					
Inhalant, systemic, and topical corticosteroids		✓	✓	✓	✓
Nonsteroidal anti-inflammatory drugs		✓			✓
Salicylates		✓			
Antibiotic medications					
Aminoglycosides		✓	✓		
Cholesterol-lowering medications					
Bile acid sequestrants	✓				
Ulcer medications					
Histamine H2 antagonists		✓			✓
Birth control medications					
Monophasic, biphasic and triphasic preparations				✓	✓
Cardiac medications					
Angiotensin-converting enzyme (ACE) inhibitors					✓
Cardiac glycosides			✓		
Vasodilators			✓		
Diuretics					
Loop diuretics			✓		
Thiazide diuretics			✓		✓

Source: Chart based on information accessed from the University of Maryland Medical Center, *Complementary and Alternative Medicine Guide,* 2011 (http://umm.edu/health/medical/altmed/supplement/copper).

Note: Limited information exists relating to chromium, iodine, and lithium depletion. These minerals have been omitted from the chart.

CHROMIUM

Although available only in trace amounts within foods, chromium is an essential nutrient that is intricately involved in major homeostatic systems within the body. This trace element is crucial for proper insulin balance and the regulation of blood cholesterol levels, in addition to its roles in providing mood stability.[66]

Historically, chromium was used in the textile industry to produce colorful dyes and applied as an anti-corrosive agent in metal manufacturing to improve the strength and durability of steel. It was not until 1959 that its nutritional benefits were recognized within the scientific community.[67] This was possible once chromium was shown to be a key player in the regulation of glucose metabolism and the potentiate action of insulin. Although chromium (Cr0) is a common trace metal in the environment, within the body it is found predominantly in the form of trivalent chromium (Cr^{3+}).

Decades of research now exists substantiating the use of the trivalent compounds chromium (III) picolinate and chromium (III) chloride in the treatment of diabetes and obesity.[14,68,69] Chromium deficiency heightens the risk of diabetes mellitus, and conversely supplementation minimizes the incidence of diabetic signs.[70] Additional evidence suggests that the incidence of depression is almost twice as high in patients with diabetes than in the general population.[71] The co-existence of diabetes and depression is associated with substantial morbidity, mortality, and inflated health-care costs.[14] Current research has focused on the interaction between chromium, insulin-sensitivity, and mood.

Intracellularly, chromium has been shown to stimulate redistribution of GLUT4, an insulin-regulated glucose transporter, to restore insulin-sensitivity in diabetic cells.[70] Recent reports have also found the GLUT4 gene within the central nervous system. In the hippocampus, impaired cellular GLUT4 activity blunts metabolic function and decreases plasticity of local neurons. The resulting glucose metabolism insufficiency and hippocampal neurodegeneration can lead to depressive behaviors and cognitive dysfunction.[72,73] Altered activity of the GLUT4 protein and consequent changes in nervous tissue may partly explain the frequent co-occurrence of chromium deficiency, diabetes, and MDD.

Other studies have suggested that chromium is involved in monoamine function. In trials with depression and anxiety-induced animals, chromium administration has been associated with increased tryptophan, serotonin (5-hydroxytryptamine, 5-HT), noradrenaline (NA), pineal melatonin, and serum corticosterone.[74] Changes in biochemical parameters have been observed primarily in discrete regions of the brain (i.e., cortex and cerebellum), while staying minimal in the periphery.[75] Chromium is thus predicted to increase selective amino acid transport to the brain, thereby enhancing the serotonergic, noradrenergic, and dopaminergic systems involved in depression.[75] It has also been suggested that chromium directly modifies 5-HT function by altering sensitivity of central 5-HT(2A) receptors.[76]

In both single- and double-blind studies, chromium has been demonstrated as an effective treatment for patients with affective disorders.[77] In a paper published in the *International Journal of Neuropsychopharmacology* (2002) eight individuals with treatment-resistant MDD, dysthymic disorder, or bipolar disorder received chromium picolinate supplementation.[78] In each case, patients enjoyed remission, reporting "dramatic improvements in their symptoms and functioning." Prior to participation in the study; all patients had received pharmaceutically accepted doses of antidepressants without noticeable benefit. Similar studies have found a reappearance of depressive symptoms in patients who discontinued treatment with chromium.[79,80]

A larger trial conducted by researchers at Duke University Medical also had promising results. Fifteen patients suffering from atypical major depressive disorder were recruited and randomly assigned to receive either 600 µg of chromium picolinate or a placebo daily for 8 weeks. At the conclusion of the study, 70% of those taking chromium responded to treatment as compared to 0% in the control group.[81]

In another study involving 110 people suffering from either MDD or dysthymia, participants were randomly assigned to take 400 µg of chromium picolinate for 2 weeks, then 600 µg per day for an additional 6 weeks, or a placebo for the 8-week duration of the study. The Hamilton Rating Scale for Depression (HDRS) was used to assess the severity of the patient's depression at the start and conclusion of the study. Among those who began the study with carbohydrate cravings, chromium was shown to be superior to the placebo in reducing both depressive symptoms and cravings.[82]

Chromium can be found in many everyday foods including fresh vegetables, meat, fish, bread, cereals, beer, and other foods. However, while available from a wide variety of sources, few of these items contain sizable amounts. A daily chromium intake requirement of 50–200 µg/day has been established, though the diet of an average American adult falls woefully short of this suggested amount.[83] Generally, men require more chromium than women, and suggested levels for both genders rise until adulthood, and then drop off in later life stages.

Stringent attempts must be made to maintain adequate chromium levels because of its sensitivity to rapid depletion by common stressors including infection, exercise, physical trauma, high sugar intake, and emotional stress. If symptomatic individuals present with low or low-normal levels of chromium, supplementation of chromium picolinate in a dose between 400 and 600 µg/day may be recommended.[79]

IRON

Iron is vital to the proper function of every cell in the body. It binds hemoglobin and myoglobin within red blood cells for oxygen transport between tissues. Iron is also essential for regulation of cell growth and hormone synthesis, yet it remains the most common nutrient deficiency worldwide.[84] Suboptimal iron intake has been associated with poor mental development, fatigue, digestive problems, and immune system malfunction.[31]

Research has shown that twice as many women as men are clinically depressed—a discrepancy that begins in adolescence and becomes more pronounced among married women between ages 25 and 45. Interestingly, women of childbearing age are also at higher risk of iron deficiency because of increased demand from menstruation, pregnancy, and lactation, suggesting a link between these occurrences.[85]

Dietary iron is absorbed across the gut lining of the small intestine within the jejunum and ileum via the iron export channel, ferroportin. Serum iron levels are regulated by the protein hepcidin, which breaks down ferroportin by binding to receptors, thus inhibiting further uptake during times of saturation. Once absorbed, the iron is then shuttled throughout the body by its carrier protein, transferrin. With adequate dietary intake the body continually repletes iron stores within the reticulo-endothelial system (e.g., bone marrow, glands) in the form of ferritin. During times of deficiency, these stores are mobilized to maintain sufficient serum levels of iron.[86]

Anemia, a condition in which the body does not have enough healthy red blood cells, can result from iron deficiency. Anemia is classified as a hemoglobin (Hb) concentration less than 13 g/dL for men and 12 g/dL for women.[86] Iron deficiency anemia (IDA) leads to fatigue, shortness of breath, chest pain, dizziness, and pallor. It has also been strongly associated with apathy, depression, and fatigue.[85] Depressed mood and the other behavioral effects associated with low iron can occur before blood levels have diminished enough for the person to be classified as iron deficient.

Several studies have reviewed the relationship between iron and neurotransmitter receptors, suggesting a potential pathway through which iron affects mood. Iron is required for the proper binding of nitric oxide, NMDA receptor functioning, and glutamate activity in the cerebellum and olfactory bulb.[87] Other studies have shown that iron is critical for gamma-aminobutyric acid (GABA) homeostasis and adequate energy metabolism.[88] Iron is also a cofactor for tyrosine hydroxylase and tryptophan hydroxylase, the enzymes that are responsible for dopamine and serotonin synthesis, respectively.[89] Furthermore, iron deficiency is associated with poor brain myelination and impaired monamine metabolism.[89] Thus, it stands that brain function and mood are highly sensitive to changes in iron status.

Studies from as early as 1975 have demonstrated the impact of iron deficiency on psychological function. A large study involving 192 women published in the *European Journal of Clinical*

Nutrition (2007) found that the average serum levels of iron were significantly lower in depressed subjects than in healthy controls.[90]

A 2005 prospective, randomized-controlled study in South African women aimed to find whether prevalence of IDA in new mothers influenced postpartum behavior and cognitive performance, as well as mother–infant interaction and development of the infant.[91] Subjects were divided into three groups: 30 nonanemic women made up the control group, 21 anemic women were given a placebo (combination of 10 μg folate and 25 mg vitamin C), and the 30 other women in the anemic group were given a combination of placebo and 125 mg of iron sulfate. The women and their babies were initially monitored for 10 weeks, with a follow-up visit at 9 months postpartum. Among the anemic women, iron supplementation resulted in a 25% improvement in measures of depression, anxiety, and stress over the course of the study.[91]

One research study evaluated the effect of iron supplementation on perceived quality of life in over 200 women with heavy menstrual bleeding. Women were divided into groups based on whether anemia was present or not, and subsequently treated with iron supplementation or placebo. Quality of life was assessed at the start of treatment, and then at 6 and 12 month intervals. Compared to controls, women who initially presented with anemia and received iron supplements showed increased biological markers for iron and scored significantly higher in areas of energy and physical function, and lower on scales of anxiety than at the start of the study.[92]

Meats, dried beans, and whole grains are common sources of iron found in a typical diet. Iron is present in two major forms within foods, which are accessed slightly differently by the body. Plants and fortified foods contain the less accessible non-heme form, whereas meat, seafood, and poultry offer a bioavailable blend of the two. Meat and ascorbic acid act to improve uptake of non-heme iron, while phytic acid and other components in dry nuts and cereals inhibit its absorption altogether.[93] According to a study conducted in 2000, high consumption of foods known to inhibit iron absorption or low consumption of foods in bioavailable forms of iron increases the risk of developing iron deficiencies.[93] Suggested dietary intake of this mineral differs according to age and gender, and ranges from 8 to 20 mg.[84]

Iron studies play a significant role in clinical evaluation and differentiating between anemias. Iron studies focus on including serum iron, serum ferritin, and transferrin. Ferritin is decreased with conditions such as IDA from lack of serum iron. Serum iron levels alone are inadequate for diagnosing deficiency, as these are initially maintained by mobilizing stored iron. Therefore, it is important for clinicians to consider the entire clinical picture when evaluating patients.

Care must be taken when supplementing with iron, as health problems can also result from too much iron intake, or hemochromatosis, sometimes called "iron overload."[94] Men and postmenopausal women should not be provided iron supplements unless there is a clear indication of deficiency, as both groups lack an ongoing mechanism to dispose of excess iron.

LITHIUM

Lithium has been widely prescribed and researched as a mood-stabilizing medication. Used primarily for chronic bipolar disorder, it has also shown promise as adjunct treatment for MDD and for suicide prevention.[95,96] Lithium is present in our environment, food, and water and is an essential nutrient for the human body.

Elemental lithium was discovered in 1817 by the Swedish chemist Johan August Arfvedson as a key component of petalite—a mineral deposit found in soils. The metal's name was derived from the Greek word *lithos,* literally meaning "from stone."[97] Research has given scientists a greater appreciation of this alkali earth metal, which is now known to be relatively common in the Earth's upper crust in concentrations of 7 and 70 parts per million (ppm). Lithium can also be found in water at varying intensities, ranging from 500 μg/L to up to 100 mg/L in certain springs.[98]

Before Arfvedson's discovery, the ancient Greeks were using mineral water with high lithium concentration to treat the sick. In ancient Greece, "taking the waters" referred to therapeutic bathing and drinking.[99] As early as 400 BC, Hippocrates advocated bathing in mineral waters, or balneo-therapy, as a treatment for disease. Asclepiades, a Greek physician who practiced in Rome at the end of the 2nd century BC, reportedly introduced hydrotherapy with a Greek mineral water for immersion and drinking.[100]

In the mid-nineteenth century, mineral water from springs in Europe and the United States was bottled and wholesaled to grocers, druggists, and wine merchants for its high lithium levels. In 1929, the inventor Charles Leiper Grigg created a beverage he called Bib-Label Lithiated Lemon-Lime Soda, now known as the popular carbonated drink "7-Up." The beverage contained lithium citrate until 1950, and was originally known and marketed for its potential to cure hangovers and its ability to uplift mood.[101] Print advertisements at the time abundantly praised lithium, describing it as "invaluable as a constant and exclusive drinking water," and "as a beautifier of the complexion, it has no equal."[102] However, a failed experiment using near-toxic levels of lithium chloride as a salt substitute for hypertensive patients in the 1940s sparked public outrage and resulted in its abrupt removal from food products across the United States.[103]

Ironically, in 1949, an Australian psychiatrist, Dr. John Cade, was experiencing great success using the carbonate form of lithium as a treatment for manic depression. As early as 1870, lithium had been used as a treatment for acute mania at New York's Bellevue Hospital Medical College.[104] Cade observed in both animal and human trials that lithium not only stabilized mood, but also restored memory and improved cognitive function. Despite these positive results, lithium continued to be viewed negatively by the U.S. Food and Drug Administration (FDA). Controversy surrounding lithium continued until 1970, when it was finally approved for clinical use, having already been in use as a therapy in 49 other countries for many years.[105]

Targeted research into lithium's antidepressant effects began in other countries as far back as the 1960s. In 1981, a paper published in the *British Journal of Psychiatry* reported that adding lithium to the standard antidepressant regimen in treating refractory depressed patients produced "remarkable relief of their depression within 48 hours."[106] Before 2010, more than 40 studies had shown great benefit of lithium augmentation in treating depression; 10 of these were large, double-blind, placebo-controlled studies.[107]

Despite such positive results, lithium has not been used nearly as often in America as in other developed countries.[108,109] Concerns have focused on toxicity risk at high levels, causing damage to the liver, thyroid, and kidneys with long-term use.[109] In recent years, lithium research has explored its possible neuroprotective effects when used in lower doses.

Several large analyses on low-dose lithium therapy have helped to shift the focus away from lithium as a pharmaceutical and into its roles as a dietary mineral. A growing collection of clinical studies has examined the effects of micro-amounts of supplemental lithium on mood.[110,111] From this research it has become evident that, similar to the other minerals discussed in this chapter, dietary lithium is important to neurological function.

Surveys have found that lithium is present in the average adult diet at amounts ranging from 650 to 3100 mcg.[105] Grains and vegetables serve as the primary food sources of lithium, with animal proteins providing less significant ratios. Particular foods with highly concentrated levels of lithium include mustard, kelp, raw pistachio nuts, and thyme.[112] By far the most potent source of lithium in the modern diet, however, is tap water.[105] In geographical locations where water levels of lithium are especially high, it has been linked to health-protective effects with minimal to no side effects.[113] Conversely, low levels of environmental lithium have been associated with increased rates of depression and suicide.[114–116]

Additional research suggests that lithium deficiency may contribute to volatile mood and aggressive behavior. One study found that violent criminals had little to no stores of lithium when tested via hair mineral analysis.[117] Another series of studies on the levels of lithium in drinking water linked low lithium levels in tap water with greater aggression. In the initial study, the levels of lithium in the water of 27 Texan counties were analyzed and compared to the rates of crime and suicide over a 9-year span. Researchers found that the incidence of suicide, homicide, and rape was significantly higher in counties where drinking water contained little or no lithium, versus those with levels ranging from 70 to 170 mcg/L.[114] This study template has been applied and repeated internationally at sites in Austria and Japan.[115,116] These experiments also supported the inverse association between suicidal mortality and crime with low environmental levels of lithium in the surrounding water supply. Higher rates of suicide and crime have been linked to low levels of lithium in the water supply.

Recent studies have suggested that low-dose lithium supplementation may help mitigate these problems. One trial found that for those with a history of aggression and impulsivity, a daily dose of 400 mcg of lithium improved perception of happiness, friendliness, and other mood-related parameters.[110] At least 11 studies reviewing the use of low-dose lithium have found that it promotes neuronal health.[111] Low-dose lithium supplementation may confer emotional balance, positive mood, tolerance of negative mood, behavioral support, decreased aggression and impulsivity, and increased neurocognitive health including memory and cognition.

Lithium functions in two central ways in the body: by repairing damaged neurons and by stimulating neuronal growth. Proposed explanations for lithium's effect on balancing mood include alteration of synaptic levels of neurotransmitters such as dopamine, glutamate, and GABA, and modulation of secondary messenger pathways including the adenylyl cyclase system, cAMP signaling pathway, and phosphoinositide system.[118] Last, lithium is also believed to stimulate the synthesis and release of BDNF to promote the survival of nerve cells.[119]

Because lithium has been generally ignored as a food source by the U.S. Department of Agriculture (USDA) and other dietetic associations, there has been little investigation into dietary requirements. A provisional RDA of 1000 µg/day has been suggested, although no official measures are in place.[105] Animal studies with use of diets deficient in lithium have revealed a severe decrease in reproductive function, life span, and lipid metabolism.[105] Moreover, communities with low levels of environmental lithium have been shown to have higher rates of physical and psychiatric disease.[114–116] It is likely that the effects of lithium deficiency in humans are also significant, yet underrecognized and often mistaken for other phenomena. Future research looking at low-lose lithium in the treatment for depression is needed.

OTHER MINERALS

There are over 25 minerals known to be essential within the human body.[120] This chapter has described five of these minerals that have been most thoroughly studied as potential contributors to treatment for depression. As research in neuroscience further uncovers the roles of minerals, it is likely more elements will be identified and found to be important in the pathophysiology of depression.

SELENIUM

Selenium is an antioxidant that supports the immune system, especially in combination with vitamin E. It is required by animals for survival and is needed to make a number of selenium-dependent enzymes, collectively known as selenoprotiens.[121] With the help of plasma selenoprotein P for transport, this mineral helps to protect pivotal areas of the nervous system from oxidative degeneration and regulates the disruptive inflammatory responses that are associated with depression.[122]

Selenium is an essential component of the glutathione peroxidase system, which works to protect lipid membranes from oxidative stress. Glutathione peroxidase enzymes are expressed in lower amounts in depressed patients and have been linked to low mood and other autonomic symptoms.[123] At serum selenium levels between 82 and 85 ug/L, however, values of glutathione peroxidase are thought to be optimal. When selenium concentrations fall below this amount, increased oxidative damage and depressive symptomatology emerge.[124] These observations suggest that the primary link between selenium and mood is through key antioxidant pathways.

Both animal model and human-based studies have found that adequate selenium levels are protective against depression.[125] Trials have shown that optimal selenium concentrations are associated with lower depression symptoms and more positive daily mood states.[124] Furthermore, research has connected selenium deficiency with higher levels of confusion, hostility, and anxiety.[126] Similar to results found in studies on groundwater lithium levels, one review indicated that areas with lower environmental selenium concentrations had higher rates of depression.[125] Paradoxically, yet other studies have demonstrated that doubling selenium levels increases depressive risk by up to 56%.[127] This evidence hints at a toxicity potential at high doses that needs to be further understood. While it is known that selenium is important for proper neurotransmission, overall more research is needed to fully elucidate its functionality in depression.

COPPER

Copper is crucial for bone formation, hemoglobin and red blood cell synthesis, collagen formation, and general immune function.[31] Together with zinc, it plays an important part in memory and stable brain activity, and acts as a potent antioxidant to rid the body of free radicals that can damage cells and DNA.[128]

In contrast to the other minerals where deficiencies are related to depression, research has correlated *elevated* serum copper with symptoms of depression.[129,130] Copper is a known inhibitor of GABA-evoked responses, notably in the large Purkinje cells of the cerebellum that control motor movement, but also in other areas.[131] Data have indicated that copper and zinc interact with one another at the GABA-A receptor complex to appropriately regulate synaptic transmission.[133] Imbalances in either mineral have been strongly associated with depression, likely due to such alterations in gabaminergic neurotransmission.

A flagship 1991 study compared copper levels in 35 depressed individuals to those of 35 healthy controls.[133] Copper levels were markedly higher in the depressed group (122 µg/dL) than in the nondepressed group (107 ug/dL). Additional studies have confirmed serum copper differences of up to 21% between depressed and nondepressed subjects.[120] Within these groups, zinc levels showed a corresponding 12% decrease, confirming the well-established antagonistic relationship of the two minerals.[134]

IODINE

Iodine is required for the synthesis, activation, and metabolism of thyroid hormone. It is a central component of the thyroid hormones, triiodothyronine (T3) and thyroxine (T4), and is thus required for normal thyroid function.[135] The thyroid gland has an elaborate mechanism for collecting and concentrating iodine from the circulation, which can then be incorporated into the thyroid hormones that are stored and released to meet physical demand.[136] Without appropriate available iodine in the body, substantial endocrine disruption will occur.

Thyroid hormone deficiencies or excesses have profound outcomes both on early brain development and ongoing adult neurological function.[137] As early as 9 weeks of gestation, human fetal brain tissues express thyroid hormone receptors and occupancy with thyroid hormone.[136] In target tissues such as the liver and the brain, active thyroid hormone in the form of T3, binds to receptors in the nuclei of cells to regulate gene expression. The most abundant form of circulating thyroid hormone, T4, is also converted into T3 by the selenium-regulated deiodinase system at these sites, contributing to the hormone's neurological influences.

Psychiatric symptoms are common with iodine deficiency and related thyroid dysfunction. Strong associations have been observed between even subclinical hypothyroidism and depressive symptoms.[138] In areas of the country with reduced levels of iodine in the soil, or lacking iodized salt, individuals presenting with signs of hypothyroidism and depression should thus be carefully monitored for iodine deficiency.[139]

TABLE 9.2

Known Neurological Functions of Select Essential Minerals

Mineral	Neurological Functions
Zinc	• Inhibits NMDA receptors • Enhances BDNF gene expression • Supports normal T cells and immune response • Increases GABA responses
Magnesium	• Inhibits NMDA receptors • Mediates stress reactions via HPA axis
Chromium	• Restores insulin sensitivity via GLUT-4 • Increases monoamine transport to brain • Alters sensitivity to 5HT(2A) receptors
Iron	• Involved in dopamine and serotonin synthesis • Supports brain myelination • Maintains GABA homeostasis
Lithium	• Stimulates synthesis and release of BDNF • Alters synaptic neurotransmitter levels • Modulates second messenger pathways: adenylyl cyclase, CAMP signaling and phosphoinositide system[119]
Selenium	• Aids in glutathione peroxidase system • Acts as antioxidant • Regulates inflammatory response
Copper	• Inhibits GABA responses • Interacts with zinc to regulate synaptic transmission
Iodine	• Synthesis, activation, and metabolism of thyroid hormones

CONCLUSION

Trace minerals are essential to many physiologic processes within the human body. Advanced testing techniques have opened up a new window of understanding into their specific influences on the pathophysiology of depression. Minerals play integral roles in our neurochemistry, contributing to the synthesis of neurotransmitters, activation of key enzymes, modulation of excitatory receptors, and regulation of the inflammatory response. The known neurological functions of key minerals are summarized in Table 9.2.

Inadequate levels of these major elements have direct, observable effects on biomarkers of mood and behavior. Yet with the rapid and irreversible loss of minerals from our soils, and subsequently foods, deficiencies have become overwhelmingly common across the population. Increased exposures to mineral-leeching chemicals have further compounded this problem.

The identification of minerals deficiencies has become an increasingly important component of treatment for mood disorders. In the literature, targeted mineral supplementation has proven to be a progressive antidepressant therapy in deficient individuals. Additional research will help to strengthen our understanding of the clinical application of minerals in the treatment of depression.

REFERENCES

1. World Health Organization. 2013. *World Health Report*. Geneva: World Health Organization Press. http://www.who.int/whr/en/
2. Darnton-Hill, I. et al. 2005. Micronutrient deficiencies and gender: Social and economic costs. *Am J Clin Nutr* 81(5): 1198S–1205S.
3. Centers for Disease Control and Prevention. Micronutrient Facts. http://www.cdc.gov/nutritionreport/pdf/Trace.pdf

4. Bertini, C. 2006. UN Standing Committee on Nutrition Chair—Thirty-third session on the standing committee on nutrition tackling the double burden of malnutrition: A global agenda, Geneva International Conference Centre, Geneva Switzerland. http://www.unsystem.org/SCN/Publications/AnnualMeeting/SCN33/FINAL%20REPORT%2033rd%20SESSION.pdf

5. Ames, B.N. 2001. DNA damage from micronutrient deficiencies is likely to be a cause of cancer. *Mutat Res* 475(1): 7–20.

6. Saramas, D. et al. 2013. Effects of widely used drugs on micronutrients: A story rarely told. *Nutrition* 29: 605–610.

7. U.S. Department of Agriculture. 2003. *Agriculture Fact Book 2001–2002.* Washington, DC: U.S. Government Printing Office.

8. Davis, D., Epp, M., and Riordan H. 2004. Changes in USDA Food Composition data for 43 garden crops, 1950 to 1999. *J Am Coll Nutr* 23(6): 669–682.

9. Thomas, D. 2007. The mineral depletion of foods available to us as a nation (1940–2002). *Nutr Health* 19: 21–55.

10. Kukreja, S., Kalra, G., Shah, N., and Shrivastava, A. 2013. Polypharmacy in psychiatry: A review. *Mens Sana Monogr* 11(1): 82–99.

11. Deans, C. 2006. *The Magnesium Miracle.* New York, NY: Ballantine Books.

12. Schiepers, O.J., Wichers, M.C., and Maes, M. 2005. Cytokines and major depression. *Prog Neuro-Phsychoph* 29(2): 201–217.

13. University of Maryland Medical Center. 2011. *Complementary and Alternative Medicine Guide.* http://umm.edu/health/medical/altmed

14. Mylenic, K. et al. 2014. Essential elements in depression and anxiety. *Pharmacol Rep* 66: 534–544.

15. Mellstrom, B., Torres, B., Link, W.A., and Naranjo, J.R. 2006. The BDNF gene: Exemplifying complexity in Ca^{2+}-dependent gene expression. *Crit Rev Neurobiol.* 16: 43–49.

16. Warner-Schmidt, J.L. and Duman, R.S. 2006. Hippocampal neurogenesis: Opposing effects of stress and antidepressant treatment. *Hippocampus* 16: 239–249.

17. Castrén, E., Võikar, V., and Rantamäki, T. 2007. Role of neurotrophic factors in depression. *Curr Opin Pharmacol* 7: 18–21.

18. Siwek, M. et al. 2009. Zinc supplementation augments efficacy of imipramine in treatment resistant patients: A double blind, placebo-controlled study. *J Affect Disord* 118(1–3): 187–195.

19. Lee, B-H. and Kim, Y-K. 2010. The roles of BDNF in the pathophysiology of major depression and in antidepressant treatment. *Psychiatry Investig* 7(4): 231–235.

20. Izumi, Y., Auberson, Y.P., and Zorumski, C.F. 2006. Zinc modulates bidirectional hippocampal plasticity by effects on NMDA receptors. *J Neurosci* 26(27): 7181–7188.

21. Polyakova, M., Stuke, K., Schuemberg, K. et al. 2014. BDNF as a biomarker for successful treatment of mood disorders: A systematic and quantitative meta-analysis. *J Affect Disord* 174C: 432–440.

22. Swardfager, W. et al. 2013. Potential roles of zinc in the pathophysiology and treatment of major depressive disorder. *Neurosci Biobehav Rev* 37(5): 911–929.

23. Maes, M. et al. 1994. Hypozincemia in depression. *J Affect Disord* 31(2): 135–140.

24. Salimi, S. et al. 2008. Lower total serum protein, albumin and zinc in depression in an Iranian population. *J Med Sci* 8: 597–590.

25. Videbech, P. and Ravnkilde, B. 2004. Hippocampal volume and depression: A meta-analysis of MRI studies. *Am J Psychiatry* 161(11): 1957–1966.

26. Lee, A.L., Ogle, W.O., and Sapolsky, R.M. 2002. Stress and depression: Possible links to neuron death in the hippocampus. *Bipolar Disord* 4(2): 117–128.

27. Slavich, G. and Irwin, M. 2014. From stress to inflammation and major depressive disorder: A social signal transduction theory of depression. *Psychol Bull* 140(3): 774–815.

28. Stefanson, A.L. and Bakovic, M. 2014. Dietary regulation of Keap1/Nrf2/ARE pathway: Focus on plant-derived compounds and trace minerals. *Nutrients* 6(9): 3777–3801.

29. Prasad, A.S. et al. 2008. Duration and severity of symptoms and levels of plasma interleukin-1 receptor antagonist, soluble tumor necrosis factor receptor, and adhesion molecules in patients with common cold treated with zinc acetate. *J Infect Dis* 197: 795–802.

30. Beck F.W. et al. 1997. Changes in cytokine production and T cell subpopulations in experimentally induced zinc-deficient humans. *Am J Physiol* 272: E1002–E1007.

31. Fallon, S. and Enig, M. 2000. Mineral primer. *Weston A Price Found J* http://www.westonaprice.org/health-topics/abcs-of-nutrition/mineral-primer/

32. Szewczyk, B. et al. 2008. Antidepressant activity of zinc and magnesium. *Pharmacol Rep* 60: 588–599.

33. Swardfager, W. et al. 2013. Zinc in depression: A meta-analysis. *Biol Psychiatry* 74(12): 872–878.

34. Irmisch, G., Schlaefke, D., and Richer, J. 2010. Zinc and fatty acids in depression. *Neurochem Res* 36(9): 1376–1383.

35. Siwek, M. et al. 2010. Serum zinc level in depressed patients during zinc supplementation of imipramine treatment. *J Affect Disord* 126(3): 447–452.

36. McLoughlin, I.J. and Hodge, J.S. 1990. Zinc in depressive disorder. *Acta Psychiatr Scand* 82(6): 451–453.

37. Wojcik, J. 2006. Antepartum/postpartum depressive symptoms and serum zinc and magnesium levels. *Pharmacol Rep* 58(4): 571–576.

38. Sawada, T. and Yokoi, K. 2010. Effect of zinc supplementation on mood states in young women: A pilot study. *Eur J Clin Nutr* 64(3): 331–333.

39. Lai, J. et al. 2012. The efficacy of zinc supplementation in depression: Systematic review of randomized controlled trials. *J Affect Disord* 136(1–2): 31–39.

40. Nowak, G., Szewczyk, B., and Pilc, A. 2005. Zinc and depression. An update. *Pharmacol Rep* 57(6): 713–718.

41. Lee, M.M., Reif, A., and Schmitt, A.G. 2013. Major depression: A role for hippocampal neurogenesis? *Curr Top Behav Neurosci* 14: 153–179.

42. National Institutes of Health. 2013. Zinc: Fact sheet for health professionals. *Office of Dietary Supplements Press.* http://ods.od.nih.gov/factsheets/Zinc-HealthProfessional/

43. Environmental Protection Agency. 2005. *Toxicological Review of Zinc and Compounds.* Washington, DC: U.S. Environmental Protection Agency. http://www.epa.gov/iris/toxreviews/0426tr.pdf

44. Bryce-Smith, D. et al. 1984. Anorexia, depression, and zinc deficiency. *Lancet* 2(8412): 1162–1163.

45. Silver, B.B. et al. 1997. A unique non-invasive intracellular magnesium assay correlating with cardiac tissues, arrhythmias and therapeutic intervention. In: *International Symposium on Magnesium. Magnesium: Current Status and New Developments Theoretical, Biological and Medical Aspects.* London, UK: Springer-Verlag.

46. Eby, G.A. and Eby, K.L. 2010. Magnesium for treatment-resistant depression: A review and hypothesis. *Med Hypotheses* 74(4): 649–660.

47. Heiden, A. et al. 1999. Treatment of severe mania with intravenous magnesium sulphate as a supplementary therapy. *Psychiatry Res* 3: 239–246.

48. Cernak, I. et al. 2000. Alterations in magnesium and oxidative stress during chronic emotional stress. *Magnes Res* 13(1): 29–36.

49. Singlewald, N. et al. 2004. Magnesium-deficient diet alters depression-and anxiety-related behavior in mice—Influence of desipramine and hypericum perforatum extract. *Neuropharmacology* 47(8): 1189–1197.

50. Imada, Y. et al. 2002 Relationships between serum magnesium levels and clinical background factors in patients with mood disorders. *Psychiatry Clin Neurosci* 56(5): 509–514.

51. Frizel, D., Coppen, A., and Marks, V. 1969. Plasma magnesium and calcium in depression. *Br J Psychiatry* 115(529): 1375–1377.

52. Jacka, F.N. et al. 2009. Association between magnesium intake and depression and anxiety in community-dwelling adults: The Hordaland Health Study. *ANZ J Psychiatry* 43(1): 45–52.

53. Nechifor, M. 2009. Magnesium in major depression. *Magnes Res* 22(3): 163S–166S.

54. Poleszak, E. 2007. Modulation of anti-depressant-like activity of magnesium by serotonergic system. *J Neural Trans* 114(9): 1129–1134.

55. Poleszak, E. et al. 2005. Enhancement of anti-depressant like activity by joint administration of imipramine and magnesium in the forced swim test: Behavioral and pharmacokinetic studies in mice. *Pharmacol Biochem Behav* 81(3): 524–529.

56. Cox, I.M., Campbell, M.J., and Dowson, D. 1991. Red blood cell magnesium and chronic fatigue syndrome. *Lancet* 337(8744): 757–760.

57. Chouinard, G., Beauclair, L., Geiser, R., and Etienne, P. 1990. A pilot study of magnesium aspartate hydrochloride (Magnesiocard) as a mood stabilizer for rapid cycling bipolar affective disorder patients. *Prog Neuropsychopharmacological Biol Psych* 14(2): 171–180.

58. Kirov, G.K. and Tsachev, K.N. 1990. Magnesium, schizophrenia and manic-depressive disease. *Neuropsychobiology* 23: 79–81.

59. Barragan-Rodriguez, L., Rodriguez-Moran, M., and Guerrero-Romero, F. 2008. Efficacy and safety of oral magnesium supplementation in the treatment of depression in the elderly with type 2 diabetes: A randomized, equivalent trial. *Magnes Res* 21(4): 218–233.

60. Jung, K.I., Ock, S.M., Chung, J.H., and Song, C.H. 2010. Association of serum Ca and Mg levels with mental health in adult women without psychiatric disorders. *Biol Trace Elem Res* 133(2): 153–161.

61. Murck, H. 2002. Magnesium and affective disorders. *Nutri Neurosci* 5(6): 375–389.
62. Combs, G.F. and Nielsen, F.H. 2009. Health significance of calcium and magnesium: Examples from human studies. In: *World Health Organization. Calcium and Magnesium in Drinking Water: Public Health Significance.* Geneva, Switzerland: World Health Organization Press.
63. Pao, E.M. and Mickle, S.J. 1981. Problem nutrients in the United States. *Food Technol* 35: 58–79.
64. Eby, G.A. and Eby, K.L. 2006. Rapid recovery from major depression using magnesium treatment. *Med Hypotheses* 67(2): 362–370.
65. National Institutes of Health. 2013. Magnesium: Fact sheet for health professionals. *Office of Dietary Supplements Press.* http://ods.od.nih.gov/factsheets/Magnesium-HealthProfessional/
66. National Institutes of Health. 2013. Chromium: Fact sheet for health professionals. *Office of Dietary Supplements Press.* http://ods.od.nih.gov/factsheets/Chromium-HealthProfessional/
67. Institute of Medicine. 2001. *DRI: Dietary Reference Intakes for Vitamin A, Vitamin K, Arsenic, Boron, Chromium, Copper, Iodine, Iron, Manganese, Molybdenum, Nickel, Silicon, Vanadium, and Zinc: A Report of the Panel on Micronutrients.* Washington, DC: National Academies Press, 2001.
68. Egede, L.E. and Ellis C. 2010. Diabetes and depression: Global perspectives. *Diabetes Res Clin Pract* 87(3): 302–312.
69. Khanain, R. and Pillai, K.K. Effect of chromium picolinate on modified forced swimming test in diabetic rats: Involvement of serotonergic pathways and potassium channels. *Basic Clin Pharmacol Toxicol* 98(2): 155–159.
70. Pattar, G.R., Tacket, L., Lui, P., and Elmendorf, J.S. 2006. Chromium picolinate positively influences glucose transporter system via affecting cholesterol homeostasis in adipocytes cultured under hyperglycemic diabetic conditions. *Mutat Res* 610(1–2): 93–100.
71. Anderson, R.J., Freedland, K.E., Clouse, R.E., and Lustman, P.J. 2001. The prevalence of comorbid depression in adults with diabetes: A meta-analysis. *Diabetes Care* 24(6): 1069–1078.
72. Grillo, C.A., Piroli, G.G., Hendry, R.M., and Reagan, L.P. 2009. Insulin-stimulated translocation of GLUT4 to plasma membrane in rat hippocampus is pl3-kinase dependent. *Brain Res* 1296: 35–45.
73. Huang, C.C., Lee, C.C., and Hsu, K.S. 2010. The role of insulin receptor signaling in synaptic plasticity and cognitive function. *Chang Gung Med J* 33(2): 115–125.
74. Franklin, M. and Odontiadis, J. 2003. Effects of treatment with chromium picolinate on peripheral amino acid availability and brain monoamine function in the rat. *Pharmacopsychiatry* 36(5): 176–180.
75. Dubey, V.K., Ansari, F., Vohara, D., and Khanam, R. 2015. Possible involvement of corticosterone and serotonin in antidepressant and antianxiety effects of chromium picolinate in chronic unpredictable mild stress induced depression and anxiety in rats. *J Trace Elem Med Bio* 29: 222–226.
76. Attenburrow, M.J., Odontiadis, J., Murray, B.J., Cowen, P.J., and Franklin, M. 2002. Chromium treatment decreases the sensitivity of 5-HT2A receptors. *Psychopharmacology* 159(4): 432–436.
77. Ioveno, N., Dalton, E.D., Fava, M., and Mischoulon, D. 2011. Second-tier natural antidepressants: Review and critique. *J Affect Disord* 130(3): 343–357.
78. McLeod, M.N. and Golden, R.N. 2002. Chromium treatment of depression. *Int J Neuropsychopharmacol* 3(4): 311–314.
79. McLeod, M.N. 1999. Method of treating depression and pre-menstrual syndrome using chromium. *U.S. Patent* US 5972390 A.
80. McLeod, M.N., Gaynes, B.N., and Golden, R.N. 1999. Chromium potentiation of antidepressant pharmacotherapy for dysthymic disorder in 5 patients. *J Clin Psychiatry* 60(4): 237–240.
81. Davidson, J.R., Abraham, K., Connor, K.M., and McLeod, M.N. 2003. Effectiveness of chromium in atypical depression: A placebo-controlled trial. *Biol Psychiatry* 53(3): 261–264.
82. Docherty, J.P., Sack, D.A., Roffman, M., Finch, M., and Komorowski, J.R. 2005. A double-blind, placebo-controlled, exploratory trial of chromium picolinate in atypical depression: Effect on carbohydrate craving. *J Psychiatr Pract* 11(5): 302–314.
83. Agency for Toxic Substances and Disease Registry. 2008. Chromium (Cr) toxicity: Where is chromium found? *Environmental Health and Medicine Education.* http://www.atsdr.cdc.gov/csem/chromium/docs/chromium.pdf
84. National Institutes of Health. 2013. Iron: Fact sheet for health professionals. *Office of Dietary Supplements Press.* http://ods.od.nih.gov/factsheets/Iron-HealthProfessional/
85. Bourre, J.M. 2006. Effect of nutrients (in food) on the structure and function of the nervous system: Update on dietary requirements for brain, Part 1: Micronutrients. *J Nutr Health Aging* 10: 377–385.
86. Citelli, M. et al. 2015. Obesity promotes alterations in iron recycling. *Nutrients* 7(1): 335–348.
87. Jaffrey, S.R. 1994. The iron-responsive element binding protein: A target for synaptic actions of nitric oxide. *Proceedings of the National Academy of Sciences* 91(26): 12994–12998.

88. Ward, K.L. et al. 2007 Gestational and lactational iron deficiency altering the development of stratal metabolome and associated behaviors in young rats. *J Nutr* 137: 1043–1049.

89. Kim, J. and Wessling-Resnick, M. 2014. Iron mechanisms of emotional behavior. *J Nutr Biochem* 25(11): 1101–1107.

90. Vahdat Shariatpanaahi, M. et al. 2007. The relationship between depression and serum ferritin level. *Eur J Clin Nutr* 64(4): 532–535.

91. Beard, J. et al. 2005. Maternal iron deficiency anemia affects postpartum emotions and cognition. *J Nutr* 135(2): 267–272.

92. Peuranpää, P. et al. 2014. Effects of anemia and iron deficiency on quality of life in women with heavy menstrual bleeding. *Acta Obstet Gynecol Scand* 93: 654–660.

93. Sandstead, H.H. 2000. Causes of iron and zinc deficiencies and their effects on the brain. *J Nutr* 130(2): 347S–349S.

94. Piperno, A. 1998. Classification and diagnosis of iron overload. *Haematologica* 83(5): 447–455.

95. Fawcett, J. 2003. Lithium combinations in acute and maintenance treatment of unipolar and bipolar depression. *J Clin Psychiatry* 64(5): 32–37.

96. Capriana, A., Pretty, H., Hawton, K., and Geddes, J.R. 2005. Lithium in the prevention of suicide and all-cause mortality in patients with mood disorders: A review of randomized trials. *Am J Psychiatry* 162(10): 1805–1819.

97. Enghag, P. 2004. *Encyclopedia of the Elements: Technical Data—History—Processing—Applications.* New York, NYL Wiley.

98. Vine, J.D. 1980. Where on earth is all the lithium? *U.S. Department of the Interior Geological Survey* 80(1234): 1–107.

99. Van Tubergen, S. and Van der Linden, A. 2002. A brief history of spa therapy. *Ann Rheum Dis* 61: 273–275.

100. Jackson, R. 1990. Waters and spas in the classical world. *Med Hist* 10: 1–13.

101. Gielen, M. and Tieking, E.R.T. 2005. *Metallotherapeutic Drugs and Metal-Based Diagnostic Agents: The Use of Metals in Medicine.* New York, NY: Wiley.

102. Strobusch, A.D. and Jefferson, J.W. 1980. The checkered history of lithium in medicine. *Pharm Hist* 22(2): 72–76.

103. Valenstein, E.S. 1998. *Blaming the Brain: The Truth about Drugs and Mental Health.* New York, NY: Free Press.

104. Shorter, E. 2009. The history of lithium therapy. *Bipolar Disord* 11(2): 4–9.

105. Schrauzer, G.N. 2002. Lithium: Occurrence dietary intakes, nutritional essentiality. *J Am Coll of Nutr* 21(2): 14–21.

106. De Montigny, C. et al. 1981. Lithium induces rapid relief of depression in tricyclic antidepressant drug non-responders. *Br J Psychiatry* 138: 252–256.

107. Bauer, M. et al. 2010. Lithium's emerging role in the treatment of refractory major depressive episodes: Augmentation of antidepressants. *Neuropsychobiology* 62(1): 36–42.

108. Fels, A. 2014. September 14. Should we all take a bit of lithium? *New York Times*, pp. SR6.

109. Young, A.H. and Hammond, J.M. 2007. Lithium in mood disorders: Increasing evidence base, declining use? *Br J Psychiatry* 191: 474–476.

110. Schrauzer, G.N. and de Vroey, E. 1994. Effects of nutritional lithium supplementation on mood. *Biol Trace Elem Res* 40: 89–101.

111. Mauer, S., Vergne, D., and Ghaemi, S.N. 2014. Standard and trace-dose lithium: A systematic review of dementia prevention and other behavioral benefits. *ANZ J Psychiatry* 48(9): 809–819.

112. Wilson, L. 1998. *Nutritional Balancing and Hair Mineral Analysis.* Prescott, AZ: L.D. Wilson Consultants, Inc.

113. Figueroa, L.T. et al. 2012. Environmental lithium exposure in the North of Chile. *Biol Trace Elem Res* 149: 280–290.

114. Schrauzer, G.N. and Shrestha, K.P. 1990. Lithium in drinking water and the incidences of crimes, suicides and arrests related to drug addictions. *Biol Trace Elem Res* 25: 105–113.

115. Kapusta, N.D. et al. 2011. Lithium in drinking water and suicide mortality. *Br J Psychiatry* 198(5): 346–350.

116. Ohgami, H., Terao, T., Siotsuki, I., and Ishii, N. 2009. Lithium levels in drinking water and risk of suicide. *Br J Psychiatry* 194: 464–465.

117. Schrauzer, G.N., Shrestha, K.P., and Flores-Acre, M.F. 1992. Lithium in scalp hair of adults, students, and violent criminals. Effects of supplementation and evidence for interactions of lithium with vitamin B12 and with other trace minerals. *Biol Trace Elem Res* 34(2): 161–176.

118. Young, W. 2009. Review of lithium effects on brain and blood. *Cell Transplant* 18: 951–975.
119. Diniz, B.S., Machado-Vieira, R.M., and Forlenza, O.V. 2013. Lithium and neuroprotection: Translational evidence and implications for the treatment of neuropsychiatric disorders. *Neuropsychiatr Dis Treat* 9: 493–500.
120. Evans, I. and Soldberg, E. 1998. Minerals for plants, animals and man. *Alberta Department of Agriculture Food and Rural Development* 531–533.
121. Linus Pauling Institute. (n.d.). Selenium. *Micronutrient Information Center, Oregon State University.* http://lpi.oregonstate.edu/infocenter/minerals/selenium/
122. Mosert, V. 2000. Selenoprotein P: Properties, functions and regulation. *Arch Biochem Biophys* 376(2): 433–438.
123. Maes, M. et al. 2011. Lower whole blood glutathione peroxidase (GPX) activity in depression, but not in myalgic encephalomyelitis/chronic fatigue syndrome: Another pathway that may be associated with coronary artery disease and neuroprogression in depression. *Neuroendocrinol Lett* 32(2): 133–140.
124. Conner, T.S., Richardson, A.C., Miller, J.C. 2014. Optimal serum selenium concentrations are associated with lower depressive symptoms and negative mood among young adults. *J Nutr* 145(1): 59–65.
125. Johnson, L.A. et al. 2013. The impact of GPX1 on the association of groundwater selenium and depression: A project FRONTIER study. *BMC Psychiatry* 13(7): 1–8.
126. Sher, L. 2001. Role of thyroid hormones in the effects of selenium on mood, behavior, and cognitive function. *Med Hypotheses* 57(4): 480–483.
127. Colangelo, L.A. et al. 2014. Selenium exposure and depressive symptoms: The coronary artery risk development in young adults trace element study. *Neurotoxicology* 41: 167–174.
128. University of Maryland Medical Center. 2011. Copper. *Complementary and Alternative Medicine Guide.* http://umm.edu/health/medical/altmed/supplement/copper
129. Manser, W.W., Khan, M.A., and Hazan, K.Z. 1989. Trace element studies on Karachi population. Part IV: Blood copper, zinc magnesium and lead levels in psychiatric patients with depression, mental retardation and seizure disorders. *J Pak Med Assoc* 39: 269–274.
130. Schlegal-Zawadzka, M. et al. 1999. Serum trace elements in animal models and human depression. Part II. Copper. *Hum Psychopharmacol* 14: 447–451.
131. Russo, A.J. 2011. Analysis of plasma zinc and copper concentration, and perceived symptoms in individuals with depression, post zinc and anti-oxidant therapy. *Nutr Metab Insights* 4: 19–27.
132. Kim, H. and Macdonald, R.L. 2003. An N-terminal histidine is the primary determinant of α subunit-dependent Cu^{2+} sensitivity of $\alpha\beta3\gamma2L$ GABAA receptors. *Mol Pharmacol* 64: 1145–1152.
133. Narang, R.L., Gupta, K.R., Narang, A.P., and Singh, R. 1991. Levels of copper and zinc in depression. *I J Physiol Pharmacol* 35(4): 373–374.
134. Nowak, G. et al. 1999. Serum trace elements in animal models and human depression. Part I. Zinc. *Hum Psychopharmacol* 14: 83–86.
135. Linus Pauling Institute. (n.d.). Iodine. Micronutrient Information Center, Oregon State University, Corvallis, OR. http://lpi.oregonstate.edu/infocenter/minerals/iodine/
136. Dunn, J.T. 1998. What's happening to our iodine? *J Clin Endocrinol Metab* 83: 3398–3400.
137. Zoeller, T.R. et al. 2002. Thyroid hormone, brain development, and the environment. *Environ Health Perspect* 110(3): 355–361.
138. Nunes, M.A., Viel, T.A., and Buck, H.S. 2013. Microdose lithium treatment stabilized cognitive impairment in patients with Alzheimer's disease. *Curr Alzheimer Res* 10(1): 104–107.
139. Demartni, B. et al. 2014. Depressive symptoms and major depressive disorder in patients affected by subclinical hypothyroidism: A cross-sectional study. *J Nerv Ment Dis* 202(8): 603–607.

10 Essential Fats and Amino Acids in Depression

Bettina Bernstein, DO

CONTENTS

INTRODUCTION

The human brain is an organ that is 60% fat by dry weight, which functions only through structural and metabolic utilization of fats: essential fatty acids (EFAs), cholesterol, and other naturally occurring fatty substances called lipids. The brain's high fat content does not resemble a steak, with chunks of fat that can be sliced off and discarded. Instead, the fat is integrated into every brain cell, where it takes different forms and performs numerous tasks.[1]

Fats belong to a larger group called lipids, which also includes sterols such as cholesterol. When we talk about fats in the body this generally refers to fatty acids, organic compounds made up of chains of carbon and hydrogen atoms that promote and maintain the health of the body in countless ways. Fatty acids are the building blocks for fat similar to how amino acids make up proteins. Amino acids can be combined to produce different proteins, and fatty acids can also be joined together in specific combinations to create different kinds of fat.[2]

The body uses numerous fatty acids, most of which it can manufacture on its own by disassembling fats from the food we eat and recombining them in different configurations (as long as the liver is able to produce cholesterol) with the exception of two fatty acids—linolenic acid and alpha linoleic acid—that the body cannot synthesize on its own, which makes them EFAs. Fatty acids, both those we can synthesize and those we must get from food, are necessary for the proper construction and maintenance of every single cell in the body. They also play roles in promoting the health of the nervous system, immune system, skin, and joints, as well as in normalizing appetite, burning body fat, manufacturing hormones, and controlling inflammation. The link between fatty acids, depression, inattention, mood regulation may have a structural marker in decreased connectivity between caudate and dorsal anterior cingulate cortex and increased connectivity between the caudate and rostral dorsal anterior cingulate cortex.[3] It is important to understand more about the basic biochemical facts regarding fatty acids before going on to the clinically relevant implications: what are fatty acids, how are they named, and what role do they play in health and illness in the body?[4]

DEFINING FATTY ACIDS

A fatty acid is basically a line of carbon atoms, much like a train, with each car hooked to two others (one in front and another in back) except for the engine and the caboose. Every carbon atom in the chain (except those on each end) has an "arm" protruding from either side, and at the end of each arm is a "hand" that can hold onto a hydrogen atom. When all of the carbons in the line are holding onto two hydrogen atoms, the fatty acid is considered saturated. Unable to hold any more hydrogen atoms, it is completely full, like a saturated sponge.

If a carbon atom should let go of a hydrogen atom, meaning that it now holds onto just one hydrogen atom, the fatty acid is considered either *monounsaturated* or *polyunsaturated*, depending on how many times this occurs in the line of carbons (mono for once; poly for more than once). If the first missing hydrogen occurs on the third carbon in the line, the configuration is called an omega-3 fatty acid. If it occurs on the sixth carbon, it is called an omega-6 fatty acid. This may not seem like much of a difference, but in the three-dimensional world of biochemistry, the position of a single atom can make a world of difference by allowing a molecule to interact with others or by preventing it from even getting close.

Omega-3 fatty acids are concentrated in fish, fish oil, flaxseed oil, and walnuts, while omega-6s are found primarily in corn, soy or sunflower oil, eggs, and meat. Both play crucial roles in brain function; thus, both are necessary components of a balanced diet. However, because omega-6 fatty acids can promote inflammation under certain circumstances, while omega-3s can help quell inflammation, it's important to have the proper ratio of omega-6s to omega-3s. The recommended ratio is 4:1. Shockingly, the Standard American Diet is not only low in omega-3s, it can contain up to 25 times more omega-6s than omega-3s, skyrocketing the ratio from 4:1 to 25:1. The omega-6 fatty acids are certainly essential, healthful, and necessary, but not in that amount, and not in a processed, distorted form.

A tremendous overload of omega-6s coupled with a deficiency in omega-3s is believed to contribute to a large number of diseases and conditions, especially depression. The imbalance between omega-6s and omega-3s is primarily due to the typical Western-style diet, which is extremely heavy in foods containing omega-6 fatty acids, especially oils used in cooking, fried foods, processed foods, and junk food. The decrease in overall levels of omega-3 fatty acids in the diet is, in part, the result of eating cage-raised cattle and farm-raised fish, which contain up to five times fewer omega-3s than their wild counterparts. Not only is the omega-6 to omega-3 ratio skewed, but we're also taking in fewer of the EFAs than we need, even though our diets are high in fats. So although fat is too plentiful in our diets, we can't seem to get the right kind of fat in the proper ratios to enjoy healthy lives.[5]

ESSENTIAL FATTY ACIDS AND DEPRESSION

Two specific omega-3 EFAs are important to brain health: eicosapentaenoic acid (EPA) and docosahexaenoic acid (DHA). Both provide fuel for the brain and help control the chronic inflammation seen in degenerative brain diseases such as Alzheimer's disease. EPA plays a major role in the maintenance of nerve cell membranes, while mildly depressed people were found to have less DHA in their fat tissue than nondepressed people. As the EPA content of red blood cells decreases, the severity of depression increases, and vice versa.[6]

Compared to healthy people, patients with bipolar mood disorder have lower levels of EPA, DHA, and alpha linolenic acid, a plant-based omega-3 that the body uses to manufacture EPA. Low blood levels of EFAs could potentially contribute to postpartum depression due to the physiological process during pregnancy when the mother transfers a significant amount of EFA to her developing fetus; thus EPA levels need to return to pre-term levels by replenishment after the birth, and if the time for EPA levels to return to normal is extended, this may increase the risk of postpartum depression. A recent randomized controlled trial looked at perceived prenatal stress among African Americans and found improved self-ratings with DHA supplementation.[7] Another recent study using a regression model confirmed the importance of nutrients and the link between low blood levels of omega-3 EFAs and depression especially in the postpartum period.[8]

Increased risk of suicide attempts may potentially correlate with lower plasma levels of DHA, and a higher ratio of omega-6s to omega-3s. Supplementation with omega-3 EFAs especially derived from fish oil appears to be a relatively safe and effective alternative that may be relatively low cost and effect to prevent depression and psychosis for populations at risk.[9]

DHA makes up a significant part of the structure as a fatty acid in the brain's gray matter and in the retina. DHA also improves the transmission of brain signals and, thus, communication between brain cells. When it comes to the brain, you are indeed what you eat, for diet affects the levels and kinds of fat that the brain contains. This is especially important for breastfeeding infants; although many studies have tried to prove that supplementation with EFAs is comparable, a meta-analysis of four trials failed to show comparability of supplements with EFAs to breast milk.[10]

Especially among women in the postpartum period, low levels of omega 3 fatty acids appeared to be associated with depressive symptoms. It is possible that depression somehow causes low levels of omega 3 or that genetic factors might account for the lower levels of omega 3; however, adequate intake and/or supplementation of EPA and possibly also DHA could prevent or improve mood during the postpartum period.[11,12]

A recent randomized controlled trial found a three times greater reduction of time of onset of depression as compared to placebo for persons treated with EPA who were receiving treatment with interferon alpha for hepatitis, supportive of its anti-inflammatory effects.[13]

Not all studies of omega 3 supplementation have shown positive results as a recent placebo-controlled, randomized, double-blind study that compared EPA and DHA as monotherapy for major depressive disorder in 196 adults failed to find superiority to placebo and one subject receiving EPA-enriched omega 3 discontinued the study due to worsening depression. Some studies of omega-3s have not yielded positive results in some cases due to lack of sufficient power related to the difficulties recruiting enough participants as well as possibly related to underdosing.[14]

In a small study done in 2010, elderly depressed women aged 66–95 years old who participated in an 8-week, randomized, double-blind, placebo-controlled trial who received 2.5 g per day of long-chain polyunsaturated fatty acid (LC PUFA) containing 1.67 g EPA and 0.83 g DHA with good compliance as confirmed by erythrocyte membrane phospholipid fatty acid concentrations, experienced a significant increase of EPA and DHA in the intervention group and a significant improvement in depressive symptoms, as evaluated by the Geriatric Depression Scale. Participants who were given the supplements also reported an improved quality of life.[15]

A meta-analysis of 11 and 8 trials conducted retrospectively on patients with a DSM-defined diagnosis of major depressive disorder (MDD) and also in patients with depressive symptoms but no diagnosis of MDD demonstrated a significant clinical benefit of omega-3 PUFA treatment compared to placebo. Supplementation with EPA appeared in some trials to explain clinical efficacy as DHA supplementation did not appear as clinically effective. Improvement in depressive symptoms was seen with the use of omega-3 PUFA as a supplement when given with other antidepressant or mood stabilizer medications as well as for adults with bipolar disorder. Omega-3 PUFA was not found as effective for depressed youth or for depression in the perinatal period as compared with efficacy for older age populations.[16]

Supplementation with omega-3 and omega-6 fatty acids may have the potential, especially in populations at risk such as the military, to reduce rates of depression, suicide, and impulsive aggression.[17] Supplementation with EFAs is more likely to be helpful if EFAs are at low levels which can be accompanied by symptoms of depression, dry skin, fatigue, allergies, and being thirsty all the time not due to a medical condition such as diabetes or hypothyroidism and potentially can be confirmed by blood tests of EFA levels.[18]

How to Add Essential Fatty Acids to the Diet

Although consuming sufficient fat is not a problem for most Americans, getting enough of the right kind of fat is. Here's what can help to ensure adequate amounts of EFAs, particularly EPA and DHA[19]:

1. Eat seafood at least twice a week, especially salmon, mackerel, herring, sardines, halibut, and albacore tuna. Grill or bake the fish without adding oils and avoid deep-frying, as this can destroy the omega-3s. Try to avoid farmed fish as farmed as well as certain types of fish can be high in mercury and industrial contaminants.
2. Eat meats from grass-fed animals whenever possible, as these contain a higher omega-3 to omega-6 ratio and if possible meats that were not fed antibiotics as antibiotics for some people may possibly increase the risk of allergic responses.
3. Eat foods that contain omega-3s, such as walnuts, pecans, pumpkin seeds, sesame seeds, tahini, hummus, tofu, and fresh spinach.
4. Check levels by a blood test for EFAs to determine proper ratios for supplementation.
5. Take an omega-3 supplement that is low or free of mercury and they have many different names: omega-3, fish oil, EPA, DHA, essential fatty acids, or cod liver oil. Be sure to read the label carefully, for it can be confusing.
6. If you have not been tested for EFA levels, look for a supplement that contains EPA, DHA, and gamma-linolenic acid, which supplies all of the EFAs.

Although omega-3 fatty acids are good for mental and physical health, overdosing is not recommended. Beyond a certain point, omega-3 fatty acids disrupt the omega-6 to omega-3 fatty acid ratio, and perhaps push certain necessary fats out of the diet. Excessive amounts of omega-3 fatty acids can cause the blood to thin, leading to excessive bleeding and delayed clotting time although still being effective as an anti-inflammatory, as a study that looked at periodontal bleeding from aspirin reported bleeding still continued with omega-3 supplementation. Consult a medical provider before taking omega-3 supplements, particularly if also taking blood-thinning medicines.

The omega-3 fatty acids are crucial for brain health, and up to 2 g/day for up to 2 months is usually relatively safe and well tolerated. Blood tests to monitor omega-3 and omega-6 levels as well as to test liver function should be done if supplementation is continued beyond that time due to the potential risk of impairment of liver function, especially if other compounds such as aspirin or acetaminophen are taken along with omega-3 fatty acids. In some situations, though, omega-3 fatty acids can actually improve liver function.[20]

Deficiencies of omega-6 fatty acids can occur in the context of supplementation if high doses of omega-3 supplements are taken for months without monitoring or testing, especially in individuals who also have some food allergies or food sensitivities that might cause a less varied dietary intake.

Omega-6 fatty acids in the form of borage oil or evening primrose oil can be rubbed right on the skin and help to soften and reduce dryness.

Scientific studies and clinical experience suggest that inadequate levels and ratios of EFAs can impact mood in a negative fashion. Clinical experience and some scientific study results support the view that inadequate levels and ratios of EFAs play a role in mood disorders and that attention to nutrition and the use of supplements is a reasonable approach when depression and unstable mood exist.[21] Intake of sufficient EFAs especially in a ratio of 4:1 omega-3 fatty acid to omega-6 fatty acid should be helpful, especially when the "typical" diet that includes red meat is consumed.[22]

LOW CHOLESTEROL LEVELS AND DEPRESSION

Cholesterol is a valuable and necessary part of human chemistry and optimal brain function. The brain is the most cholesterol-rich organ in the body. Cholesterol is a waxy steroid metabolite that is found in body cells and is transported through the body in the bloodstream. It is absolutely essential for life. Cholesterol ensures that cell walls function properly, is converted into vitamin D, is used to make sex and stress hormones, and serves as a major part of the coating of nerve cells, making it essential for smooth and efficient function.

The body manufactures cholesterol as necessary, with the bulk of the production occurring in the liver. Relatively little cholesterol, about 15%, comes from the food we eat. The body responds to cholesterol absorbed from food. If more is consumed, less is made internally. If less is consumed, the body produces more. Cholesterol is essential for the synthesis of all steroid and sex hormones, including DHEA, testosterone, and estrogen. Vitamin D is synthesized with the help of cholesterol and ultraviolet light and essential for a healthy nervous system.[23]

The lipid hypothesis, proposed by the German pathologist Rudolf Virchow in 1856, received renewed attention in the latter half of the twentieth century: Elevated levels of total cholesterol and low-density lipoprotein (LDL), "bad" cholesterol, set the stage for cardiovascular disease by damaging the interior linings of the arteries. But high-density lipoprotein (HDL), "good" cholesterol, can protect the arterial linings by carrying cholesterol away, so higher levels of HDL are considered to be good. Current guidelines for total cholesterol are as follows:

Desirable less than 200 mg/dL
Borderline 200–239 mg/dL
High Risk 240-plus mg/dL

There has been a major effort to reduce these numbers in recent years, despite the fact that our understanding of the causes of cardiovascular disease has grown more sophisticated since cholesterol was singled out as the chief cause of heart attacks several decades ago. Many studies have shown, for example, that medications to lower cholesterol levels are effective; however, it is not universally correct to assume that elevated cholesterol levels will cause heart attacks or strokes in everyone, as many people who do have heart attacks or strokes do not have elevated cholesterol.[24] Depression and lower cholesterol levels may not be a cause-and-effect relationship, but may instead be reflective of other potentially interactive factors due to the impact of aging on cholesterol levels in older people, especially males.[25]

LOW CHOLESTEROL AND SUICIDE

Recent studies suggest that low cholesterol, especially in the context of severe stressors such as posttraumatic stress disorder (PTSD), may be associated with higher levels of aggression and suicide.[26] Unusually low serum cholesterol levels, especially when achieved through pharmacological intervention, may not be as desirable from a mental health standpoint due to the correlation of lower levels of total cholesterol to depression and suicide.[27]

In a recent cross-sectional study, 73 outpatient depressed persons who had received antidepressant treatment were divided into those with and without suicide ideation. Triglyceride levels differed significantly between the two groups, separating out those with suicide ideation as having lower levels even though body mass index (BMI), total cholesterol, LDL, HDL, and Auditory Processing for the Loudness Dependence of Auditory Evoked Potentials (LDAEP), did not differ between the two groups.[28]

The psychological impact of long-lasting depression can result in suicidal ideation and even death due to suicide. A 2010 study of suicide attempters found a correlation between low cholesterol and lower cerebrospinal fluid levels of 5-HIAA, a precursor to serotonin.[29]

VITAMIN D, INFLAMMATION, CHOLESTEROL, AND DEPRESSION

Low vitamin D levels have been associated with the development of metabolic syndrome possibly due to increased inflammation, especially, in a study of obese Australians.[30] A recent study showed reduction of potentially harmful lipids such as triglycerides with vitamin D supplementation in postmenopausal women with diabetes.[31] A recent cross-sectional study showed that low 25 hydroxy-vitamin D (25OHVD) levels are associated with depression in women with and without polycystic ovarian syndrome.[32]

Lower hormone levels may result when there is insufficient cholesterol. This is an important potential factor impacting mental health, as higher hormone levels may play a protective role in depression, especially for older males. A study of older Japanese males showed that normal dehydroepiandrosterone sulfate levels were protective of depression.[33]

Cholesterol and EFAs are intimately linked to depression, although the links are not always linear and thus may require further elucidation. Understanding the consequences of deficiencies in essential fats and cholesterol is important for the effective treatment of depression. Whether it is drug induced, genetic, or a result of dietary patterns, low cholesterol prevents our brains from functioning optimally. Low plasma total cholesterol occurs after a suicide attempt and remains low when followed up. Therefore, measuring cholesterol levels in the context of depression and ensuring a diet that provides good-quality fats high in omega-3 fatty acids may be helpful in preventing or reducing depression.[34]

AMINO ACID PRECURSORS

Amino acids are important due to their potential effect on neurotransmitters. The underlying mechanisms of antidepressants are complex and involve both circulating levels of neurotransmitters as well as feedback systems between neurotransmitters as they interact with neurochemical receptors. Selective serotonin reuptake inhibitors (SSRIs) such as fluoxetine (Prozac®), for example, should increase the amount of serotonin available in the brain by decreasing reuptake—as the serotonin remains in the receptors instead of being broken down as would normally occur.[35]

Other antidepressant medications may influence not just serotonin neurotransmitter levels but also the levels of other compounds such as glutamate, norepinephrine, and nicotine—important compounds that regulate mood and behavior. A well-done meta-analysis of two antidepressant medications—fluoxetine and venlafaxine—found that for a 6-week period, although average differences were small for adults treated with fluoxetine, 55.1% of treated patients achieve a 50% reduction in the severity of depression compared with only 33.7% of controls.[36]

When depression fails to respond to treatment, this may be due to a lack of sufficient amino acid precursors to produce adequate levels of neurotransmitters. One approach is to use amino acid precursors, either through intake of foods or by taking supplements that supply the body with extra amounts of the amino acids that influence neurotransmitter levels or activity. Amino acids, when present through dietary sources as well as when supplements are given, work alone or in a synergistic manner to antidepressants to improve depressed mood.[37]

Amino acids are the building blocks of protein. These molecules, which contain carbon, hydrogen, oxygen, and nitrogen atoms in specific configurations, can be strung together in unique sequences to form a huge variety of proteins. In addition to building proteins, amino acids build and repair muscle tissue, form enzymes and hormones (which are also proteins) crucial to the regulation of body processes, and provide the "raw material" for the production of neurotransmitters.[38]

The liver manufactures 11 of the 20 amino acids necessary for human health, while the remaining nine must be obtained through the diet. These nine are called the "essential" amino acids, since consumption of them is essential to good health and cannot be produced by the body. The nine essential amino acids are as follows: histidine, isoleucine, leucine, lysine, methionine, phenylalanine, threonine, tryptophan, and valine. The other amino acids are considered "nonessential." Since the body makes them, consuming them is not necessarily crucial to health.[39]

AMINO ACIDS AND MOOD

Certain amino acids, including gamma-aminobutyric acid (GABA), glutamine, phenylalanine, taurine, tryptophan, and tyrosine, have been shown to influence mood.[40] Some are converted into neurotransmitters that are critical to brain function and disposition, others affect the way the brain works, and one is actually a neurotransmitter itself.

GABA

GABA is a neurotransmitter—one of the main substances that helps brain cells communicate with each other. GABA helps brain cells calm down and become less excited, aids in the control of muscle activity, and plays an important part in vision. Because it reduces brain-cell excitability, GABA acts as a natural tranquilizer, reducing stress and anxiety while increasing alertness and helping to keep other neurotransmitters in check. People with low levels of GABA often experience anxiety, depression, irritability, headaches, and hypertension.[41]

GLUTAMINE

The most abundant amino acid in the body, glutamine, increases GABA levels in the brain. Glutamine also helps remove excess ammonia from the body, improves immune-system function, protects the intestinal lining, and appears to be needed for normal brain function. Although the body usually makes enough glutamine on its own, extreme stress (e.g., heavy exercise or an injury) can increase the need for this amino acid beyond the amount naturally manufactured. Some experts believe that low levels of glutamine may contribute to depression, fatigue, and alcohol cravings.[42]

PHENYLALANINE

The endorphins, natural substances that help modulate mood and block chronic pain, occur naturally in the body and are continually built and destroyed. Phenylalanine appears to protect the endorphins from routine destruction, increasing their levels and improving depressed moods. This essential amino acid also plays a part in creating the neurotransmitters dopamine and norepinephrine; however, abnormally elevated serum phenylalanine levels with abnormal ratios of phenylalanine to tyrosine may be seen in a subgroup of patients with Alzheimer's dementia due to immune activation and impaired conversion of phenylalanine as well as other amino acids.[43]

TAURINE

A nonessential amino acid, taurine works with GABA to help prevent overactivity of neurotransmitters, to decrease anxiety and excessive motor activity. Taurine can function as a neurotransmitter to help prevent the reuptake of serotonin and other neurotransmitters such as dopamine, epinephrine, and norepinephrine, thus preserving their levels in the brain.[44]

TRYPTOPHAN

Tryptophan is the amino acid from which serotonin and melatonin are created in the brain. Some studies have shown that taking 5-HTP, a form of tryptophan, boosts brain levels of serotonin and can be an important adjunct in treating depression. Normally, the body uses tryptophan to manufacture 5-HTP, which easily crosses the blood-brain barrier to enhance the synthesis of serotonin. Giving 5-HTP saves a step and, because 5-HTP is not incorporated into various proteins, more is available to increase brain serotonin levels.[45]

Mild depression symptoms can improve with supplementation of a combination of 5-HTP and other amino acids such as tyrosine which should be done under close monitoring for those who are already prescribed a serotonin reuptake or norepinephrine/serotonin reuptake inhibitor due to the risk of serotonin syndrome, a situation in which toxic levels of serotonin result in a potentially life-threatening reaction.[46,47]

The 5-HTP can trigger some side effects, including gastrointestinal distress, gas, and cramping. These symptoms may be minimized by starting slowly in divided dosages as well as when excessive doses of tryptophan are given to elderly people with urinary tract infections, the syndrome of a "purple" urine due to the interaction of tryptophan, bacteria, and low output in a catheterized patient.[48,49] Providing more L-tryptophan naturally via the diet should increase available levels of serotonin in the brain, and recent studies show that it improves mood and decreases depression.

TYROSINE

Tyrosine is a precursor of the neurotransmitters norepinephrine and dopamine. When levels of tyrosine are optimal, energy, alertness, and improved moods may follow.[49]

AMINO ACIDS AND DEPRESSION

Low or abnormally high levels of amino acids can be linked to depression, anxiety, and impaired cognitive function; however, at this time, it appears to be complex to be able to predict neural cell function and what the level needs to be to be sure functioning is abnormal.[42] Recent research has shown that supplementation with SAMe (S-adenylmethionine) has been shown to be effective to reduce symptoms of depression possibly as effectively as SSRIs in the first few weeks of treatment.

In one study with 144 adults diagnosed with MDD, SAMe was found to be superior to escitalopram during weeks 2, 4, and 6, although no significant effect was found from weeks 8–12.[50]

MALABSORPTION OF PROTEIN

A lack of sufficient amino acids can result from a lack of absorption of protein that occurs because a lack of hydrochloric acid in the stomach fails to convert pepsinogen in the stomach to pepsin needed to digest proteins, including absorbing vitamins such as B12 and other minerals in the gastrointestinal tract. Additionally, a lack of hydrochloric acid can result in a failure to destroy bacteria and the reduced ability to perceive satiety signals in the gastrointestinal tract.[51]

WHO'S AT RISK FOR DECLINING HYDROCHLORIC ACID LEVELS?

The amount of gastric acid produced by the stomach falls sharply with age, dropping by roughly 40% from the teens to the thirties, and almost half again by the time a person reaches the seventies. This means that the ability to digest protein also decreases markedly with age as well as when hypothyroidism has been caused by autoimmunity.[52]

Stomach acid levels are also lower in those who regularly use antacids and other medicines that interfere with acid production, whether prescription or over the counter. Lower stomach acid can result in lower nutrient absorption, and digestive capabilities can decrease not just in older people.[53] Low hydrochloric acid levels are associated with many chronic digestive complaints, including pain or discomfort after eating, gas, bloating, and food sensitivities and allergies. Low hydrochloric acid levels can also contribute to iron-deficiency anemia, osteoporosis, gallstones, skin conditions, rheumatoid arthritis, periodontal disease, asthma, and chronic stress. Extremely low levels of vitamin B12 may result in severe depression with psychotic features.[54]

LOW ACID LEVELS

We generally think of acid indigestion, heartburn, or gastroesophageal reflux disease (GERD) as problems caused by excess acid in middle-aged and older adults. What many people (including quite a few health professionals) don't realize is that commonly mechanical problems such as motor dysfunction of the lower esophageal sphincter (LOS) and, possibly, the proximal stomach are a major cause of the increase in the number of reflux episodes and can trigger symptoms of GERD, which include burning pain in the middle of the chest, nausea, and regurgitation.[55]

Rather than avoiding the foods that seem to cause the problem as well as changing eating habits, such as determining if there are foods that are triggering an autoimmune reaction, such as the commonly allergenic foods like wheat, milk, egg, soy, peanut, and corn, most people are inclined to pop a pill to "cool the burn."[56] Thanks to ongoing advertising campaigns by pharmaceutical companies on television, radio, and in person to doctors, millions of prescriptions for GERD medicines are written every year, in addition to the sale of a vast array of over-the-counter remedies to reduce stomach acid.[57]

Millions of people may be attempting to treat symptoms of low stomach acid by lowering it even further, exacerbating problems with protein digestion and poor nutrient absorption. Low levels of stomach acid can also impair absorption of zinc, magnesium, and other minerals, as well as vitamin C and certain B vitamins. Poor absorption of zinc plays an important role, as zinc is involved in more than 200 different enzyme reactions, including several having to do with digestion.[58] All of the digestive enzymes, including hydrochloric acid, depend on zinc to function properly, and low zinc levels have been associated with depression.[58]

POOR ABSORPTION OF NUTRIENTS CAN CONTRIBUTE TO DEPRESSION

When proteins are not broken down efficiently into their components, sufficient levels of key amino acids may not be released into the bloodstream. Among the amino acids that may not be present in sufficient amounts are tryptophan, tyrosine, and phenylalanine, all of which play an important role in mood regulation.

Tryptophan is a precursor molecule needed by the body in order to form serotonin. Phenylalanine is a precursor molecule that is required by the body to produce dopamine and norepinephrine. In addition, in order to create neurotransmitters, ample supplies of zinc, copper, magnesium, folic acid, vitamin B6, vitamin B12, and other nutrients are required for optimal functioning, and adequate amounts of stomach acid and digestive enzymes should be considered first to normalize neurotransmitter levels.[59]

142 Integrative Therapies for Depression

MAINTAINING PROPER AMINO ACID AND PROTEIN LEVELS

Sometimes amino acid levels are low for dietary reasons, especially in diets that include no meat or exclude all animal products. Other fad diets or crash weight-loss diets can also be protein deficient. Depression itself may play a role in amino acid deprivation, as some depressed people lose interest in food, eat fewer kinds of foods, and eat less food overall. Sometimes food sensitivities interfere with being able to absorb certain sources of protein such as from milk (whey), egg, or even for those people with sensitivities or intolerance to fish, chicken, poultry, or other animal sources. Sometimes cooking proteins lessens the severity of the food sensitivity or intolerance; however, sometimes it is the very nature of contact with the protein that is the problem due to the abnormal autoimmune reaction.[60]

WHEN SHOULD PROTEIN BE CONSUMED?

Instead of a diet that contains protein only at night, a more even delivery of protein can be helpful. Although many people do not have time or aren't hungry for a breakfast containing protein in the morning, high-quality protein that contains all the essential amino acids that the body cannot manufacture should be consumed in the morning to start the day, as the body disassembles the protein from food into amino acids, absorbs them, and then recombines them in new ways to create proteins.[61]

CONCLUSION

Clinically, when depression is a concern and other physical symptoms such as dry skin and brittle or dull hair are present and are not due to hypo- or hyperthyroidism or other physical illness, it is reasonable to try supplements such as omega-3 and SAMe, while awaiting results of blood tests to determine if there are deficiencies on testing. Do not forget that supplementation with vitamin D can be helpful for some people suffering depression.

It is important to keep in mind that supplements are not bioequivalent to the health benefits of consuming a healthy balanced diet that consists of mostly vegetables, legumes, and some good sources of proteins such as fish. Some groups of people such as adolescents, the elderly, and those on a restricted or limited diet may require supplementation to obtain needed building blocks for normal mood and brain functioning when standard nutritional intake is not optimal, such as in situations where restricted calorie intake is crucial to health, such as the ketogenic diet for seizure control or when weight loss is needed.[62]

Diets that are lower in carbohydrates may facilitate weight loss due to the lower total calories consumed; however, for some people, these diets can result in initial worsening of depression and anxiety as well as increased irritability and possibly nutritional deficiencies. The importance of a nutritionally sound diet that does not include excessive calorie intake should not be overlooked.[53]

REFERENCES

1. Clark, D. and Sokoloff, L. 1999. Circulation and energy metabolism of the brain. In *Basic Neurochemistry: Molecular, Cellular and Medical Aspects*, Ed. G.J. Siegel, B.W. Agranoff, R.W. Albers et al. Philadelphia, PA: Lippincott-Raven, pp. 637–669.
2. Brosnan, J.T. and Brosnan, M.E. 2006. The sulfur-containing amino acids: An overview. *J Nutr* 136: 1636S–1640S.
3. Admon, R., Nickerson, L.D., Dillon, D.G., Holmes, A.J., Bogdan, R., Kumar, P., Dougherty, D.D. et al. 2015. Dissociable cortico-striatal connectivity abnormalities in major depression in response to monetary gains and penalties. *Psychol. Med.* 45(1): 121–131.
4. Das, U.N. 2006. Essential fatty acids—A review. *Curr Pharm Biotechnol* 7(6): 467–482.
5. Gibbs, R.A. and Gibbs, R.A. 2008. Current intakes of EPA and DHA in European population. *Proceedings of the Nutrition Society* 67(3): 273–280.

6. Su, K.P., Lai, H.C., Yang, H.T. et al. 2014. The role of nutrients in protecting mitochondrial function and neurotransmitter signaling: Implications for the treatment of depression, PTSD, and suicidal behaviors. *Crit Rev Food Sci Nutr* 2014: 3.

7. Keenan, K., Hipwell, A.E., Bortner, J., Hoffmann, A., and McAloon, R. 2014 Association between fatty acid supplementation and prenatal stress in African Americans: A randomized controlled trial. *Obstet Gynecol* 124(6): 1080–1087.

8. Markhus, M.W., Skotheim, S., Graff, I.E. et al. 2013. Low omega-3 index in pregnancy is a possible biological risk factor for postpartum depression. *PLoS One* 8(7): e67617.

9. Schlogelhofer, M., Amminger, G.P., Schaefer, M.R. et al. 2014. Polyunsaturated fatty acids in emerging psychosis: A safer alternative? *Early Intervention Psychiatry* 8(3): 199–208.

10. Beyerlein, A., Hadders-Algra, M., Kennedy, K. et al. 2010. Infant formula supplementation with long-chain polyunsaturated fatty acids has no effect on Bayley developmental scores at 18 months of age— IPD meta-analysis of 4 large clinical trials. *J Pediatr Gastroenterol Nutr* 50(1): 79–84.

11. Beydoun, M.A., Fanelli Kuczmarski, M.T., Beydoun, H.A. et al. 2013. Omega-3 fatty acid intakes are inversely related to elevated depressive symptoms among United States women. *J Nutr* 143(11): 1743–1752.

12. Bloch, M.H. and Qawasmi, A. 2011. Omega-3 fatty acid supplementation for the treatment of children with attention-deficit/hyperactivity disorder symptomatology: Systematic review and meta-analysis. *J Am Acad Child Adolesc Psychiatry* 50(10): 991–1000.

13. Su, K.P., Pai, H.C., Yang, H.T. et al. 2014. Omega-3 fatty acids in the prevention of interferon-alpha-induced depression: Results from a randomized controlled trial. *Biol Psychiatry* 76(7): 559–566.

14. Mischoulon, D., Nierenberg, A.A., Schettler, P.J. et al. 2014. A double-blind, randomized controlled clinical trial comparing eicosapentaenoic acid versus docosahexaenoic acid for depression. *J Clin Psychiatry* 75(4): 370–376.

15. Rondanelli, M., Giacosa, A., Opizzi, A. et al. 2010. Effect of omega-3 fatty acids supplementation on depressive symptoms and on health-related quality of life in the treatment of elderly women with depression: A double-blind, placebo-controlled, randomized clinical trial. *J Am Coll Nutr* 29(1): 55–64.

16. Sallis, H., Steer, C., Paternoster, L. et al. 2014. Perinatal depression and omega-3 fatty acids: A Mendelian randomization study. *J Affect Disord* 166: 124–131.

17. Hibbeln, J.R. and Gow, R.V. 2014. The potential for military diets to reduce depression, suicide, and impulsive aggression: A review of current evidence for omega-3 and omega-6 fatty acids. *Military Med* 179(11 Suppl): 117–128.

18. Sinn, N., Milte, C., and Howe, P.R. 2010 Oiling the brain: A review of randomized controlled trials of omega-3 fatty acids in psychopathology across the lifespan. *Nutrients* 2(2): 128–170.

19. Meyer, B.J.l., Mann, N.J., Lewis, J.L. et al. 2003. Dietary intakes and food sources of omega-6 and omega-3 polyunsaturated fatty acids. *Lipids* 38(4): 391–398.

20. Naqvi, A.Z., Hasturk, H., Mu, L. et al. 2014. Docosahexaenoic acid and periodontitis in adults: A randomized controlled trial. *J Dent Res* 93(8): 767–773.

21. Grosso, G., Pajak, A., Marventano, S. et al. 2014. Role of omega-3 fatty acids in the treatment of depressive disorders: A comprehensive meta-analysis of randomized clinical trials. *PLoS One*, 9(5): e96905.

22. Bae, S.H., Park, H.S., Han, H.S. et al. 2014. Omega-3 polyunsaturated fatty acid for cholestasis due to bile duct paucity. *Pediatr Gastroenterol Hepatol Nutr* 17(2): 121–124.

23. Lotrich, F.E., Sears, B., and McNamara, R.K. 2013. Elevated ratio of arachidonic acid to long-chain omega-3 fatty acids predicts depression development following interferon-alpha treatment: Relationship with interleukin-6. *Brain Behav Immun* 31: 48–53.

24. Martin, S.S., Abd, T.T., Jones, S.R. et al. 2014. 2013 ACC/AHA cholesterol treatment guideline: What was done well and what could be done better. *J Am Coll Cardiol* 63(24): 2674–2678.

25. Boden, W.E. 2000. High-density lipoprotein cholesterol as an independent risk factor in cardiovascular disease: Assessing the data from Framingham to the Veterans Affairs High-Density Lipoprotein Intervention Trial. *Am J Cardiol* 86(12A): 19L–22L.

26. Atmaca, M., Kuloglu, M., Tezcan, E. et al. 2008. Serum leptin and cholesterol values in violent and nonviolent suicide attempters. *Psychiatry Res* 158(1): 87–91.

27. Vilibić, M., Jukić, V., Pandžić-Sakoman, M. et al. 2014. Association between total serum cholesterol and depression, aggression, and suicidal ideations in war veterans with posttraumatic stress disorder: A cross-sectional study. *Croat Med J* 55(5): 520–529.

28. Park, Y.M., Lee, B.H., and Lee, S.H. 2014. The association between serum lipid levels, suicide ideation, and central serotonergic activity in patients with major depressive disorder. *J Affect Disord* 159: 62–65.

29. Asellus, P., Nordström, P., and Jokinen, J. 2010 Cholesterol and CSF 5-HIAA in attempted suicide. *J Affect Disord* 125(1–3): 388–392.

30. Gagnon, C., Lu, Z.X., Magliano, D.J. et al. 2012. Low serum 25-hydroxyvitamin D is associated with increased risk of the development of the metabolic syndrome at five years: Results from a national, population-based prospective study (The Australian Diabetes, Obesity and Lifestyle Study: AusDiab). *J Clin Endocrinol Metab* 97(6): 1953–1961.

31. Muñoz-Aguirre, P., Flores, M., Macias, N. et al. 2014. The effect of vitamin D supplementation on serum lipids in postmenopausal women with diabetes: A randomized controlled trial. *Clin Nutr* 2014: Article ID S0261–5614(14)00254-4. doi:10.1016/j.clnu.2014.10.002.

32. Moran, L.J., Teede, H.J., and Vincent, A.J. 2015. Vitamin D is independently associated with depression in overweight women with and without PCOS. *Gynecol Endocrinol* 31(3): 179–182. doi:10.3109/095135 90.2014.975682.

33. Michikawa, T., Nishiwaki, Y., Nakano, M. et al. 2013. Higher serum dehydroepiandrosterone sulfate levels are protectively associated with depressive symptoms in men, but not in women: A community-based cohort study of older Japanese. *Am J Geriatr Psychiatry* 21(11): 1154–1163.

34. Papadopoulou, A., Markianos, M., Christodoulou, C. et al. 2013. Plasma total cholesterol in psychiatric patients after a suicide attempt and in follow-up. *J Affect Disord* 148(2–3): 440–443.

35. Bari, A., Eagle, D.M., Mar, A.C. et al. 2009. Dissociable effects of noradrenaline, dopamine, and serotonin uptake blockade on stop task performance in rats. *Psychopharmacology* (Berlin) 205(2): 273–283.

36. Gibbons, R.D., Hur, K., Brown, C.H. et al. 2012. Benefits from antidepressants: Synthesis of 6-week patient-level outcomes from double-blind placebo-controlled randomized trials of fluoxetine and venlafaxine. *Arch Gen Psychiatry* 69(6): 572–579. doi:10.1001/archgenpsychiatry.2011.2044.

37. Mischoulon, D., Price, L.H., Carpenter, L.L. et al. 2014. A double-blind, randomized, placebo-controlled clinical trial of S-adenosyl-L-methionine (SAMe) versus escitalopram in major depressive disorder. *J Clin Psychiatry* 75(4): 370–376.

38. Pegg, A.E. and McCann, P.P. 1988. Polyamine metabolism and function in mammalian cells and protozoans. *ISI Atlas of Sci: Biochem* 1: 11–18.

39. Holecek, M. 2002. Relation between glutamine, branched-chain amino acids, and protein metabolism. *Nutrition* 18(2): 130–133.

40. Ruhé, H.G., Mason, N.S., and Schene, A.H. 2007 Mood is indirectly related to serotonin, norepinephrine and dopamine levels in humans: A meta-analysis of monoamine depletion studies. *Mol Psychiatry* 12(4): 331–359.

41. Stan, A.D., Schirda, C.V., Bertocci, M.A. et al. 2014. Glutamate and GABA contributions to medial prefrontal cortical activity to emotion: Implications for mood disorders. *Psychiatry Res* 223(3): 253–260.

42. Pålsson, E., Jakobsson, J., Södersten, K. et al. 2015. Markers of glutamate signaling in cerebrospinal fluid and serum from patients with bipolar disorder and healthy controls. *Eur Neuropsychopharmacol* 25(1): 133–140. doi:10.1016/j.euroneuro.2014.11.001.

43. Wissmann, P., Geisler, S., Leblhuber, F. et al. 2013. Immune activation in patients with Alzheimer's disease is associated with high serum phenylalanine concentrations. *J Neurol Sci* 329(1–2): 29–33. doi:10.1016/j.jns.2013.03.007.

44. Luckose, F., Pandey, M.C., and Radhakrishna, K. 2015. Effects of amino acid derivatives on physical, mental and physiological activities. *Crit Rev Food Sci Nutr* 55(13): 1793–1807.

45. Iovieno, N., Dalton, E.D., Fava, M. et al. 2011. Second-tier natural antidepressants: Review and critique. *J Affect Disord* 130(3): 343–357. doi: 10.1016/j.jad.2010.06.010.

46. Papakostas, G.I., Petersen, T., Mischoulon, D. et al. 2004. Serum folate, vitamin B12, and homocysteine in major depressive disorder, Part 1: Predictors of clinical response in fluoxetine-resistant depression. *J Clin Psychiatry* 65(8): 1090–1095.

47. Gude, M.F., Bjerre-Kristensen, L., and Jensen, L.T. 2014. Fatal outcome after overdosage with antidepressants. *Ugeskr Laeger* 176(7A): 2–4.

48. Kang, K.H., Jeong, K.H., Baik, S.K. et al. 2011. Purple urine bag syndrome: Case report and literature review. *Clin Nephrol* 75(6): 557–559.

49. Papakostas, G.I., Petersen, T., Mischoulon, D. et al. 2004. Serum folate, vitamin B12, and homocysteine in major depressive disorder, Part 2: Predictors of relapse during the continuation phase of pharmacotherapy. *J Clin Psychiatry* 65(8): 1096–1098.

50. Sarris, J., Papakostas, G.I., Vitolo, O. et al. 2014. S-adenosyl methionine (SAMe) versus escitalopram and placebo in major depression RCT: Efficacy and effects of histamine and carnitine as moderators of response. *J Affect Disord* 164: 76–81.

51. Axon, A.T. 1986. Potential hazards of hypochlorhydria in the treatment of peptic ulcer. *Scand J Gastroenterol Suppl* 122: 17–21.

52. Pannala, A.S., Mani, A.R., Rice-Evans, C.A. et al. 2006. pH-dependent nitration of para-hydroxyphen-ylacetic acid in the stomach. *Free Radic Biol Med* 41(6): 896–901.

53. Penagini, R., Carmagnola, S., and Cantu, P. 2002. Review article: Gastro-oesophageal reflux disease—Pathophysiological issues of clinical relevance. *Aliment Pharmacol Ther* 16(Suppl 4): 65–71.

54. Ness-Abramof, R., Nabriski, D.A., Braverman, L.E. et al. 2006. Prevalence and evaluation of B12 defi-ciency in patients with autoimmune thyroid disease. *Am J Med Sci* 332(3): 119–122.

55. Boettcher, E. and Crowe, S.E. 2013. Dietary proteins and functional gastrointestinal disorders. *Am J Gastroenterol* 108(5): 728–736. doi: 10.1038/ajg.2013.97.

56. Park, H. 2014. An overview of eosinophilic esophagitis. *Gut Liver* 8(6): 590–597.

57. Hamzat, H., Sun, H., Ford, J.C. et al. 2012. Inappropriate prescribing of proton pump inhibitors in older patients. *Drugs Aging* 29(8): 681–690.

58. Grønli, O., Kvamme, J.M., Friborg, O. et al. 2013. Zinc deficiency is common in several psychiatric disorders. *PLoS One* 8(12): e82793.

59. Mosienko, V., Beis, D., Pasqualetti, M. et al. 2015. Life without brain serotonin: Reevaluation of serotonin function with mice deficient in brain serotonin synthesis. *Behav Brain Res* 277C: 78–88. doi:10.1016/j.bbr.2014.06.005.

60. Sato, S., Yanagida, N., Ogura, K. et al. 2014. Clinical studies in oral allergen-specific immunotherapy: Differences among allergens. *Int Arch Allergy Immunol* 164(1): 1–9.

61. Brown, D. and Wyon, M. 2014. The effect of moderate glycemic energy bar consumption on blood glu-cose and mood in dancers. *Med Probl Perform Art* 29(1): 27–31.

62. Shabbir, F., Patel, A., Mattison, C. et al. 2013. Effect of diet on serotonergic neurotransmission in depression. *Neurochem Int* 62(3): 324–329. doi:10.1016/j.neuint.2012.12.014.

11 Sex Steroids and Mood in Women

Ann Hathaway, MD

CONTENTS

INTRODUCTION

Integrative functional medicine incorporates a search for all factors impacting each individual's optimal health, and all factors that interfere are sought out and addressed. Included are social and psychological factors, genetic predispositions, optimal nutrient levels, as well as considerations of gastrointestinal (GI), immune, cardiovascular and mitochondrial function, metabolic and hormonal balancing, and infectious issues. In this chapter we narrow our focus to sex steroids in women— estrogen, progesterone, and testosterone—because these hormones are powerful tools that are often overlooked as potential therapies in both conventional and integrative medicine.

Clinical research demonstrates a significantly increased rate of depression in women compared to men beginning at puberty. While girls and boys suffer from mood disorders at the same rate, once a female passes through menarche her relative risk increases to approximately 2:1 compared with males.[1-4] Hence, many experts have hypothesized a relationship between female hormones and mood disorders, and a significant number of clinical trials and review papers have attempted to examine and elucidate this relationship. Clinicians know and research verifies that women are more vulnerable to mood disorders at three specific times of dramatic flux in sex steroid hormones[5]: (1) in the late luteal phase of the menstrual cycle, some women experience premenstrual syndrome (PMS) or the more severe premenstrual dysphoric disorder (PMDD); (2) immediately following childbirth, a significant number of women suffer from postpartum depression (PPD); (3) finally, at the climacteric, a significant subset of women experience perimenopausal depression and then postmenopausal depression (PMD).

One characteristic of all these events is a rapid fall in the estradiol level. It is further known that women who have suffered from PMS, PMDD, or PPD are at much greater risk of major depression at menopause.[6,7]

ESTROGEN AND PROGESTERONE

Multiple data streams suggest that lack of estrogen is implicated in the pathobiology of mood disorders. Basic science supports and clinical research demonstrates marked improvement in symptoms of depression, anxiety, irritability, cognitive impairment, and sleep deprivation when estradiol is supplemented at these times of rapid estrogen decline.[8-13]

A consensus of researchers conclude that progesterone is implicated as a cause in the pathophysiology of mood disorders in PMS and PMDD. However, some data show sleep benefits with progesterone, and some clinicians report benefits for their clients with high-dose progesterone use. Clinical trials will be reviewed later in this chapter showing benefit with estradiol treatment in PMS, PPD, and menopausal depression; benefits with testosterone; and potential negative and positive outcomes with progesterone. These data are particularly important because the extension of the human life span means that many women will live almost half of their lives in a postmenopausal state characterized by low estrogen, low progesterone, and reduced testosterone levels that may increase their risk of depression.

ALL HORMONES ARE NOT EQUAL

Research, the U.S. Food and Drug Administration (FDA) and popular press articles about estrogen, progesterone, and testosterone often have a major flaw. The type of hormone and the significant differences between them is obscured. Estrogen could be a synthetic, such as ethinyl estradiol found in oral contraceptives, or an animal product, such as conjugated equine estrogens used in oral menopausal formulations, or identical to human estradiol, the form most often used in transdermal patches for menopause. Conjugated equine estrogen (CEE) is derived from the urine of pregnant mares (Premarin and Prempro) and consists of 50%–70% estrone, 22%–32% equilin, and 7 or more other poorly characterized estrogens, none of which are found in the human female.[14] Estrogens behave very differently in the body, yet they are often lumped together for a risk or benefit discussion.

The method of delivery is also significant. If the estrogen is oral, its risk profile is higher; for example, oral estrogen will increase the risk of a blood clot or a stroke, whereas transdermal estrogen demonstrates no increased risk. Yet the method of delivery, or type of estrogen, is often omitted from conventional media pieces as well as the theoretically more precise research abstracts or FDA policy statements. Furthermore, the term *progesterone* will often be used when in fact a synthetic progestogen was studied. Conclusions that should only be applied to one particular synthetic will be applied to all synthetics and most unfortunately to progesterone, which refers only to that hormone that is identical to human progesterone. Testosterone has been available as a low-dose oral methyltestosterone (in combination with Premarin) for women in the United States for many years. However, methyltestosterone is known to have liver toxicity even in low doses.[15] Analysis of health issues potentially caused by methyltestosterone have delayed the availability of a topical bioidentical testosterone for women in the United States, while women in Canada and the European Union currently have access to an approved topical testosterone.

ENDOGENOUS ESTROGENS

There are three major human estrogens: estradiol, estrone, and estriol. Estradiol is the most potent estrogen, and it is important to note that women's estrogen brain receptors are specific to estradiol. Most estrogen-related basic research is done with estradiol, and it is the most significant estrogen with regard to mood. Estradiol, produced primarily in the theca and granulosa cells of the ovary, enters the brain through the blood-brain barrier. The highly lipophilic molecule crosses the lipid bilayer cell membrane and attaches to intracellular estrogen receptors. These estradiol-estrogen receptor complexes then diffuse into the cell nucleus and bind to specific estrogen-responsive DNA, thereby altering transcription. Estrogen receptors are of two known types—ER alpha and ER beta—both widely distributed in brain regions associated with mood and depression. ER alpha and ER beta have both overlapping and distinct functions, but the medical literature is not consistent in reporting on the specialized function of alpha versus beta receptors.

ESTROGEN AND MOOD

There are many evidence streams that point to a robust relationship between falling estrogen and depression or other negative mood effects. Additionally, a chronically lower level of estradiol is likely to be related to mood disorders in some premenopausal and postmenopausal women. For example, women with major depressive disorder (MDD) show 25% lower levels of estradiol at the midpoint of the menstrual cycle in a study by Holsen et al.,[16] and in another study women with MDD had a 30% lower estradiol level during the follicular phase of the menstrual cycle.[17]

Multiple researchers have found marked and rapid improvement in depressive symptoms with estradiol treatment in the postpartum[9,18] and menopausal phase of life.[8,19] Though there are only a few studies, improvement in PMS mood symptoms or PMDD symptoms with estradiol has been demonstrated.[10] We will review research in more detail for each of these estrogen-depleted phases. A significant body of research, some studies over 30 years old and others current work, demonstrates the neurobiological underpinnings that support these clinical findings.

NEUROBIOCHEMISTRY OF ESTROGEN AND MOOD

Basic science and mammalian animal models demonstrate that estradiol's impact on mood is mediated via multiple mechanisms. Virtually every neural pathway—serotonergic, dopaminergic (DA), noradrenergic, cholinergic, and gamma-aminobutyric (GABA)nergic—responds to estrogen.[20] The major mediator of estrogen's impact in the central nervous system (CNS) is the neurotransmitter serotonin. Although not fully addressing the heterogeneous nature of major depressive disorder, serotonin deficiency with other monoamine deficiencies comprise the oldest, most well-established causal theory of depression.[21] Estradiol is known to increase serotonin availability in the synapse and thereby enhance mood by several complex mechanisms, several of which will be described in the next section.

SEROTONIN AND ESTROGEN

A brief review of the pertinent neuroanatomy is helpful. Most of the brain's serotonin is produced in the dorsal raphe nuclei located in the brainstem. The dorsal raphe has a very high density of estrogen receptors identified on the serotonergic neurons in mammalian species.[22] Activation of estrogen receptors causes increased serotonin release.[22] Estradiol both increases the production and slows the breakdown of serotonin. First, it upregulates production of tryptophan hydroxylase (TPH), the rate-limiting enzyme in the synthesis of serotonin.[23] Both TPH and TPH mRNA levels are increased in the dorsal raphe nucleus.[24] Estradiol also diminishes serotonin catabolism by decreasing mono-amine oxidase-A, the enzyme that breaks down serotonin.[25]

Serotonin is transported from the dorsal raphe via multiple neural projections extending to cortical and limbic structures important in mood regulation, including the hippocampus, amygdala, anterior cingulate cortex, dorsolateral prefrontal cortex, and ventromedial cortex.[22] E2 stimulates a significant increase in the density of the serotonin-binding site known as 5-hydroxytryptamine2A (5-HTP2A) in various frontal cortical and limbic brain areas concerned with mood and emotion.[26]

Evidence suggests estradiol has a direct tonic effect through its receptors on the neurons in multiple brain regions highly associated with mood. The highest density of estradiol receptors in the brain are found in the amygdala, hippocampus, and hypothalamus in human postmortem studies.[27,28] Micro-anatomical growth is stimulated in these areas by estradiol. In animal models with low estrogen, estradiol administration increases the number of dendritic synapses in the amygdala[29] and the density of dendritic spines in hippocampal pyramidal neurons.[30] The evidence for serotonergic mechanisms for estradiol's positive mood effect is robust.

ADRENERGIC SYSTEM AND ESTROGEN

The adrenergic and dopaminergic neurotransmitter systems, well known to be involved in mood control, are also favorably impacted by estradiol. Estradiol positively modulates the norepinephrine (NE) brain system originating in the locus coeruleus (LC) with projections to multiple cortical and limbic structures implicated in mood.[20,27] NE neurons in the LC express moderate levels of both types of estrogen receptors, ER alpha and ER beta,[31] and estrogen increases the concentration of NE receptors.[32]

Estrogen is known to increase activity of the dopamine system both by upregulation of dopamine receptors[33] and by stimulating the synthesis and release of dopamine,[34] in some instances within seconds of estradiol exposure. Serotonin receptors populate dopamine neurons and create multiple points of interaction between estrogen, serotonin, and dopamine neurotransmission.

Estrogen also modulates the hypothalamic-pituitary-adrenal (HPA) axis and our physiologic response to stress. The hypothalamus has a high concentration of estradiol receptors and receives input from the serotonergic and other neurotransmitter systems. Other authors in this publication will more fully address the HPA axis and mood.

PROGESTERONE AND NEUROCHEMISTRY

Progesterone, produced in the ovaries, adrenals, and CNS, exerts neuropsychological and neuroprotective functions.[35,36] Progesterone's impact appears contradictory, as it can be beneficial or detrimental, possibly depending on concentration of progesterone, concentration of progesterone metabolites, progesterone-to-estradiol ratios, or variations in individual neurochemistry and other unknowns.[37–39] Progesterone is known to have anxiolytic and sleep-enhancing beneficial effects, but has also been shown to have paradoxical anxiogenic and dysphoric effects in multiple well-controlled studies.[37,40] A highly lipid soluble molecule, progesterone has multiple metabolites. The major mediator of CNS effects is not the classic progesterone molecule, rather the progesterone metabolites, allopregnanolone (ALLO) and pregnenolone, are responsible.[41] The most neuroactive metabolite, ALLO, is a GABA agonist. The primary inhibitory neurotransmitter system, the GABAnergic, is widely distributed in the CNS and is an important regulator of stress, anxiety, vigilance, alertness, and seizures.[42] The action of ALLO on GABA receptors has been shown to mediate both the calming, insomnia-reducing effects, and also the anxiety and negative mood effects.[37,41,43] ALLO binds to the GABA receptor and changes its configuration, thus rendering it resistant to further activation, which can decrease central GABA-mediated inhibition and result in anxiety, depression, and irritability.[37,43] Additional mechanisms for progesterone-related negative mood impact involve the serotonergic system. Progesterone decreases platelet serotonin uptake, which decreases serotonin availability and can lower mood.[44,45] It is also observed that increased luteal phase ALLO inhibits serotonin release in the dorsal raphe, amygdala, and hippocampus, which can result in dysphoria and increased anxiety.[46–48] Progesterone also lowers serotonin and potentially diminishes mood by increasing monoamine oxidase (MAO), the enzyme that breaks down serotonin.[39,49]

PREMENSTRUAL SYNDROME

Premenstrual syndrome (PMS), occurring during the luteal phase of the menstrual cycle, often includes depression, mood swings, anxiety, irritability, self-deprecation, aggression, poor impulse control, and decreased pain threshold, and affects up to 20% of women between menarche and menopause.[39,50,51] PMS symptoms peak in the last 5 days of the luteal phase and often resolve at the onset of menses, but may persist until day 4 of the next cycle. Premenstrual dysphoric disorder (PMDD), a moderately to severely disabling mood disorder, as defined by the American Psychiatric Association, impacts 3%–8% of women.[50,52]

Following ovulation, progesterone is produced in the corpus luteum of the ovary, and production continues until the end of the menstrual cycle when it rapidly declines. Estradiol levels peak in late follicular phase and fall throughout the luteal phase, and both estradiol and progesterone may be important in the pathophysiology of PMS and PMDD. There are divergent opinions on the hormonal cause(s) of PMS, and it is possible that subgroups of women have PMS symptoms related to different hormonal imbalances. Low estrogen may be the cause in some women, progesterone the cause in others, and the ratio of estrogen to progesterone the cause in others.

PROGESTERONE AS A CAUSE OF PMS

A consensus of peer-reviewed published research concludes that endogenous progesterone is implicated in the pathophysiology of diminished mood in PMS and PMDD.[53] Multiple valid trials support the theory that progesterone or its metabolites are the cause of mood disruption in women with enhanced sensitivity to progesterone.[38–40] During anovulatory cycles when a corpus luteum fails to develop, PMS symptoms do not occur.[54] A Swedish study demonstrated a strong relationship between increased symptom severity in an individual woman and a higher progesterone concentration in that specific month, as well as decreased severity of symptoms associated with a lower progesterone concentration for the same woman in another specific month.[55] Women with PMS are also intolerant of the synthetic progestins in oral contraceptives and can develop continuous rather than cyclical depressive symptoms on oral contraceptive pills (OCPs).[56,57] Some research suggests that oral contraceptives containing the synthetic progestogen drospirenone are better tolerated by some women with PMS, which emphasizes the point that all progestins are not the same, and synthetic progestins are very different from progesterone. Very minor differences in a molecule can result in major changes in outcome.[58]

Estradiol peaks in late follicular phase, then drops substantially, next increases by a lesser degree, and then a second drop occurs as luteal phase progresses,[59,60] reaching the lowest levels at menses, resulting in decreases in serotonin activity via multiple previously described mechanisms. Van Goozen et al. studied estradiol and progesterone levels in women with and without PMS symptoms, and found significant differences among them. The no PMS group had higher estradiol levels during all segments of their cycle and higher estradiol-to-progesterone ratios during follicular, ovulatory, and mid-luteal phases. Progesterone levels did not differ significantly in this study.[61]

A placebo-controlled trial of a high-dose estradiol patch (200 mcg) in women with severe PMS substantially reduced premenstrual anxiety, irritability, and depression on validated questionnaires for three cycles. In this study the women were also given 8 days of a synthetic progestin, norethindrone, during each cycle to provoke shedding of the endometrium, and mood changes were not noted during the progestin phase.[62] Mood improvement is thought to result from the suppression of ovulation preventing the progesterone surge. Also, given the known mood-enhancing effects of estradiol, beneficial mood effects directly due to increased estradiol or increased estradiol-to-progesterone ratio must be considered. It is biologically plausible that a smaller increase in estradiol, such as 50 mcg transdermal, may result in relief from PMS in some women, via mechanisms previously described resulting in increased CNS serotonin effect.

PROGESTERONE MAY IMPROVE PMS

The opposite point of view, that progesterone insufficiency causes PMS, has been proposed since the 1970s by some authors and clinicians. Progesterone supplementation by skin cream application has been recommended, and many thousands of women have purchased progesterone cream, available over the counter, and many have noted benefits.[63] Some practitioners and well-known online sites continue to recommend treatment of PMS with topical progesterone, sometimes in very high doses, and report significant benefits for their patients.[64,65] A Cochrane database systems review published in 2009 determined that there is no reliable evidence to support this claim and stated that the research to date neither proves nor disproves progesterone's efficacy.[66] This is still true: there are no controlled trials that meet criteria for a valid study, meaning that the hypothesis has not been effectively examined. This is an area where there is marked disagreement between practitioners.

Progesterone's potential benefits do have biological plausibility given that basic research demonstrates anxiolytic and sleep-enhancing benefits via progesterone's metabolites at certain doses. Swedish research on progesterone/ALLO effects demonstrates anxiety-generating effects at concentrations seen in luteal phase, whereas higher concentrations show beneficial calming effects.[67] The mood symptoms are related to the allopregnanolone and progesterone serum concentrations in a manner similar to an inverted U-shaped curve. Negative mood symptoms occur when the serum concentration of allopregnanolone is similar to endogenous luteal phase levels, while at both very low and high concentrations there is less effect or improvement.[38,68]

The doses recommended by Women to Women's website and others for PMS are high; for example, doses are suggested up to 100 mg applied topically three times daily.[64] Others recommend only 20–40 mg topically once or twice daily.[65] A study comparing oral and topical progesterone in postmenopausal women showed similar plasma levels in women on 200 mg oral progesterone per day and women on 80 mg daily of topical progesterone.[69] A well-controlled Swedish study demonstrated negative mood and anxiety effects in postmenopausal women on 400 mg vaginal progesterone per day for a portion of each month; however, no negative mood effects were experienced by the same women at 800 mg/day, lending some credence to the position that some women with PMS may respond positively to doses higher than those usually recommended or studied in research trials.[67]

Another possible mechanism to consider for progesterone's beneficial effects at higher doses is the effects of downstream metabolites in the steroid synthesis pathway (see Figure 11.1). Progesterone metabolizes into cortisol and cortisone, which may counter some of the negative effects, and progesterone also can metabolize into testosterone, which can further metabolize into estradiol and estrone. The possible downstream steroid metabolites have not been measured in these studies. Estradiol and testosterone may improve mood and lower anxiety via previously discussed mechanisms.

ESTROGEN DOMINANCE

The term *estrogen dominance*, commonly used by integrative practitioners, has no precise definition and is of complex origin. A consensus of authors in the integrative health community view this as a relative lack of progesterone with any estrogen level, high, normal, or low, resulting in adverse symptoms such as breast tenderness, fatigue, and low mood or anxiety, which may be continuous or confined to the luteal phase.[70]

Excess estrogen activity may be a valid aspect of the problems in the complex known as estrogen dominance. For some premenopausal women, cycles become anovulatory characterized by

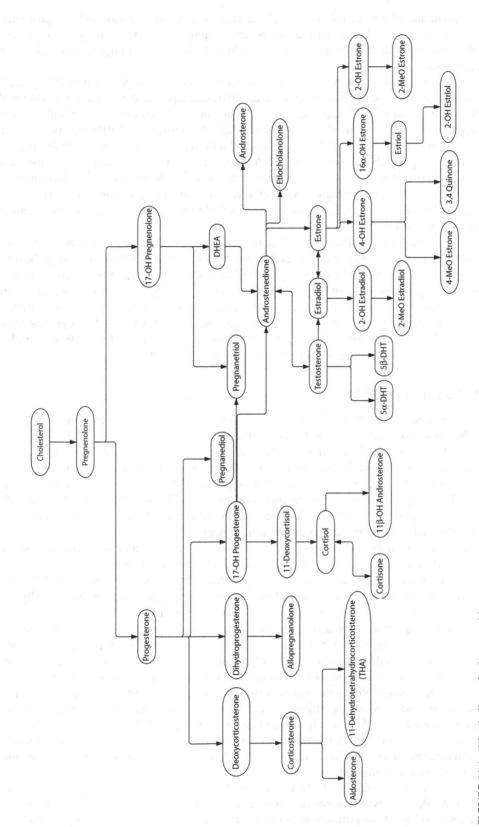

FIGURE 11.1 Metabolism of select steroids.

persistent ovarian and adipose estrogen production and the absence of ovulation-induced progesterone production. Mid-luteal plasma estrogen levels remain high with very low progesterone levels. Some of these women will develop insomnia or anxiety, which will often improve with topical or oral progesterone.

Excess estrogenic activity can result from xenoestrogens such as Bisphenol A (BPA), phthalates, and other chemical additives found in food, cosmetics, and packaging. They are in a class of chemicals known as endocrine disrupters, can act as ongoing abnormal estrogenic stimulants, and are implicated in excess estrogenic effects.[71] Recent studies demonstrate that BPA may be as potent as estradiol in stimulating some cellular responses,[72–74] and that these effects occur at levels at or below the currently acceptable daily exposure. BPA has been shown to bind to nonclassical estrogen membrane receptors and to act through nongenomic pathways.[74–76] Some phthalates, including di-n-butyl phthalate (DBP), act as estrogens in cell cultures, and can bind to estrogen receptors (ERs), induce estrogen-appropriate cellular responses, and act additively with endogenous estrogens in altering biological systems.[77,78]

Xenoestrogens may be one of the causes of the increased rate of premature menarche in girls and the feminization of some male animal species. Excess reabsorption of estrogens from an unhealthy GI tract, due to dysbiosis-induced high beta-glucuronidase activity, may also create an imbalance with relative estrogen to progesterone excess in some women. Again, this may lend weight to the proposal that some women with PMS or excess estrogenic effects may benefit from natural progesterone in various doses. However, many important questions remain, such as, Does progesterone help a subset of PMS women? How do we identify the women most likely to benefit from estradiol or progesterone? What dosage ranges or plasma levels should be targeted?

POSTPARTUM DEPRESSION

In pregnancy estrogens are produced in very high concentrations. Postpartum estradiol levels drop dramatically, and this decrease is believed to play a role in postpartum depression (PPD). Depression impacts 10%–16% of women in the first 3 months and up to 22% in the first 6 months postpartum.[79] Cox et al. found a threefold increase in risk of depression in the first month after childbirth compared to nonchildbearing women.[80] Although most postnatal depression resolves spontaneously within 6 months, longitudinal studies show that approximately 25% of affected mothers are still depressed at the child's first birthday. Follow-up of children of women with postnatal depression shows delayed social development and cognitive impairment.[81–83]

Selective serotonin reuptake inhibitors (SSRIs) are considered an acceptable treatment by some, yet they have a delayed onset of 2–3 weeks and limited long-term safety data. SSRIs are excreted into breast milk, and some studies suggest increased behavioral problems in exposed children.[84] Despite methodological problems in some studies, there is evidence that estradiol successfully and rapidly resolves depressive symptom in a significant number of women with PPD.

In Gregoire's 1996 study, 61 women with postpartum depression were randomly assigned to 6 months of placebo or 3 months of 200 mcg transdermal estradiol patches, followed by 3 months with added cyclical synthetic progestin. Statistically significant reductions in depressive symptoms were apparent after 1 month and continued at 3 months of topical estradiol treatment compared with placebo.[9] Abatement of symptoms was rapid, with many women reporting resolution in the first week of treatment, and response was sustained over 5 months. Nearly half of the women had been on antidepressant medication for 6 weeks with no benefit prior to estradiol therapy and had the same significant improvement on estradiol as the women not on antidepressants. The placebo group did improve with time; however, their scores did not drop below the range for major depressive disorder until after a minimum of 4 months.

In 2001 Ahokas et al. studied 23 women recruited from a psychiatric emergency unit with major depressive disorder with postpartum onset. Serum estradiol concentrations were measured at baseline and weekly. Mean estradiol level before treatment was very low, 21 pg/mL, and 16 of

23 women met criteria for gonadal failure. Sublingual estradiol was administered for 8 weeks at the dose necessary to increase the serum estradiol level to 109 pg/mL, approximately 30%–50% of the mean peak levels seen in normal menstrual cycles. The average sublingual dose given was 4.8 mg. Depressive symptoms diminished rapidly and significantly in the first week, and depression scores were consistent with clinical recovery in 19 of 23 of the patients.[18]

Successful resolution of postpartum depression has been demonstrated with both topical and sublingual estradiol at doses that approximate physiologic menstrual cycle subpeak levels. These studies were done in 1996 and 2001, and in 2015 estradiol is still considered a novel treatment; unfortunately, further research has not been pursued. Further safety and efficacy studies are needed to determine optimal dose and serum levels and to pursue more rigorous safety data. This promising therapy may improve quality of life for mothers and their children and may be life-saving for some women.

MENOPAUSAL HORMONE REPLACEMENT AND MOOD

Perimenopausal women report mood disturbances three times more often than premenopausal women.[85,86] The proportion of women experiencing depressive symptoms ranges from 15% to 50%[87] and depressive disorders such as major depression and bipolar disorder from 15% to 30%.[88,89] Anxiety is also increased.[90,91] Women who have experienced severe PMS, PMDD, or postpartum depression are at higher risk for significant mood problems at menopause.[6,7,92] However, there is also a risk for a first time episode of depression or severe anxiety.[94] Depression that begins at menopause may be persistent.[95] Depression is associated not only with a decreased quality of life but also with cognitive decline and other functional disabilities.[17,95,96]

A majority of women experience some degree of climacteric symptoms such as hot flashes, night sweats, palpitations, and sleep disturbances, all of which can take a toll on quality of life and impact mood. Negative psychological changes at menopause may not be appreciated as depression or anxiety by some women or their clinicians. Symptoms such as loss of motivation, loss of self-esteem, or loss of interest in sex, may be interpreted as the normal impact of losses or aging. Some have speculated that depression at menopause comes from a domino effect: hot flashes and night sweats cause discomfort, sleep disturbance, and fatigue, resulting in diminished quality of life, and then diminished mood as a natural consequence. While this may be a plausible mechanism, research shows that even when sleep and hot flashes are normalized, an increased incidence of depression persists.[89,92]

For most women in the reproductive phase of life, plasma estradiol seldom drops below 90 and averages above 200 pg/mL, with variation from 70 to 490 pg/mL. After menopause, E2 levels generally drop below 30 pg/mL and are often below 10 pg/mL. Levels are often less than 10% of premenopausal levels, and the levels trend lower in depressed women.[97–99] Estrone (E1) diminishes but does not drop as precipitously, because aromatase enzymes continue to convert adrenal androgens to estrone in adipose tissue, making estrone the dominant form of estrogen following menopause.[98] Estradiol, however, is more favorable for mood and cognition, not estrone, because the central nervous system receptors are sensitive to the estradiol form of estrogen.

Studies examining estrogen and progesterone replacement for menopausal mood disorders show variable results. As many authors point out, the problem with interpretation of the human clinical studies is that there are a great number of variables: the type and dose of estrogen, the route of delivery, the addition of a synthetic progestin or actual progesterone, the dose of the progestin, the continuous or sequential use of a progestin, and the stage of menopause when a woman is treated. All of these questions will require a great deal more research for full elucidation.

For menopausal therapy estrogens are most commonly delivered as topical estradiol, oral estradiol, or oral conjugated equine estrogens (CEEs). E2 is available as an oral tablet, transdermal patch, gel, or cream. Transdermal estradiol has many advantages over oral estrone-dominant preparations. Oral estrogens are subject to extensive hepatic metabolism with increased medical risks, and transdermal E2 preparations are not. Because transdermal estradiol is not subject to first-pass liver effects, it does not markedly increase the estrogen carrier protein, sex hormone binding globulin (SHBG) as oral E1 does, so the resultant free E2 concentrations are higher and the favorable impact on mood is more pronounced and more stable.[98,99] Furthermore, due to bypassing hepatic circulation, a more favorable ratio of about 1:1 of estradiol to estrone results from topical E2, which is closer to the premenopausal ratio. Conversely, oral high estrone preparations, such as CEE, result in E1 to E2 ratios of about 5–7:1.[97] Multiple trials have shown successful mood improvement with transdermal E2, while most studies utilizing oral CEE failed to demonstrate a positive mood effect.

Studies consistently point to the fact that estradiol delivered topically results in improvements in mood in both peri- and postmenopausal women with depression and anxiety.[100] Topical estradiol alleviates depressive symptoms even when depression is the only symptom. Oral estradiol has far fewer studies, and mood results are inconsistent. Oral conjugated equine estrogens, a high estrone combination, as well as other estrone sources, show mood benefit in a few studies, but most results are negative.[99] Of 16 studies summarized by Toffol et al. in a 2014 review testing efficacy of estrogen therapy for treatment of menopausal mood disorders of varying severity, transdermal estradiol, without a progestin, showed the greatest benefit, with four out of five studies showing improvement or resolution.[12,99] In two studies using oral estradiol, one showed improvement in depressive symptoms, and one did not.[102,103] Oral conjugated equine estrogens, a high estrone combination, and other oral estrone sources demonstrated mood benefit in only three out of nine studies reviewed by Toffol et al.[99]

The transdermal estradiol studies include a 2000 trial by Schmidt et al. with depressed perimenopausal women randomized in a double-blind parallel design, administered estradiol 50 mcg or placebo for 3 weeks, then crossed over to the other treatment. After 3 weeks there was partial or full remission of depressive symptoms observed in 80% of the treatment group, independent of its effects on vasomotor symptoms, but only 22% of the placebo group.[100] In 2001 Soares et al. demonstrated similar findings using a prospective placebo-controlled double-blind design with estradiol by transdermal patch, 100 mcg, in 50 perimenopausal women diagnosed with a varied severity of mood disorders, major depression, minor depression, and dysthymia. After 12 weeks there was resolution of depressive symptoms in 60% of the women treated with estradiol and in only 20% of the control group. Similar results were seen with oral estradiol at 0.3 mg per day in another well-controlled study of perimenopausal women with major depressive disorder.[8] An oral estradiol study in women over 70 years old with depression and anxiety symptoms failed to show benefit, and it may be important to initiate estrogen treatment in the earlier phase of menopause to obtain benefit.[103] However, it is also possible that transdermal application, higher doses, or longer treatment would have had a positive outcome in older women.

Topical estradiol appears to be the better choice for estrogen replacement. However, dosing is a complex issue with each woman. Individuals will absorb and metabolize estradiol at rates that may vary significantly. In addition, because of neurochemical and hormonal variations between women, it is highly probable, though not well researched, that individual women will have optimal well-being at different doses and serum levels. Hence, an optimal approach relies on patients being well-educated about their hormonal choices, self-monitoring the effects of a given dose, and reporting back to the physician who can then make ongoing adjustments to maximize benefit and minimize risk.

PROGESTERONE IN MENOPAUSE

Progesterone, in either a synthetic or a natural form, is a required component of menopausal hormone replacement unless a woman has undergone hysterectomy, to prevent uterine endometrial hyperplasia that can progress to endometrial cancer. Estrogens stimulate the growth of the endometrium, and progesterone reverses the possible overstimulation and decreases the cancer risk.

Most menopausal research has been done on a single synthetic progestin, medroxyprogesterone (Provera®), because it has been the most prescribed menopausal progestin in the United States and in many other developed countries. Most studies confirm a negative effect for mood when MPA or one of several other synthetic progestins is part of the menopausal hormone treatment.[104–106]

In the review by Toffol et al., seven out of nine studies that included a progestin showed no benefit or worsening of mood.[99] In mood studies when progestins are given continuously, the beneficial effects of estrogen often are negated, and when given part time, the benefits are most often seen to decline during the progestin phase of treatment and improvement in mood is most marked during the phase off of progestin.[108,109]

Unfortunately, there is a deficiency of research utilizing supplementation identical to human progesterone. In some women, progesterone supplementation results in lower anxiety and improves sleep.[67,106] Eighty percent of women experienced improvement in anxiety and depressive symptoms when switched from medroxyprogesterone to oral micronized progesterone.[107] However, in some studies bioidentical progesterone used orally or topically has been demonstrated to result in a depressed mood in a subset of women.[67,68] This is consistent with the previously mentioned studies reporting that PMS mood changes are due to progesterone produced in the luteal phase of the menstrual cycle.

It is well known that during the progesterone phase of sequential hormone replacement therapy (HRT) many women experience negative mood changes and unpleasant physical symptoms, similar to those encountered in premenstrual syndrome.[109–113] In women who have a history of PMS, there is increased sensitivity to the negative impact of synthetic progestins.[114] For some women, even a bioidentical progesterone replacement at menopause prescribed in low doses can result in negative mood effect.[67,68] Hence, it is important to consider different dosage and sequencing strategies for individual women.

In women with poor progesterone tolerance, some authors have used vaginal suppositories at very high doses, 800 mg per day, and found no diminished mood in the same women who did not tolerate 200 to 400 mg vaginal suppository doses.[67] This may support recommendations by some physicians who advise a trial of very high dose topical progesterone for treatment of PMS. This seemingly paradoxical effect may be based on the steroid biosynthesis pathway (see Figure 11.1), and the possibility that the downstream products of very high dose progesterone could be very different from those of the low or moderate dose products. High-dose progesterone may produce significant increases in cortisone, testosterone, and estrogen, and this could then negate the negative GABAnergic mood impact.

Alternatively, for women intolerant of progesterone, a strategy of a very limited number of days of moderate dose progesterone, such as 200 mg per day for 12 days every 3 months, may provide a solution for those women with poor progesterone tolerance who need reversal of the endometrial proliferative effects of estrogen. Because of poorly understood hormonal and neurochemical interactions and their uniqueness in individual women, various treatment strategies should be considered and instituted on a trial basis and then adjusted over time. Again, patient education about the possible positive or negative impacts of treatment, with self-monitoring of results, and regular readjustments of dose are required for maximum benefits and quality of life.

TESTOSTERONE, MOOD, AND SEXUAL FUNCTION

Some evidence supports the theory that testosterone's mood impact is optimal in a mid-range concentration, with negative effects at both the very high or very low end of the range in women.[115,116] There is a substantial consensus in research and reviewers of the clinical literature that many late reproductive age and postmenopausal women experience symptoms caused by androgen deficiency, and that these symptoms are alleviated by testosterone therapy.[117,118] Affected women complain of fatigue, low libido, fewer satisfactory sexual experiences, and diminished well-being, symptoms easily and frequently attributed to psychosocial and environmental factors. When such symptoms occur in the setting of low circulating bioavailable testosterone, testosterone replacement results in significant improvement in symptomatology and, hence, quality of life for a majority of women.[118–120]

Androgens refer to a group of related hormones including testosterone, dihydrotestosterone, andro-stenedione, and androstenediol. Testosterone is the most prevalent of the androgens in both males and females, and testosterone and androgen deficiency or administration will be used interchange-ably in this chapter.

Although symptoms associated with low testosterone are reported in 52% of menopausal women and 39% of premenopausal women, there is no approved testosterone therapy for women available in the United States.[122,123,125] Approved topical testosterone products have been available for women in Canada since 2002 and in the European Union since 2007. The FDA cites safety concerns regard-ing breast cancer and cardiovascular risk as the reasons for nonapproval of the testosterone patches and testosterone gels proposed for treatment of women. In 2011 the FDA advisory committee to the division of Reproductive and Urologic Drug Products stated that hypoactive sexual desire disorder (HSDD) is a significant medical condition for women, opening the door for medical treatments to be considered a higher priority. HSDD is defined as a persistent deficiency of sexual desire resulting in marked personal distress or interpersonal difficulty.[124] The prevalence of HSDD is estimated to be between 8% and 26% and is highest among surgically menopausal women.[126]

Total and free testosterone levels decline with age in premenopausal women such that women in their forties have half the circulating hormonal levels of women in their twenties.[127]

There is not a dramatic drop at menopause, but levels continue to decline with diminishing adre-nal and ovarian androgen production with increasing age.[128,129] Approximately 99% of circulating testosterone is bound to sex hormone-binding globulin (SHBG), and estrogen therapy, especially oral estrogen, will increase SHBG resulting in lower free and bioavailable testosterone, while insu-lin, obesity, and menopause can each result in lower SHBG and slightly increased free testosterone. In the decade preceding menopause, there is loss of the mid-cycle surge of free testosterone and androstenedione.[130] Thus the proposed clinical manifestations of female androgen insufficiency—namely, loss of libido, lowered mood, fatigue—may precede menopause, and decline may continue after natural menopause.[117,127] Women who undergo bilateral oophorectomy sustain a 40%–50% decline in total and free testosterone levels compared to age-matched pre- and postmenopausal controls.[131]

Published studies demonstrate beneficial effects of testosterone on sexual function,[132–134] includ-ing a Cochrane Review meta-analysis,[134] and improved mood and well-being in surgically or naturally postmenopausal women, as well as in premenopausal women in their later reproductive years.[117–119,134,135]

In the 1980s Sherwin demonstrated improved mood and sexual satisfaction in post-oophorec-tomy women using intramuscular injections of testosterone and estrogen, testosterone alone, or estrogen alone.[131] Several other trials in the 1980s showed psychological and sexual benefit in natu-rally menopausal women using implants of estrogen and testosterone.[134,135] The disadvantages of this method were the supra-physiologic levels in the early weeks of treatment followed by a gradual decrease to subtherapeutic levels and loss of benefit over the duration of the trial, as well as the need to return to a medical provider for repeated and painful injections. Further trials with implant and oral testosterone, when added to estrogen, confirmed benefits for libido and sexual function. A 2005 Cochrane Review meta-analysis concurred.[134]

Shifren et al. conducted the first randomized, double-blinded placebo-controlled study of a trans-dermal testosterone patch.[117] Surgically induced menopausal women aged 31–56 years with self-reported impaired sexual function and taking oral estrogen therapy were the study group. Women with a previously active and satisfying sex life who reported a decrease in sexual satisfaction follow-ing surgery, and who preferred their preoperative state, were identified as having impaired sexual function. The 75 participants were randomly assigned to one of three 12-week treatment condi-tions: 150 mcg/day testosterone patch, 300 mcg/day testosterone patch, or placebo. Women receiv-ing 300 mcg/day of testosterone reported significantly higher scores for libido, pleasure and orgasm with sex, and greater frequency of sexual activity, than those in the lower testosterone group and placebo. The higher testosterone group also showed significant improvement in well-being, vitality, depressed mood, and anxiety compared with placebo. Because of aromatization of testosterone to estradiol and estrone, it is possible that the improvements in psychological well-being were in part due to an increase in estradiol levels.

In Goldstat's 2003 double-blind placebo-controlled crossover study of premenopausal women with low sexual desire and low sexual function, both psychological well-being and sexual satisfaction were examined endpoints.[119] Validated questionnaires were used for the assessments. The mean baseline testosterone was 30 ng/dL, falling in the lower third of the normal range. Administered was 10 mg of 1% topical testosterone for two 12-week periods with a 4-week washout between groups on testosterone versus placebo. The testosterone levels increased by a mean of 44 ng/dL in the treatment group, staying in the normal premenopausal range; testosterone increased by 6.2 ng/dL in the placebo group. Significant improvements were seen in all variables scored for the Psychological General Well-Being Index, including improved mood, lower anxiety, and increased positive well-being, self-confidence, vitality, and general health in the group on testosterone. By comparison there was a significant decrease in the well-being index for the women on placebo. On an established Sexual Self-Rating Scale, 46% of women achieved a 50% increase in their sexual satisfaction rating on the testosterone treatment, compared with 19% in the placebo group. No increased hirsutism, acne, or deepening of voice occurred. Davis's 2008 study of late reproductive age women showed only a small increase in satisfactory sexual events in the treatment group compared to the placebo group. However, in this self-reported study there was a large beneficial placebo effect making interpretation challenging. Hypertrichosis at the application site was the only side effect of any significance.[120] Women in the United States need access to a long awaited reliable and safe testosterone therapy for sexual dysfunction.

TESTOSTERONE SAFETY CONCERNS

Safety concerns are responsible for the lack of available testosterone replacement for women in the United States. Long-term studies demonstrating no increased cardiovascular and breast cancer risks are required and underway. In lieu of approved testosterone, women are prescribed lower doses of topical testosterone products designed for men and compounded formulations of topical testosterone.

A large case-controlled study reported a substantial increased breast cancer risk in women using a fixed-dose oral CEE 1.25 mg plus methyltestosterone 2.5 mg. This is an additional case where the replacement molecule, methyltestosterone, is distinctly altered from endogenously produced testosterone, yielding less favorable results. Methyltestosterone not only is subject to first-pass liver effects but is also known to be hepatotoxic, even in low doses, when given over a long period of time.[136] In contrast there is a large body of work of various kinds demonstrating reduced risk or unchanged breast cancer risk profiles for implants, injections, and topical testosterone.[137–139] In an Australian study of 508 postmenopausal women on HRT, participants using testosterone reported a lower incidence of breast cancer than women on HRT without testosterone.[138] Data from in vitro studies show androgens have apoptotic and antiproliferative effects on breast tissue, and in animal models androgens inhibit breast cancer growth.[139] Patients with polycystic ovary syndrome (PCOS) and high testosterone do not have an increased breast cancer risk, and in female-to-male transgenderism where large doses of testosterone are given to genetic females, there is no increase in breast cancer or cardiovascular disease.[139] Prospective studies do not support a causal role for testosterone in cardiovascular events.[140] A 12.3-year population-based study suggests optimal health at mid ranges and that very low or very high bioavailable testosterone levels may increase cardiovascular risk.[141] Oral forms of testosterone reduce HDL levels, whereas transdermal T has no effect.[142] No increase in fibrinogen, other pro-coagulants, viscosity, or polycythemia was seen in transdermal T, or T implant studies.[142] An ongoing large safety study, in preliminary reports, shows no significant increased risks to date with transdermal testosterone, and this may resolve residual safety concerns and allow approval of a women's testosterone supplement.[143]

SAFETY AND RISK BENEFIT WITH HORMONES

The Women's Health Initiative Study of 2002 and 2004 and many subsequent reports have dramatically changed the face of menopausal hormone replacement.[144,145] Because of the double-blind placebo-controlled high quality, the size (approximately 16,000 women and 16,000 controls in arm one, and approximately 8000 women and 8000 controls in arm two), the scope of end-points examined (breast cancer, osteoporosis, stroke, deep vein thrombosis [DVT] and other cardiovascular risks), this study has had a major impact on all estrogen- and progesterone-related risk benefit analyses and has changed the way major portions of the public think about hormones. Arm one of the study was carried out with Premarin (equine estrogens), with Provera (medroxy-progesterone) as Prempro versus placebo, and was halted early at 5.2 years for ethical reasons, due to an increased rate of adverse outcomes. The headlines were big and bold: hormones cause breast cancer and do not protect against heart disease. Arm two of the study continued for an additional 2 years, and the decrease in breast cancer on Premarin alone, and other additional benefits, were barely noted by the media. The gynecological community and the pharmaceutical companies did pay attention, and some benefits followed in new forms of menopausal replacement hormones. Oral bioidentical progesterone began to replace synthetic MPA. Estradiol patches and gels for the skin proliferated because evidence mounted that topical estradiol, by avoiding first-pass liver effects, did not increase risk of clotting, DVTs, strokes, or other cardiovascular risks. Unfortunately, the vast majority of women and the nongynecologic physician community are not well-versed in these important distinctions. The FDA requires the same warning label on all estrogens whether horse-derived, synthetic, or identical to human, whether oral, topical, or vaginal. This denies women accurate risk-to-benefit information.

BREAST CANCER

It has become axiomatic in the general public and some of the medical community that estrogen replacement at menopause causes increased risk of breast cancer. Some women choose to avoid estrogen replacement at menopause or are advised to avoid it because of this fear; however, this fear may be unfounded. Three studies were very influential in creating this belief. The Million Woman Study,[146] The Women's Health Initiative (WHI) Estrogen plus Progestin trial,[144] and the Collaborative Study.[147] In an exhaustive four-part review of the scientific validity of these studies, Shapiro and colleagues found major methodological flaws in all three and reported that they neither prove nor disprove that estrogen or estrogen plus progesterone increases risk of breast cancer.[148–150] Shapiro states that significant detection bias was not excluded, that the statistical data was inconclusive for both lack of stability and strength, that confounding of variables was present, and that biological plausibility was not established in any of the studies. In Shapiro's evaluation of the unopposed estrogen (oral CEE) arm of the WHI, he agrees with the WHI's conclusion that oral CEE alone does not increase the risk of breast cancer, and may even reduce it.[151] WHI's researchers found that estrogen (CEE) used alone by postmenopausal women with prior hysterectomy decreased the risk of breast cancer by 7 women per 10,000 per year compared with women on placebo. An updated WHI report in 2012, after tracking women for an additional 10.7 years, found that women in the conjugated equine estrogen only group showed a statistically significant 23% lower risk of invasive breast cancer than those who took a placebo.[152]

Additionally, CEE alone did not interfere with mammography screening by increasing breast density as seen in the CEE + MPA arm of WHI.[145,152] The WHI reports that the CEE plus MPA arm of the study showed an increase in breast cancer of 8 women per 10,000 per year compared to women on placebo.[144] If there is a causal agent for breast cancer based on the WHI data, medroxy-progesterone (Provera®), Provera, appears the likely candidate. A recent smaller study, the Kronos Early Estrogen Prevention Study (KEEPS), shows that bioidentical oral progesterone (commercially available as Prometrium® or generic progesterone) is likely to be safer than MPA and that topical estradiol is a safer choice than oral.[153]

In 2012 KEEPS reported their finding on a 4-year double-blind placebo-controlled trial of approximately 730 postmenopausal women, most of them in the early stages of menopause, on low-dose oral CEE (0.45 mg) or transdermal estradiol 50 mcg with 200 mg of oral progesterone, and found no increased risk of breast cancer. KEEPS was a high-quality trial and an excellent first step in recalibrating the risks and benefits of hormone replacement. However, by virtue of its smaller numbers, KEEPS lacks the statistical power to contradict the WHI study. Hormone replacement and risk of breast cancer continue to be an important area for study. We can conclude that avoidance of MPA appears advisable.

ESTROGEN METABOLITES AND BREAST CANCER RISK

Important work is ongoing on the metabolic breakdown products of estradiol and estrone, showing that there may be a relationship between the estrogen metabolites and breast cancer risk. The activity of the estrogen metabolizing enzymes, such as 1B1 and 1A1 cytochrome 450 enzymes, catechol-O-methyl transferase (COMT) and glutathione S transferase enzyme, is impacted by genetic single nucleotide polymorphisms (SNPs).[154–156] The 1B1 cytochrome 450 pathway creates the less favorable 4-OH estrogens, which can then be metabolized to the 3,4-quinones, and these are thought to act as carcinogens via the formation of depurinating DNA adducts (i.e., by products of breakage of DNA).[157,158] But, if estrone and estradiol metabolize via the 1A1 enzyme, resulting in 2-OH estrogens, COMT may then convert those 2-OH metabolites to 2-methoxy estrogens which have protective antiproliferative apoptotic and antiangiogenic properties.[159]

Hence, some authors propose that production of increased 2-OH metabolites and less 4-OH metabolites will reduce breast cancer risk.[160] The enzyme activity controlling these metabolites may be altered by diet and lifestyle factors. It is possible to enhance 1A1 activity and hence production of 2-methoxy estradiol with cruciferous vegetables or indole-3-carbinol.[161,162] Research is ongoing utilizing 2-methoxy estradiol as a treatment for multiple cancer types including end-stage ovarian cancer.[163,164] COMT activity is increased by methylcobalamin, methyl folate, and other B vitamins. Exercise, a low normal BMI, low alcohol intake, and adequate vitamin D levels have all been shown to decrease the risk of breast cancer.

CARDIOVASCULAR RISKS

Women treated with oral estrogen have an increased risk of developing venous thromboembolism, a serious and potentially fatal complication of HRT. However, multiple studies, including placebo-controlled trials as well as large observational studies, show no such increased risk with topical estradiol.[165–167] The transdermal form of estrogen avoids the digestive tract and first-pass hepatic metabolism which results in an unfavorable imbalance between pro-coagulant factors and antithrombotic mechanisms. An increase in CRP, a known cardiac risk factor, increased pro-thrombin activation protein, F1+F2, decreased antithrombin activity, lower plasminogen, all factors that aggravate thromboembolic risk, have been demonstrated with oral but not with topical estrogen.[168,169]

Although the WHI study demonstrated increased stroke risk in both the unopposed oral conjugated equine estrogen (CEE) arm and the CEE plus medroxyprogesterone (MPA) arm, the MPA conferred additional cardiac risk. With CEE alone a decreased risk for heart disease events and cardiac-related deaths was found, while in the CEE plus MPA arm there was an increase in heart disease deaths and cardiac events.[144,145] Therefore, oral estrogen confers a mixture of benefit and risk in cardiovascular disease. Some biological plausibility for oral estrogen's protective effects has been shown, include lowering LDL and Lp(a) while raising HDL.[170]

The 1997 PEPI study demonstrated the superiority of oral micronized progesterone over medroxyprogesterone for glucose control and a greater increase in HDL.[170] Estradiol, but not estrone, has been shown to decrease and delay the oxidation of LDL.[171] LDL exposure to estradiol enhances resistance to oxidation and slows the development of arterial plaque, another means by which estradiol lowers coronary artery disease in women.[172] Overall, the risk-to-benefit data support the superior safety and benefits of topical estradiol over oral and of oral micronized progesterone over MPA for cardiovascular health.

ESTROGEN AND PREVENTION OF COGNITIVE DECLINE AND ALZHEIMER'S DISEASE

There is compelling evidence that the steep drop in estrogen levels that begins with the menopausal transition is closely linked to an increased risk of cognitive decline and subsequent dementia in women.[173] A large upsurge in Alzheimer's disease (AD) is expected with the continuing demographic shift to a larger elderly population and incidence rates are predicted to increase from 4.5 million in 2000 to 13.2 million in 2050.[174] As of 2010, women make up 68% of those living with Alzheimer's disease.[175,176] In a 2009 review summarizing the clinical studies using estrogen and measuring cognitive benefit, transdermal estradiol showed benefit in 15 out of 20 studies.[177] Conjugated equine estrogen resulted in less favorable outcomes, and when combined with medroxyprogesterone, outcomes were even less favorable.[178] Basic science and some researchers suggest a critical period hypothesis, where neurological response to estrogen is beneficial if initiated within a few years after menopause but deleterious if treatment is initiated after long-term estrogen deprivation.[173] However, two small randomized studies showed benefit in older women with Alzheimer's disease when treated with a 0.1 transdermal patch.[178,179] An issue facing many clinicians is the question of continuing or discontinuing estrogen at age 60 or 65. An important 2014 study examined fPET scans of postmenopausal women with increased Alzheimer's disease risk who had been on HRT for an average of 10 years.[180] After the initial scan, half the women went off the HRT, while half continued for an additional 2 years at which time the fPET scans were repeated. They found that continuation of unopposed transdermal estradiol but not oral CEE, and not if a progestin was added, preserved the posterior cingulate cortex, the area known to undergo the most significant deterioration in early Alzheimer's.

A GUIDE TO PRACTICE

1. Take a full history, past and current, physical and psychological.
2. Consider interventions to improve diet, stress, sleep, toxin exposure, GI and detoxification function, insulin, weight and blood sugar management, nutrient optimization, immune and mitochondrial function, and genomic and epigenetic factors.
3. Measure hormone levels before and after. For most postmenopausal women, estradiol levels between 25 and 40 pg/mL will give the mood and cognitive benefits desired, along with bone and cardiovascular protection without significant risk of postmenopausal bleeding, or excess estrogen symptoms such as breast tenderness. In menopause prior to age 45, consider much higher levels of replacement up to 120–130 pg/mL E2 with high cycled P4, up to 6–8 ng/mL.
4. There is a range for optimal progesterone. A minimum is needed to protect the endometrium. For women who feel better on a higher progesterone level, a much higher level is fine. These are minimum levels based only on the author's experience.
   E2 = 25–30 pg/mL P4 = 1–1.7 ng/mL at peak level
   E2 = 30–40 P4 = 1.5–2
   E2 = 40–50 P4 = 2.5–3.5
   E2 = 50–100 P4 = 3.5–6.5
5. Consider increased cruciferous vegetables, B12, methyl folate, other Bs, and D3 and testing for estrogen metabolites.

CONCLUSION

In this chapter the profound impact of estrogen, testosterone, and progesterone on mood and well-being were reviewed. Carefully managed, these hormones could prevent suffering and create an improved quality of life. Their clinical use is poorly understood and underutilized in part because of insufficient research or clear guidelines for their use, in part due to safety concerns, and in part because they fall out of the purview of any particular specialty for the treatment of mood disorders. Gynecologists are comfortable with hormones but not with the treatment of depression, while psychiatrists are unfamiliar with hormones and are very comfortable with the antidepressant, anti-anxiety, and insomnia medications. This chapter summarizes some of the scientific data in order to move the discussion forward, increase awareness and utilization, and improve psychological health for women in all stages of life.

REFERENCES

1. Weissman, M.M. 1985. Gender and depression. *Trends Neurosci* 8: 416–420.
2. Weissman, M.M. 1995. Depression in women: Implications for health care research. *Science* 269: 799–808.
3. Piccinelli, M. 2000. Gender differences in depression: Critical Review. *Brit J Psych* 177: 486–493.
4. Kessler, R.C. et al. 1993. Sex and depression in the National Comorbidity Survey 1: Lifetime prevalence, chronicity, and recurrence. *J of Affective Disorders* 29(2–3): 85–86.
5. Arpels, J.C. 1996. The female brain hypoestrogenic continuum from the premenstrual syndrome to menopause. A hypothesis and review of supporting data. *J Reprod Med* 41(9): 633–639.
6. Stewart, D.E. and Boydell, K.M. 1993. Psychological distress during menopause: Associations across the reproductive life cycle. *Int J Psychiatry Med* 23: 157–162.
7. Payne, J.L. et al. 2007. Reproductive cycle-associated mood symptoms in women with major depression and bipolar disorder. *J Affect Disord* 99(1–3): 221–229.
8. Soares, C. et al. 2001. Efficacy of estradiol for the treatment of depressive disorders in perimenopausal women: A double blind, randomized, placebo-controlled trial. *Arch Gen Psychiatry* 58(6): 529–534.
9. Gregoire, A.J.P. et al. 1996. Transdermal oestrogen for treatment of severe postnatal depression. *Lancet* 347(9006): 930–933.
10. Watson, N.R., Studd, J.W., Savvas, M., Garnett, T., and Baber, R.J. 1989. Treatment of severe premenstrual syndrome with oestradiol patches and cyclical oral norethisterone. *Lancet* 2: 730–732.
11. Rasgon, N.L., Altshuler, L.L., and Fairbanks, L. 2001. Estrogen-replacement therapy for depression. *Am J Psychiatry* 158(10): 1738.
12. Cohen, L.S. et al. 2003. Short-term use of estradiol for depression in perimenopausal and postmenopausal women. *Am J Psychiatry* 160(8): 1519–1522.
13. Halbreicht, U. 2001. Role of estrogen in the aetiology and treatment of mood disorders. *CNS Drugs* 15(10): 797–817.
14. FDA Backgrounder on Conjugated Estrogens. 2005. FDA Backgrounder on Conjugated Estrogens. July 1. http://www.fda.gov/Drugs/DrugSafety/InformationbyDrugClass/ucm168838.htm (accessed February 27, 2015).
15. Westaby, D. and Ogle, S.J. 1977. Liver damage from long-term methyltestosterone. *Lancet* 2(8032): 262–263.
16. Holsen, L.M. et al. 2011. Stress response circuitry hypoactivation related to hormonal dysfunction in women with major depression. *J Affect Disord* 131: 379–387.
17. Young, E.A. et al. 2000. Hormonal evidence for altered responsiveness to social stress in major depression. *Neuropsychopharmacology* 23(4): 411–418.
18. Ahokas, A. et al. 2001. Estrogen deficiency in severe postpartum depression: Successful treatment with sublingual physiologic 17beta-estradiol: A preliminary study. *J Clin Psychiatry* 62(5): 332–336.
19. Schmidt, P.J. et al. 2000. Estrogen replacement in perimenopause-related depression: A preliminary report. *Am J Obstet Gynecol* 183(20): 414–420.
20. McEwan, B.S. et al. 1999. Estrogen actions in the central nervous system. *Endocr Rev* 20: 279–307.
21. Krishnan, V. et al. 2008. The molecular neurobiology of depression. *Nature* 455: 894–902.
22. Borrow, A.P. et al. 2014. Estrogenic mediation of serotonergic and neurotrophic systems: Implications for female mood disorders. *Prog Neuro-Psychopharm Biol. Psychiatry* 54: 13–25.

23. Bethea, C.I. et al. 2000. Steroid regulation of tryptophan hydroxylase protein in the dorsal raphe of macaques. *Biol Psychiatry* 47: 562–576.
24. Donner, N. et al. 2009. Estrogen receptor beta regulates the expression of tryptophan hydroxylase 2 mRNA within the serotonergic neurons of the rat dorsal raphe nuclei. *Neuroscience* 163: 705–718.
25. Carretti, N. et al. 2005. Serum fluctuations of total and free serum tryptophan levels during the menstrual cycle are related to gonadotropins and reflect brain serotonin utilization. *Human Reprod* 20(6): 1548–1553.
26. Fink, G. et al. 1996. Estrogen control of central neurotransmission: Effect on mood, mental state, and memory. *Cell Mol Neurobiol* 16(3): 325–344.
27. Ostlund, H. et al. 2003. Estrogen receptor gene expression in relation to neuropsychiatric disorders. *Ann NY Acad Sci* 1007: 54–63.
28. Merchenthaler, I. et al. 2004. Distribution of estrogen receptor alpha and beta in the mouse central nervous system. *J Compar Neurol* 473(2): 270–291.
29. Nishizuka, M. et al. 1982. Synapse formation in response to estrogen in the medial amygdala. *Proc Natl Acad Sci USA* 79(22): 7024–7026.
30. Brinton, R.D. 2009. Estrogen-induced plasticity from cells to circuits: Predictions for cognitive function. *Trends Pharmacol Sci* 30(4): 212–222.
31. Serova, L. et al. 2002. Estradiol stimulates gene expression of norepinephrine biosynthetic enzymes in rat locus coeruleus. *Neuroendocrinology* 75: 193–200.
32. Pau, K.Y. et al. 2000. Oestrogen upregulates noradrenaline release in the mediobasal hypothalamus and tyrosine hydroxylase gene expression in the brainstem of ovarectomized rhesus macaques. *J Neuroendocrinol* 12: 899–909.
33. Lee, S.H. et al. 1999. Up-regulation of D1A dopamine receptor gene transcription by estrogen. *Mol Cell Endocrinol* 156(1–2): 151–157.
34. Becker, J.B. 1999. Differences in dopaminergic function in striatum and nucleus accumbens. *Pharmacol Biochem Behav* 64(4): 803–812.
35. Andersen, M.L. et al. 2006. Effects of progesterone on sleep: A possible pharmacological treatment for sleep-breathing disorders? *Curr Med Chem* 13(29): 3575–3582.
36. Jiang, C. et al. 2009. Progesterone exerts neuroprotective effects by inhibiting inflammatory response after stroke. *Inflamm Res* 58(9): 619–624.
37. Andréen, L., Nyberg, S., Turkmen, S., van Wingen, G., Fernández, G., and Bäckström, T. 2009. Sex steroid induced negative mood may be explained by the paradoxical effect mediated by GABAA modulators. *Psychoneuroendocrinology* 34(8): 1121–1132.
38. Bäckström, T. et al. 2003. Pathogenesis in menstrual cycle-linked CNS disorders. *Ann NY Acad Sci* 1007: 42–53.
39. Rapkin, A.J. et al. 2012. Pathophysiology of premenstrual syndrome and premenstrual dysphoric disorder. *Menopause Int* 18: 52–59.
40. Hammarbäck, S., Bäckström, T., Holst, J., von Schoultz, B., and Lyrenäs, S. 1985. Cyclical mood changes as in the premenstrual tension syndrome during sequential estrogen-progestagen postmenopausal replacement therapy. *Acta Obstet Gynecol Scand* 64(5): 393–397.
41. Bitran, D. 1995. Anxiolytic effect of progesterone is mediated by the neurosteroid allopregnanolone at brain GABAA receptors. *J Neuroendocrinol* 7(3): 171–177.
42. Rupprecht, R. 2003. Neuroactive steroids: Mechanism of action and neuropsychological properties. *Psychoneuroendocrinology* 28: 139–168.
43. Bäckström, T. 2014. Allopregnanolone and mood disorders. *Prog Neurobiol* 113: 88–94.
44. Rapkin, A.J. 1992. The role of serotonin in premenstrual syndrome. *Clin Obstet Gynecol* 35(3): 629–636.
45. Ashby, C.R. 1988. Alteration of platelet serotonergic mechanisms and monoamine oxidase activity in premenstrual syndrome. *Biol Psychiatry* 24(2): 225–233.
46. Agís-Balboa, R.C., Pinna, G., Zhubi, A., Maloku, E., Veldic, M., Costa, E., and Guidotti, A. 2006. Characterization of brain neurons that express enzymes mediating neurosteroid biosynthesis. *Proc Natl Acad Sci USA* 103(39): 14602–14607.
47. Gao, B., Fritschy, J.M., Benke, D., and Mohler, H. 1993. Neuron-specific expression of GABAA-receptor subtypes: differential association of the alpha 1- and alpha 3-subunits with serotonergic and GABAergic neurons. *Neuroscience* 54(4): 881–892.
48. Michopoulos, V. 2011. Estradiol and progesterone modify the effects of the serotonin reuptake transporter polymorphism on serotonergic responsivity to citalopram. *Exp Clin Psychopharmacol* 19(6): 401–408.
49. Biegon, A. 1982. Modulation by estradiol of serotonin receptors in the brain. *J Neurosci* 2: 199–205.

50. Halbreich, U. 2003. The prevalence, impairment, impact, and burden of premenstrual dysphoric disorder (PMS/PMDD). *Psychoneuroendocrinology* 28(3): 1–23.

51. 2001. American College OBGYN practice bulletin No. 15: Premenstrual syndrome. *Int J Gynecol Obstet*, 2001: 1–9.

52. American Psychiatric Association. 2000. Premenstrual dysphoric disorder. In *Diagnostic and Statistical Manual of Mental Disorders*. 4th ed. Alexandria, VA: American Psychiatric Press, pp. 771–774.

53. Bäckström, T. et al. 1983. Mood, sexuality, hormones, and the menstrual cycle. II. Hormone levels and their relationship to the premenstrual syndrome. *Psychosom Med* 43: 505–507.

54. Hammarback, S. 1991. Spontaneous anovulation causing disappearance of cyclical symptoms in women with the premenstrual syndrome. *Acta Endocrinol* 125: 132–137.

55. Hammarbäck, S., Damber, J.E., and Bäckström, T. 1989. Relationship between symptom severity and hormone changes in women with premenstrual syndrome. *J Clin Endocrinol Metab* 68(1): 125–130.

56. Graham, C.A. and Sherwin, B.B. 1992. A prospective treatment study of premenstrual symptoms using a triphasic oral contraceptive. *J Psychosom Res* 36(3): 257–266.

57. Joffe, H., Cohen. L.S., and Harlow, B.L. 2003. Impact of oral contraceptive pill use on premenstrual mood: Predictors of improvement and deterioration. *Am J Obstet Gynecol* 189(6): 1523–1530.

58. Rapkin, A.J., McDonald, M., Sharon, A., and Winer, S.A. 2007. Ethinyl estradiol/drospirenone for the treatment of the emotional and physical symptoms of premenstrual dysphoric disorder. *Women's Health* 3(4): 395–408.

59. Gruber, C. et al. 2002. Production and actions of estrogens. *N Engl J Med* 346: 340–352.

60. Michaud, D.S. et al. 1999. Reproducibility of plasma and urinary sex hormone levels in premenopausal women over a one year period. *Cancer Epidemiol Biomarkers Prev* 8(12): 1059–1064.

61. Van Goozen, S.H. et al. 1997. Psychoendocrinological assessment of the menstrual cycle: The relationship between hormones, sexuality, and mood. *Arch Sex Behav* 26(4): 359–382.

62. Watson, N.R., Studd, J.W., Savvas, M., and Garnett, T. 1989. Treatment of severe premenstrual syndrome with oestradiol patches and cyclical oral norethisterone. *Lancet* 2: 730–732.

63. Lee, J.R. 1998. Use of Pro-Gest cream in postmenopausal women. *Lancet* 352(9131): 905.

64. Pick, M. Advanced premenstrual syndrome (PMS) and premenstrual dysphoric disorder (PMDD) treatment. Women to Women. https://www.womentowomen.com/pms/severe-pms-and-pmdd-treatment (accessed February 26, 2015).

65. Northup, C. 2007. Estrogen dominance. February 5. http://www.drnorthrup.com/estrogen-dominance (accessed February 25, 2015).

66. Ford, O., Lethaby, A., Roberts, H., and Mol, B.W. 2012. Progesterone for premenstrual syndrome. *Cochrane Database Syst Rev* 14(3): CD003415, doi: 10.1002/14651858.CD003415.pub4.

67. Andréen, L. et al. 2003. Progesterone effects during sequential hormone replacement therapy. *Eur J Endocrinol* 148: 571–577.

68. Andreen, L. et al. 2005. Relationship between allopregnanolone and negative mood in postmenopausal women taking sequential hormone replacement therapy with vaginal progesterone. *Psychoneuroendocrinology* 30(2): 212–224.

69. Hermann, A.C. et al. 2005. Over-the-counter progesterone cream produces significant drug exposure compared to an FDA-approved, oral progesterone product. *J Clin Pharmacol* 45(6): 614–619.

70. Pick, M. Estrogen dominance—Is it real? Women to Women. https://www.womentowomen.com/hormonal-health/estrogen-dominance/ (accessed February 26, 2015).

71. Rubin, B.S. 2011. Bisphenol A: An endocrine disruptor with widespread exposure and multiple effects. *J Steroid Biochem Mol Bio* 127(1–2): 27–34.

72. Alonso-Magdalena, P. 2005. Low doses of bisphenol A and diethylstilbestrol impair $Ca2+$ signals in pancreatic alpha-cells through a nonclassical membrane estrogen receptor within intact islets of Langerhans. *Environ Health Perspect* 113(8): 969–977.

73. Alonso-Magdalena, P. et al. 2008. Pancreatic insulin content regulation by the estrogen receptor ER alpha. *PLoS One* 3(4): e2069, doi: 10.1371/journal.pone.0002069.

74. Zsarnovszky, A. et al. 2005. Ontogeny of rapid estrogen-mediated extracellular signal-regulated kinase signaling in the rat cerebellar cortex: Potent nongenomic agonist and endocrine disrupting activity of the xenoestrogen bisphenol A. *Endocrinology* 146(12): 5388–5396.

75. Ropero, A.B. et al. 2006. Rapid endocrine disruption: Environmental estrogen actions triggered outside the nucleus. *J Steroid Biochem Mol Biol* 102(1–5): 163–169.

76. Leranth, C. et al. 2008. Bisphenol A prevents the synaptogenic response to estradiol in hippocampus and prefrontal cortex of ovariectomized nonhuman primates. *Proc Natl Acad Sci USA* 105(37): 14187–14191.

77. Jobling, S. 1995. A variety of environmentally persistent chemicals, including some phthalate plasticizers, are weakly estrogenic. *Environ Health Perspect* 103(6): 582–587.
78. Oh, B.S. 2006. Application of ozone, UV and ozone/UV processes to reduce diethyl phthalate and its estrogenic activity. *Sci Total Environ* 367(2–3): 681–693.
79. Ahokas, A. et al. 2001. Estrogen deficiency in severe postpartum depression: Successful treatment with sublingual physiologic 17 beta-estradiol: A preliminary study. *J Clin Psychiatry* 62(5): 332–336.
80. Cox, J.L. et al. 1993. A controlled study of the onset duration and prevalence of postpartum depression. *Br J Psychiatry,* 163, 27–31.
81. Murray, L. 1992. The impact of postnatal depression on infant development. *J Child Psychol Psychiatry* 33: 543–561.
82. Cummings, E.M. et al. 1995. Maternal depression and child development. *J Child Psychol Psychiatry* 35: 73–112.
83. Sharp, D. et al. 1995. The impact of postnatal depression on boys' intellectual development. *J Child Psychol Psychiatry* 36: 1315–1336.
84. Sie, S.D. et al. 2012. Maternal use of SSRIs, SNRIs and NaSSAs: Practical recommendations during pregnancy and lactation. *Arch Dis Child Fetal Neonatal Ed* 97(6): F472–F476.
85. Freeman, E.W. et al. 2006. Associations of hormones and menopausal status with depressed mood in women with no history of depression. *Arch Gen Psychiatry* 63: 375–382.
86. Bromberger, J.T. et al. 2007. Depressive symptoms during the menopausal transition: The Study of Women's Health Across the Nation (SWAN). *J Affect Disord* 103: 267–272.
87. Bromberger, J.T. et al. 2003. Persistent mood symptoms in a multiethnic community cohort of pre- and postmenopausal women. *Am J Epidemiol* 158: 347–356.
88. Cohen, L.S. et al. 2006. Risk for new onset of depression during the menopausal transition: The Harvard Study of Moods and Cycles. *Arch Gen Psychiatry* 63: 385–390.
89. Bromberger, J.T. et al. 2009. Predictors of first lifetime episodes of major depression in midlife women. *Psychol Med* 39: 55–64.
90. Paoletti, A.M. et al. 2001. Evidence that cyproterone acetate improves psychological symptoms and enhances the activity of the dopaminergic system in postmenopause. *J Clin Endocrinol Metab* 86(2): 608–612.
91. Studds, J.W. 2011. A guide to the treatment of depression in women by estrogen. *Climacteic* 14: 637–642.
92. Schmidt, P.J. et al. 2004. A longitudinal evaluation of the relationship between reproductive status and mood in perimenopausal women. *Am J of Psychiatry* 161(12): 2238–2244.
93. Maki, P.M. et al. 2010. Summary of the National Institute on Aging-sponsored conference on depressive symptoms and cognitive complaints in the menopausal transition. *Menopause* 17: 815–822.
94. Judd, L.L. et al. 1996. Socioeconomic burden of subsyndromal depressive symptoms and major depression in a sample of the general population. *Am J Psychiatry* 153(11): 1411–1417.
95. Judd, L.L. et al. 2000. Delineating the longtitudinal structure of depressive illness: Beyond clinical subtypes and duration thresholds. *Pharmacopsychiatry* 33(1): 3–7.
96. Rapaport, M.H. et al. 1998. Minor depressive disorder and subsyndromal depressive symptoms: Functional impairment and response to treatment. *J Affect Disord* 48(2–3): 227–232.
97. Gruber, C. et al. 2002. Production and actions of estrogens. *N Engl J Med* 346: 340–352.
98. Wharton, W. et al. 2012. Neurobiological underpinnings of the estrogen-mood relationship. *Curr Psychiatry Rev* 8(3): 247–256.
99. Toffol, E. et al. 2014. Hormone therapy and mood in perimenopausal and postmenopausal women: A narrative review. *J N Am Menopause Soc* 22(5): 1–15.
100. Schmidt, P.J. et al. 2000. Estrogen replacement in perimenopause-related depression: A preliminary report. *Am J Obstet Gynecol* 183: 414–420.
101. Joffe, H. et al. 2011. Increased estradiol and improved sleep, but not hot flashes, predict enhanced mood during the menopausal transition. *J Clin Endocrinol Metab* 96(7): E1044–E1054.
102. Ragson, N.L. et al. 2002. Estrogen replacement therapy in the treatment of major depressive disorder in perimenopausal women. *J Clin Psychiatry* 63 Suppl 7: 45–48.
103. Almeida, O.P. et al. 2006. A 20-week randomized controlled trial of estradiol replacement therapy for women aged 70 years and over: Effect on mood, cognition and quality of life. *Neurobiol Aging* 27: 141–149.
104. Zweifel, J.E. et al. 1997. A meta-analysis of the effects of hormone replacement therapy upon depressed mood. *Psychoneuroendocrinology* 22: 189–212.
105. Sherwin, B.B. 1991. The impact of different doses of estrogen and progestin on mood and sexual behavior in postmenopausal women. *J Clin Endocrinol Metab* 72: 336–343.

106. Bjorn, I. et al. 2000. Negative mood changes during hormone replacement therapy: A comparison between 2 progestogens. *Am J Obstet Gynecol* 183: 1419–1426.
107. Fitzpatrick, L.A. et al. 2000. Comparison of regimens containing oral micronized progesterone or medroxyprogesterone acetate on quality of life in postmenopausal women: A cross-sectional survey. *J Womens Health Gend Based Med* 9(4): 381–387.
108. Magos, A.L. et al. 1986. The effects of norethisterone in postmenopausal women on oestrogen replacement therapy: A model for the premenstrual syndrome. *Br J Obstet Gynaecol* 93: 1290–1296.
109. Holst, J. et al. 1989. Progestogen addition during oestrogen replacement therapy—Effects on vasomotor symptoms and mood. *Maturitas* 11: 13–20.
110. Klaiber, E.L. et al. 1997. Relationship of serum estradiol levels, menopausal duration, and mood during hormone replacement therapy. *Psychoneuroendocrinology* 22: 549–558.
111. Girdler, S.S. et al. 1999. A comparison of the effects of estrogen with and without progesterone on mood and physical symptoms in postmenopausal women. *J Womens Health Gend Based Med* 8: 637–646.
112. Hammarback, S. et al. 1985. Cyclical mood changes as in the premenstrual tension syndrome during sequential estrogen-progestagen postmenopausal replacement therapy. *Acta Obstet Gynecol Scand* 64: 393–397.
113. Panay, N. et al. 1997. Progesterone intolerance and compliance with hormone replacement therapy in menopausal women. *Human Reprod Update* 3: 159–171.
114. Schmidt, P.J. et al. 1998. Differential behavioral effects of gonadal steroids in women with and in those without premenstrual syndrome. *N Engl J Med* 338: 209–216.
115. Weiner, C.L., Primeau, M., and Ehrmann, D.A. 2004. Androgens and mood dysfunction in women: Comparison of women with polycystic ovarian syndrome to healthy controls. *Psychosom Med* 66(3): 356–362.
116. Davis, S. 1999. Androgen replacement in women: A commentary. *J Clin Endocrinol Metab* 84(6): 1886–1891.
117. Shifren, J.L. et al. 2000. Transdermal testosterone treatment in women with impaired sexual function after oophorectomy. *N Engl J Med* 343: 682–688.
118. Krapf, J. et al. 2009. The role of testosterone in the management of hypoactive sexual desire disorder in postmenopausal women. *Maturitas* 63(3): 213–219.
119. Goldstadt, R. et al. 2003. Transdermal testosterone therapy improves well-being, mood, and sexual function in premenopausal women. *Menopause* 10(5): 390–398.
120. Davis, S. et al. 2008. Safety and efficacy of a testosterone metered-dose transdermal spray for decreased sexual satisfaction in premenopausal women. *Ann Int Med* 148: 569–577.
121. Lauman, E.O. et al. 1999. Sexual dysfunction in the United States: Prevalence and predictors. *JAMA* 281: 537–544.
122. Lindau, S.T. et al. 2007. A study of sexuality and health among older adults in the United States. *N Engl J Med* 357: 762–774.
123. West, S.L. et al. 2008. Prevalence of low sexual desire and hypoactive sexual desire disorder in a nationally representative sample of US women. *Arch Intern Med* 168: 1441–1449.
124. American Psychiatric Association (APA). 2000. Hypoactive Sexual Desire Disorder. *Diagnostic and Statistical Manual of Mental Disorders*. Revised 4th ed. Alexandria, VA: APA, pp. 496–498.
125. Longcope, C. 1990. Hormone dynamics at the menopause. *Ann NY Acad Sci* 595: 21–30.
126. Zumoff, B. et al. 1995. Twenty-four hour mean plasma testosterone concentration declines with age in normal premenopausal women. *J Clin Endocrinol Metab* 80: 1492–1430.
127. Burger, H.G. et al. 2000. A prospective longitudinal study of serum testosterone, dehydroepiandrosterone sulfate, and sex hormone-binding globulin levels through the menopause transition. *J Clin Endocrinol Metab* 84: 2832–2838.
128. Labrie, F. et al. 1997. Marked decline in serum concentrations of C19 sex steroid precursors and conjugated androgen metabolites during aging. *J Clin Endocrinol Metab* 82: 2396–2402.
129. Mushayandebvu, T. et al. 1996. Evidence for diminished midcycle ovarian androgen production in older reproductive aged women. *Fertil Steril* 65: 721–723.
130. Davison, S.L. et al. 2005. Androgen levels in adult females: Change with age, menopause and oophorectomy. *J Clin Endocrinol Metab* 90: 3847–3853.
131. Sherwin, B.B. et al. 1987. The role of androgen in the maintenance of sexual functioning in oophorectomized women. *Psychosom Med* 49: 397–409.
132. Sarrel, P. et al. 1998. Estrogen and estrogen-androgen replacement in postmenopausal women dissatisfied with estrogen-only therapy. *J Reprod Med* 43, 847–856.

133. Davis, S.R. et al. 2012. Efficacy and safety of testosterone in the management of hypoactive sexual desire disorder in postmenopausal women. *J Sex Med* 9: 1134–1148.

134. Somboonporn, W., Davis, S., Seif, M., and Bell, R. 2005. Testosterone for peri- and postmenopausal women. *Cochrane Database Syst Rev* 19(4): CD004509.

135. Montgomery, J. et al. 1987. Effect of oestrogen and testosterone implants on psychological disorders in the climacteric. *Lancet* 1: 297–299.

136. Westaby, D. et al. 1977. Liver damage from long-term methyltestosterone. *Lancet* 2(8032): 262–263.

137. Davis, S.R. et al. 2009. The incidence of invasive breast cancer among women prescribed testosterone for low libido. *J Sex Med* 6: 1850–1856.

138. Dimitrakakis, C. et al. 2004. Breast cancer incidence in postmenopausal women using testosterone in addition to usual hormone therapy. *Menopause* 11: 531–535.

139. Shufelt, C.L. and Braunstein, G.D. 2008. Testosterone and the breast. *Menopause Int* 14(3): 117–122.

140. Laughlin, G.A. et al. 2010. Extremes of endogenous testosterone are associated with increased risk of incident coronary events in older women. *J Clin Endocrinol Metab* 95: 740–747.

141. Shifren, J.L. et al. 2006. Testosterone patch for the treatment of hypoactive sexual desire in naturally postmenopausal women: Results from the INTIMATE NMI study. *Menopause* 13: 770–779.

142. Buckler, H.M. et al. 1998. The effect of low-dose testosterone treatment on lipid metabolism, clotting factors and ultrasonographic ovarian morphology in women. *Clin Endocrinol* 49: 173–178.

143. Swanson, S. et al. 2007. Treatment of HSDD in surgically menopausal women: A newly initiated Phase III, randomized double-blind, placebo-controlled, multi-center study of the safety and efficacy of LibiGel. Presented at the annual meeting of the International Society for the Study of Women's Sexual Health. February 22–25, Orlando, FL.

144. Rossouw, J.E. et al. 2002. Risks and benefits of estrogen plus progestin in healthy postmenopausal women: Principal results from the Women's Health Initiative randomized controlled trial. *JAMA* 288(3): 321–333.

145. Anderson, G.L. et al. 2004. Effects of conjugated equine estrogen in postmenopausal women with hysterectomy: The Women's Health Initiative randomized controlled trial. *JAMA* 291(14): 1701–1712.

146. Beral, V. 2003. Breast cancer and hormone-replacement therapy in the Million Women Study. *Lancet* 362(9382): 419–427.

147. Collaborative Group on Hormonal Factors in Breast Cancer. 1997. Breast cancer and hormone replacement therapy: Collaborative reanalysis of data from 51 epidemiological studies of 52,705 women with breast cancer and 108,411 women without breast cancer. Collaborative Group on Hormonal Factors in Breast Cancer. *Lancet* 350(9084): 1047–1059.

148. Shapiro, S. 2011. Does hormone replacement therapy cause breast cancer? An application of causal principles to three studies: Part 1. The collaborative reanalysis. *J Fam Plann Reprod Health Care* 37(2): 103–109.

149. Shapiro, S. 2011. Does hormone replacement therapy cause breast cancer? An application of causal principles to three studies: Part 2. The Women's Health Initiative: Estrogen plus progestogen. *J Fam Plann Reprod Health Care* 37(3): 165–172.

150. Shapiro, S. et al. 2012. Does hormone replacement therapy cause breast cancer? An application of causal principles to three studies part 4 the million women study. *J Fam Plann Reprod Health Care* 38(2): 102–109.

151. Shapiro, S. 2011. Does hormone replacement therapy cause breast cancer? An application of causal principles to three studies: Part 3. The Women's Health Initiative: Unopposed estrogen. *J Fam Plann Reprod Health Care* 37(4): 225–230.

152. Chlebowski, R.T., and Anderson, G.L. 2012. Changing concepts: Menopausal hormone therapy and breast cancer. *J Natl Cancer Inst* 104(7): 517–527.

153. KEEPS Results Give New Insight Into Hormone Therapy. 23rd Annual Meeting of the North American Menopause Society October 3–6, 2012, Orlando, FL. Available at: http://www.menopause.org/annual-meetings/2012-meeting/keeps-report

154. Hanna, I.H. 2000. Cytochrome P450 1B1 (CYP1B1) pharmacogenetics: Association of polymorphisms with functional differences in estrogen hydroxylation activity. *Cancer Res* 60(13): 3440–3444.

155. Ambrosone, C.B. 1995. Cytochrome P4501A1 and glutathione S-transferase (M1) genetic polymorphisms and postmenopausal breast cancer risk. *Cancer Res* 55(16): 3483–3485.

156. Lakhani, N.J. 2003. 2-Methoxyestradiol, a promising anticancer agent. *Pharmacotherapy* 23(2): 165–172.

157. Cavalieri, E. 2006. Catechol estrogen quinones as initiators of breast and other human cancers: Implications for biomarkers of susceptibility and cancer prevention. *Biochim Biophys Acta* 1766(1): 63–78.

158. Cavalieri, E.L. 1997. Molecular origin of cancer: catechol estrogen-3,4-quinones as endogenous tumor initiators. *Proc Natl Acad Sci USA* 94(20): 10937–10942.
159. Pribluda, V.S. et al. 2000. 2-methoxyestradiol: An endogenous antiangiogenic and antiproliferative drug candidate. *Cancer Metastasis Rev* 19(1–2): 173–179.
160. Fuhrman, B.J. 2012. Estrogen metabolism and risk of breast cancer in postmenopausal women. *J Natl Cancer Inst* 104: 326–339.
161. Keck, A.S. and Finley, J.W. 2004. Cruciferous vegetables: Cancer protective mechanisms of glucosinolate hydrolysis products and selenium. *Integr Cancer Ther* 3(1): 5–12.
162. Lee, S.A. 2008. Cruciferous vegetables, the GSTP1 Ile105Val genetic polymorphism, and breast cancer risk. *Am J Clin Nutr* 87(3): 753–760.
163. Tinley, T.L. et al. 2003. Novel 2-methoxyestradiol analogues with antitumor activity. *Cancer Res* 63: 1538–1549.
164. Golebiewska, J. et al. 2002. Dual effect of 2-methoxyestradiol on cell cycle events in human osteosarcoma 143 B cells. *Acta Biochemica Polonica* 49(1): 59–65.
165. Olié, V., Canonico, M., and Scarabin, P.Y. 2010. Risk of venous thrombosis with oral versus transdermal estrogen therapy among postmenopausal women. *Curr Opin Hematol* 217(5): 457–463.
166. Laliberté, F. et al. 2011. Does the route of administration for estrogen hormone therapy impact the risk of venous thromboembolism? Estradiol transdermal system versus oral estrogen-only hormone therapy. *Menopause* 18(10): 1052–1059.
167. Høibraaten, E. et al. 2000. Increased risk of recurrent venous thromboembolism during hormone replacement therapy results of the randomized, double-blind, placebo-controlled estrogen in Venous Thromboembolism Trial (EVTET). *Thromb Haemost* 84(6): 961–967.
168. Eilertsen, A.L., Høibraaten, E., Os, I., Andersen, T.O., and Sandvik, L. 2005. The effects of oral and transdermal hormone replacement therapy on C-reactive protein levels and other inflammatory markers in women with high risk of thrombosis. *Maturitas* 52(2): 111–118.
169. Scarabin, P.Y. 1997. Effects of oral and transdermal estrogen/progesterone regimens on blood coagulation and fibrinolysis in postmenopausal women. *Arterioscler Thromb Vasc Biol* 17: 3017.
170. Barrett-Connor, E., Slone, S., Greendale, G., Kritz-Silverstein, D., and Espeland, M. 1997. The Postmenopausal Estrogen/Progestin Interventions Study: Primary outcomes in adherent women. *PEPI Maturitas* 27(3): 261–274.
171. Rifici, V.A. and Khachadurian, A.K. 1992. The inhibition of low-density lipoprotein oxidation by 17-beta estradiol. *Metabolism* 41(10): 1110–1114.
172. Shwaery, G.T., Vita, J.A., and Keaney, J.F. 1997. Antioxidant protection of LDL by physiological concentrations of 17β-estradiol. *Circulation* 95(6): 1378–1385.
173. Daniel, J.M. and Bohacek, J. 2010. The critical period hypothesis of estrogen effects on cognition: Insights from basic research. *Biochim Biophys Acta* 1800: 1068–1076.
174. Hebert, L.E., Scherr, P.A., Bienias, J.L., and Bennett, D.A. 2003. Alzheimer disease in the US population: Prevalence estimates using the 2000 census. *Arch Neurol* 60: 1119–1122.
175. Gao, S., Hendrie, H.C., Hall, K.S., and Hui, S. 1998. The relationships between age, sex, and the incidence of dementia and Alzheimer disease: A meta-analysis. *Arch Gen Psychiatry* 55(9): 809–815.
176. de la Fuente-Fernandez, R. 2006. Impact of neuroprotection on incidence of Alzheimer's disease. *PLoS One* 1: e52.
177. Wharton, W. et al. 2009. Potential role of estrogen in the pathobiology and prevention of Alzheimer's disease. *Am J Transl Res* 1(2): 131–147.
178. Asthana, S. et al. 2001. High dose estradiol improves cognition for women with AD: Results of a randomized study. *Neurology* 57: 605–612.
179. Asthana, S. et al. 1999. Cognitive and neuroendocrine response to transdermal estrogen in postmenopausal women with Alzheimer's disease: Results of a placebo-controlled, double-blind, pilot study. *Psychoneuroendocrinology*, 24: 657–677.
180. Rasgon, N.L. et al. 2014. Prospective randomized trial to assess effects of continuing hormone therapy on cerebral function in postmenopausal women at risk for dementia. *PLoS One* 9(3): e89095.

12 The Hypothalamic-Pituitary-Adrenal Axis in Mood Disorders

Sara Gottfried, MD

CONTENTS

INTRODUCTION

We release hormones such as adrenaline and cortisol in response to stress—a smart evolutionary adaptation that triggers rapid physiologic changes such as increased heart rate and blood pressure, and redirects blood flow to your muscles so that you may fight or flee. For more than 50 years, scientists have agreed that psychosocial stressors are the most potent activators of the stress feedback loop, known as the hypothalamic-pituitary-adrenal (HPA) axis.[1] However, the alarm can backfire:

The HPA is more vulnerable than once realized under the threat of chronic psychosocial stress, which may cause HPA dysregulation and thereby significantly compromise mood and health.[2] Untangling what we know about the HPA and its positive and negative levers is key to skillful and integrative care of people suffering with mood disorders.

Over the past decade, there's been a paradigm shift in how we think about the role of stress, the HPA axis, and mood. There is a complex, bidirectional relationship between the serotonergic and stress systems of the human body.[3] Various research threads—genetic, molecular, endocrinological, and psychosocial—have converged in support of improving and maintaining mental health by reducing stress reactivity, targeting the correction of HPA dysfunction. Additionally, most scientists have thought that chronic stress caused or worsened disease via HPA dysfunction and that the level of dysfunction was measurable in the levels of stress hormones, such as cortisol—but this premise lacks integration of a greater level of complexity.

While ambient levels of cortisol may be an important marker of HPA dysfunction, emerging evidence suggests that there's also a problem of glucocorticoid receptor activity and resistance.[4] Similar to insulin resistance, where cells become increasingly insensitive to insulin and hyperinsulinemia occurs, one can develop glucocorticoid resistance. Beyond absolute hormone levels, epigenetic factors such as methylation of the glucocorticoid receptor gene (NR3C1) may influence cortisol sensitivity and risk of mood disorders.[5]

Additionally, there are important sex and gender differences in the role of the HPA axis in mental health, which may relate to the sex differences in prevalence of common conditions such as anxiety, depression, posttraumatic stress disorder (PTSD), and insomnia. In this chapter, we'll review the existing literature on mental health and the role of the HPA axis with a functional medicine perspective, and create a framework with which to understand the role of the HPA axis in creating hormone resistance, particularly glucocorticoid resistance.

Most integrative clinicians appreciate the role of stress in hormonal imbalance but are vague on the specifics. The main reason is that the HPA axis regulates the functions of sex steroid hormones through interaction with corticotropin-releasing hormone (CRH) and gonadotropin-releasing hormone (GnRH). As a result, unlocking the entire stress system or HPA axis is crucial to long-term mental and physical health. A multimodal functional medicine approach of addressing the underlying causes of mood problems as they relate to HPA axis dysregulation by applying a systems approach is cogent and proven. As you read this chapter, please consider the interactions among the genetic, environmental, and lifestyle factors that may influence the stress response, and how these interactions may present actionable therapeutic and preventive possibilities for your patients.

NORMAL REGULATION OF HPA FUNCTION

Stress enters your body via certain parts of your brain, including the hypothalamus, amygdala, and hippocampus. The response is coordinated by a hormonal-control system called the HPA axis, which sets off a chain reaction of fear and response.

The HPA axis is a hierarchical feedback loop, which operates in the central nervous system according to the following simplified schema:

- Emotional input is processed by the limbic system, which includes the amygdala and the hippocampus.
- A signal is then sent to the locus coeruleus, which releases norepinephrine—and the norepinephrine stimulates the hypothalamus to produce CRH from the paraventricular nucleus.
- The hypothalamus communicates the stress message to the pituitary via CRH and also produces norepinephrine.
- Norepinephrine from the hypothalamus increases activity of the sympathetic nervous system.
- CRH stimulates the anterior pituitary to synthesize and release adrenocorticotropic hormone (ACTH), also known as corticotropin, a polypeptide tropic hormone. ACTH travels

to the adrenal glands to stimulate production of corticosteroids. CRH effects on ACTH release are potentiated by vasopressin, which is also produced in increasing amounts when the hypothalamic paraventricular neurons are chronically activated. While vasopressin stimulates ACTH release, oxytocin inhibits it.

- Adrenal glands respond to ACTH with release of corticosteroids, such as cortisol, which raises blood glucose and blood pressure, and activates the immune system and inflammatory cascade. Heart rate increases, and blood is shunted away from the digestive tract toward your muscles—so you can fight or flee. Cortisol output from the adrenal glands is approximately 15–20 mg/day.
- Finally, cortisol and other glucocorticoids regulate the CRH-producing neurons in a negative feedback loop through the limbic system and pituitary, particularly the hippocampus.

This antiquated system determines how you deal with stress and regulates such crucial tasks as digestion, immune function, sex drive, energy use, and storage. When working properly, you experience *allostasis,* which literally means maintaining stability (homeostasis) through change. In the normal sequence of events, the HPA induces the adrenal glands to increase cortisol production, and then, via a feedback loop, the increased cortisol inhibits the HPA pending a future trigger.

On a molecular level, mechanisms of genetic regulation are emerging. For instance, the FK506 binding protein 5 (FKBP5) modulates glucocorticoid receptor sensitivity and signaling, which is age dependent.[6] Additionally, the T polymorphism in the gene causes increased FKBP5 induction by cortisol, increased suppression of cortisol, and greater risk for PTSD symptoms.

ALLOSTATIC LOAD

Of particular interest is the hippocampus, which contains high levels of glucocorticoid receptors, and as a result, is more vulnerable to increased allostatic load, the physiological aggregate effects of chronic stressors.[7]

HPA dysregulation occurs when allostatic load exceeds reserves. More important than the amount of stress is one's reaction to it or perception of it. Excess allostatic load and high perception of stress have been shown to shorten telomeres, the caps on chromosomes that serve as a proxy of biological aging as opposed to chronological aging.[8] There is a critical length of telomere shortness that results in genomic instability, apoptosis, and cell senescence, often with degraded transcriptional programming and mitochondrial dysfunction.[9] Left unchecked, chronic stress leads to adverse outcomes such as insulin resistance, hypertension, visceral fat deposition, weakened immunity, decreased protein synthesis, less DNA repair, and relevant to this chapter, mood disorders. Reduced allostatic load improves longevity.[10]

PREGNENOLONE STEAL

High allostatic load may perturb other sex hormone signaling, a pattern called "pregnenolone steal" or "cortisol steal." The body adapts to produce more cortisol in times of high need by stealing or diverting the mother hormone, pregnenolone—a building block of all adrenal hormones—from its other functions. As a result, the body has a ready supply of cortisol as needed, which may cause other hormones levels, such as dehydroepiandrosterone (DHEA), progesterone, and testosterone, to drop.

HPA DYSREGULATION IN MOOD DISORDERS

The problem of HPA dysregulation can be conceptualized as an excessive or insufficient stress response. There's a biological cost to chronically elevated heart rate, blood pressure, and muscular blood flow, shunting blood away from your gut—and sometimes the cost is affective problems in vulnerable populations, particularly women.

The HPA controls our response to actual, anticipated, and *perceived* danger. Many of us are so accustomed to unremitting stress—whether from long work hours, or a difficult marriage, or demanding children—that we've actually rewired our brains to perceive danger when it's no longer a threat, or when it's relatively minor. Perpetual activation of the HPA leads to overactivity, followed over time by underactivity associated with a greater susceptibility to contagious illness, decreased sex drive, low blood pressure, orthostatic hypotension, and cortisol resistance.

In the classic work of Hans Selye, there are three stages that ultimately lead to HPA dysregulation, which he called the general adaptation syndrome.

GENERAL ADAPTATION SYNDROME

Stage 1: Arousal

- Cortisol and dehydroepiandrosterone sulfate (DHEA(S)) increase in response to stressors, with recovery to baseline.

Stage 2: Adaptation

- Chronic hypercortisolism is seen, but DHEA declines along with other sex hormones.
- Symptoms include dysphoria, depression, mood swings, feeling "stressed," anxiety, and vasomotor symptoms.

Stage 3: Exhaustion

- Hypocortisolism and low DHEA, and low gonadal sex hormones are found.
- Depression, fatigue, PTSD, and fibromyalgia develop.

Selye's model has its detractors, but the general adaptation model provides a suitable paradigm from which to understand the connection between HPA dysregulation and mood disorders. Stage 1 is the normal stress response of a resilient individual, which is typically transient. Depending on genetic, environmental, and lifestyle factors, some people progress to Stage 2, whereby stressors, usually psychosocial, cause sustained high cortisol, and DHEA production is diminished. Some individuals have a problem of persistent stressors and high perceived stress, which may lead to Stage 3 or Exhaustion. This stage is characterized by low cortisol and DHEA, which put an individual at risk for depression, fatigue, PTSD, and fibromyalgia.

The limitation of the model is that symptoms don't always correlate with stage, which means that biomarker testing becomes important. Additionally, there are single nucleotide polymorphisms (SNPs) associated with differential responses to stress, such as the serotonin transporter gene.[11]

In the functional medicine paradigm, there are several steps for patient assessment.

EVALUATION OF HPA

GATHERING THE PATIENT'S STORY

Typically, when you have a problem such as an overactive HPA axis, you can trace it back to a predisposing factor, known as an antecedent. For additional information about the HPA, consider using the questionnaire developed by WholePsychiatry.com.[12]

Triggers involved in HPA dysregulation include the following:

- Stress
- Aging
- Inflammatory and/or infectious conditions
- Toxins

- Food sensitivity and intolerance
- Nutritional insufficiencies and excesses, including prenatal ethanol exposure[13]
- Sex differences

Chronic perceived stress. Early life stress, such as physical or sexual abuse, sets patients up for future HPA over- or underactivity.[14] In one study, women with a history of childhood abuse and a current diagnosis of depression had a sixfold increased stress response.[15] Traumatic stress causes greater relative hippocampal atrophy in humans compared with the rest of the brain.[16] Hippocampal atrophy has been documented in severe depression.[17] Under normal conditions, the HPA axis shows circadian and ultradian rhythms with pulsed glucocorticoid secretion greater in amplitude during waking hours. The suprachiasmatic nucleus (SCN), located in the hypothalamus, maintains the circadian rhythms in the body and is mainly entrained by light. Dyscircadianism, or desynchronization of the circadian rhythm, is common in major depression, particularly disruption of the sleep-wake system. In animals, chronic stress and cortisol cause oxidative damage to mitochondria, which play an important role in neurotransmitter signaling and represent another key target of functional medicine treatment.

Aging. In general, hyperactivation of the HPA axis occurs as a consequence of aging. Several pathophysiologic changes may occur, including increased baseline ACTH and cortisol secretion; decreased glucocorticoid negative feedback at the level of the hypothalamus, hippocampus, and prefrontal cortex; decreased sensitivity of the adrenal glands to ACTH; and flattening of the diurnal pattern of cortisol release. Increased cortisol secretion is secondary to peripheral conversion from cortisone. There is also a decline in pregnenolone levels and C-19 steroids (DHEA) associated with aging, but overall, the workings of the HPA axis and aging remain a complex area with conflicting studies.[18]

Inflammatory and/or infectious conditions. Stress has been shown to induce replication of certain viruses, such as cytomegalovirus (CMV), a beta-herpesvirus commonly found within the general population.[19] In one study of Detroit, Michigan, residents, those with the highest quartile of CMV IgG antibody levels had a fourfold increase in incident depression.[20] In the Whitehall II cohort, participants with positive CMV serostatus were significantly associated with lower telomerase among women, and higher CMV IgG antibody levels were associated with lower telomerase overall.[21] Although mostly CMV infection is asymptomatic, affected patients show increased serum concentrations of cytokines such as TNF-α and IL-6, which are linked to mood and well-being. CMV viral load is associated in older adults with depression and anxiety.[22]

Toxins. The exposome is the aggregate environmental exposure over one's lifetime, including both the exogenous and endogenous toxins that are sometimes worse than the original exogenous exposure.[23] Environmental toxins may act as endocrine disruptors and modulate hormonal activity, contributing to HPA dysregulation. External toxins can become an issue for patients with impaired clearance of metabolic wastes. One example is lead, which increases conversion of cortisone, a weaker glucocorticoid, into cortisol, a stronger glucocorticoid. Bisphenol A has a similar effect in children.[24]

Sex differences. There are substantial sex differences in the etiology and epidemiology of mood disorders with incidence in females two to three times the incidence in males for psychiatric conditions such as depression, anxiety, and insomnia. Women have double the prevalence of major depressive disorder.[25] Substantial evidence exists to show that women have more HPA dysregulation compared with men, perhaps because estrogen and progesterone disrupt negative feedback.[26] There is also a role for HPA axis maladaptation postpartum, posited to contribute to an inflammatory model of postpartum depression. [27]

LABORATORY INVESTIGATION

Various laboratory tests are used to track the HPA, including diurnal cortisol, DHEA, DHEA(S), ACTH stimulation test, and telomeres. The most common tests are listed in Table 12.1. For the sex steroid cascade that occurs in the adrenal glands, refer to Figure 12.1.

TABLE 12.1

HPA Laboratory Reference Ranges

Biomarker	Range for Normal Population	Optimal Range
Cortisol (morning)	Saliva: 3.7–9.5 ng/mL Serum: 7–28 µg/dL	Saliva: mid-range Serum: 10–15 µg/dL
Cortisol (noon)	Saliva: 1.2–3.0 ng/mL	Same
Cortisol (5 p.m.)	Saliva: 0.6–1.9 ng/mL	Same
Cortisol (10 p.m.)	Saliva: 0.4–1.0 ng/mL	Same
ACTH stimulation	Two to three times increase in serum cortisol, 30 min after injection	Same
DHEA(S)	Saliva: 2–23 µg/dL Serum: 65–380 µg/dL	Age dependent; generally top half of normal range

The feedback system of the HPA reflects the following quote from Robert Sapolsky, professor of biology, neurology, and neurological sciences at Stanford University, California, and author of *Why Zebras Don't Get Ulcers: The Acclaimed Guide to Stress, Stress-Related Diseases, and Coping*: "Everything in physiology follows the rule that too much can be as bad as too little. There are optimal points of allostatic balance".[28] By way of caveat and as mentioned in the introduction, we have spent decades following absolute levels of hormonal mediators, such as cortisol and DHEA, but the role of glucocorticoid resistance is emerging as equally, if not more, important than absolute hormone levels.

Under normal conditions, cortisol secretion follows a diurnal pattern with a negative slope—characterized by high concentrations at wakening, a morning peak shortly after waking up, a decline over the day, and lowest levels in the evening. Deviations from this diurnal cycle can occur, though, and these altered dynamics have been implicated in several adverse health consequences including depression, cardiovascular disease, breast cancer, and PTSD.[29]

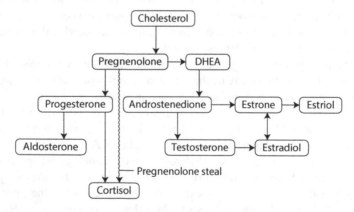

FIGURE 12.1 Hormone tree: sex hormones. In the adrenals and ovaries (as well as in the fetus/placenta), cholesterol is converted into several sex steroid hormones. The hormones listed in this figure are called sex steroid hormones because they are derived from cholesterol's characteristic chemical structure and influence the sex organs. One may further subclassify adrenal hormones as follows. Progesterone is part of the *mineralocorticoid* subclass (affects salt, mineral, and water balance in the body), whereas cortisol is a member of the *glucocorticoid* subclass (*glu*cose + *cor*tex + ster*oid*; made in the cortex of the adrenal glands, binds the glucocorticoid receptor, and raises glucose, among other tasks). Testosterone is a member of the *androgen* subclass (responsible for hair growth, repair, and sex drive); estradiol, estriol, and estrone are members of the *estrogen* subclass (sex steroid hormones produced primarily in the ovaries to promote female characteristics such as breast growth and menstruation).

There are distinct biomarkers that reflect cortisol signaling and HPA function, including the following:

- *Dysregulated cortisol.* One of the best ways to measure the pattern of cortisol release over the course of the day is with a diurnal saliva test. Commercially available kits measure cortisol at four time points throughout the day—usually upon awakening, before lunch, before dinner, and before bedtime. Commonly observed patterns include chronically high cortisol, chronically low cortisol, and a combination of high and low.
- *Dysregulated DHEA(S).* DHEA and DHEA sulfate—collectively referred to as DHEA(S)—may be dysregulated in many patients with mood and anxiety disorders, particularly in major depressive disorder and PTSD. Several large-scale studies show lower serum DHEA levels in depression,[30] although one study indicated that DHEA(S) is higher in patients with depression compared to healthy controls, and may be an biomarker of remission during standard antidepressant therapy.[31] DHEA(S) are important regulators of glucocorticoid activity.[32] Bioidentical hormone substrates are hormonal precursors that the body may use to adjust downstream hormone levels. In one study of 32 women with undetectable DHEA(S), there were significantly higher rates of depression compared with those with detectable DHEA(S) and higher rates of depression (21.7% compared with 4.6%, $p = .001$).[33]
- *Testosterone.* In male patients with major depression, a significant negative correlation exists between testosterone levels and the "retardation" score of a depression scale (Hamilton Rating Scale for Depression, HAM-D). However, endogenous levels of testosterone are not different in men and women with major depression compared with controls.[34] Estradiol but not testosterone improves negative feedback to the HPA in older men and women.[35]
- *Receptor activity.* The glucocorticoid receptor plays an important role in the HPA and mood disorders, including bipolar.[36] Mineralocorticoid receptor activity is impaired in depression.[37]
- *Shorter telomeres.* Telomere length is a marker of cumulative stress exposure, and excess stress activity is an established cause of depression and anxiety disorders. Telomere length and telomerase activity track with depression: Depressed younger patients have shorter telomeres, which is related to adverse childhood experiences.[38] However, decreased telomere length has not been found in late-life depression, suggesting a differential effect by age.[39]

With the foundational understanding of biomarkers of normal and dysregulated HPA function, the physician may review the range of evidence of HPA problems in mood disorders.

SUMMARY OF HPA DYSREGULATION IN MENTAL HEALTH

Depression is associated with a dysregulated HPA. The cause is a combination of genetic factors interacting with negative environmental stimuli. Endogenous cortisol levels are just one marker, and hypercortisolism occurs in 25%–50% of patients, and 24% of premenopausal women[40]:

- One study showed that depressed people have the same cortisol levels at baseline as nondepressed people, but when stressed, depressed people produce more cortisol, and it stays high.[41] Another study linked hypercortisolism in major depression in younger adults, and both hypocortisolism and hypercortisolism to major depression in older adults.[42] Additionally, depressed people don't "recover" to normal cortisol levels the way that other people do.[43]
- Data shows significantly elevated cortisol levels among people with major depression that is recurrent (on average, six episodes) compared to controls.[44] The high cortisol levels

were both in the morning and before bedtime, and were high regardless of daily stress and hassles, and childhood trauma.

- Patients with Cushing's syndrome have problems with emotion perception, processing, and regulation, similar to mood disorder found in major depressive disorder.[45]
- Flatter diurnal cortisol slopes and glucocorticoid resistance are documented in premenopausal women with depression.[46]
- Approximately 27%–66% of depressed patients show nonsuppression of cortisol to dexamethasone.
- As humans age in a normal fashion, activation of CRH neurons is mild in comparison to the activation in major depression. Increased CRH is linked to depression.[47]
- Traumatic stress causes greater relative hippocampal atrophy in humans compared with the rest of the brain.[48] Hippocampal atrophy has been documented in severe depression.[49]
- Mineralocorticoid receptors are impaired.[50]
- There are increased glucocorticoid receptor levels in the amygdala of depressed patients, but not in bipolar patients.[51]
- Hyper- and hypocortisolism are linked to depression and poor quality of life among patients with bipolar disorder.[52]
- High cortisol is linked to suicide risk. From autopsy studies we know that people who commit suicide ("completers") have high cortisol levels and larger adrenal glands as a result of chronic, high output of cortisol. Relatives of completers have altered HPA activity too, although it's unclear if this is from grief or a heritable trait.[53] Relatives show blunted response to stress as measured with salivary cortisol, which is consistent with cortisol resistance.

OTHER CONDITIONS LINKED TO HPA DYSREGULATION

- *Poor sleep.* Insomniacs have higher 24-hour cortisol levels.[54]
- *Posttraumatic stress disorder (PTSD).* Maladaptation of the HPA is documented in PTSD, including altered DHEA(S) and hippocampal atrophy.[55,56]
- *Premenstrual syndrome (PMS).* PMS is linked to altered HPA activity.[57]
- *Polycystic ovary syndrome (PCOS).* PCOS, the top reason for infertility in the United States, has been linked to hyperactivity of the HPA axis, which makes sense since high DHEA(S) is associated with Stage 1 of the general adaptation syndrome.[58]
- *Alzheimer's disease.* This is linked to higher levels of CRH and greater activation of the paraventricular nucleus.[59]
- *Multiple sclerosis (MS).* Both development and progression of MS are linked to stress and HPA reactivity. In particular, hyperactivity of the HPA axis has been linked to neurodegeneration (breakdown of the nerves) and increased disability.[60] People with all stages of MS have high cortisol levels; early stage patients have increased morning cortisol.[61]

LIFESTYLE INTERVENTIONS

In the final step of a functional medicine approach to mood disorders and the dysregulated HPA, develop a functional medicine protocol. There are several points of intervention for resetting the HPA, including diet, lifestyle, and supplements. Because of pregnenolone steal, addressing cortisol first allows a patient to develop more behavioral flexibility and improve the cascade and function of other sex steroids.

DIETARY

Food consumption, especially at lunch, induces HPA axis activation. Subjects with abdominal obesity demonstrate hyperactivation of the HPA axis. Skipping meals raises cortisol.[62] The suprachiasmatic nucleus (SCN) of the hypothalamus maintains the circadian clock. Peripheral oscillators exist as well in other tissues, and are entrained by various factors, most importantly, feeding and fasting. Altering the timing of food intake can desynchronize the central (SCN) and peripheral clocks and can lead to their uncoupling, which has been linked to the development of metabolic disorders, including obesity and type 2 diabetes. High-sugar and high-fat diets have been shown to alter circadian rhythms, and the researchers in this study discuss the influence of these nutrients (fatty acids and glucose) and how they are able to alter normal circadian rhythms in the SCN and peripheral clocks.[63] Food timing changes circadian rhythm in animals.[64] When an animal's food availability is disrupted, for example, limiting access to food during its normal sleep period, the animal can shift its circadian rhythm to a new pattern to be awake and alert when food is available. An oscillator in the dorsomedial hypothalamus can determine food training of circadian rhythms.

CARBOHYDRATE TIMING

When your blood sugar drops, the body produces cortisol to raise blood glucose. Likewise, eating carbohydrates lowers cortisol. Consequently, researchers have been investigating the timing of carbohydrate consumption and how it may reset the HPA and diurnal cortisol rhythm. Glucose increases retinal reaction to light, and evening carb-rich meals may help phase delay the circadian rhythm. Recent data show that eating low carbs at breakfast and more carbs at dinner, known as carb cycling, may reset a flattened diurnal cortisol slope.[65]

ALCOHOL

Paradoxically, alcohol simultaneously reduces anxiety and stimulates stress hormone production via the HPA axis. In other words, alcohol makes you feel more relaxed in the short term, but raises cortisol and may disrupt sleep and circadian rhythm.[66] Studies indicate that rats exposed to daily high alcohol levels can develop tolerance for alcohol's stimulatory effect on glucocorticoid production and therefore produce smaller increases in glucocorticoid levels. It is unclear if this phenomenon develops in humans as well. In some humans, excessive alcohol consumption leads to extremely elevated cortisol production. Most humans, however, develop some sort of tolerance to the HPA axis's response to alcohol, which may detrimentally affect the system's ability to perform its normal functions. Alcohol's stimulatory effect on the HPA axis is dependent on genetic factors. Though it isn't certain how alcohol stimulates the HPA axis and cortisol production, the researchers maintain that one possibility is that alcohol dis-inhibits the HPA axis, or that the HPA axis might be activated in response to alcohol's stimulating property as part of a "whole-body" stress response.[67] HPA axis dysregulation is associated with alcohol abuse and dependence. Cortisol can interact with the brain's reward system and contribute to the reinforcing effects of alcohol. Some researchers have found that measuring cortisol levels during alcohol abstinence is a useful indication of the likelihood of relapse.[68] Other researchers discovered that long-term exposure to alcohol in rats causes significant dysregulation of the HPA axis.[69] Excessive alcohol consumption stimulated the release of corticosterone and adrenocorticotropic hormone; however, chronic exposure and dependence led to a weakened HPA axis response. This suggests that a level of tolerance had been reached prior to dependence, and is related to the amount of alcohol consumed.

EXERCISE

One of the known benefits of exercise is that it improves stress adaptation and resilience. In one study, highly trained and sedentary young men either exercised on a treadmill at moderate intensity or performed a placebo exercise. After 90 minutes, they underwent a standardized stress test. The first group showed a significantly reduced cortisol response to the stress test, and showed higher bilateral hippocampus and lower prefrontal cortex activity and showed lower cortisol response to the stress test. The authors concluded that exercise has a stress buffering effect, which relies on HPA negative feedback.[70] In another study, women treated for breast cancer in the previous months were allocated to two groups: 6 months of exercise and reduced calorie diet, or usual care (control group). The exercise and hypocaloric group showed a reduction in depressive symptoms, as well as a significant impact on diurnal salivary cortisol rhythm, with an increase in morning salivary cortisol, indicating a change in HPA axis regulation.[71]

MEDITATION

We've known about the benefits of meditation for regulating the stress-response system and retraining the mind for centuries, and it has been documented for decades starting first with transcendental meditation and leading to most recently with mindfulness-based stress reduction and other forms.[72] Cortisol levels are modulated by meditation in a dose-dependent manner.[73] Mindfulness is arguably the most thoroughly studied form of meditation, and a recent meta-analysis of 47 trials and 3500 participants of mindfulness for stress-related conditions showed it improves anxiety, depression, and pain. Either low or no effect or lack of evidence exists for improving mood, attention, substance use, eating, sleep, and weight. However, the majority of studies were subject to bias, had too much heterogeneity in the clinical spectrum of participants, had too much variability in controls, or had too much heterogeneity of the treatment (dose, frequency, duration, and technique).[74]

The benefit doesn't take long: Short- and long-term meditators enrolled in a 9-week mindfulness-based stress reduction course show reduced morning cortisol and improved sleep.[75] Mindfulness-based stress reduction has been shown to reduce anxiety, depression, and suicidal ideation.[76] Mindfulness reduces serum cortisol levels in second-year medical students.[77] Among older patients with depression, a randomized trial of Buddhist walking meditation demonstrated improved depression scores.[78]

There are limited data indicating that meditation for pregnant women creates a more positive and resilient temperament in their offspring, including a randomized trial of 64 pregnant women and 59 controls with follow-up Carey Infant Temperament Questionnaire at 5 months performed in infants.[79]

RELIGION AND SPIRITUALITY

Religiosity and/or spirituality are important and unique realms of quality of life that demonstrate positive outcomes. Prayer has been shown to reduce depression scores.[80] Preservation of the diurnal cortisol pattern, and thereby regulation of the HPA, has been associated with religiosity among women with stress-related conditions.[81] In one quantitative review of 69 studies in healthy populations and 22 studies in diseased populations, religion and/or spirituality had a protective effect. In the healthy populations, improved outcomes were independent of positive behaviors such as smoking, exercise, drinking, and socioeconomic factors, as well as social support and negative mood—and organized religion as measured by church attendance is linked to improved survival and reduced cardiovascular mortality.[82] Indeed, religiosity and/or spirituality as indicated by frequency of prayer and attendance at service shows lower cortisol responses. However, there may be a gender effect as males show lower blood pressure related to composite religiosity/spirituality composite scores, whereas women show higher blood pressure.[83] Even intercessory (remote prayer for another) prayer has been shown to improve significantly spiritual well-being in cancer patients.[84]

SLEEP

Sleep debt is associated with elevated basal cortisol release and an excessive cortisol response to a stressor, which suggests hyperactive HPA axis responses even in healthy adults. A patient's individual response may represent a risk factor for psychological and physical health consequences linked to excess cortisol exposure.[85]

YOGA

Yoga practitioners downregulate their HPA axis and modulate their cortisol levels.[86] The mechanisms that are involved in the effect of yoga on stress response include the following: positive affect, self-compassion, inhibition of the posterior hypothalamus, and salivary cortisol.[87] Yoga has been shown to have long-term benefits for people with major depression. In breast cancer survivors, yoga reduces morning and 5 p.m. salivary cortisol.[88] One recent trial of yoga as an add-on treatment in major depression suggested that it doesn't significantly change cortisol, perhaps because pharmacological treatment downregulates the HPA to a greater extent than yoga—reduction of HPA axis overactivity was detected after 1 week of treatment with either quetiapine fumarate extended release (300 mg/day) or escitalopram (10 mg/day).[89]

SUPPLEMENTS

Various natural therapies affect the HPA. They act at different points mechanistically. Hormonal treatments include DHEA, discussed below, and estrogen, progesterone, and testosterone (discussed in previous chapters). Neurotransmitter substrates include 5-hydroxytryptophan, L-tryptophan, acetyl-L-carnitine, phosphatidylserine, St. John's wort (*Hypericum perforatum*), and tyrosine. Several substrates, such as L-tryptophan and 5-HTP, allow the clinician to shift the equilibrium of tryptophan metabolism, and impact production and function of serotonin and melatonin. Specific nutrients such as omega-3 fatty acids, antioxidants (vitamin C and zinc), vitamin B (including vitamin B12 and folic acid), and magnesium improve mitochondrial function.[90]

DEHYDROEPIANDROSTERONE

DHEA and its sulfated version, DHEA(S), are the most common steroid hormones in humans. DHEA impacts the growth, differentiation, normal and abnormal physiology, and aging of the central nervous system (CNS) in ways that are still being elucidated.[91] In humans, DHEA levels decrease with age beginning in the late twenties, with a drop by more than half by age 50.[92] Researchers have hypothesized that restoring levels may slow down aging, protect the brain, and perhaps extend life.[93] In modulating the body's hormone function, such as DHEA, one should consider not just production but also transport, conversion, cellular sensitivity, and detoxification/metabolism. Endogenous DHEA(S) levels correlate negatively with depression in older women.[94] Given that DHEA(S) levels drop with age, and cortisol either remains the same or rises, some consider tracking the DHEA(S)-to-cortisol ratio to be important.[95]

Studies of DHEA treatment for depression are limited and small, but suggest benefit. One study in six patients with major depression at a DHEA dose of 30–90 mg/day for 4 weeks showed benefit.[96] One randomized trial of 22 patients with major depression indicated that DHEA at a dose up to 90 mg/day, either as monotherapy or added to a stable antidepressant dose, improves symptoms as measured by the Hamilton Depression Rating Scale.[97] Another randomized trial of DHEA at 90 mg for 3 weeks, followed by 450 mg for 3 weeks, compared to placebo for 6 weeks, reduced symptoms of major depression in 55 subjects.[98] Finally, one randomized trial of 24 healthy men showed that DHEA administration at 150 mg for 1 week improved mood and memory.[99] Data on safety and long-term effectiveness are limited, and quality control of DHEA (as well as other supplements) remains a concern.[100] In women participating in long-term trials, side effects are mainly acne and hirsutism. Recommended dosages are between 10 and 90 mg/day, with lower doses in women.

KETOCONAZOLE

Limited data on the use of inhibitors of glucocorticoid synthesis, such as ketoconazole, a widely used antifungal, exist for patients with depression. Ketoconazole inhibits 11-hydroxylase, and can treat hypercortisolism at central (hippocampus) and peripheral (hepatic, adipose tissues) sites.[101] In one clinical trial of 20 patients with depression, those with hypercortisolemia responded to keto-conazole with improved symptoms after 4 weeks of treatment (400–800 mg/day) compared with controls.[102] Side effects of ketoconazole include nausea, pruritus, and elevations of liver enzymes, which limit its use. Recommended dosage is between 400 and 800 mg/day.

MELATONIN

Melatonin and melatonin agonists have chronobiotic effects, which mean that they can readjust the circadian system and HPA, and may improve mood.[103] However, meta-analyses show no benefit in doses of 0.5 to 6 mg over a duration of 2 weeks to 3.5 years.[104] Another strategy that this author has used successfully is microdosage of melatonin at 0.3 mg orally, 4 hours prior to bedtime to reset the melatonin rhythm and augment endogenous production.[105] The recommended dosage is 0.3 mg, 4 hours before bedtime.

PHOSPHATIDYLSERINE (OR PHOSPHORYLATED SERINE)

Phosphatidylserine (PS) targets the hippocampus, the set point for basal cortisol secretion.[106] Given the effect of phosphorylated serine on the hippocampus and cortisol rhythm, it's not surprising to learn that it may improve depression[107] and age-related cognitive impairment, including Alzheimer's disease. PS is a phospholipid that occurs endogenously in cell membranes, particularly in the brain, and functions to maintain signaling, secretory vesicles, and cell growth. The exact mechanism of action beyond effects on cortisol signaling is not clear. Efficacy occurs at 6 to 12 weeks of treatment with improved attention, arousal, verbal fluency, and memory,[108] but may wane in Alzheimer's disease after 16 weeks.[109] PS reduces cortisol levels in humans.[110] The recommended dosage is 100 mg three times daily.

S-ADENOSYL METHIONINE (SAMe)

SAMe is used orally to treat depression, anxiety, premenstrual syndrome (PMS), premenstrual dys-phoric disorder (PMDD), lead poisoning, dementia, and Alzheimer's disease, and also to slow the aging process. Studies vary in quality, but the number needed to treat (NNT) is seven—meaning that seven people need to be treated for 6 weeks for one additional nonresponder to reach remission, which is remarkably low.[111] Recommended dosage is between 400 and 800 mg, twice daily.

CONCLUSION

In summary, psychological stress and depression are associated with HPA axis dysregulation. The HPA represents an important but underutilized target for treatment, especially within a functional medicine context. HPA dysregulation has been well documented in depression, anxiety, PTSD, PMS, PMDD, PCOS, obesity, metabolic syndrome, diabetes, and cardiovascular disease.

Therapeutic modalities that address root causes—such as nutrition, exercise, meditation, yoga, other epigenetic influences, and natural therapies including neurotransmitter substrates, enzyme modulators, and bioidentical neurohormone substrates—are novel approaches to affective regulation and dysregulation. Functional medicine therapies that act as glucocorticoid agonists, antagonists, and steroid synthesis modulators (such as ketoconazole) are promising and warrant further investigation.

Conceptual and therapeutic strategies that treat all parts of the person, from micronutrient defi-ciencies to excess stress activation to neurohormonal imbalance, are most likely to succeed. While glucocorticoid modulation may not yet be proven to be superior to existing and conventional treat-ments, they warrant the attention of psychiatrists and primary care clinicians who treat mood, fatigue, and sleep problems in their patients.

ACKNOWLEDGMENTS

Special thanks to Rachel Jurkowicz and Sumeet Brar for their invaluable research and editorial assistance.

REFERENCES

1. Mason, J.W. 1968. A review of psychoendocrine research on the pituitary-adrenal cortical system. *Psychosom Med* 30: 576–607.
2. McEwen, B.S. 1998. Protective and damaging effects of stress mediators. *N Engl J Med* 338: 171–179.
3. McIsaac, S.A. and Young, A.H. 2009. The role of hypothalamic pituitary-adrenal axis dysfunction in the etiology of depressive disorders. *Drugs Today (Barcelona)* 45: 127–133.
4. Ingawale, D.K., Mandlik, S.K., and Patel, S.S. 2014. An emphasis on molecular mechanisms of anti-inflammatory effects and glucocorticoid resistance. *J Complement Integr Med* 12(1): 1–13.
5. Perroud, N., Paoloni-Giacobino, A., Prada, P. et al. 2011. Increased methylation of glucocorticoid receptor gene (NR3C1) in adults with a history of childhood maltreatment: A link with the severity and type of trauma. *Transl Psychiatry* 2011: e59.
6. Fujii, T., Hori, H., Ota, M. et al. 2014. Effect of the common functional FKBP5 variant (rs1360780) on the hypothalamic-pituitary-adrenal axis and peripheral blood gene expression. *Psychoneuroendocrinology* 42: 89–97.
7. Joels, M. 2008. Functional actions of corticosteroids in the hippocampus. *Eur J Pharmacol* 583: 312–321.
8. Zalli, A., Carvalho, L.A., Lin, J., Hamer, M., Erusalimsky, J.D., Blackburn, E.H., and Steptoe, A. 2014. Shorter telomeres with high telomerase activity are associated with raised allostatic load and impoverished psychosocial resources. *Proc Natl Acad Sci USA* 111: 4519–4524.
9. Blackburn, E.H., Greider, C.W., and Szostak, J.W. 2006. Telomeres and telomerase: The path from maize, tetrahymena and yeast to human cancer and aging. *Nature Med* 12: 1133–1138.
10. Karlamangla, A.S., Singer, B.H., and Seeman, T.E. 2006. Reduction in allostatic load in older adults is associated with lower all-cause mortality risk: MacArthur studies of successful aging. *Psychosom Med* 68(3): 500–507.
11. Bredemeier, K., Beevers, C.G., and McGeary, J.E. 2014. Serotonin transporter and BDNF polymorphisms interact to predict trait worry. *Anxiety Stress Coping* 27: 712–721.
12. HPA Axis Questionnaire. 2011. *AFMCP Webinar Series Description*. Case Template. Federal Way, WA: Institute for Functional Medicine. Available at: www.functionalmedicine.org
13. Glavas, M.M., Ellis, L., Yu, W.K., and Weinberg. J. 2007. Effects of prenatal ethanol exposure on basal limbic-hypothalamic-pituitary-adrenal regulation: Role of corticosterone. *Alcohol Clin Exp Res* 31: 1598–1610.
14. Voellmin, A., Winzeler, K., Hug, E. et al. 2015. Blunted endocrine and cardiovascular reactivity in young healthy women reporting a history of childhood adversity. *Psychoneuroendocrinology* 51C: 58–67.
15. Heim, C., Newport, D.J., Heit, S., Graham, Y.P., Wilcox, M., Bonsall, R., Miller, A.H., and Nemeroff, C.B. 2000. Pituitary-adrenal and autonomic responses to stress in women after sexual and physical abuse in childhood. *J Am Med Assoc* 284: 592–597.
16. Fu, W., Sood, S., and Hedges, D.W. 2010. Hippocampal volume deficits associated with exposure to psychological trauma and posttraumatic stress disorder in adults: A meta-analysis. *Prog Neuropsychopharmacol Biol Psychiatry* 34: 1181–1188.
17. Kempton, M.J., Salvador, Z., Munafò, M.R., Geddes, J.R., Simmons, A., Frangou, S., and Williams, S.C. 2011. Structural neuroimaging studies in major depressive disorder: Meta-analysis and comparison with bipolar disorder. *Arch Gen Psychiatry* 68: 675–690.
18. Gupta, D. and Morley, J.E. 2014. Hypothalamic-pituitary-adrenal (HPA) axis and aging. *Compr Physiol* 4(4): 1495–1510.
19. Rector, J.L., Dowd, J.B., Loerbroks, A. et al. 2014. Consistent associations between measures of psychological stress and CMV antibody levels in a large occupational sample. *Brain Behav Immun* 38: 133–141.
20. Simanek, A.M., Cheng, C., Yolken, R., Uddin, M., Galea, S., and Aiello, A.E. 2014. Herpesviruses, inflammatory markers and incident depression in a longitudinal study of Detroit residents. *Psychoneuroendocrinology* 50: 139–148.
21. Dowd, J.B., Bosch, J.A., Steptoe, A., Blackburn, E.H., Lin, J., Rees-Clayton, E., and Aiello, A.E. 2013. Cytomegalovirus is associated with reduced telomerase activity in the Whitehall II cohort. *Exp Gerontol* 48: 385–390.

22. Phillips, A.C., Carroll, D., Khan, N., and Moss, P. 2008. Cytomegalovirus is associated with depression and anxiety in older adults. *Brain Behavior Immun* 22: 52–55.

23. Wild, C.P. 2005. Complementing the genome with an "exposome": The outstanding challenge of environmental exposure measurement in molecular epidemiology. *Cancer Epidemiol Biomarkers Prev* 14: 1847–1850.

24. Wang, J., Sun, B., Hou, M., and Pan, X, and Li, X. 2013. The environmental obesogen bisphenol A promotes adipogenesis by increasing the amount of 11β-hydroxysteroid dehydrogenase type 1 in the adipose tissue of children. *Int J Obes (Lond)* 37: 999–1005.

25. Fernandez-Gausti, A., Fiedler, J.L., and Herrera, L. 2012. Sex, stress, and mood disorders: At the intersection of adrenal and gonadal hormones. *Horm Metab Res* 44: 607–618. doi:10.1055/s-0032–1312592.

26. Panagiotakopoulos, L., and Neigh, G.N. 2014. Development of the HPA axis: Where and when do sex differences manifest? *Front Neuroendocrinol* 35: 285–302.

27. Thomson, M. 2013. The physiological roles of placental corticotropin releasing hormone in pregnancy and childbirth. *J Physiol Biochem* 69: 559–573.

28. Sapolsky, R. 2004. *Why Zebras Don't Get Ulcers: The Acclaimed Guide to Stress, Stress-Related Diseases, and Coping.* New York, NY: Holt Paperbacks, p. 123.

29. Hatzinger, M. 2000. Neuropeptides and the hypothalamic-pituitary-adrenocortical (HPA) system: Review of recent research strategies in depression. *World J Biol Psychiatry* 1: 105–111.

30. Barrett-Connor, E., von Mühlen, D., Laughlin, G.A., and Kripke, A. 1999. Endogenous levels of dehydroepiandrosterone sulfate, but not other sex hormones, are associated with depressed mood in older women: The Rancho Bernardo Study. *J Am Geriatr Soc* 47: 685–691.

31. Morita, T., Senzaki, K., Ishihara, R. et al. 2014. Plasma dehydroepiandrosterone sulfate levels in patients with major depressive disorder correlate with remission during treatment with antidepressants. *Hum Psychopharmacol* 29: 280–286.

32. Maninger, N., Wolkowitz, O.M., Reus, V.I., Epel, E.S., and Mellon, S.H. 2009. Neurobiological and neuropsychiatric effects of dehydroepiandrosterone (DHEA) and DHEA sulfate (DHEAS). *Front Neuroendocrinol* 30: 65–91.

33. Yaffe, K., Ettinger, B., Pressman, A. et al. 1998. Neuropsychiatric function and dehydroepiandrosterone sulfate in elderly women: A prospective study. *Biol Psychiatry* 43: 694–700.

34. Matsuzaka, H., Maeshima, H., Kida, S. et al. 2013. Gender differences in serum testosterone and cortisol in patients with major depressive disorder compared with controls. *Intl J Psychiatry Med* 46: 203–221.

35. Sharma, A.N., Aoun, P., Wigham, J.R. et al. 2014. Estradiol, but not testosterone, heightens cortisol-mediated negative feedback on pulsatile ACTH secretion and ACTH approximate entropy in unstressed older men and women. *Am J Physiol Regul Integr Comp Physiol* 306: R627–R635.

36. Ceulemans, S., De Zutter, S., Heyrman, L. et al. 2011. Evidence for the involvement of the glucocorticoid receptor gene in bipolar disorder in an isolated northern Swedish population. *Bipolar Disord* 13: 614–623.

37. Baes, C., Martins, C., Tofoli, S. et al. 2014. Early life stress in depressive patients: HPA axis response to GR and MR agonist. *Front Psychiatry* 5: 2.

38. Karabatsiakis, A., Kolassa, I.T., Kolassa, S., Rudolph, K.L., and Dietrich, D.E. 2014. Telomere shortening in leukocyte subpopulations in depression. *BMC Psychiatry* 14: 192.

39. Schaakxs, R., Verhoeven, J.E., Voshaar, R.C.O., Comijs, H.C., and Penninx, B.W. 2014. Leukocyte telomere length and late-life depression. *Am J Geriatr Psychiatry* 23(4): 423–432.

40. Jarcho, M.R., Slavich, G.M., Tylova-Stein, H., Wolkowitz, O.M., and Burke, H.M. 2013. Dysregulated diurnal cortisol pattern is associated with glucocorticoid resistance in women with major depressive disorder. *Biol Psychol* 93: 150–158.

41. Römer, B., Lewicka, S., Kopf, D. et al. 2009. Cortisol metabolism in depressed patients and healthy controls. *Neuroendocrinology* 90: 301–306.

42. Bremmer, M., Deeg, D., Beekman, A. et al. 2007. Major depression in late life is associated with both hypo- and hypercortisolemia. *Biol Psychiatry* 62: 479–486.

43. Burke, H.M., Davis, M.C., Otte, C., and Mohr, D.C. 2005. Depression and cortisol responses to psychological stress: A meta-analysis. *Psychoneuroendocrinology* 30: 846–856.

44. Lok, A., Mocking, R.J., Ruhé, H.G., Visser, I., Koeter, M.W., Assies, J., and Schene, A.H. 2012. Longitudinal hypothalamic–pituitary–adrenal axis trait and state effects in recurrent depression. *Psychoneuroendocrinology* 37: 892–902.

45. Langenecker, S.A., Weisenbach, S.L., Giordani, B. et al. 2012. Impact of chronic hypercortisolemia on affective processing. *Neuropharmacology* 62: 217–225.

46. Rush, A.J., Giles, D.E., Schlesser, M.A. et al. 1996. The dexamethasone suppression test in patients with mood disorders. *J Clin Psychiatry* 57: 470–484.

47. Swaab, D.F., Bao, A.M., and Lucassen, P.J. 2005. The stress system in the human brain in depression and neurodegeneration. *Ageing Res Rev* 4: 141–194.
48. Fu, W., Sood, S., and Hedges, D.W. 2010. Hippocampal volume deficits associated with exposure to psychological trauma and posttraumatic stress disorder in adults: A meta-analysis. *Prog Neuropsychopharmacol Biol Psychiatry* 34: 1181–1188.
49. Kempton, M.J., Salvador, Z., Munafò, M.R., Geddes, J.R., Simmons, A., Frangou, S., and Williams, S.C. 2011. Structural neuroimaging studies in major depressive disorder: Meta-analysis and comparison with bipolar disorder. *Arch Gen Psychiatry* 68: 675–690.
50. Baes, C., Martins, C., Tofoli, S. et al. 2014. Early life stress in depressive patients: HPA axis response to GR and MR agonist. *Front Psychiatry* 5: 2. doi:10.3389/fpsyt.2014.00002.
51. Wang, Q., Verweij, E.W.E., Krugers, H.J., Joels, M., Swaab, D. F., and Lucassen, P.J. 2013. Distribution of the glucocorticoid receptor in the human amygdala; changes in mood disorder patients. *Brain Struct Funct* 219: 1615–1626.
52. Maripuu, M., Wikgren, M., Karling, P. et al. 2014. Relative hypo- and hypercortisolism are both associated with depression and lower quality of life in bipolar disorder: A cross-sectional study. *PLoS One* 9: e98682
53. McGirr, A., Diaconu, G., Berlim, M.T., Pruessner, J.C., Sablé, R., Cabot, S., and Turecki, G. 2010. Dysregulation of the sympathetic nervous system, hypothalamic-pituitary-adrenal axis and executive function in individuals at risk for suicide. *J Psychiatry Neurosci* 35: 399–408.
54. Vgontzas, A.N., Bixler, E.O., Lin, H.M., Prolo, P., Mastorakos, G., Vela-Bueno, A., Kales, A., and Chrousos, G.P. 2001. Chronic insomnia is associated with nyctohemeral activation of the hypothalamic-pituitary-adrenal axis: Clinical implications. *J Clin Endocrinol Metab* 86: 3787–3794.
55. Deppermann, S., Storchak, H., Fallgatter, A.J. et al. 2014. Stress-induced neuroplasticity: (Mal)adaptation to adverse life events in patients with PTSD—A critical overview. *Neuroscience* 283C: 166–177.
56. Karl, A., Schaefer, M., Malta, L.S., Dörfel, D., Rohleder, N., and Werner, A. 2006. A meta-analysis of structural brain abnormalities in PTSD. *Neurosci Biobehav Rev* 30: 1004–1031.
57. Roca, C., Schmidt, P., Altemus, M. et al. 2003. Differential menstrual cycle regulation of hypothalamic-pituitary-adrenal axis in women with premenstrual syndrome and controls. *J Clin Endocrinol Metab* 88: 3057–3063.
58. Milutinovic, D.V., Macut, D., Božić, I., Nestorov, J., Damjanović, S., and Matić, G. 2011. Hypothalamic-pituitary-adrenocortical axis hypersensitivity and glucocorticoid receptor expression and function in women with polycystic ovarian syndrome. *Exp Clin Endocrinol Diabetes* 119: 636–643.
59. Swaab, D.F., Bao, A.M., and Lucassen, P.J. 2005. The stress system in the human brain in depression and neurodegeneration. *Ageing Res Rev* 4: 141–194.
60. Heesen C., Mohr, D.C., Huitinga, I., Bergh, F.T., Gaab, J., Otte, C., and Gold, S.M. 2007. Stress regulation in multiple sclerosis: Current issues and concepts. *Mult Scler* 13: 143–148.
61. Kern, S., Schultheiss, T., Schneider, H., Schrempf, W., Reichmann, H., and Ziemssen, T. 2011. Circadian cortisol, depressive symptoms and neurological impairment in early multiple sclerosis. *Psychoneuroendocrinology* 36: 1505–1512.
62. Mitrakou, A., Ryan, C., Veneman, T., Mokan, M., Jenssen, T., Kiss, I., Durrant, J., Cryer, P., and Gerich, J. 1991. Hierarchy of glycemic thresholds for counterregulatory hormone secretion, symptoms, and cerebral dysfunction. *Am J Physiol* 260: E67–E74.
63. Oosterman, J.E., Kalsbeek, A., la Fleur, S.E., and Belsham, D.D. 2014. Impact of nutrients on circadian rhythmicity. *Am J Physiol Regul Integr Comp Physiol* 308(5): R337–R350.
64. Patton, D.F., Katsuyama, Â.M., Pavlovski, I. et al. 2014. Circadian mechanisms of food anticipatory rhythms in rats fed once or twice daily: Clock gene and endocrine correlates. *PLoS One* 9: e112451.
65. Sofer, S., Eliraz, A., Kaplan, S., Voet, H., Fink, G., Kima, T., and Madar, Z. 2013. Changes in daily leptin, ghrelin and adiponectin profiles following a diet with carbohydrates eaten at dinner in obese subjects. *Nutr Metab Cardiovasc Dis* 23: 744–750.
66. Thakkar, M.M., Sharma, R., and Sahota, P. 2014. Alcohol disrupts sleep homeostasis. Alcohol; Roehrs, T., and Roth, T. 2001. Sleep, sleepiness, and alcohol use. *Alcohol Res Health* 25: 101–109.
67. Spencer, R.L. and Hutchison, K.E. 1999. Alcohol, aging, and the stress response. *Alcohol Res Health* 23: 272–283.
68. Stephens, M.A.C. and Wand, G. 2012. Stress and the HPA axis: Role of glucocorticoids in alcohol dependence. *Alcohol Res Curr Rev* 34: 468.
69. Richardson, H.N., Lee, S.Y., O'Dell, L.E., Koob, G.F., and Rivier, C.L. 2008. Alcohol self-administration acutely stimulates the hypothalamic-pituitary-adrenal axis, but alcohol dependence leads to a dampened neuroendocrine state. *Eur J Neurosci* 28: 1641–1653.

70. Zschucke, E., Renneberg, B., Dimeo, F., Wüstenberg, T., and Ströhle, A. 2014. The stress-buffering effect of acute exercise: Evidence for HPA axis negative feedback. *Psychoneuroendocrinology* 51C: 414–425.

71. Saxton, J.M., Scott, E.J., Daley, A.J., Woodroofe, M.N., Mutrie, N., Crank, H., Powers, H.J., and Coleman, R.E. 2014. Effects of an exercise and hypocaloric healthy eating intervention on indices of psychological health status, hypothalamic-pituitary-adrenal axis regulation and immune function after early-stage breast cancer: A randomised controlled trial. *Breast Cancer Res* 16: R39.

72. MacLean, C.R., Walton, K.G., Wenneberg, S.R. et al. 1997. Effects of the transcendental meditation program on adaptive mechanisms: Changes in hormone levels and responses to stress after 4 months of practice. *Psychoneuroendocrinology* 22(4): 277–295.

73. Fan, Y., Tang, Y.Y., and Posner, M.I. 2014. Cortisol level modulated by integrative meditation in a dose-dependent fashion. *Stress Health* 30: 65–70.

74. Goyal, M., Singh, S., Sibinga, E.M. et al. 2014. Meditation programs for psychological stress and well-being: A systematic review and meta-analysis. *JAMA Intern Med.* 174(3): 357–368.

75. Brand, S., Holsboer-Trachsler, E., Naranjo, J.R., and Schmidt, S. 2012. Influence of mindfulness practice on cortisol and sleep in long-term and short-term meditators. *Neuropsychobiology* 65: 109–118.

76. Serpa, J.G., Taylor, S.L., and Tillisch, K. 2014. Mindfulness-based stress reduction (MBSR) reduces anxiety, depression, and suicidal ideation in veterans. *Med Care* 52: S19–S24.

77. Turakitwanakan, W., Mekseepralard, C., and Busarakumtragul, P. 2013. Effects of mindfulness meditation on serum cortisol of medical students. *J Med Assoc Thai* 96 Suppl 1: S90–S95.

78. Prakhinkit, S., Suppapitiporn, S., Tanaka, H., and Suksom, D. 2004. Effects of Buddhism walking meditation on depression, functional fitness, and endothelium-dependent vasodilation in depressed elderly. *J Altern Complement Med* 20(5): 411–416.

79. Chan, K.P. 2014. Prenatal meditation influences infant behaviors. *Infant Behav Dev* 37(4): 556–561.

80. Boelens, P.A., Reeves, R.R., Replogle, W.H., and Koenig, H.G. 2012. The effect of prayer on depression and anxiety: maintenance of positive influence one year after prayer intervention. *Int J Psychiatry Med* 43: 85–98.

81. Dedert, E.A., Studts, J.L., Weissbecker, I., Salmon, P.G., Banis, P.L., and Sephton, S.E. 2004. Religiosity may help preserve the cortisol rhythm in women with stress-related illness. *Int J Psychiatry Med* 34: 61–77.

82. Chida, Y., Steptoe, A., and Powell, L.H. 2009. Religiosity/spirituality and mortality. A systematic quantitative review. *Psychother Psychosom* 78(2): 81–90.

83. Tartaro, J., Luecken, L.J., and Gunn, H.E. 2005. Exploring heart and soul: Effects of religiosity/spirituality and gender on blood pressure and cortisol stress responses. *J Health Psychol* 10(6): 753–766.

84. Olver, I.N. and Dutney, A. 2012. A randomized, blinded study of the impact of intercessory prayer on spiritual well-being in patients with cancer. *Altern Ther Health Med* 18(5): 18–27.

85. Minkel, J., Moreta, M., Muto, J. et al. 2014. Sleep deprivation potentiates HPA axis stress reactivity in healthy adults. *Health Psychol* 33: 1430–1434.

86. Sieverdes, J.C., Mueller, M., Gregoski, M.J., Brunner-Jackson, B., McQuade, L., Matthews, C., and Treiber, F.A. 2014. Effects of Hatha yoga on blood pressure, salivary α-amylase, and cortisol function among normotensive and prehypertensive youth. *J Altern Complement Med.* 20(4): 241–2450.

87. Riley, K.E. and Park, C.L. 2015. How does yoga reduce stress? A systematic review of mechanisms of change and guide to future inquiry. *Health Psychol Rev* 3: 1–30.

88. Rao, N.P., Varambally, S., and Gangadhar, B.N. 2013. Yoga school of thought and psychiatry: Therapeutic potential. *Indian J Psychiatry* 55: S145.

89. Sarubin, N., Nothdurfter, C., Schüle, C. et al. 2014. The influence of Hatha yoga as an add-on treatment in major depression on hypothalamic-pituitary-adrenal-axis activity: A randomized trial. *J Psychiatr Res* 53: 76–83.

90. Du, J., Zhu, M., and Bao, H. in press. The role of nutrients in protecting mitochondrial function and neurotransmitter signaling: Implications for the treatment of depression, PTSD, and suicidal behaviors. *Crit Rev Food Sci Nutr* PMID 25365455.

91. Pluchino, N. 2015. Neurobiology of DHEA and effects on sexuality, mood and cognition. *J Steroid Biochem Mol Biol* 145: 273–280.

92. Labrie, F., Bélanger, A., Bélanger, P. et al. 2006. Androgen glucuronides, instead of testosterone, as the new markers of androgenic activity in women. *J Steroid Biochem Mol Biol* 99: 182–188.

93. Maninger, N., Wolkowitz, O.M., Reus V.I. et al. 2009. Neurobiological and neuropsychiatric effects of dehydroepiandrosterone (DHEA) and DHEAsulfate (DHEAS). *Front Neuroendocrinol* 30: 65–91.

94. Barrett-Connor, E., von Muhlen, D., Laughlin, G.A. et al. 1999. Endogenous levels of dehydroepiandrosterone sulfate, but not other sex hormones, are associated with depressed mood in older women: The Rancho Bernardo Study. *J Am Geriatr Soc* 47: 685–691.

95. Guazzo, E.P., Kirkpatrick, P.J., Goodyer, I.M. et al. 1996. Cortisol, dehydroepiandrosterone (DHEA), and DHEA sulfate in the cerebrospinal fluid of man: Relation to blood levels and the effects of age. *J Clin Endocrinol Metab* 81: 3951–3960.

96. Wolkowitz, O.M., Reus, V.I., Roberts, E. et al. 1997. Dehydroepiandrosterone (DHEA) treatment of depression. *Biol Psychiatry* 41: 311–318.

97. Wolkowitz, O.M., Reus, V.I., Keebler, A. et al. 1999. Double-blind treatment of major depression with dehydroepiandrosterone (DHEA). *Am J Psychiatry* 156: 646–649.

98. Schmidt, P.J., Daly, R.C., Bloch, M. et al. 2005. Dehydroepiandrosterone monotherapy in midlife-onset major and minor depression. *Arch Gen Psychiatry* 62: 154–162.

99. Alhaj, H. 2006. Effects of DHEA administration on episodic memory, cortisol and mood in healthy young men: A double-blind placebo-controlled study. *Psychopharmacology* 188: 541–551.

100. Olech, E. 2005. DHEA supplementation: The claims in perspective. *Cleve Clin J Med* 72: 965–966, 968, 970–971.

101. Martocchia, A., Stefanelli, M., Falaschi, G.M. et al. 2013. Targets of anti-glucocorticoid therapy for stress-related diseases. *Recent Pat CNS Drug Discov* 8: 79–87.

102. Wolkowitz, O.M., Reus, V.I., Chan, T. et al. 1999. Antiglucocorticoid treatment of depression: Double-blind ketoconazole. *Biol Psychiatry* 45: 1070–1074.

103. Quera Salva, M.A., Hartley, S., Barbot F. et al. 2011. Circadian rhythms, melatonin and depression. *Curr Pharm Des* 17: 1459–1470.

104. Hansen, M.V., Danielsen, A.K., Hageman, I. et al. 2014. The therapeutic or prophylactic effect of exogenous melatonin against depression and depressive symptoms: A systematic review and meta-analysis. *Eur Neuropsychopharmacol* 24: 1719–1728.

105. Breslow, E.R., Phillips, A.J.K., Huang, J.M. et al. 2004. A mathematical model of the circadian phase-shifting effects of exogenous melatonin. *J Biol Rhythms* 28: 78–89.

106. Buchanan, T.W., Kern, S., Allen, J. S. et al. 2004. Circadian regulation of cortisol after hippocampal damage in humans. *Biol Psychiatry* 56: 651–656.

107. Maggioni, M., Picotti, G.B., Bondiolotti, G.P., Panerai, A., Cenacchi, T., Nobile, P., and Brambilla, F. 1990. Effects of phosphatidylserine therapy in geriatric patients with depressive disorders. *Acta Psychiatrica Scand* 81: 265–270.

108. Cenacchi, T., Bertoldin, T., Farina, C., Fiori, M.G., and Crepaldi, G. 1993. Cognitive decline in the elderly: A double-blind, placebo-controlled multicenter study on efficacy of phosphatidylserine administration. *Aging Clin Exp Res* 5: 123–133.

109. Heiss, W.D., Kessler, J., Mielke, R., Szelies, B., and Herholz, K. 1994. Long-term effects of phosphatidylserine, pyritinol, and cognitive training in Alzheimer's disease. *Dementia* 5: 88–98.

110. Monteleone, P., Beinat, L., Tanzillo, C. et al. 1990. Effects of phosphatidylserine on the neuroendocrine response to physical stress in humans. *Neuroendocrinology* 52: 243–248.

111. Papakostas, G.I., Mischoulon, D., Shyu, I. et al. 2010. S-adenosyl methionine (SAMe) augmentation of serotonin reuptake inhibitors for antidepressant nonresponders with major depressive disorder: A double-blind, randomized clinical trial. *Am J Psychiatry* 167: 942–948.

13 Adrenal, Reproductive, and Thyroid Hormone Testing for Depression

Dean Raffelock, DC, Dipl. Ac., DAAIM
and Lara Pizzorno, MAR, MA, LMT

CONTENTS

INTRODUCTION

It is often helpful to look at hormones from a functional, hierarchical perspective when considering their potential roles in causing or contributing to depression. When we look at lab assessments for adrenal and reproductive steroids and thyroid hormones, we are looking at extremely important information because these are *genomic* hormones; they directly switch "on and off" the body's

DNA programs. We could call this class of hormones the "supreme commanders," because they significantly impact protein synthesis and can have a profound effect on moods, behavior, and inflammatory cytokines.

Other categories of hormones, such as amino acid chains (i.e., hypothalamic releasing hormones, pituitary trophic hormones, insulin, glucagon, IGF-1 and -ll), structurally modified amino acids (i.e., neurotransmitters, neuropeptides, cytokines, endothelin, and bradykinin), and local-acting signaling hormones (i.e., eicosanoids and nitric oxide), are clearly quite important. Neurotransmitter imbalances have been associated with mood disorders for decades now. However, only the genomic hormones have the ability to direct the DNA programs that control protein synthesis including the manufacturing and sensitizing of neurotransmitter receptors. It can be quite helpful to keep this important hierarchical distinction in mind when evaluating lab assessments for adrenal and reproductive steroids along with thyroid hormones.

This chapter focuses on the three most widely available laboratory mediums for evaluating hormones. Specific advantages and disadvantages of testing hormones in blood, saliva, and urine are discussed. It is hoped that this information will provide the integrative physician with expanded diagnostic and treatment options for patients suffering from depression.

A FUNCTIONAL ENDOCRINOLOGY APPROACH TO DEPRESSION

The symptoms of depression could be simplified into two fundamental categories. The first is a form of depression in which the person finds him- or herself in a lowered energy state in which it is very difficult to be motivated to take positive action for him- or herself or others. These patients tend to have difficulty stringing together multiple positive thoughts and feelings. They often report feeling as if they have fallen into a deep, dark hole from which they cannot climb out because there is not the available psychic or physiologic energy to do so. This is often labeled a "sluggish" or "melancholic" depression.

From a neurochemical perspective, this first type of depression is often thought of as a low norepinephrine or low dopamine mediated form of depression. Serotonin-norepinephrine reuptake inhibitors (SNRIs), norepinephrine-dopamine reuptake inhibitors (NDRIs), norepinephrine reuptake inhibitors (NRIs), and tricyclic antidepressants (TCAs) are frequently prescribed for this type of depression. However, this type of depression may be caused or exacerbated by either pathological or *suboptimal* levels of thyroid, adrenal, and/or reproductive hormones. Suboptimal levels mean that the lab numbers fall within the "normal" reference range but the patient has symptoms of hormone deficiency.

The second symptomatic category of depression is a form in which there is despondency or despair *coupled* with significant anxiety. These individuals may experience frequent agitation and insomnia and at times various forms of addictive or compulsive behavior. This second group might be generally classified as low serotonin or low GABA individuals or as having an "agitated" or "anxious" type of depression. Often SSRIs and GABA-related drugs are utilized. The low serotonin or GABA person's body may, in fact, be deficient in these neurotransmitters due to trying to keep up with elevated levels of catecholamines or cortisol brought on by prolonged hypothalamus-pituitary-adrenal (HPA) axis stress. Alternatively, the body may be producing an adequate amount of serotonin or GABA but have a pathological or suboptimal deficiency in one or more of the hormones necessary to manufacture or sensitize their receptors. For instance, adequate progesterone is required to sensitize GABA receptors and adequate estrogen, testosterone, and thyroid levels are required to sensitize serotonin receptors.

Blood serum laboratory tests can reveal pathologically low levels of these hormones, but a *functional* endocrinology approach can reveal less obvious deficiencies that may be the underlying cause or a complicating factor in depression. The laboratory numbers can be within the lower "normal" or nonpathological reference range, but the patient may still present with the symptoms of one or more hormone deficiencies. One example of this would be too much reliance on a "normal" blood TSH test to fully rule out hypothyroidism as a physiological cause of depression. These patients may report any of the following symptoms: feeling sluggish, fatigued, or depressed; having cold hands and feet, chronic constipation, hoarse voice, unexplained weight gain, scalloping on the sides of the tongue, dry skin, and/or thin brittle hair and nails. These are all possible symptoms of hypothyroidism. The importance of knowing the signs and symptoms of *functional hypothyroidism* along with assessing lab results but not relying on them as the only diagnostic tool better assures that the patient will not fall through the diagnostic "cracks" and fail to receive the assistance he or she is seeking.

In the above example, requesting a 24-hour urine collection that includes free T3 and T4 would be a better diagnostic tool than serum because it measures thyroid hormone production and excretion for a whole day, not just levels at the precise moment the patient's blood was drawn.

The knowledgeable integrative physician can make a distinction between a fully developed Addison's disease and a *functional hypoadrenia* in which the patient has a number of psychological and physical symptoms of suboptimal adrenal gland functioning, even though lab results fall within the normal reference ranges. Such individuals may present with depression, fatigue, orthostatic hypotension, hypoglycemia, musculoskeletal pain (especially lower back and knees), chronic allergies, food hypersensitivities, trouble waking from sleep, and/or significant energy drops in the afternoon, but not the unrelenting symptoms of untreated Addison's disease. This patient may be on the way to developing Addison's, but the clinician may intervene and help avoid the inevitable if he or she is aware that there is a somewhat predictable continuum of adrenal stress that closely follows the three stages of adrenal stress described in Hans Selye's perennial book *The Stress of Life*[1]: (1) the alarm stage (high cortisol, high catecholamines, high DHEA [dehydroepiandrosterone], high aldosterone), (2) the resistance stage (high cortisol, fluctuating catecholamines, variable DHEA and aldosterone, and (3) the exhaustion stage (low cortisol, low catecholamines, low DHEA, variable aldosterone). This example illustrates the importance of knowing which labs to request to help differentiate these three stages of adrenal stress so the most effective treatment strategy can be implemented. For this example, measuring 24-hour adrenal steroid production with metabolites or diurnal saliva testing of cortisol would provide better information than solely assessing morning serum cortisol and adrenocorticotropic hormone (ACTH).

Difficult-to-treat depression will often have a hormone deficiency component, no matter how apparent the psychological diagnosis may be. Replenishing needed genomic hormones can often enhance and hasten the psychotherapeutic process by helping the individual cope with his or her stresses with more resilience.

TESTING ADRENAL STEROIDS, REPRODUCTIVE STEROIDS, AND THYROID HORMONES IN BLOOD, URINE, AND SALIVA: ADVANTAGES AND DISADVANTAGES

SALIVARY HORMONE TESTING: ADVANTAGES

Saliva testing may be helpful for monitoring the four-point (6 a.m., 12 p.m., 6 p.m., and 12 a.m.) cortisol assay to evaluate cortisol circadian rhythm. It may also be helpful to monitor the cyclical pattern of estradiol and progesterone throughout the menstrual cycle in a premenopausal woman. Saliva testing is a more practical option than blood draws to assess the cyclical estrogen and progesterone pattern throughout the month in a cycling or perimenopausal woman. Saliva samples have been demonstrated to enable differentiation between the follicular and luteal phase for both estradiol and progesterone. Saliva collected daily throughout the menstrual cycle shows a specific pattern, with a mid-cycle rise and a peak in the early luteal phase. Mean salivary progesterone concentrations in the follicular phase range from 20 to 100 pmol/L, whereas peak concentrations during the periovulatory period may attain 300 pmol/L. This significant difference is consistently reported and allows for an assessment of ovarian function.[1] The clinician can see if the patient is cycling, determine where hormone levels are off during the cycle, and get an overview of the cycle's pattern.

Assessing free cortisol four times throughout the day (usually 8 a.m., noon, 4 p.m., and 8 p.m.) provides better information than a "one-catch" morning serum cortisol.

SALIVARY HORMONE TESTING: DISADVANTAGES

None of the reproductive or adrenal steroid metabolites discussed in the urine testing section can be tested in saliva, and thyroid hormones cannot be tested. These are major disadvantages when evaluating for possible physical etiologies of depression.

Saliva test readings may be generally unreliable.[2] Evaluation of saliva samples obtained from the same subject at the same time and sent to two different labs has been shown to produce results with rates of variation from 35% to 75% for estradiol, 8%–103% for progesterone, and 13%–40% for testosterone.[3]

Salivary testing has repeatedly been shown to be highly unreliable for testosterone. Salivary testing of postmenopausal women receiving transdermal testosterone supplementation found no correlation with salivary testosterone levels for any of the serum testosterone subtypes (total testosterone, bioavailable testosterone [free and albumin-bound testosterone], and free testosterone.[4]

It has been well documented that salivary testosterone measurements, more so than other commonly measured salivary analytes (i.e., cortisol), can be substantially influenced during the process of sample collection. Materials commonly used to absorb the saliva sample (cotton and polyester swabs) or stimulate saliva flow (powdered drink-mix crystals and/or chewing gum) can artificially inflate testosterone results as much as two- to threefold.[5]

Salivary testosterone levels are also susceptible to distortion resulting from the leakage of blood (plasma) into saliva as a result of micro-injury to the oral mucosa. In one study confirming this, the micro-injury group donated a baseline saliva sample, then manually brushed their teeth for 2 minutes using an American Dental Association (ADA) recommended medium bristle brush without toothpaste. Saliva samples were collected immediately after brushing and then every 15 minutes for 1 hour. A control group provided saliva samples without brushing teeth. In the toothbrushing group, the resulting micro-injury elevated the presence of blood and its components in saliva within minutes, and correspondingly, testosterone levels in saliva increased and remained elevated over baseline well after micro-injury, even in samples that did not appear visually contaminated with blood. The effect of micro-injury was specific for testosterone; neither salivary cortisol nor DHEA levels differed from baseline after brushing.[5]

In addition to possible blood contamination, the presence of both corticosteroid-binding globulin and sex hormone binding globulin (SHBG) in uncontaminated saliva renders questionable whether salivary steroids can accurately reflect circulating free steroid levels, particularly in the older patient since SHBG levels increase with age.

Another potential confounder is the presence of the enzyme that converts cortisol to cortisone, 11β-hydroxysteroid dehydrogenase II (11β-HSD II), in salivary glands. Significant conversion of cortisol to cortisone (the inactive/storage form) may occur in the salivary glands via the activity of 11β-HSD II. This enzymatic conversion is often underappreciated in salivary cortisol measurements with the result that the data reflect not cortisol, but falsely increased measurements of both glucocorticoids together.[2] Furthermore, ascertaining the ratio of cortisol:cortisone (the ratio of active hormone:hormone reserves) provides significant insight into the patient's adrenal health. The cortisol:cortisone ratio is easily determined using the 24-hour urine tests.

Storage temperatures can also contribute to error in the values estimated for salivary testosterone. One group of researchers evaluating the reliability of salivary testosterone found a striking linear increase in testosterone levels across 4 weeks for samples stored at 4°C. On average, after one week of storage at 4°C, measured testosterone levels increased 20.59% (9.1 pg/mL). By 4 weeks, testosterone levels had increased 330.77% (150.5 pg/mL) over baseline.[5]

Artificially elevated results have been reported not only for testosterone, but DHEA, progesterone, and estradiol using cotton-absorbent materials. On the other hand, salivary cortisol values are reduced by more than 50% when saliva is not retrieved immediately from cotton buds.[6,7]

In an effort to mitigate the numerous problems with saliva sample reliability, a recent review recommends collection of unstimulated saliva into small plain tubes and storage at −20°C as the best method to avoid known pitfalls. If long-term storage is anticipated, storage at −80°C is advised.[7]

However, there are additional problems for which no recourse is currently available. As we age, we produce less saliva, fewer hormones, and more SHBG. Since saliva tests reflect only the metabolic process of salivary glands and a limited passive diffusion of the hormones from the bloodstream, levels may be below detection limits in elderly patients.

On the other hand, saliva testing has repeatedly been found to indicate significantly higher than physiological levels of hormones assayed in samples from patients using transdermal creams to deliver bio-identical hormone replacement therapy. This gives a false impression of overdosing.[7] A possible explanation may be that red blood cells passing through capillaries rapidly uptake steroid hormones, which are lipophilic, and quickly transport them to salivary glands and other tissues. This results in elevated hormone concentrations in saliva, while serum and urine levels remain low.[8-10]

Saliva tests cannot capture hormone metabolites, so they do not provide the clinician with information essential to safe hormone replacement therapy, for example, what percentage of estrogens are being converted into carcinogenic (4-OH estrone) rather than protective compounds; the extent of adrenal fatigue; and the activity level of 5α-reductase (the enzyme that converts testosterone to the more potent [and potentially prostate-carcinogenic] DHT; DHT also promotes benign prostatic hypertrophy and male pattern baldness in men, and hirsutism and polycystic ovarian syndrome [PCOS] in women). The 24-hour urine test reports all of these variables.

Like serum testing, saliva tests also offer only a "snapshot" look at hormones that ebb and flow throughout a 24-hour period. Testing cortisol in saliva four times during the day gives a general indication of production patterns but still provides only four snapshots, not a 24-hour overview. Due to this fact, the conclusion drawn in a 2009 review entitled, "Salivary steroid assays—research or routine?" was, "The diagnostic value of salivary estradiol, progesterone, testosterone, DHEA, and aldosterone testing is compromised by rapid fluctuations in salivary concentrations of these steroids. Multiple samples are required to obtain reliable information, and at present the introduction of these assays into routine laboratory testing is not justified."[11]

One prominent lab, for example, has a salivary test and lists its postmenopausal range as higher than its premenopausal range for estradiol. Common sense tells us this cannot be true. A quality blood or urine test will show premenopausal levels of estrogens as being around 10 times higher than those of postmenopausal women. Most saliva labs show at most a difference of two- or threefold difference (and some show no difference at all). This is troubling.

Another problem that plagues saliva testing is assay cross-reactivity. This happens when the presence of one hormone increases the lab value of a different (but similar) hormone. For example, 7-keto-DHEA (a common supplement) can falsely increase DHEA, DHEA-S, and testosterone levels in many commonly used assays. Another example is the ability of estriol to increase the assay levels of estradiol. When patients take transdermal estriol, salivary levels can increase astronomically. These levels can artificially increase salivary estradiol values significantly. This causes a false impression that circulating levels of estradiol are much higher than they actually are. When using methods like gas chromatography-mass spectrometry (GC-MS), gas chromatography-tandem mass spectrometry (GC-MS/MS), or liquid chromatography-tandem mass spectroscopy (LC-MS/MS) are used in urine testing (some labs use these methods for serum testing as well), estriol will not change the analytical value of estradiol, so the providers can accurately assess the estradiol status with more confidence.

Saliva testing is not a reliable option for even a snapshot evaluation of androgen levels or for monitoring the absorption of sex hormones from transdermal creams, which are likely to show elevated salivary hormone levels, while plasma and urinary levels remain low.[2] There is now at least one lab claiming to be able to assay pituitary trophic hormones via saliva. This does not appear to make clinical sense given that trophic hormones are peptides too large to pass through salivary glands.

In summary, salivary steroid testing may be useful for assessing circadian patterns for free cortisol and for evaluating estrogen and progesterone *patterns* (ovarian function) in cycling and perimenopausal women. For these indications, collection of unstimulated saliva into small plain tubes and storage at $-20°C$ are recommended to avoid known pitfalls.

BLOOD (SERUM) HORMONE TESTS: ADVANTAGES

Serum testing offers a reliable and preferred option for testing a number of hormones, including

- All pituitary trophic hormones including follicle stimulating hormone (FSH), luteinizing hormone (LH), growth hormone (GH), adrenocorticotrophic hormone (ACTH), prolactin (PL)
- Thyroid panels including TSH, T3, T4, free T3, free T4, reverse T3, thyroid antibodies
- Insulin
- All hypothalamic releasing hormones

Measurement of these compounds in serum is the best choice because most of these hormones are longer-chain proteins and therefore do not easily pass through salivary glands or show up in urine in significant quantities if the kidneys are functioning normally. Others, for example, reverse T3, are extremely small, so are more easily measured in serum than in urine.

It should be mentioned that thyroid antibody testing is significantly underutilized. There is significant thyroid autoimmunity because of food hypersensitivities and cross-reactants and ever-increasing sensitivities to environmental toxins, especially heavy metals. Many physicians do not test thyroid antibodies, erroneously assuming that there is no reason to do so because thyroid hormone replacement therapy (HRT) treatment will remain the same. However, if thyroid auto-immunity is present, a progressive destruction of thyroid tissue takes place that will require increasing dosages of thyroid HRT. Also, rarely is only the thyroid involved in autoimmunity, so further laboratory exploration is encouraged to ascertain if other tissues are involved and which lifestyle changes may be helpful.

This test is typically covered by most insurance companies and is a commonly recognized method of testing for most physicians.

BLOOD (SERUM) HORMONE TESTS: DISADVANTAGES

Blood (serum) hormone tests directly assess the amount of hormones in the circulation; however, significant limitations must be noted. Most important is that measurement of hormones in serum is necessarily a "snapshot in time" peek at hormones that fluctuate significantly during the day within normal circadian rhythms and in individuals using any form of HRT. Blood drawn at 8:15 a.m. reflects levels for only that time of day and does not reflect changes throughout the day. In premenopausal women, the ovaries secrete hormones in pulses. In men, the testes, in which Leydig cells produce 95% of the body's testosterone, perform similarly with pulses that closely approximate 8 a.m. and 4 p.m. Postmenopausal women using bioidentical hormone replacement therapy (BHRT) or patented, pharmaceutical hormone replacement therapy (HRT), typically take their replacement hormones once or twice daily, as do men using BHRT.

Adding to the "snapshot" limitation is the fact that most serum tests report only "total" hormone values—that is, the sum of free, conjugated, and bound forms of the hormones—again, with the exception of testosterone, for which both free and total values are typically reported. Free estrone, free estradiol, and free progesterone are rarely measured in serum. Serum hormone tests typically include measurements only of total estradiol (E2), although total estrone (E1, the most potent and potentially oncogenic estrogen) may be available. Since bound estradiol and estrone are inactive, serum tests do not provide feedback regarding the levels of active hormone.

Another distinction often not taken into consideration in serum tests is differentiation among the free, conjugated, and protein-bound forms. Unlike bound forms, which have been completely inactivated, conjugated steroids, which have combined with simple molecules—glucuronic acid or sulfates in phase II liver conjugation—can be reactivated by glucuronidases and sulfatases. Sulfatases are not only highly prevalent in breast tissue, but are also found in numerous other tissues including the endometrium, ovaries, bone, brain, and prostate. Quantitative data show that the sulfatase pathway, which transforms estrogen sulfates into bioactive unconjugated estradiol, is actually 100–500 times more active than the aromatase pathway, which converts androgens into estrogens. Thus, the distinction between conjugated and bound forms of estradiol is clinically important since the sulfatase pathway is a significant contributor to body load of bioactive estradiol. Conjugated estradiol cannot be discounted as a factor in estrogen-related oncogenesis.[12]

In addition, conjugated estrogens can be reactivated in the intestines and returned to circulation via the action of beta-glucuronidase enzymes, which are produced by *Escherichia coli, Clostridium,* and *Bacteroides*, thus intestinal dysbiosis may increase circulating levels of active estrogens.[13] For these reasons, HRT assessment (whether bioidentical HRT or molecularly altered, patented HRT) should incorporate both free and conjugated estrogens. The 24-hour urine test does; serum tests do not.

Levels of unconjugated estriol (E3, considered protective and the weakest form of estrogen) are sometimes available in serum tests. While measurement of unconjugated estriol may be helpful in terms of evaluating a woman's risk of cancer, its usefulness is significantly hampered because 90% of estriol is conjugated.

As a consequence of all of the above, serum testing does not provide the clinician with adequate information to safely prescribe and evaluate the effects of hormone replacement therapy (BHRT or HRT). For example, a menopausal woman whose serum test results indicate total estradiol at normal levels may still be experiencing hot flashes and other common climacteric symptoms if most of her estrogen is bound, which it likely is, as levels of SHBG increase with age.[14]

Prescribing estradiol to this patient to alleviate her symptoms may result in increasing her levels of estrone since estradiol readily converts to estrone. This may not be advisable since estrone may be metabolized to the relatively safe 2-hydroxyestrone (2-OH), 2-methoxyestrone (2-CH3O), or estriol (E3) or into pro-carcinogenic 4-hydroxyestrone (4-OH estrone) and 16α-OH estrone. There is some controversy about the validity of 16α-OH estrone being indicated with cancer, but the research is clear about elevated 4-OH estrone levels increasing cancer risk. Serum testing will not indicate which pathways are capturing estrogens, so will not provide the clinician with the insight necessary to safely alleviate a woman's symptoms. Furthermore, BHRT typically involves using a compounded bi-test containing a combination of estriol and estradiol (often 80% and 20%, respectively). Yet serum testing does not usually measure estriol.

To be able to safely and effectively prescribe hormone replacement therapy (BHRT or HRT) will necessitate knowing not only how much estrone, estradiol, and estriol are in circulation, but how much is active (free plus conjugated [potentially active]), and into what forms each estrogen is being metabolized: Is her body predominantly producing protective or carcinogenic estrogen metabolites? These data are provided by the 24-hour urine test. Testing genomic hormone levels via blood samples is the most common form of testing and, in all likelihood, the form with which the average clinician is most familiar.

24-HOUR URINE HORMONE TESTING: ADVANTAGES

Urine hormone testing is well established in medical literature as a reliable method of assessing levels of active (mostly conjugated, approximately 2% free) hormones and their metabolites, and has been shown in clinical settings to correlate well with patient symptoms and reflect the beneficial impact (or lack of benefit and potentially oncogenic effect) of therapeutic interventions.[15,16] Since these tests offers a wealth of information that cannot be assessed within blood or saliva, a significant amount of detail is contained in this section. The immense value of some of the below-mentioned hormone metabolites relative to cancer risks are included to help BHRT or pharmaceutically patented hormone replacement therapy (HRT) strategies be as safe as possible. Few things in life are as depressing as the words, "You have cancer."

The 24-hour urine samples may be relied upon to accurately evaluate and monitor the following:

- Total daily production of hormones
- Overall anabolic to catabolic hormonal balance (sex hormones, glucocorticoids, mineralocorticoids)
- Levels of active (free plus conjugated) estrogens (estrone, estradiol, and estriol)
- Progesterone (indirectly using pregnanediol)
- Female and male sex hormone balance and metabolites
- Free androgens (DHEA and testosterone)
- Androgen balance
- Androgen metabolites
- Glucocorticoid balance and metabolites
- Activity of the 5α-reductase and aromatase enzymes
- Breast and prostate cancer hormonal risk factors (e.g., in women the 2:16α ratio, 4-OH estrone, the estrogen quotient; in men, the 2:16α ratio, the testosterone:estrogen ratio [low T:E suggests insulin resistance which correlates with increased risk for prostate cancer])
- Liver function as indicated by assessment of phases I and II metabolites
- Human growth hormone
- Adrenal health/adrenal reserves
- Response to and safety of hormone replacement therapy (BHRT or patent HRT)
- Free T3 and free T4

Measuring steroid hormones via urine testing using GS-MS, LC-MS/MS, or GC-MS/MS. Of these GC-MS/MS appears to yield the most accurate results. Radioimmunoassay (RIA) and enzyme-linked immunosorbent assay (ELISA, also known as enzyme immunoassay [EIA]) analysis may not be accurate. Comparisons of RIA and ELISA (methods routinely used to measure estrogen metabolites in blood and urine due to efficiency and low cost) with GS-MS and LC-MS/MS have shown RIA and ELISA estrogen metabolite measures to be much less accurate, especially at the low estrogen metabolite levels characteristic of postmenopausal women.[17–19]

A 24-hour urine sample is practical (collection is noninvasive) and provides a more accurate indication of hormonal output since it averages out the hour-to-hour fluctuations seen in both serum and salivary measurements. Urinary spot testing that measures urine four times per day on strips has come and gone over the years due to inconsistencies in results and difficulty accurately extracting hormones from the collection paper. At the time of this writing there is not enough evidence to recommend this form of urine testing. If the technology can be perfected it will have the advantage of offering diurnal cortisol plus metabolites and be preferable to diurnal salivary cortisol testing.

The 24-hour urine test captures numerous metabolites that are not measurable in saliva and cannot be reliably measured by a single, or even multiple, blood draws. Besides the necessity of adequate estrogen to help sensitize serotonin receptors, some estrogen metabolites have been shown to impact estrogen-related cancers, so the type of estrogen is very important clinically. This is a prime example of information offered in a 24-hour urine comprehensive hormone profile not offered in blood or saliva.

A number of glucocorticoid and mineralocorticoid metabolites measured in a 24-hour urine hormone profile, but not in a serum or saliva assay, provide greater insight into long-term adrenal health, short-term stress response, the cortisol/cortisone balance, and other measures of adrenal health and function than assessment of cortisol alone. These include cortisone, tetrahydracortisone, allo-tetrahydrocortisol, tetrahydrocortisol, aldosterone, allo-tetrahydrocorticosterone, tetrahydocorticosterone, and 11-dehydrotetrahydrocorticosterone. It is well documented that low adrenal hormones can cause fatigue that can mimic many of the symptoms of depression.

The glucocorticoid metabolites are especially important in assessing overall cortisol production. Free cortisol measurements (as in saliva) tend to be preferred by physicians using saliva assessments; however, the free fraction of cortisol is only about 1% of the total produced. Many patients show increased or decreased cortisol clearance. In these cases, free hormone measurements are important, but they can be grossly misleading when used to assess overall cortisol secretion. A common example of this is when hypothyroid patients present with high free cortisol with co-occurring symptoms of depression, insomnia, and weight gain. Hypothyroidism correlates with sluggish cortisol clearance, and often these patients make very little cortisol. Their free cortisol levels are high because they are not properly clearing cortisol and the metabolized cortisol levels (tetrahydrocortisol, tetrahydrocortisone, etc.) can actually be low in these cases, even though free cortisol is elevated. More metabolite explanations are noted under the specific headings below. Figure 13.1 depicts a steroid metabolism flowchart by one of the reputable 24-hour comprehensive hormone labs.

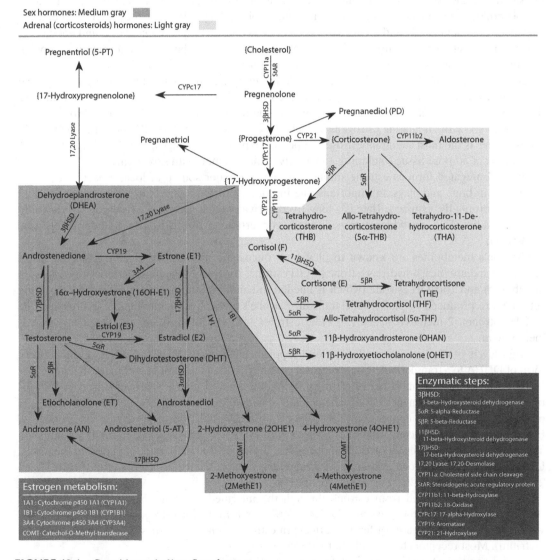

FIGURE 13.1 Steroid metabolism flowchart.

24-HOUR URINE HORMONE TESTING: DISADVANTAGES

Circadian fluctuation of cortisol cannot be measured using 24-hour urine collection, and it cannot show the monthly cyclical pattern in estrogen and progesterone production in a menstruating or perimenopausal woman. Twenty-four hour urine collections for each of the days (as many as 11) tested in a saliva panel may also be doable, although the logistics and out-of-pocket expenses make this an unattractive option.

It should be mentioned that there is a genetic defect in phase II metabolism of testosterone that is quite common in people of Asian descent, and it can register false lows in urine. If this defect is suspected, it is better to rely on serum testing to help monitor changes in testosterone levels.

24-HOUR URINE TEST ANALYTES: SEX HORMONES

ESTROGENS

Physicians should confirm that patients have a clear understanding of collection instructions because sample collection should occur during the mid-luteal phase (days 19–21) if the patient is premenopausal, or postmenopausal and on hormone replacement therapy; if postmenopausal and not on hormone replacement therapy, sample collection may be taken on any day. Different urine labs provide varying instructions, so it is best to follow the directions of the lab being used.

Levels of all steroids reported indicate predominantly the conjugated forms. The most potent estrogen, estrone is synthesized from androstenedione by aromatase in the ovaries and adipose tissue in premenopausal women, and in adipose tissue in postmenopausal women. Estrone, which constitutes ~33% of circulating estrogens in cycling women (compared to 44% for estradiol and 10% for estriol),[20] is the most abundant estrogen in postmenopausal women, especially those with a high percentage of adipose tissue (including apparently "lean" women with sarcopenia).

In its conjugated form as estrone sulfate, estrone is a major source of local bioactive estrogen formation in bone and plays an important role in bone maturation and homeostasis, especially in elders. Additionally, estrone sulfate is a long-lived derivative that serves as a reservoir for the more active estradiol (E2), into which estrone is easily converted via 17β-hydroxysteroid dehydrogenase (17β-HSD).

Estrone's metabolites are known to play both oncogenic and anti-oncogenic roles. Estrone's oncogenic metabolites, 4-hydroxyestrone (4-OH estrone, considered the most carcinogenic estrogen metabolite) and 16α-OH estrone (which is needed in small amounts because of its bone-building actions), are produced by phase I metabolism. Estrone's protective metabolites, 2-hydroxyestrone (2-OH estrone), 2-methoxyestrone (2-CH3O-estrone), and estriol (E3), are produced in phase II metabolism.

High levels of estrone may result from oral supplementation with DHEA. Switching the delivery form of DHEA to a transdermal or transmucosal cream will often lower EI to within normal range.[21,22]

Estradiol (E2) is the most active estrogen. Estradiol is the primary "estrogen" used in conventional hormone replacement (HRT) whether the delivery form is oral or patch. In humans, it is produced both from the conversion of estrone by 17β-HSD and from testosterone via aromatase. Estradiol is also readily converted to estrone via 17β-HSD, which is reversible. Small amounts are also produced in the adrenal cortex, adipose tissue, brain, arterial wall, and, in males, in the testes. Unless converted to estrone, estradiol is metabolized into protective 2-OH estradiol (phase I) and 2-methoxyestradiol ([2-CH3O estradiol], phase II).

Estriol (E3) is derived from estrone through the intermediate (bone-building but potentially oncogenic) 16α-OH estrone, estriol has 20%–30% less affinity for estrogen receptors and is the weakest estrogen, with antiproliferative effects in estrogen-sensitive tissues (e.g., breast and endometrium). Most receptors for estriol are found in the vagina.

Estriol has been found to have beneficial immune-modulating effects in patients with multiple sclerosis, increasing protective immune responses and decreasing the number and volume of lesions seen in cerebral MRIs.[23] Estriol is the primary estrogen produced during pregnancy, when it is made by placenta from 16α-OH DHEA sulfate (DHEA-S), an androgen made in the fetal liver and in the adrenal glands.[24]

In relation to breast cancer prevention, the amount of estriol relative to estradiol and estrone (the EQ, which should be >1), appears to be more important than the absolute amount of estriol.

An estrone metabolite, 4-OH estrone (4-OH E1), can be enzymatically oxidized to catechol estrogen quinones, which can damage DNA by forming predominantly depurinating adducts. This results in the accumulation of mutations and promotes transformation into malignant cells.[25]

Measurement of urinary estrogens also provides insight into liver and gut function, both of which may cause or contribute to depression when dysfunctional. Urinary levels of phase I and phase II estrogen metabolites serve as a functional indication of liver detoxification capability. Abnormal levels may indicate exposure to compounds that stress liver function, such as heavy metals, environmental chemicals, or pharmaceuticals including conjugated equine estrogens and progestins.

Urinary estrogen levels outside the reference range may also be suggestive of intestinal dysbiosis since beta-glucuronidase enzymes, which are produced by *E. coli, Clostridium,* and *Bacteroides* in the intestines, can deconjugate conjugated estrogens, enabling their return to the circulation.[13] For these reasons, interventions that improve liver and gut function may assist in gradual normalization of estrogen levels and improve mood and vitality.

Metabolites 2-methoxyestradiol (2-CH3OE2) and 2-methoxyestrone (2-CH3O E1) are phase II metabolites of estradiol and estrone. Metabolite 2-CH3O E2 has generated a lot of research excitement because it not only has anti-angiogenic and antitumor effects, but it has been shown to inhibit bone resorption, both by inhibiting osteoclast differentiation and by being cytotoxic to osteoclasts, while it is harmless to most normal cells.[26–29] Methoxy estrogens are difficult to measure, so it is recommended that the clinician become comfortable with the measuring methods of the lab he or she utilizes.

PROGESTERONES

Progesterone is the major naturally occurring member of a class of structurally similar hormones. It is produced by the ovaries, brain, and during pregnancy, the placenta. Progesterone opposes, modulates, and balances estrogen's effects, not only in the uterus but in numerous other tissues including the breast, brain, bones, urinary tract, and skin. Unopposed estrogen ("estrogen dominance") can excessively stimulate cell growth in the breast, uterine lining, and endometrium, leading to hyperplasia and cancer.[30] Levels of progesterone are low during the preovulatory (follicular) phase of the menstrual cycle, rise at ovulation, and are elevated during the luteal phase.

The body's innate awareness of the importance of balance between the estrogens and progesterone is illustrated by the fact that estrogen increases the expression of progesterone receptors.[31–33] Adequate progesterone is necessary to sensitize GABA receptors. Among its numerous other beneficial functions, progesterone also acts as a natural antidepressant[34,35] and diuretic agent,[36,37] activates osteoblasts to build bone,[38–40] normalizes blood clotting,[41] prevents blood-brain barrier breakdown after stroke by reducing expression of metalloproteinases and inflammation,[42] and plays a significant role among factors contributing to thyroid-stimulating hormone (TSH) and free thyroxine (T4) regulation.[43]

Symptoms of progesterone deficiency include depression, agitation, irritability, anxiety, anger, weight gain, water retention, headaches, swollen or tender breasts, fibrocystic breasts, breakthrough bleeding, spotting, prolonged cycles, mood swings, insomnia, achy joints, excessive bleeding, and endometriosis. Because progesterone is the precursor of the glucocorticoids (e.g., cortisol), low levels can significantly contribute to adrenal fatigue and the symptoms of depression.

Progesterone is an aromatase inhibitor,[44] so it may also help improve libido via increasing testosterone levels by preventing its aromatization to estradiol in women. (In men, progesterone's inhibition of aromatase may be useful for treating benign prostatic hyperplasia [BPH]. In men, progesterone levels should be similar to women's levels during the follicular phase).

Pregnanediol, an inactive progesterone metabolite, is used to provide an indirect (but accurate) measure of progesterone levels in the body, because progesterone's structure prevents it from being eliminated in urine in significant quantities.[45,46]

ANDROGENS

DHEA is produced in the adrenals and is the most abundant steroid in the human body. Levels peak between 25 to 30 years of age and then decline. After conversion into androstenedione, DHEA may be used to produce testosterone and its metabolites (for which reason DHEA replacement may boost libido in women) or estrone, and thus other estrogens.[47]

DHEA helps build new bone tissue, primarily through its indirect elevation of serum levels of estradiol, and has been shown to significantly improve bone mineral density in older adults.[47–50] Low levels are associated with increased risk of fracture and osteoporosis.[51]

DHEA and its metabolite etiocholanolone (also reported by the 24-hour urine test), inhibit glucose-6-phosphate dehydrogenase (G6PD), an enzyme that plays a key role in anaerobic glycolysis, the major route of energy production for cancer cells.[52,53] DHEA has significant immune-modulatory functions—both immune-stimulatory and antiglucocorticoid effects. Evidence is accumulating that DHEA may be effective as a treatment for the immunological abnormalities that arise in subjects with low circulating levels of this hormone, including the impaired immune response of older individuals and immune dysregulation in patients with chronic autoimmune disease.[54]

Etiocholanolone is one of two DHEA metabolites reported on the 24-hour urine test. As noted above, it has cancer-preventive antiproliferative effects via its inhibition of G6PD. Etiocholanolone is produced from androstenedione by the enzyme 5β-reductase followed by 3α-hydroxysteroid dehydrogenase (3α-HSD). Excessive DHEA supplementation (>25 mg/day in females; >50 mg/day in males) may be the cause of high etiocholanolone levels.

Androsterone is a DHEA metabolite derived from androstenedione via the activity of 5α-reductase followed by 3α-hydroxysteroid dehydrogenase (3α-HSD), and is therefore useful for monitoring 5α-reductase activity. If androsterone is high in relation to etiocholanolone, 5α-reductase activity may be elevated, resulting in increased conversion of testosterone to dihydrotestosterone (5α-DHT).

5α-DHT is many times more powerful than testosterone, and unlike testosterone, cannot be aromatized to estradiol. Thus, in women, elevated 5α-reductase may contribute to PCOS. (In men, excess 5α-reductase is associated with male pattern baldness). Excessive DHEA supplementation (>25 mg/day in females; >50 mg/day in males) is a possible cause of high androsterone levels. However, if androsterone is low in relation to etiocholanolone in men, then 5α-reductase activity may be low as well, leaving more testosterone to be aromatized to estradiol.

Testosterone is primarily secreted by the testes in men and the ovaries in women but is also produced in the adrenals, liver, skin, and brain. It helps to sensitize serotonin receptors and is important for its effects on female and male libido,[55,56] and on bone mineral density. In a yearlong double-blind study, postmenopausal women were given either sublingual micronized estradiol and micronized progesterone alone or with the addition of micronized testosterone. Bone mineral density in the lumbar spine increased by +2.2 ± 0.5% the HRT alone group and by +1.8 ± 0.6% in the HRT+T group. Total hip bone mineral density was maintained in the HRT alone group (+0.4 ± 0.4%) and increased in the HRT+T group (+1.8 ± 0.5%).[57] It would be much safer to use a topical delivery form for these hormones as there are serious problems with taking either estrogen or testosterone orally. Unlike topical estrogens, oral estradiol increases risk of heart attack, stroke, and deep vein thrombosis.[58–70] Transmucosal delivery of both these hormones is preferred.

In addition to its positive effects on BMD, testosterone significantly lessens the age-related decline in, and preserves, lean body mass and muscle strength in postmenopausal women as well as in men.[71]

Since women as well as men metabolize DHEA to testosterone, DHEA replacement in a female patient may render testosterone replacement unnecessary; however, if the 24-hour urine test shows insufficient conversion of DHEA to testosterone, replacement (at a fraction of the male dose—an adult male produces 40–60 times more testosterone than an adult female) may be indicated if depression, flagging libido, or excessive bone loss is an issue.

5α-Androstanediol is a testosterone/5α-DHT metabolite produced via the activity of 5α-reductase. High levels indicate testosterone is primarily being metabolized through 5α-DHT, especially if levels of 5β-androstanediol are low. As noted above, 5α-DHT is highly potent—anywhere from 3 to 10 times more powerful than testosterone. In women, elevated 5α-reductase activity is linked to acne, hirsutism, hair loss, hypothyroidism, PCOS, insulin resistance, and obesity.

24-HOUR URINE TEST ANALYTES: GLUCOCORTICOIDS

PREGNANETRIOL

Pregnanetriol is a progesterone metabolite and indicator of sufficient substrate for the cortisol pathway. Progesterone supplementation may increase pregnanetriol levels, but very high levels, while rare, are suggestive of 21-hydroxylase deficiency, which is the proximate underlying cause of adrenal hyperplasia. When 21-hydroxylase is dysfunctional, conversion of progesterone to both glucocorticoids and mineralocorticoids is blocked. Disorders resulting from glucocorticoid and mineralocorticoid deficiency as well as androgen excess can result in depression, PCOS, and infertility. DHEA may also be elevated.[72,73]

CORTISOL

Cortisol is the second most plentiful steroid in a healthy person. Cortisol increases gluconeogenesis, affects protein and fat metabolism, and affects thyroid metabolism. Both excess and insufficient cortisol inhibit, while normal levels promote the conversion of T4 to T3.[74,75] Cortisol has potent immunosuppressive and anti-inflammatory activity.

In excess, cortisol promotes insulin resistance and many features of the metabolic syndrome (e.g., glucose intolerance, hypertension, dyslipidemia). High levels of cortisol also decrease the ability of osteoblasts to synthesize new bone and interfere with absorption of Ca^{2+} from the gastrointestinal tract.

In twenty-first century life, cortisol is often elevated due to unremitting stress and sleep deprivation, and in "Catch 22" fashion, elevated cortisol promotes both. Elevated cortisol (or cortisone, see below) is associated with Cushing disease, unipolar depression, anxiety, panic disorder, PTSD in its early stages, sleep deprivation, exogenous cortisol supplementation, high-dose licorice root supplementation, intense physical exercise, and acute ingestion of alcohol.

Clinical signs of adrenal excess include insomnia, anxiety, insulin resistance, obesity (especially truncal adiposity), hyperglycemia, hypertension, easy bruising in the extremities due to loss of subcutaneous adipose and connective tissue, bone loss, muscle weakness, and sarcopenia. If causes are not addressed, adrenal fatigue and cortisol insufficiency is the likely outcome.

CORTISONE

Cortisone is the inactive metabolite of cortisol and serves as a "cortisol reserve," in the body. Cortisone is produced by the action of 11β-hydroxysteroid dehydrogenase (11β-HSD), an enzyme with two isoforms, the first of which, 11β-hydroxysteroid dehydrogenase I (11β-HSD I), catalyzes cortisone into cortisol, enabling rapid supply of the active hormone as needed. The second isoform, 11β-HSD II, inactivates cortisol to cortisone (an action that is reversible via the activity of 11β-HSD I).

Decreased cortisol or cortisone seen with adrenal insufficiency is associated with late stage panic disorder, chronic fatigue syndrome, fibromyalgia, and rheumatoid arthritis. The clinical signs of adrenal insufficiency include depression, insomnia, irritability, fatigue, exercise intolerance, hypoglycemia, salt craving, positive Hippus test (greater light exposure should result in pupil contraction), and low blood pressure. The ideal cortisol:cortisone ratio is 0.7 (i.e., cortisone should be ~30% higher than cortisol), as this indicates slightly more storage (cortisone) than active (cortisol) hormone. Sleep problems are common when this ratio gets to ≥1.

A ratio greater than 1.4 is considered possibly suspicious for the hypertensive syndrome "Apparent Mineralocorticoid Excess Type 2." (AME Type 2 is a much milder version of AME Type 1, a severe and lethal congenital deficiency of 11β HSD II.)

Tetrahydrocortisone, Tetrahydrocortisol, and Allo-tetrahydrocortisol

Tetrahydrocortisone, tetrahydrocortisol, and allo-tetrahydrocortisol are metabolites of cortisone (tetrahydrocortisone) and cortisol (tetrahydrocortisol and allo-tetrahydrocortisol), and can be used to determine daily cortisol output.

When their 24-hour urine test values are added together, these three metabolites account for approximately half of daily cortisol output. Taking the sum of the three, doubling it, and moving the decimal three points to the left will give, in milligrams, about how much cortisol is being made each day. For a female, these three metabolites should add up to 5000 to 7000, which translates to a cortisol output of 10–14 mg/day. For a male, the three metabolites should add up to between 8000 and 10,000, which corresponds to a cortisol output of 16–20 mg/day.

Low levels are a very strong indication of weak adrenal function and may cause fatigue and the low moods of depression. If allo-tetrahydrocorticosterone (5α-THB), tetrahydrocorticosterone (THB), and 11-dehydrotetrahydrocorticosterone (THA) levels are also low, this is a very strong indication of long-term adrenal insufficiency.

11β-OH Androsterone and 11β-OH Etiocholanolone

11β-OH androsterone and 11β-OH etiocholanolone are terminal metabolites of cortisol. Their values will confirm if cortisol production is excessive or insufficient. Often, as patients become insufficient, cortisol levels may still appear within normal range, but downstream metabolites will be low.

24-HOUR URINE TEST ANALYTES: MINERALOCORTICOIDS

Aldosterone

Aldosterone is the major mineralocorticoid. Aldosterone is part of the renin-angiotensin system and acts on the distal tubules and collecting ducts of the nephron (the functional unit of the kidney) to cause conservation of sodium, secretion of potassium, increased water retention, and increased blood pressure. Aldosterone levels are usually a reliable indication of whether a person is on a normal, low-, or high-salt diet.

Allo-tetrahydrocorticosterone, Tetrahydrocorticosterone, and 11-Dehydrotetrahydrocorticosterone

Allo-tetrahydrocorticosterone (5α-THB), tetrahydrocorticosterone (THB), and 11-dehydrotetrahydrocorticosterone (THA) are metabolites of aldosterone that serve as sensitive markers for monitoring acute adrenal stress. These metabolites are the first to rise in the ACTH stimulation test; high levels suggest acute stress at the time of collection. Low levels are a good indication of chronic adrenal fatigue.

THYROID HORMONES

Upon stimulation by thyroid-stimulating hormone (TSH), the thyroid produces two main hormones: thyroxine (T4), the major form of thyroid hormone in the blood, and triiodothyronine (T3), the active hormone (three to four times more potent than T4), which primarily regulates the metabolic machinery inside cells. (The ratio of T4 to T3 released into the blood is roughly 20 to 1.) Thyroid hormones' effects include controlling the speed of protein synthesis, mitochondrial energy production, and sensitivity to other hormones.

Both thyroid hormones combine tyrosine with iodine (T4 with four iodine molecules, and T3 with three iodine molecules); thus, iodine insufficiency prevents adequate thyroid hormone formation. Even if TSH is effectively signaling the thyroid gland, and iodine is present in sufficient amounts for adequate production of T4 and T3 (blood test levels thus appearing normal), intracellular conversion to T3 may not occur for several reasons. T4 is converted to the T3 within cells by deiodinases (5'-iodinase), enzymes for which selenium is the required cofactor. Cortisol is also required for the conversion of T4 to T3; long-term stress, which depletes adrenal reserves of cortisone, will therefore cause inhibition of the T4 to T3 conversion. Inflammatory cytokines (notably interleukin-2) can promote formation of autoantibodies to the thyroid, again inhibiting the T4 to T3 conversion.[76] Thus, a patient can have hypothyroid symptoms despite normal serum levels of thyroid hormones. The 24-hour urine test gives a better indication of what is happening inside the cell.[77]

Ideally, one wants to see higher levels of free T3 than free T4. The richest food source of selenium, Brazil nuts, may help improve conversion of T4 to T3, and may also help lessen inflammation since selenium is a cofactor for reduction of glutathione peroxidases. One caveat here, a person should consume no more than two Brazil nuts daily, 5 days each week. One Brazil nut provides ~100 mcg of selenium; 200 mcg is the recommended dosage. Excessive selenium can interfere with enzyme systems related to sulfur metabolism and can be toxic in amounts greater than 900 mcg/day.[78–81]

URINARY MINERALS (SODIUM AND POTASSIUM)

Urinary levels of sodium and potassium clearly reflect dietary intake. The ideal ratio of sodium:potassium is 1.5. Due to the typical Western diet, which contains a disproportionate amount of high-sodium processed foods and few servings of potassium-rich green leafy and other vegetables, the ratio of sodium:potassium is typically elevated. Bringing this ratio into ideal range is well recognized to be of vital importance in the prevention of hypertension, myocardial infarction, stroke, and kidney failure.[82–85] When salt intake is high, even a modest reduction for a duration of 4 or more weeks has a significant and important beneficial effect on blood pressure in individuals with normal as well as elevated blood pressure. A modest and long-term reduction in population salt intake could significantly reduce strokes, heart attacks, and heart failure.[86] Decrease sodium by avoiding processed foods, and increase potassium by increasing green leafy vegetable intake.

On the other hand, 24-hour urine sodium on the low end of the reference range is not uncommon in people with low adrenal function. Many people have heard that it is beneficial to reduce salt and are overzealous about it, and thus they are not getting the sodium they require for good adrenal function.

ENZYME ACTIVITY

5α-Reductase is the enzyme that converts testosterone to the more potent (and potentially prostate-carcinogenic) 5α-DHT. In men, excessive 5α-DHT activity promotes BPH and male pattern baldness. In women, excessive 5α-DHT activity is associated with hirsutism, acne, and PCOS. In both sexes, upregulated 5α-reductase is associated with insulin resistance and obesity. 5α-Reductase activity is reflected by two ratios on the 24-hour urine test: (1) androsterone/etiocholanolone ratio and (2) allo-tetrahydrocortisol/tetrahydrocortisol ratio.

If excessive, 5α-reductase can be inhibited by zinc, gamma-linolenic acid (GLA), saw palmetto, progesterone, green tea extract, finasteride, and dutasteride. However, dutasteride, and presumably finasteride, can overinhibit 5α-reductase. In the Prostate Cancer Prevention Trial, a study involving more than 18,000 men, subjects taking dutasteride had a lower rate of prostate cancer, but a significantly higher rate of aggressive prostate cancers than the placebo group. This resulted in a higher absolute number of aggressive prostate cancers in the dutasteride group than in the placebo group—even though the placebo group had a higher rate of prostate cancer.[87] Thus, as we have seen elsewhere (e.g., rofecoxib [Vioxx®], celecoxib [Celebrex®]), balance in biological processes is more beneficial than absolute interruption.

11β-Hydroxysteroid dehydrogenase I converts cortisone to cortisol. 11β Hydroxysteroid dehydrogenase II converts cortisol to cortisone. 11β HSD I is inhibited by estradiol and HGH. 11β HSD II is inhibited by licorice and cadmium; this latter inhibition explains some of the hypertensive effects of these two substances.

11β-HSD I is highly expressed in key metabolic tissues including the liver, adipose tissue, and the central nervous system, where it reduces cortisone into the active hormone, cortisol. 11β-Hydroxysteroid dehydrogenase II (11β-HSD II) is found in salivary glands and aldosterone-selective tissues, for example, kidneys, where it oxidizes cortisol to cortisone to prevent activation of the mineralocorticoid receptor. The presence of 11β-HSD II in salivary glands can invalidate salivary cortisol measurements.[1]

Activity of 11β-hydroxysteroid dehydrogenase I and II is reflected by two ratios provided by the 24-hour urine test: (1) cortisone to cortisol ratio; (2) tetrahydrocortisol + allo-tetrahydrocortisol/tetrahydrocortisone ratio.

The ratio of hormone reserve (cortisone) to active hormone (cortisol) shows enzyme activity in adipose tissue and kidneys and provides significant insight into the patient's adrenal health. The ideal ratio is 0.7. Licorice, which contains glycyrrhetinic acid, can inhibit 11 β-HSD II, causing increased conversion of (storage) cortisone to (active) cortisol.

Low ratios for tetrahydrocortisol + allo-tetrahydrocortisol/tetrahydrocortisone ratio are associated with obesity and insulin resistance, while elevated ratios are associated with low-renin hypertension, high-dose licorice, and exogenous cortisol. The ideal ratio is 0.9.

In patients with essential hypertension, elevated ratios may also be a sign of primary aldosteronism (PA), for which recent reports suggest incidence may be as high as 10%–15% in hypertensive patients. PA may be missed in these patients because it can exist for many years before hypokalemia is demonstrable. Such patients are often misplaced on antihypertensive medications, which do not prevent progression of the hypertensive vascular complications induced by hyperaldosteronemia (i.e., heart attack, stroke, and kidney failure). If 11β-HSD ratios are elevated, hyperproduction of aldosterone will be detectable by ACTH-stimulated venous sampling.[88]

CONCLUSION

Deficiencies in any of the adrenal steroids, reproductive steroids, and/or thyroid hormones can contribute to the symptoms of depression. These hormones are *genomic* in that they direct DNA programs within the cell's nucleus. The integrative psychiatrist is encouraged to become familiar with the importance of looking for hormone imbalances as the possible cause or contributing factor when evaluating treatment strategies for depression and other mood disorders. Knowing the advantages and disadvantages of hormone lab assays (serum, saliva, and 24-hour urine) can help the physician initiate more informed treatment strategies.

REFERENCES

1. Selye, H. 1978. *The Stress of Life*. USA: McGraw-Hill.
2. Gröschl, M. 2008. Current status of salivary hormone analysis. *Clin Chem* 54(11): 1759–1769.
3. Hagen, J., Gott, N., and Miller, D.R. 2003. Reliability of saliva hormone tests. *J Am Pharm Assoc* 43(6): 724–726.
4. Flyckt, R.L., Liu, J., Frasure, H. et al. 2009. Comparison of salivary versus serum testosterone levels in postmenopausal women receiving transdermal testosterone supplementation versus placebo. *Menopause* 16(4): 680–688.
5. Granger, D.A., Shirtcliff, E.A., Booth, A. et al. 2004. The "trouble" with salivary testosterone. *Psychoneuroendocrinology* 29(10): 1229–1240.
6. Mörelius, E., Nelson, N., and Theodorsson, E. 2006. Saliva collection using cotton buds with wooden sticks: A note of caution. *Scand J Clin Lab Invest* 66(1): 15–18.
7. Lewis, J.G. 2006. Steroid analysis in saliva: An overview. *Clin Biochem Rev* 27(3):139–146.
8. Stanczyk, F.Z., Paulson, R.J., and Roy, S. 2005. Percutaneous administration of progesterone: Blood levels and endometrial protection. *Menopause* 12(2): 232–237.
9. Lewis, J.G., McGill, H., Patton, V.M. et al. 2002. Caution on the use of saliva measurements to monitor absorption of progesterone from transdermal creams in postmenopausal women. *Maturitas* 41(1): 1–6.
10. Wren, B.G., McFarland, K., Edwards, L. et al. 2000. Effect of sequential transdermal progesterone cream on endometrium, bleeding pattern, and plasma progesterone and salivary progesterone levels in postmenopausal women. *Climacteric* 3(3): 155–160.
11. Wood, P. 2009. Salivary steroid assays—research or routine? *Ann Clin Biochem* 46(Pt 3): 183–196.
12. Pasqualini, J.R. and Chetrite, G.S. 2005. Recent insight on the control of enzymes involved in estrogen formation and transformation in human breast cancer. *J Steroid Biochem Mol Biol* 93(2–5):221–236.
13. Lyon, M., Bland, J., and Jones, D. 2005. Chapter 31: Clinical approaches to detoxification and biotransformation. In *Textbook of Functional Medicine*. Perkins, H., Benum, S., Larson-Irwin, D., and Eury, T. (eds.). Gig Harbor, WA: Institute for Functional Medicine, p. 564.
14. Maggio, M., Lauretani, F., Basaria, S. et al. 2008. Sex hormone binding globulin levels across the adult lifespan in women—The role of body mass index and fasting insulin. *J Endocrinol Invest* 31(7): 597–601.
15. Eliassen, A.H., Ziegler, R.G., Rosner, B. et al. 2009. Reproducibility of fifteen urinary estrogens and estrogen metabolites over a 2- to 3-year period in premenopausal women. *Cancer Epidemiol Biomarkers Prev* 18(11): 2860–2868.
16. Falk, R.T., Xu, X., Keefer, L. et al. 2008. A liquid chromatography-mass spectrometry method for the simultaneous measurement of 15 urinary estrogens and estrogen metabolites: Assay reproducibility and interindividual variability. *Cancer Epidemiol Biomarkers Prev* 17(12): 3411–3418.
17. Faupel-Badger, J.M., Fuhrman, B.J., Xu, X. et al. 2010. Comparison of liquid chromatography-tandem mass spectrometry, RIA, and ELISA methods for measurement of urinary estrogens. *Cancer Epidemiol Biomarkers Prev* 19(1): 292–300.
18. Wolthers, B.G. and Kraan, G.P. 1999. Clinical applications of gas chromatography and gas chromatography-mass spectrometry of steroids. *J Chromatogr A* 843(1–2): 247–274.
19. Moon, J.Y., Jung, H.J., Moon, M.H. et al. 2009. Heat-map visualization of gas chromatography-mass spectrometry based quantitative signatures on steroid metabolism. *J Am Soc Mass Spectrom* 20(9): 1626–1637.
20. Xu, X., Roman, J.M., Issaq, H.J. et al. 2007. Quantitative measurement of endogenous estrogens and estrogen metabolites in human serum by liquid chromatography-tandem mass spectrometry. *Anal Chem* 79(20): 7813–7821.
21. Wright, J.V. 2005. Bio-identical steroid hormone replacement: Selected observations from 23 years of clinical and laboratory practice. *Ann N Y Acad Sci* 1057: 506–524.
22. Wright, J.V. 2010. Bio-identical HRT risks you need to know about and the simple solutions that will solve them—naturally. *Nutrition and Healing*. Available at: http://wrightnewsletter.com/2010/01/01/january-2010/
23. Gold, S.M. and Voskuhl, R.R. 2009. Estrogen treatment in multiple sclerosis. *J Neurol Sci* 286(1–2): 99–103.
24. Touchstone, J.C., Greene, J.W. Jr, McElroy, R.C. et al. Blood estriol conjugation during human pregnancy. *Biochemistry* 2: 653–657.
25. Saeed, M., Rogan, E., Fernandez, S.V. et al. 2007. Formation of depurinating N3Adenine and N7Guanine adducts by MCF-10F cells cultured in the presence of 4-hydroxyestradiol. *Int J Cancer* 120(8): 1821–1824.

26. Mooberry, S.L. 2003. New insights into 2-methoxyestradiol, a promising antiangiogenic and antitumor agent. *Curr Opin Oncol* 15(6): 425–430.

27. Ricker, J.L., Chen, Z., Yang, X.P. et al. 2004. 2-Methoxyestradiol inhibits hypoxia-inducible factor 1alpha, tumor growth, and angiogenesis and augments paclitaxel efficacy in head and neck squamous cell carcinoma. *Clin Cancer Res* 10(24): 8665–8673.

28. Chua, Y.S., Chua, Y.L., and Hagen, T. 2010. Structure activity analysis of 2-methoxyestradiol analogues reveals targeting of microtubules as the major mechanism of antiproliferative and proapoptotic activity. *Mol Cancer Ther* 9(1): 224–235.

29. Maran, A., Gorny, G., Oursler, M.J. et al. 2006. 2-Methoxyestradiol inhibits differentiation and is cytotoxic to osteoclasts. *J Cell Biochem* 99(2): 425–434.

30. Kim, J.J. and Chapman-Davis, E. Role of progesterone in endometrial cancer. 2010. *Semin Reprod Med* 28(1): 81–90.

31. Kastner, P., Krust, A., Turcotte, B. et al. 1990. Two distinct estrogen-regulated promoters generate transcripts encoding the two functionally different human progesterone receptor forms A and B. *EMBO J* 9(5): 1603–1614.

32. Micevych, P. and Sinchak, K. 2008. Estradiol regulation of progesterone synthesis in the brain. *Mol Cell Endocrinol* 290(1–2): 44–50.

33. Micevych, P., Soma, K.K., and Sinchak, K. 2008. Neuroprogesterone: Key to estrogen positive feedback? *Brain Res Rev* 57(2): 470–480.

34. Andrade, S., Silveira, S.L., Arbo, B.D. et al. 2010. Sex-dependent antidepressant effects of lower doses of progesterone in rats. *Physiol Behav* 99(5): 687–690.

35. Morita, K. and Her, S. 2008. Progesterone pretreatment enhances serotonin-stimulated BDNF gene expression in rat c6 glioma cells through production of 5α-reduced neurosteroids. *J Mol Neurosci* 34(3): 193–200.

36. Komukai, K. and Mochizuki, S., and Yoshimura M. 2010. Gender and the renin-angiotensin-aldosterone system. *Fundam Clin Pharmacol* 24(6): 687–698.

37. Fronius, M., Rehn, M., Eckstein-Ludwig, U. et al. 2001. Inhibitory non-genomic effects of progesterone on Na+ absorption in epithelial cells from Xenopus kidney (A6). *J Comp Physiol B* 171(5): 377–386.

38. Quinkler, M., Kaur, K., Hewison, M. et al. 2008. Progesterone is extensively metabolized in osteoblasts: Implications for progesterone action on bone. *Horm Metab Res* 40(10): 679–684.

39. Trémollières, F., Pouilles, J.M., and Ribot, C. 1992. Postmenopausal bone loss. Role of progesterone and androgens. *Presse Med* 21(21): 989–993.

40. Seifert-Klauss, V. and Prior, J.C. 2010. Progesterone and bone: Actions promoting bone health in women. *J Osteoporos* 2010: 845180.

41. Gee, A.C., Sawai, R.S., Differding, J. et al. 2008. The influence of sex hormones on coagulation and inflammation in the trauma patient. *Shock* 29(3): 334–341.

42. Ishrat, T., Sayeed, I., Atif, F. et al. 2010. Progesterone and allopregnanolone attenuate blood-brain barrier dysfunction following permanent focal ischemia by regulating the expression of matrix metalloproteinases. *Exp Neurol* 226(1): 183–190.

43. Zagrodzki, P. and Przybylik-Mazurek, E. 2010. Selenium and hormone interactions in female patients with Hashimoto disease and healthy subjects. *Endocr Res* 35(1): 24–34.

44. Shimizu, Y., Mita, S., Takeuchi, T. et al. 2010. Dienogest, a synthetic progestin, inhibits prostaglandin E(2) production and aromatase expression by human endometrial epithelial cells in a spheroid culture system. *Steroids*. 76(1–2): 60–67.

45. Fabres, C., Zegers-Hochschild, F., and Altieri, E. et al. 1993. Validation of the dual analyte assay of the oestrone: Pregnanediol ratio in monitoring ovarian function. *Hum Reprod* 8(2): 208–210.

46. Collins, W.P., Collins, P.O., Kilpatrick, M.J. et al. 1979. The concentrations of urinary oestrone-3-glucuronide, LH and pregnanediol-3α-glucuronide as indices of ovarian function. *Acta Endocrinol (Copenh)* 90(2): 336–348.

47. Labrie, F., Luu-The, V., Labrie, C. et al. 2001. DHEA and its transformation into androgens and estrogens in peripheral target tissues: Intracrinology. *Front Neuroendocrinol* 22(3): 185–212.

48. Jankowski, C.M., Gozansky, W.S., Kittelson, J.M. et al. 2008. Increases in bone mineral density in response to oral dehydroepiandrosterone replacement in older adults appear to be mediated by serum estrogens. *J Clin Endocrinol Metab* 93(12): 4767–4773.

49. von Mühlen, D., Laughlin, G.A., Kritz-Silverstein, D. et al. 2008. Effect of dehydroepiandrosterone supplementation on bone mineral density, bone markers, and body composition in older adults: The DAWN trial. *Osteoporos Int* 19(5): 699–707.

50. Weiss, E.P., Shah, K., Fontana. L. et al. 2009. Dehydroepiandrosterone replacement therapy in older adults: 1- and 2-y effects on bone. *Am J Clin Nutr* 89(5): 1459–1467.
51. Garnero, P., Sornay-Rendu, E., Claustrat, B. et al. 2000. Biochemical markers of bone turnover, endogenous hormones and the risk of fractures in postmenopausal women: The OFELY study. *J Bone Miner Res* 15(8): 1526–1536.
52. Yoshida, S., Honda, A., Matsuzaki, Y. et al. 2003. Anti-proliferative action of endogenous dehydroepiandrosterone metabolites on human cancer cell lines. *Steroids* 68(1): 73–83.
53. Matsuzaki, Y. and Honda, A. 2006. Dehydroepiandrosterone and its derivatives: Potentially novel anti-proliferative and chemopreventive agents. *Curr Pharm Des* 12(26): 3411–3421.
54. Hazeldine, J., Arlt, W., and Lord, J.M. 2009. Dehydroepiandrosterone as a regulator of immune cell function. *J Steroid Biochem Mol Biol* 120(2–3): 127–136.
55. Kingsberg, S.A., Simon, J.A., Goldstein, I. et al. 2008. The current outlook for testosterone in the management of hypoactive sexual desire disorder in postmenopausal women. *J Sex Med* 5(Suppl 4): 182–193.
56. Kingsberg, S. 2007. Testosterone treatment for hypoactive sexual desire disorder in postmenopausal women. *J Sex Med* 4(Suppl 3): 227–234.
57. Miller, B.E., De Souza, M.J., Slade, K. et al. 2000. Sublingual administration of micronized estradiol and progesterone, with and without micronized testosterone: Effect on biochemical markers of bone metabolism and bone mineral density. *Menopause* 7(5): 318–326.
58. Kuhl, H. 2005. Pharmacology of estrogens and progestogens: Influence of different routes of administration. *Climacteric* 8(Suppl 1): 3–63.
59. Buster, J.E. 2010. Transdermal menopausal hormone therapy: Delivery through skin changes the rules. *Expert Opin Pharmacother* 11(9): 1489–1499.
60. Eilertsen, A.L., Høibraaten, E., Os, I. et al. 2005. The effects of oral and transdermal hormone replacement therapy on C-reactive protein levels and other inflammatory markers in women with high risk of thrombosis. *Maturitas* 52(2): 111–118.
61. Lacut, K., Oger, E., Le Gal, G. et al. 2003. Differential effects of oral and transdermal postmenopausal estrogen replacement therapies on C-reactive protein. *Thromb Haemost* 90(1): 124–131.
62. Post, M.S., Christella, M., Thomassen, L.G. et al. 2003. Effect of oral and transdermal estrogen replacement therapy on hemostatic variables associated with venous thrombosis: A randomized, placebo-controlled study in postmenopausal women. *Arterioscler Thromb Vasc Biol* 23(6): 1116–1121.
63. Miller, V.M. and Duckles, S.P. Vascular actions of estrogens: Functional implications. *Pharmacol Rev* 60(2): 210–241.
64. Canonico, M., Fournier, A., Carcaillon, L. et al. 2010. Postmenopausal hormone therapy and risk of idiopathic venous thromboembolism: Results from the E3N cohort study. *Arterioscler Thromb Vasc Biol* 30(2): 340–345.
65. Oger, E., Alhenc-Gelas, M., Lacut, K. et al. 2003. Differential effects of oral and transdermal estrogen/progesterone regimens on sensitivity to activated protein C among postmenopausal women: A randomized trial. *Arterioscler Thromb Vasc Biol* 23(9): 1671–1676.
66. Abbas, A., Fadel, P.J., Wang, Z. et al. 2004. Contrasting effects of oral versus transdermal estrogen on serum amyloid A (SAA) and high-density lipoprotein-SAA in postmenopausal women. *Arterioscler Thromb Vasc Biol* 24(10): e164–e167.
67. Canonico, M., Oger, E., Plu-Bureau, G. et al. 2007. Hormone therapy and venous thromboembolism among postmenopausal women: Impact of the route of estrogen administration and progestogens: The ESTHER study. *Circulation* 115(7): 840–845.
68. Straczek, C., Oger, E., Yon de Jonage-Canonico, M.B. et al. 2005. Prothrombotic mutations, hormone therapy, and venous thromboembolism among postmenopausal women: Impact of the route of estrogen administration. *Circulation* 112(22): 3495–3500.
69. Friel, P.N., Hinchcliffe, C., and Wright, J.V. 2005. Hormone replacement with estradiol: Conventional oral doses result in excessive exposure to estrone. *Altern Med Rev* 10(1): 36–41.
70. Chen, F.P., Lee, N., Soong, Y.K. et al. 2001. Comparison of transdermal and oral estrogen-progestin replacement therapy: Effects on cardiovascular risk factors. *Menopause* 8(5): 347–352.
71. van Geel, T.A., Geusens, P.P., Winkens, B. et al. 2009. Measures of bioavailable serum testosterone and estradiol and their relationships with muscle mass, muscle strength and bone mineral density in postmenopausal women: A cross-sectional study. *Eur J Endocrinol* 160(4): 681–687.
72. Dauber, A., Kellogg, M., and Majzoub, J.A. 2010. Monitoring of therapy in congenital adrenal hyperplasia. *Clin Chem* 56(8): 1245–1251.
73. Merke, D.P., Bornstein, S.R., and Avila, N.A. 2002. Future directions in the study and management of congenital adrenal hyperplasia due to 21-hydroxylase deficiency. *Ann Intern Med* 136(4): 320–334.

74. Kelly, G.S. 2000. Peripheral metabolism of thyroid hormones: A review. *Altern Med Rev* 5(4): 306–333.
75. Pizzorno, L. and Ferril, W. 2005. Clinical approaches to hormonal and neuroendocrine imbalances: Thyroid (Chapter 32). In *Textbook of Functional Medicine*. Jones, D. and Quinn, S. (eds.). Gig Harbor, WA: Institute of Functional Medicine, p. 645.
76. Jones, D. 2005. Clinical approaches to hormonal and neuroendocrine imbalances (Chapter 32). *Textbook of Functional Medicine*. Jones, D. and Quinn, S. (eds.). Gig Harbor, WA: Institute for Functional Medicine, pp. 644–668.
77. Ristic-Medic, D., Piskackova, Z., Hooper, L. et al. 2009. Methods of assessment of iodine status in humans: A systematic review. *Am J Clin Nutr* 89(6): 2052S–2069S.
78. Thomson, C.D., Chisholm, A., McLachlan, S.K. et al. 2008. Brazil nuts: An effective way to improve selenium status. *Am J Clin Nutr* 87(2): 379–384.
79. Gladyshev, V.N. 2006. Selenoproteins and selenoproteomes. In *Selenium: Its Molecular Biology and Role in Human Health*, 2nd ed., Ed. D.L. Hatfield, M.J. Berry, and V.N. Gladyshev. New York, NY: Springer, pp. 99–114.
80. Rayman, M.P. 2000. The importance of selenium to human health. *Lancet* 356(9225): 233–241.
81. Burk, R.F. 2002. Selenium, an antioxidant nutrient. *Nutr Clin Care* 5(2): 75–79.
82. [No authors listed]. 2009. High sodium-to-potassium ratio increases cardiac event risk. Study underscores the importance of balanced mineral intake. *Heart Advis* 12(4): 5.
83. Suter, P.M., Sierro, C., and Vetter, W. 2002. Nutritional factors in the control of blood pressure and hypertension. *Nutr Clin Care* 5(1): 9–19.
84. Hooper, L., Bartlett, C., Davey Smith, G. et al. 2003. Reduced dietary salt for prevention of cardiovascular disease. *Cochrane Database Syst Rev* 3: CD003656.
85. Hooper, L., Bartlett, C., Davey Smith, G. et al. 2002. Systematic review of long term effects of advice to reduce dietary salt in adults. *BMJ* 325(7365): 628.
86. He, F.J., Li, J., and Macgregor, G.A. 2013. Effect of longer-term modest salt reduction on blood pressure. *Cochrane Database Syst Rev* (4): CD004937. doi:10.1002/14651858.CD004937.pub2.
87. Thompson, I.M., Goodman, P.J., Tangen, C.M. et al. 2003. The influence of finasteride on the development of prostate cancer. *N Engl J Med* 349(3): 215–224.
88. Nishikawa, T., Saito, J., and Omura, M. 2007. Prevalence of primary aldosteronism: Should we screen for primary aldosteronism before treating hypertensive patients with medication? *Endocr J* 54(4): 487–495.

14 Exposure to Toxic Chemicals as a Cause of Depression

William Shaw, PhD

CONTENTS

INTRODUCTION

Because the human brain is so metabolically active, it is exquisitely vulnerable to any toxic chemical that causes depressed metabolic activity. There are good reasons that psychiatrists and family physicians dealing with psychiatric patients should be focusing on toxic exposures. Although many of the organs in the human body are subject to environmental toxic chemicals, the human brain and the brains of marine mammals such as whales and dolphins are especially vulnerable. These large animals have larger physical brains in absolute terms, but when measured using the brain-to-body-weight ratio (which compensates for body size), the human ratio is almost twice as large as the ratio of the bottlenose dolphin, and three times as large as the ratio of a chimpanzee. Therefore, the brain is a very vulnerable target in humans and large marine mammals because of its large size compared to total body weight and its high concentrations of fats (including cholesterol and unsaturated essential fatty acids) present in myelin and neuron cell membranes.[1] Many fat-soluble environmental chemicals deposit readily into this fatty tissue. Due to the fact that the brain is an extremely metabolically active organ (generating high quantities of free radicals), any amount of toxic chemical exposure only further increases the production of free radicals beyond baseline levels, quickly causing oxidative damage to the unsaturated fatty acids so important to brain function. The brain consumes up to 20% of the energy used by the human body, more than any other organ. Although the human brain represents only 2% of the body weight, it receives 15% of the cardiac output, consumes 20% of total body oxygen, and utilizes 25% of total body glucose.

There is a direct relationship between the amount of sulfur-containing amino acids in the brain and phylogenetic brain development. Birds' brains possess the lowest percentages, followed by those of rodents and then cows. The brains of primates contain higher levels of sulfur-containing amino acids, while those of humans and cetacean (whale-like) mammals have the highest percentage.[2] This high amount of sulfur in the brain makes it much more susceptible to binding a variety of toxic metals such as lead, mercury, and arsenic and toxic drug metabolites such as the acetaminophen metabolite *N*-acetyl-*p*-benzoquinone imine (NAPQ I) that binds to sulfhydryl (-SH) groups in the brain. Hair has a very high percentage of sulfur amino acids. It is tempting to hypothesize that the dramatic loss of human body hair (compared to our ape ancestors) with its high stores of sulfur was an evolutionary sacrifice in order to put more sulfur-containing amino acids into the brain. Therefore, it is conceivable that depression and other psychiatric disorders can be considered signals that may indicate toxic exposures to the brain.

ENVIRONMENTAL HISTORY AS AN IMPORTANT ASPECT OF PSYCHIATRIC WORKUP

A clinical strategy for complete history taking would include an inquiry into environmental factors that may have changed since the patient last seemed mentally healthy. Another key question should be what happened just before any of the patient's symptoms got worse. If the person is exposed to chemicals on the job, this exposure may be important in determining the cause of mental illness as well as in the provision of workman's compensation. A list of professions and common exposures are listed in Table 14.1. Even office workers may be exposed to a variety of indoor toxic chemicals that can cause what is known as "sick building syndrome," which is discussed in one of the most comprehensive and readable books on the effects of toxic chemicals on health, *Our Toxic World: A Wake Up Call*, by Doris Rapp.[3]

Various studies confirm that some chemical toxicants which modify brain physiology have the potential to affect mood, affect cognitive function, and provoke socially undesirable outcomes. With pervasive concern about the myriad chemical agents in the environment and resultant toxicant bioaccumulation, human exposure assessment has become a clinically relevant area of medical investigation. Adverse exposure and toxicant body burden should routinely be explored as an etiological determinant in assorted health afflictions including disordered thinking, moods, and

---

TABLE 14.1

Common Chemical Exposures in Different Occupations

Occupation	Common Chemical Exposures
Painter	Lead, mercury, solvents
Policeman, fireman	Carbon monoxide
Taxi, truck, bus driver	Carbon monoxide
Bicycle messenger	Carbon monoxide
Plumber	Lead, solvents
Lawn service, exterminator, golf course maintenance	Herbicides, pesticides, solvents
Welder	Toxic metals
Beautician	Solvents used in hair styling, nails
Home renovation	Lead, solvents, mold toxins
Farmer	Pesticides, herbicides, mold toxins
Manufacturing	Depends on processes and products
Airline baggage handlers	Carbon monoxide, diesel fuel
Medical workers, restaurant workers	Antibacterial soaps

behavior. In cases involving exposure to toxic air, water, or food, exploration of the history of the individual may require considerable effort. Some of the most common toxic chemicals in the environment are associated with depression and other psychiatric disorders and will now be examined.

CARBON MONOXIDE

One of the first accounts of depression caused by carbon monoxide exposure was presented to the author in an introductory biochemistry class by a professor at the Medical University of South Carolina in Charleston. A lawyer friend of the professor recounted to him that he had experienced bouts of severe depression during the work week but not on the weekends. Every weekday morning he would get in his older car and commute from an outlying island to his office downtown. Feeling bright and cheerful at the beginning of the commute, he would invariably feel quite depressed when he arrived at his downtown office about 30 minutes later. He was beginning to entertain the notion that perhaps the legal profession was not for him, given that the depression began just about the time he was unlocking his firm's front door. The professor told him that it might be a bit premature to take up a new profession and asked him to stop at the chemistry lab near his law firm at the end of his next morning commute. The professor requested that a test for carboxyhemoglobin be performed, which is a good indicator of carbon monoxide poisoning. The test result revealed severe carbon monoxide poisoning. His lawyer friend took the car to a nearby garage where a large hole in his muffler was found. The car was repaired. The depression no longer occurred, and his friend continued in his legal profession.

A study of 127 patients exposed to carbon monoxide who were treated with oxygen therapy revealed that 43% of the patients had symptoms of anxiety and depression as long as one year after exposure.[4] Individuals with carbon monoxide poisoning who were treated with hyperbaric oxygen had significantly fewer delayed neurologic sequelae.[5] In some cases, patients may completely recover and after a short recovery period, neurological and/or psychiatric symptoms appear again. This condition is known as *delayed encephalopathy,* and its occurrence rate is between 0.06% and 11.8%. In one case,[6] delayed encephalopathy began after carbon monoxide intoxication and included neurological symptoms as well as obsessive-compulsive disorder, depression, kleptomania, and psychotic disorder.

MERCURY

Virtually all occupational toxic exposures can also be a factor in individuals with hobbies. This author consulted with a physician who had a patient with severely increasing memory loss (suspected Alzheimer's disease) who was having difficulty dealing with his complex financial affairs. The patient had very elevated mercury following a chelation challenge test in which a chelating agent was given just before urine collection to assess toxic elements. Since the individual had a large number of amalgams (alloy dental fillings), which contain high amounts of mercury, he was advised to remove the amalgams and replace them with composites. After doing this, he was given chelation treatment for several months. Periodic tests revealed that mercury levels in the urine steadily declined until only small amounts of mercury were present following subsequent chelation treatments. At that point, however, the physician noticed high amounts of lead showing up in the urine tests. Further questioning revealed that the man had a hobby of making toy soldiers using melted lead from bullets taken from his father's ammunition provisions. Evidently, the lead vapor that he inhaled was likely stored in his bones for more than 40 years. After additional chelation treatment to remove the lead, the memory of the man returned to normal, and he was able to easily handle his financial matters again. This case is interesting in that the elevated lead in his body was not detected until his considerable mercury had been excreted, indicating that follow-up testing is essential in monitoring the progress of heavy metal detoxification.

Stephen Genuis[7] describes a case where a schoolteacher became increasingly depressed and eventually began having obsessive thoughts about murdering his students. A family physician immediately instituted therapy with a selective serotonin reuptake inhibitor (SSRI) antidepressant (fluvoxamine)—which, after 16 weeks of increasing doses made little difference to his depression or intrusive thoughts. At that time, he was referred to a psychiatrist, who failed to benefit him despite pharmacotherapeutic interventions including a second SSRI medication (paroxetine), a serotonin-norepinephrine reuptake inhibitor (SNRI) drug (venlafaxine), a tricyclic antidepressant (clomipramine), combination therapy of paroxetine and clomipramine, as well as augmentation therapy with antipsychotic medications (risperidone and olanzapine). In response to these drug therapies, however, the patient experienced assorted side effects including marked weight gain, persistent nightmares, debilitating drowsiness, and intractable constipation with no significant improvement of psychiatric symptoms. Suicidal thoughts became an increasingly prominent feature of his presentation. At this point, he was examined by a physician who was skilled in toxic exposures. The physician found that the psychiatric symptoms began after the patient read that omega-3 fatty acids from fish were good for health. The individual started eating large portions of tuna fish daily, but instead of feeling healthy, he became increasingly depressed. As a result of becoming depressed, he began to eat even more tuna. When his blood was tested, high mercury was found, and he was treated with a chelating agent, dimercaptosuccinic acid (DMSA), for 8 months to remove the mercury. In addition, the patient was advised to eliminate fish from the diet. All conventional medications were discontinued, all psychiatric symptoms disappeared, and the patient returned to his work at the school.

METAL TOXICITY DUE TO MULTIPLE EXPOSURES TO TOXIC METALS

In some cases, medical history may be unproductive even though toxic chemical exposure is the main cause of psychiatric symptoms. In such cases, extensive screening for toxic chemicals, infectious disease, and other biochemical causes of psychiatric disease may be necessary. The author consulted on a case in Mexico in which toxic exposure was the cause of a variety of neurological and psychiatric symptoms. A 20-year-old female college student with an excellent academic record, and no significant medical history, complained of a wide range of symptoms after a trip to a rural area of Mexico with her boyfriend. Her symptoms included disturbances in visual field, slow thinking, memory loss, difficulty forming words and sentences, inability to understand what her professors were saying, failure of arms and legs to respond to her wishes, shaking episodes, seizures, difficulty walking, chronic constipation, abnormal emotional responses with a "flat affect," extended crying spells, and severe joint pain in elbows, knees, right hip, and lower back. She denied the use of any recreational drugs. She was seen by a family physician and psychiatrist in Mexico City and was prescribed a number of psychiatric drugs and psychiatric counseling, which were not helpful. She was then sent to the teaching hospital of a preeminent medical school in the northeastern United States for further evaluation. She was given a computed tomography (CT) scan and three magnetic resonance imaging (MRI) scans of her brain without finding any abnormality. However, an electroencephalogram (EEG) revealed an abnormal brain wave pattern. Potential diagnoses at the hospital were multiple sclerosis, measles infection of the brain, tertiary syphilis, HIV infection of the brain, or prion disease (even though there have been no reports to date of cannibalism, a major cause of prion disease, in Mexico). She was treated with glucocorticoids to reduce inflammation, Klonopin® and Depakene® for the seizures, and the antiviral Acyclovir® in case she had a viral brain infection. However, her symptoms continued to worsen. After consultation with the girl's mother, the author recommended hair metals testing and referred her to an integrative physician in Mexico City for follow-up. The results of the test are indicated in Figure 14.1. Arsenic, barium, mercury, and uranium are somewhat elevated. Uranium is a toxic metal in addition to being radioactive. Figure 14.2 illustrates the nutritional elements. The girl had a variety of abnormal results in both the toxic element group and the essential element group that are summarized in Table 14.2. Figure 14.2 and

Toxic elements	Result µg/g	Reference range	Percentile 68th	95th
Aluminum	3.2	<7.0		
Antimony	0.046	<0.050		
Arsenic	0.12	<0.060		
Barium	3.3	<2.0		
Beryllium	<0.01	<0.020		
Bismuth	0.096	<2.0		
Cadmium	0.043	<0.050		
Lead	0.43	<0.60		
Mercury	3.1	<0.80		
Platinum	<0.003	<0.005		
Thallium	0.001	<0.002		
Thorium	<0.001	<0.002		
Uranium	0.22	<0.060		
Nickel	0.16	<0.30		
Silver	0.10	<0.15		
Tin	0.24	<0.30		
Titanium	0.42	<0.70		
Total toxic representation				

FIGURE 14.1 Toxic elements in hair sample of young woman with a number of neuropsychiatric symptoms. Units are micrograms per gram hair.

Table 14.2 indicate a marked excess of the essential element manganese, which is present in the hair sample at six times the upper limit of normal, a value at which manganese becomes toxic.

Most of the scientific literature focuses on toxic exposures due to a single toxic chemical. The author's experience, however, is that many toxic exposures are similar to the current case study and may involve exposures to multiple toxic chemicals as well as excesses and deficiencies of essential metals.

The patient was treated with ethylenediaminetetraacetic acid (EDTA) suppositories and oral dimercaptosuccinic acid (DMSA) for 2 weeks with complete remission of all symptoms, without the use of any other pharmaceuticals.

Elements	Result µg/g	Reference range
Calcium	2120	300–1200
Magnesium	280	35–120
Sodium	16	20–250
Potassium	5	8–75
Copper	56	11–37
Zinc	220	140–220
Manganese	2.9	0.08–0.60
Chromium	0.42	0.40–0.65
Vanadium	0.13	0.018–0.065
Molybdenum	0.045	0.020–0.050
Boron	0.33	0.25–1.5
Iodine	2.3	0.25–1.8
Lithium	0.007	0.007–0.020
Phosphorus	174	150–220
Selenium	1.0	0.55–1.1
Strontium	9.5	0.50–7.6
Sulfur	47200	44,000–50,000
Cobalt	0.015	0.005–0.040
Iron	17	7.0–16
Germanium	0.038	0.030–0.040
Rubidium	0.007	0.007–0.096
Zirconium	0.24	0.020–0.042

FIGURE 14.2 Nutritional elements in young woman with neuropsychiatric symptoms. Units are micrograms per gram hair.

TABLE 14.2

Summary of Abnormally Elevated Metals in Hair Sample of Young Woman with Neuropsychiatric Symptoms

Manganese—an essential element	6× upper limit of normal (most abnormal result)
Mercury—a toxic element	4× upper limit of normal
Arsenic—a toxic element	2× upper limit of normal
Uranium—a toxic and radioactive element	4× upper limit of normal

EDTA and DMSA bind a variety of metals including arsenic, mercury, and manganese. It is unclear whether uranium can be cleared with EDTA or DMSA. Undoubtedly, the symptoms of this woman were due to toxicity of several of the metals to which she was exposed. However, many of her symptoms were those often reported with manganese toxicity. In the case of this young woman, her lead was only slightly elevated, and the cause of her symptoms might never have been diagnosed if a blood test for lead was the only toxic analysis performed.

Although the use of lead in gasoline and paint has been banned in many countries throughout the world, lead exposure has been implicated as a cause of depression,[8] developmental delay,[9] crime,[10] attention deficit with hyperactivity,[11] and Alzheimer's disease.[12] Studies indicate that values of blood lead in the "normal" range that are 40%–60% *below* the current upper limit of common laboratory normal ranges (5–10 mcg/dL) are associated with significantly increased incidence of kidney damage,[13] depression,[8] developmental delays,[9] and panic attacks.[8] Due to the fact that excesses and deficiencies of metals are such a common factor in neurological and psychiatric disorders, the author recommends that metal screening be a part of the evaluation of every person with a significant psychiatric or neurological disorder.

Toxic metals that have been implicated in a variety of psychiatric disorders include aluminum, antimony, arsenic, lead, mercury, uranium, cadmium, and nickel. If any of these elements are in the highest concentration category (Figure 14.1) or if the total toxic representation (an indicator that takes into account all the toxic metals) is elevated, the author generally recommends chelation treatment. In addition, all possible efforts should be made to identify and eliminate well-known sources of toxic chemicals. For example, silver dental amalgams are almost 50% mercury. Chelation will not be effective until the amalgams are removed and replaced with less toxic fillings. Chelation should also be considered if there are elevated levels of copper and manganese, accompanied with severe clinical symptoms.

Figures 14.1 and 14.2 indicate that both deficiencies and excesses of many nutritional elements can cause psychiatric illness. Copper and zinc are two common elements for which both deficiencies and excesses are common. These heavy metal exposures are not rare.

TESTING FOR METAL TOXICITY

Hair metal testing is based on the transfer of metals from the blood perfusing the hair follicles to sulfur groups in the amino acids of nascent hair proteins. It is doubtful that this transfer should be thought of as a detoxification reaction. Humans have only a tiny amount of hair compared to most of our mammalian cousins, so it is doubtful that such reactions achieve a significant reduction in body metal load. It may be better to consider such reactions as coincidental rather than physiological systems honed to perfection by evolution. The author has found hair metals to be an excellent indicator of metal toxicity. Hair testing is analogous to hemoglobin A1c (glycohemoglobin) testing for assessing long-term glucose control. Blood glucose testing is the test of choice for monitoring daily control of glucose metabolism. In the same way, blood and urine tests of metals are essential for monitoring acute metal toxicity and to measure success of chelation in stimulating the removal of toxic elements, but hair metals indicate average toxic metal exposure over a long time period. Measurement of Napoleon's hair more than a century after his death[14] indicates that he may have been poisoned with arsenic by his British captors to prevent a new return to power. Hair metal testing of many of the victims of industrial mercury pollution near Minamata Bay in Japan who subsequently died revealed hair mercury values between 500 and 1000 µg/g hair, more than 100 times higher than the hair mercury of the young woman in Mexico City. Interestingly, The Great Plains Laboratory found amounts of mercury in hair samples of a number of women in Mexico similar to those who died in Minamata Bay. The Mexican women had used beauty cream that was 10% mercury, and they still had high hair mercury (levels similar to those exposed at Minamata Bay) years after the exposure stopped. The women had a variety of symptoms including multiple sclerosis, depression, and amyotrophic lateral sclerosis. Studies indicate that hair mercury provides an excellent estimate of total body burden of mercury[15] and that hair mercury is an excellent indicator of brain mercury exposure in humans.[16] Some studies indicating low mercury values in children with autism may have been due to the fact that many children with autism were exposed to acetaminophen; a major toxic metabolite of acetaminophen (NAPQI) may bind to hair sulfhydryl groups so that heavy metals are not able to bind to those same groups.[17] Thus, individuals who use acetaminophen on a regular basis may not be able to be adequately tested for heavy metals using the hair test; a drug history is essential to determine prior acetaminophen exposure. The chelation challenge test described below seems more suitable in such cases.

Blood and urine testing of metals are most suitable for the evaluation of acute exposures to toxic metals since several weeks may need to elapse after acute toxic exposure before a significant amount of heavy metals accumulates in the hair follicles, and then the hair grows sufficiently to be harvested. In cases where there is insufficient clinical history to differentiate acute and chronic exposure, the author recommends that hair metal testing be combined with blood or urine metals testing. Another option is the chelation challenge test in which a chelating agent such as DMSA, EDTA, or 2,3-dimercaptopropanesulfonic acid (DMPS) is given orally, and the amount of metals in the urine is measured for a period of time after the administration of the chelating agent. A baseline urine test is sometimes collected prior to the use of the chelation challenge but is sometimes omitted to reduce the cost of testing.

CLINICAL USEFULNESS OF CHELATION TREATMENT FOR METAL TOXICITY

The three chelating agents mentioned above (DMSA, DMPS, and EDTA) are widely used for chelation treatment. The use of oral chelation agents is widespread and is safe and effective overall. Intravenous chelation treatment requires much more training and caution before using this modality for treatment. Psychiatrists or family physicians who are nervous about the use of chelation for treatment of metal toxicity should know that the suppositories of EDTA and oral DMSA have an excellent safety record and are not difficult to use.[18] However, if uncomfortable with using this therapy for their patients, they should refer them to a physician who performs metal detoxification on a regular basis. An even better situation would be to enter into a formal agreement or a combined practice with an environmental physician. The American Academy of Environmental Medicine (www.aaemonline.org) has a referral database that will yield physician experts in this field in the United States and some other countries as well.

COPPER AND ZINC

Copper and zinc are both trace metals and only minute amounts of these metals are found in the entire human body. Copper and zinc have the ability to form positively charged ions in the body called *cations*. Virtually all of the copper and zinc in the body is in the form of these cations. Zinc ions always have an electrical charge of +2, whereas copper ions may have a charge of +1 or +2. This variable charge of copper ions is extremely important since it makes copper ions able to form free radicals by the Fenton reaction. (Iron is another ion that has this property and thus is suspected of playing an important role in free radical production.) Copper is sometimes found in cookware and is the major element in electrical wire. Copper salts are commonly used to control algae in swimming pools and water reservoirs used for drinking water. Algae overgrowth in our water reservoirs may be more severe due to global warming, and there is a concern that the use of even "safe" amounts of copper may expose us to excessive amounts. Copper salts are also sprayed on fruits and vegetables to control fungus overgrowth. Although it is an essential nutrient, even a slight increase in copper supplementation can be harmful to one's health.[19–22] Most individuals receive adequate copper in the diet and do not require supplementation. The only exception is when excessive amounts of zinc supplements are taken, which can reduce copper absorption and cause copper deficiency.[23] Therefore, copper is a nutrient in which there is not a wide margin of safety for intake. A little too much and a bit too little can both be very harmful. Adult vitamin preparations usually contain 2 mg of copper per capsule intended for daily use. However, some studies indicate that copper in excess of 1.3 mg per day is excessive even for adults.[19] Most individuals take in about 25% more copper than they need in the diet even without copper supplementation. Therefore, the body must have a mechanism for removing this excess copper. This important mechanism will be discussed later in this chapter.

BIOCHEMICAL FUNCTIONS OF COPPER AND ZINC

Both copper and zinc act as catalysts for enzymatic reactions in the body, and both metals are essential elements. Copper has about a dozen essential functions[24] but zinc has a much higher number of functions, perhaps as many as 200 different functions.[25] As a result, it is nearly impossible to state that a particular symptom of zinc deficiency is due to any of its specific biochemical functions. Zinc is an essential cofactor for enzymes such as alkaline phosphatase, alcohol dehydrogenase, and the digestive enzymes carboxypeptidase A, aminopeptidase, and phospholipase C. The synthesis of both DNA and RNA requires adequate zinc supplementation. Copper is required for cytochrome C oxidase in the mitochondria in order to produce energy, for the biochemical reaction needed to produce the skin pigment melanin, and for collagen cross-linking.[24] Copper has an effect on several biochemical reactions that regulate neurotransmitters and thus can be a major factor in psychiatric disorders. For example, the copper-dependent enzyme tyrosinase shunts tyrosine away from dihydroxyphenylalanine (DOPA) production. Copper inhibits dopa-decarboxylase, thereby inhibiting dopamine production while the copper-dependent enzyme dopamine beta-hydroxylase catalyzes the conversion of dopamine into norepinephrine. The copper-dependent enzyme monoamine oxidase (MAO) catalyzes the breakdown of dopamine into other metabolites.[26]

Zinc deficiency is common in depression and in anorexia nervosa. Almost all the signs of zinc excess are due to its inhibition of copper absorption and subsequent copper deficiency. Premature gray hair after excessive zinc supplementation is an obvious clinical sign of zinc excess that may occur with supplementation of more than 100 mg of zinc per day. Excessive copper has been found in a variety of psychiatric disorders. One of the most common causes of excess copper is Wilson's disease. The symptoms of Wilson's disease include neurological, psychiatric, and hepatic dysfunctions.[27,28] However, the types of symptoms that appear first are highly variable so that some patients with psychiatric symptoms may not have hepatic symptoms. The psychiatric symptoms include temper tantrums, inability to focus and concentrate, loss of emotional control, depression, and insomnia. Neurological symptoms include drooling, speech impairment, hypoactivity, difficulties in controlling facial muscles, tremors, and spasms of the limbs and face. In addition, abnormal copper metabolism has been reported in both obsessive compulsive disorder and schizophrenia.[26]

WILSON'S DISEASE

Wilson's disease is a genetic disease on chromosome 13 in which there is excess accumulation of copper, leading to deposits of copper in the liver and the brain.[29,30] It is estimated that the incidence of Wilson's disease is 1 in 40,000 people.[29,30] However, the true incidence might be much higher due to the high variability of symptoms that may be easily overlooked, and due to the fact that the immunoassay for ceruloplasmin may yield false-positive results in samples that have mutant protein sequences but deficient enzyme activity. Many individuals may have died before symptoms of Wilson's disease were diagnosed, or some may have had a less severe form of the disease that was never diagnosed. Individuals with Wilson's disease have two affected genes and must have received a copy of the defective gene from each of his or her parents. The gene for Wilson's disease has been cloned, and the dysfunctional protein has been identified as an ATPase copper pump[30] whose function is to remove copper from the cells. Over 200 different mutations in this gene have been identified,[27] so a simple DNA test is not yet possible. The high number of mutations probably also accounts for the wide variety of symptoms that occur in patients with Wilson's disease. With just 200 different mutations, there are at least 40,000 different Wilson's disease genotypes with somewhat different symptoms for each genotype. In addition, there would be a wide range of individuals with the heterozygous condition or with low activity polymorphisms, who might only be affected under certain environmental stresses. Copper is excreted mainly in the bile, where it is excreted from the liver into the bile duct and into the intestine to be removed in the stool. The copper pump in the person with Wilson's disease does not function correctly; therefore, not enough copper is transferred from the liver into the bile.

High serum copper is considered by many physicians to be a confirmation for Wilson's disease; however, high, normal, and low values can commonly occur. Biopsy of the liver for copper content is considered the definitive test for this, but most individuals would probably prefer to skip this invasive procedure and determine if treatment of excess free copper is valuable. An elevated 24-hour urine copper is also considered a good confirmation test for Wilson's disease, which is much less invasive than a liver biopsy. Since collection of a 24-hour urine may be difficult or impossible for many children with autism, the measurement of both copper and creatinine for 4–6 hours might serve as a less-definitive test in such children. And last, another useful test is a slit-lamp exam of the eyes by an ophthalmologist to check for corneal copper deposits, the so-called Kayser-Fleischer rings.

Ceruloplasmin is the main copper binding protein in serum. Six atoms of copper are bound to each molecule of ceruloplasmin, a large protein with a molecular weight of 132,000 Daltons. It is the non-ceruloplasmin or free copper that is elevated in virtually all untreated patients with Wilson's disease, regardless of whether total serum copper is high, low, or normal. High values of ceruloplasmin are found with pregnancy, estrogen or antiseizure drug use, infections, inflammation, tissue necrosis, and trauma. Since low values for ceruloplasmin in serum are characteristic for Wilson's disease, some patients who potentially have Wilson's disease may also concurrently have infections or inflammation, so the diagnosis might be missed unless the effects of infection and inflammation on ceruloplasmin values are considered.

MANGANESE

Manganese is used for the production of dry batteries, stainless steel, and ceramics and is an essential element.[31–34] It is being increasingly used as an anti-knock compound (methylcyclopentadienyl manganese tricarbonyl, MMT) in gasoline in many countries and is also present in the pesticide Maneb, as well as in paint. Water and tea are contaminated with manganese in different parts of the world. Manganese is present as a significant contaminant in the illegal production of cocaine and methcathinone. (The patient in the previously mentioned case study, the young woman in Mexico, denied the use of any illicit drugs.) Welders are also commonly exposed to manganese vapors in the materials used for welding. Manganese toxicity has been associated with Parkinson's disease, disorientation, loss of memory, anxiety, bipolar symptoms, hallucinations, mental confusion, loss of appetite, mask-like facial expression and monotonous voice, violent or abnormal behavior, reduced response speed, irritability, mood changes, compulsive behaviors, apathy, bradykinesia, gait disorder with postural instability, spastic hypokinetic dysarthria, and attention deficit.

Manganese toxicity has sometimes been diagnosed as multiple sclerosis or amyotrophic lateral sclerosis (ALS). The toxicity of manganese is attributed to increased conversion of dopamine to its semiquinone which can lead to increased free radical damage and neuron death.[32] Each molecule of dopamine semiquinone initiates the production of thousands of molecules of oxygen superoxide free radicals.[35]

Low manganese values in hair are associated with alopecia. Supplementation with manganese improves hair growth. Low manganese values are also associated with ataxia, low cholesterol, hearing loss, myasthenia gravis, and epilepsy. Dark hair dyes can contain manganese and thus falsely elevate hair levels. In the case of extremely high manganese levels obtained from scalp hair, pubic hair could be used as a confirmation test.

Cesium deficiency has been associated with depression, and values in the blood return to normal levels after supplementation, along with relief from depression.[36]

OTHER TOXIC CHEMICALS

In addition to toxic metals, there are tremendous quantities of other toxic chemicals that can likely cause psychiatric disorders. According to Doris Rapp,[3] in 1998, there were at least 1.2 billion pounds of chemicals released into the environment, with 80,000 different types. Only about 7500 of these chemicals have been safety tested and primarily on young, healthy males. In this author's experience, a wide range of toxic chemicals such as pesticides, herbicides, rodenticides, plasticizers, and antimicrobial compounds can cause severe depression. It is likely that any substance that can cause death at very high levels could also cause psychiatric illness at more moderate levels.

Organophosphates are a group of insecticides or nerve agents containing organic phosphorus that act on the enzyme acetylcholinesterase, a critical enzyme in insects and most other higher life forms. Forty different types of organophosphates are in use in the United States. Symptoms associated with exposure to organophosphates include personality change, destabilization of mood, impaired exercise tolerance, reduced tolerance to alcohol, and heightened sensitivity to organophosphates. The disorder associated with these symptoms has been termed *chronic organophosphate-induced neuropsychiatric disorder* (COPIND).[37] Additional symptoms may also include exacerbation of flu-like symptoms, impulsive suicidal thinking, language disorder, heightened sense of smell, and deterioration of handwriting. The most common clinical symptoms include impairment in memory, concentration, and learning; anxiety; depression; psychotic symptoms; chronic fatigue; peripheral neuropathy; and autonomic dysfunction. In addition, there are extrapyramidal symptoms such as dystonia, resting tremor, bradykinesia, postural instability and rigidity of face muscles, along with nonresponsiveness to levodopa treatment.

Decreased cholinesterase is the hallmark finding in acute organophosphate poisoning. However, it is interesting that in a study of a group of 25 Brazilian patients exposed to high levels of organophosphates with psychiatric symptoms,[38] none of these patients had decreased cholinesterase values. Decreased cholinesterase is the hallmark finding in acute organophosphate poisoning. Failure to find decreased values of cholinesterase leads one to the conclusion that other biochemical causes of organophosphate toxicity are in play in these disorders. In the group of workers exposed to organophosphates in Brazil, 48% were found to have psychiatric diagnoses: 13 with generalized anxiety disorder, 8 with major depression, and 3 with both, for a total of 24 psychiatric patients with one or more diagnoses. After removal from organophosphate exposure for 3 months, the number of psychiatric diagnoses dropped to 13. In addition, extrapyramidal symptoms were present in nearly half the workers, and that decreased considerably after organophosphate exposure removal. Therefore, it is critically important to remove all existing exposure as the first step toward treating chemical toxicity. The use of the Hubbard protocol (discussed below) appears to be a good choice for those exposures in which a specific antidote is not available.

One of the most common groups of toxic chemicals is pharmaceutical drugs, both prescription and over the counter. While we may be exposed to environmental chemicals in microgram amounts, we may be exposed to pharmaceutical drugs in the gram amounts on a frequent or even daily basis. Therefore, it is possible to be exposed to pharmaceutical drugs at amounts a million times higher than environmental chemicals. The drug acetaminophen, commonly used as an analgesic by millions of people throughout the world, causes marked reduction of glutathione in a variety of tissues. The use of this drug has been associated with increased incidence of autism, attention deficit, asthma, and testicular birth defects.[17] Glutathione deficiency and deficiency of other antioxidants are associated with both depression and manic depression.[39]

Another patient discussed by Genuis[40] is relevant as an example of exposure to multiple toxic chemicals. This patient reported experiencing excellent health until 2 years before, when she began to feel increasingly "emotionally unstable, irritable, and very depressed." The patient also complained of an 18-month history of debilitating fatigue, severe headaches, recurring dizziness, frequent bouts of apparently unprovoked palpitations associated with marked nausea and occasional vomiting, and intermittent visual changes, which she described as a "blinding blurriness." The main factor that had changed concurrently with the mood disorder was going to work in a hair salon where she was exposed to a variety of chemicals such as hair sprays, dyes, bleaches, permanent wave solutions, shampoos, and conditioners. The patient had previously seen two different family physicians and an internist who had conducted a complete neurological examination. Each physician concluded that the patient had a mood disorder and recommended antidepressant therapy. She was placed on a 6-month course of a SSRI (40 mg/day paroxetine) and then a subsequent 6 month trial of venlafaxine (150 mg/day). Neither of the treatments significantly relieved the symptoms of the patient. She was referred to a physician familiar with environmental causes of mental illness who recommended that she find an occupation with less toxic chemical exposure. She changed jobs, and as a result, her symptoms rapidly improved. At her follow-up visits, 12 and 24 months later she reported no longer having any of the previous psychiatric symptoms she had experienced as a hairdresser. In addition, despite a history of deteriorating health prior to being a hairdresser, both her nonpsychiatric (including visual, neurological, cardiovascular, and gastrointestinal complaints) as well as psychiatric symptoms resolved when exposure to the potentially hazardous chemicals was eliminated. This case study is important in that, in this case, the patient was able to be treated by a thorough medical history without laboratory testing. The other important factor illustrated here is that other somatic symptoms are common in psychiatric illness. One study found that a wide range of symptoms commonly found in major depression included fatigue, headaches, gastrointestinal symptoms, psychomotor slowing, insomnia, irritability, arthralgia, musculoskeletal pain, abdominal pain, and anorexia.[41]

Testing for a wide range of environmental chemicals is available from a first morning urine sample. The chemicals include the widespread plasticizers phthalates, pesticides, herbicides, and toxic gasoline additives. Metal testing for hair, blood, and urine and free serum copper is also available.

DETOXIFICATION METHODS FOR A WIDE RANGE OF TOXIC CHEMICALS

The Hubbard protocol has been widely used to detoxify a wide range of different chemicals. For example, large numbers of emergency workers and the general public were exposed to a variety of chemicals following the terrorist attack on the World Trade Center, including asbestos, radionuclides, benzene, dioxins, polychlorinated biphenyls, fiberglass, mercury, lead, silicon, and sulfuric acid.[42] Many of these individuals were successfully treated with the Hubbard protocol. *This protocol must be performed under the supervision of a physician.* An overview of the protocol follows[43]:

- Daily physical exercise, immediately followed by forced sweating in a sauna at 140°F–180°F for two-and-a-half to five hours with short breaks for hydration to offset the loss of body fluids and to cool down. The extended periods of time in the sauna were tolerated very well. Individuals with heat intolerance adapted quickly to the sauna temperatures, and after a few days were able to comfortably stay for 30 minutes to an hour at a time with no clinically observed adverse effects. The average length of the regimen was about 31 days, with time spent on the program varying from 11 to 89 days. Subjects take frequent showers, both to cool down and to remove substances from the skin and prevent their reabsorption. Water, sodium chloride, and potassium salts are taken as needed to avert dehydration or salt depletion due to the concentrated sweating.

- Nutritional supplementation centered on gradually increasing doses of crystalline niacin to promote lipid mobilization of stored toxicants and stimulate circulation. The flushing reaction commonly follows niacin and is associated with redness, heat, and itching. The typical starting dose is 100 mg niacin, increasing the dose up to 5000 mg as tolerance to the niacin flush reaction increases, and is continued for a period of 30–60 days. Time-release niacin or nicotinamide are not recommended. It is unclear if flush-free niacin like inositol hexaniacinate is effective for this protocol. The mechanism of flush-type niacin involves suppression of fatty acid release from adipose tissue followed by a rebound effect in which generation of fatty acids by lipolysis of triglycerides in adipose tissue is increased with concomitant release of toxic chemicals.

- Administration of additional vitamins, minerals, electrolytes, and oils includes vitamins A, D, C, E, B complex, and B1; multiminerals including calcium, magnesium, iron, zinc, manganese, copper, and iodine; sodium and potassium; and a blend of oils are administered in high quantities to prevent enterohepatic circulation of toxic chemicals excreted in the bile.

- A fireman exposed to a variety of chemicals during the 9/11 attacks described himself as "depressed, angry, and sullen," and said that he had "just no enjoyment out of life anymore." He started the Hubbard detoxification program "hoping to regain some sense of normalcy." After completion of the process, he reported the following to the supervising personnel:

> While on the program I experienced a change in my overall attitude and my mood. The best description I can give is that I feel more comfortable in my own skin. I no longer feel tired, depressed, weak, angry, or sullen. I sleep like a baby now. My future looks bright, and I am not overwhelmed by life like I was prior to the detox and after 9/11. I had no idea how this program could have renewed every aspect of who I am! This includes physically, spiritually, and emotionally. I am at a place where I never thought I would get back to again.

CONCLUSION

Due to their prevalence in our environment today, it is important that treating physicians be aware of the impact of toxic chemicals on human physiology. The extreme metabolic activity of the human brain and its very high concentrations of fats and sulfur amino acids make the brain a substantial target for a wide variety of toxic chemicals. Depression and other psychiatric disorders are commonly associated with a wide range of exposures to toxic chemicals. A complete medical history including work-related and leisure exposures to toxic chemicals should be included in every psychiatric history. Both toxic and essential metals are a common cause of depression and other psychiatric illnesses. Since toxic chemicals also affect other illnesses as well, a resolution of toxic exposures triggering mental illness will frequently lead to an overall health improvement. Testing for toxic and essential elements has been well established and is very reliable and relatively inexpensive. Such testing should be used on a frequent basis since abnormalities are so common. The physician treating patients with depression and other psychiatric disorders can provide simple oral chelation treatments or refer patients with significant toxicity to specialists. Some patients with a variety of toxic chemical exposures may need to be treated with broad-spectrum detoxification methods such as those employing sauna treatments.

ACKNOWLEDGMENTS

The author thanks Lori Knowles-Jimenez and Heather Getz for their assistance in editing the content of this chapter.

REFERENCES

1. Shaw, W. 2010. The unique vulnerability of the human brain to toxic chemical exposure and the importance of toxic chemical evaluation and treatment in orthomolecular psychiatry. *J Orthomol Med* 25(3): 125–134.
2. Frimpter, G.W., Haymovitz, A., and Horwith, M. 1963. Cystathioninuria. *N Engl J Med* 268: 333–339.
3. Rapp, D. 2004. *Our Toxic World: A Wake Up Call. Chemicals Damage Your Body, Brain, Behavior, and Sex.* Buffalo, NY: Environmental Medical Research Foundation.
4. Jasper, B.W., Hopkins, R.O., Duker, H.V. et al. 2005. Affective outcome following carbon monoxide poisoning: A prospective longitudinal study. *Cogn Behav Neurol* 18(2): 127–134.
5. Thom, S.R., Taber, R.L., Mendiguren, I. et al. 1995. Delayed neuropsychologic sequelae after carbon monoxide poisoning: Prevention by treatment with hyperbaric oxygen. *Ann Emerg Med* 25(4): 474–480.
6. Gürlek, Y.E., Taşkin, E.O., Yilmaz, O.G. et al. 2007. Case report: Kleptomania and other psychiatric symptoms after carbon monoxide intoxication. *Turkish J Psychiatry* 18(1): 1–6.
7. Genuis, S.J. 2009. Toxicant exposure and mental health—Individual, social, and public health considerations. *J Forensic Sci* 54: 474–477.
8. Bouchard, M., Bellinger, D., Weuve, J. et al. 2009. Blood lead levels and major depressive disorder, panic disorder, and generalized anxiety disorder in U.S. young adults. *Arch Gen Psychiatry* 66: 1313–1319.
9. Jedrychowski, W., Perera, F., Jankowski. J. et al. 2009. Very low prenatal exposure to lead and mental development of children in infancy and early childhood. Krakow prospective cohort study. *Neuroepidemiology* 32: 270–278.
10. Nevin, R. 2000. How lead exposure relates to temporal changes in IQ, violent crime, and unwed pregnancy. *Environ Res* 83: 1–22.
11. Roy, A., Bellinger, D., Hu, H. et al. 2009. Lead exposure and behavior among young children in Chennai, India. *Env Health Persp* 117: 1607–1611.
12. Wu, J., Basha, M.R., Brock, B. et al. 2008. Alzheimer's disease (AD)-like pathology in aged monkeys after infantile exposure to environmental metal lead (Pb): Evidence for a developmental origin and environmental link for AD. *J Neurosci* 28: 3–9.
13. Fadrowski, J., Navas-Acien, A., Tellez-Plaza, M. et al. 2010. Blood lead level and kidney function in U.S. adolescents. The third national health and nutrition examination survey. *Arch Intern Med* 170: 75–82.
14. Lin, X. and Henkelmann, R. 2003. Contents of arsenic, mercury and other trace elements in Napoleon's hair determined by INAA using the k0-method. *J Radioanal Nucl Chem* 257(3): 615–620.
15. Al-Shahristani, H., Shibab, K., and AL-Haddad, I. 1976. Mercury in hair as an indicator of total body burden. *Bull World Health Org* 53: 105–112.
16. Hac, E., Krzyzanowski, M., and Krechniak, J. 2000. Total mercury in human renal cortex, liver, cerebellum and hair. *Sci Total Environ* 248(1): 37–43.
17. Shaw, W. 2013. Evidence that increased acetaminophen use in genetically vulnerable children appears to be a major cause of the epidemics of autism, attention deficit with hyperactivity, and asthma. *J Restor Med* 2: 1–16.
18. Chisolm Jr., J.J. 2000. Safety and efficacy of meso-2,3-dimercaptosuccinic acid (DMSA) in children with elevated blood lead concentrations. *J Clin Toxicol* 38(4): 365–375.
19. Knobeloch, L., Ziarnik, M., Howard, J. et al. 1994. Gastrointestinal upsets associated with ingestion of copper-contaminated water. *Environ Health Perspect* 102(11): 958–961.
20. Eife, R., Weiss, M., Barros, V. et al. 1999. Chronic poisoning by copper in tap water: I. Copper intoxications with predominantly gastrointestinal symptoms. *Eur J Med Res* 4(6): 219–223.
21. Eife, R., Weiss, M., Muller-Hocker, M. et al. 1999. Chronic poisoning by copper in tap water: II. Copper intoxications with predominantly systemic symptoms. *Eur J Med Res* 4(6): 224–228.
22. Araya, M., Olivares, M., Pizarro, F. et al. 2003. Gastrointestinal symptoms and blood indicators of copper load in apparently healthy adults undergoing controlled copper exposure. *Am J Clin Nutr* 77(3): 646–650.

23. Hein, M.S. 2003. Copper deficiency anemia and nephrosis in zinc-toxicity: A case report. *S D J Med* 56(4): 143–147.

24. Groff, J. and Gropper, S. 2000. *Advanced Nutrition and Human Metabolism*, 3rd ed. Belmont, CA: Wadsworth, pp. 430–440.

25. Groff, J. and Gropper, S. 2000. *Advanced Nutrition and Human Metabolism*, 3rd ed. Belmont, CA: Wadsworth, pp. 419–430.

26. Osman, V., Salih, S., Mahmut, B. et al. 2008. High ceruloplasmin levels are associated with obsessive compulsive disorder: A case control study. *Behav Brain Funct* 4: 52.

27. Hermann, W., Caca, K., Eggers, B. et al. 2002. Genotype correlation with fine motor symptoms in patients with Wilson's disease. *Eur Neurol* 48(2): 97–101.

28. Schoen, R.E. and Sternlieb, I. 1990. Clinical aspects of Wilson's disease. *Am J Gastroenterol* 85: 1453–1457.

29. Brewer, G. 1998. Wilson disease and canine copper toxicosis. *Am J Clin Nutr* 6: 1087S–1090S.

30. Johnson, S. 2001. Micronutrient accumulation and depletion in schizophrenia, epilepsy, autism and Parkinson's disease. *Med Hypotheses* 56(5): 641–645.

31. Bouchard, M., Laforest, F., Vandelac, L. et al. 2007. Hair manganese and hyperactive behaviors: Pilot study of school-age children exposed through tap water. *Environ Health Perspect* 115(1): 122–127.

32. Sistrunk, S.C., Ross, M.K., and Filipov, N.M. 2007. Direct effects of manganese compounds on dopamine and its metabolite dopac: An *in vitro* study. *Environ Toxicol Pharmacol* 23(3): 286–296.

33. Blaurock-Busch, E. 1998. The clinical effects of manganese (Mn). Townsend Letter for Doctors and Patients 180. http://www.tldp.com/issue/180/Clinical%20Effects%20of%20Mn.html (accessed June 20, 2014).

34. Kondakis, X.G., Makris, N., Leotsinidis, M. et al. 1989. Possible health effects of high manganese concentration in drinking water. *Arch Environ Health* 44: 175–178.

35. Baez, S., Segura-Aguilar, J., Widersten, M. et al. 1997. Glutathione transferases catalyse the detoxication of oxidized metabolites (*o*-quinones) of catecholamines and may serve as an antioxidant system preventing degenerative cellular processes. *Biochem J* 324: 25–28.

36. Ali, S.A., Peet, M., and Ward, N.I. 1985. Blood levels of vanadium, caesium, and other elements in depressive patients. *J Affect Disord* 9(2): 187–191.

37. Davies, R., Ahmed, G., and Freer, T. 2000. Psychiatric aspects of chronic exposure to organophosphates: Diagnosis and management. *Adv Psychiatr Treat* 6: 356–361.

38. Salvi, R.M., Lara, D.R., Ghisolfi, E.S. et al. 2003. Neuropsychiatric evaluation in subjects chronically exposed to organophosphate pesticides. *Toxicol Sci* 72: 267–271.

39. Siwek, M., Sowa-Kućma, M., Dudek, D. et al. 2013. Oxidative stress markers in affective disorders. *Pharmacol Rep* 65(6):1558–1571.

40. Genuis, S.J. and Genuis, S.K. 2004. Human exposure assessment and relief from neuropsychiatric symptoms: Case study of a hairdresser. *J Am Board Fam Pract* 17: 136–141.

41. Su, K.P. 2009. Biological mechanism of antidepressant effect of omega-3 fatty acids: How does fish oil act as a "mind-body interface." *Neurosignals* 17: 144–152.

42. Cecchini, M.A., Root, D.E., Rachunow, J.R. et al. 2006. Chemical exposures at the World Trade Center. *Townsend Lett Doctors Patients* 273: 58–65.

43. Schnare, D.W., Denk, G., Shields, M. et al. 1982. Evaluation of a detoxification regimen for fat stored xenobiotics. *Med Hypotheses* 9: 265–282.

15 Dietary Peptides and the Spectrum of Food Hypersensitivities

Cynthia Gariépy, ND

CONTENTS

INTRODUCTION

Current therapies for depression and related disorders focus on the treatment of the symptoms associated with depression under the neurotransmitter model of depression, which does not answer the question, "if there is an imbalance in neurotransmitters, where does it come from?" The root cause of depression is, thus, never assessed. Immunological, biochemical, and epidemiological evidence gives us indications that depression, a mental illness, develops in certain individuals with a specific history. Those evidences now point to the new theory of depression, the Cytokine Model of Depression. In line with this model, the work of several pioneers is now revisited to highlight the relationship between inflammation and immune-mediation and depression. The role of dietary peptides, gluten and casein being the two proteins that have yielded the most research, has now become increasingly important for their potential in triggering an inflammatory and immunological cascade of events leading to depression. In a time where the sequencing of the human genome and microbiome in addition to all the research in epigenetics, it has become paramount to recognize that any genetic disposition or epigenetic processes have underlying physiological, biochemical, and functional foundations. Dietary peptides, in their immune-balancing and inflammatory-modulating role, have their place in the treatment of depression.

Food hypersensitivities have increased everywhere, and so have the rates of depression. The role of the intestine has shifted from being basically a digestive tube to being an immune-cataloguing entity with functional mechanisms having repercussions on the neurological system and the brain, among others. This chapter explains the wide spectrum of food hypersensitivity in relation to depression and focuses mainly on two dietary peptides, gluten and casein, to illustrate the importance of specific nutrition in the treatment of depression.

DEFINING FOOD HYPERSENSITIVITIES

A worldwide shift away from traditional lifestyles has been linked to increased rates of depression.[1] One area that has changed is certainly the way we eat.

Very few people in the medical community, yet alone in society, appreciate the connection between nutrition and physical illness, even if most modern diseases could dramatically be decreased by simple lifestyle changes. On a deeper level, there are nutritional deficiencies leading to physical illnesses, but that area also seems to be forgotten. We still associate scurvy with vitamin C deficiency, but we rarely see a screening being performed on a psychiatric population to look for possible deficiencies. We know that psychiatric populations often skip meals because of lack of structure or economic difficulties. People suffering from depression often forget to eat, but nutrition can play a key role in the onset as well as severity and duration of depression.[2] The underlying mechanisms linking nutrition and depression are numerous yet often intertwined among themselves.

Dietary patterns have changed over the past 50 years. Industrialized, ready-to-eat meals tend to be the preferred form of feed for an ever-increasing part of the population. The obesity epidemic is prevailing, and there has been an increase in diabetes and cardiovascular disease. Even if those diseases are lifestyle diseases, society still has a difficult time changing dietary patterns that they have grown accustomed to. The medical establishment also has to face a huge paradigm shift that has become increasingly needed: we can no longer exclude nutrition from the health equation. This need is even more urgent in the psychiatric population, because this portion of the population has a very distinctive food pattern where eating more in depressed periods is true,[3] but eating and craving more carbohydrates is also indubitable.[4]

According to different sources, food allergy prevalence estimates vary greatly. Between perceived allergies and confirmed allergies, the gap is often enormous. If we pay close attention when we ask the depressed patient if he or she has issues related to food, most will remark when eating certain foods, they feel worse. They are tired, less focused, and feel like their brain is foggy. When screened, these patients usually come back as "nonallergic." One of the reasons explaining this gap between what is perceived and the reality is the very definition of allergies.

Great confusion inhabits the world of food hypersensitivities. When talking about food hypersensitivities, one has to readily define the term *hypersensitivity*. One could define food hypersensitivity as undesirable reactions triggered by foods. Food hypersensitivities can further be classified into food allergies, food intolerances, and adverse reactions to foods due to other causes (Figure 15.1).

Yet, when in a clinic or a hospital setting, the presence of IgE-mediated food allergies is often tested, but the path of food allergies should not be left too swiftly. Psychiatry has a history of research done around the concept linking food allergies and depression. In the early mid-1900s, psychiatry had a branch called ecological psychiatry which was interested in the environment surrounding a psychiatric patient and the effect of the environment on the pathology. As early as 1961, Randolph, an ecological psychiatrist, noticed that many of his patients had allergic symptoms co-occurring with depression.[5] This led others such as Sheinkin, Schacter, Hutton,[6] as well as Philpott[7] to look into the possible connections. Orthomolecular medicine and functional medicine will look into food reactions when faced with a patient presenting symptoms of depression. Multiple chemical sensitivity is also an avenue to explore in front of a depression diagnostic. Abraham Hoffer wrote a position paper in 1979 where he also makes a connection between different classes of antidepressants, namely, tricyclic antidepressants, and their antihistaminic properties reinforcing the link between food allergies and depression.[8]

Type-1 food allergies are considered true allergies or classic allergies. They can produce an anaphylactic reaction leading to death. True immunoglobulin-E (IgE) reactions are part of the atopic march; the array of symptoms presents with allergy, whether it be food allergies or environmental allergies.

The oral allergy syndrome is considered part of the IgE-mediated food allergies category, because the proteins found in some fruits and vegetables are similar to those found in particular

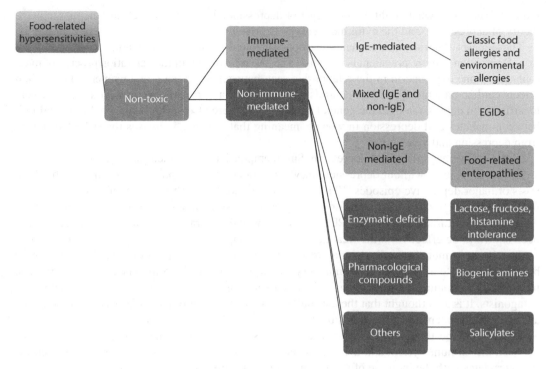

FIGURE 15.1 The various mechanisms of immune-mediated allergies versus intolerances where the immune system is not driving the symptoms. Even though the different symptoms could seem identical, the underlying mechanisms are entirely different and the consequences in the long run are also different.

pollens. These proteins can confuse the immune system in people with food or outdoor allergies.[9] The result is called *oral allergy syndrome* (OAS).

The eosinophilic gastrointestinal disorders stand in between the IgE-mediated food allergies and the non-IgE-mediated food allergies as both mechanisms are in action. Eosinophilic esophagitis and gastritis are closer to IgE-mediated food allergies, and eosinophilic gastroenteritis and colitis seem to be more T-cell mediated.

The non-IgE food allergies are referred to as such since the reaction is not caused by the production of IgE but rather by T cells and other immune mediators. IgE food allergies, mixed food allergies, and the dietary protein enteropathy, enterocolitis syndrome, and proctitis mostly affect children, where the gluten trilogy seems to affect mostly adults, in the mind of the medical system, at least, for now.

ATOPY AND DEPRESSION

For a while now, a new theory to explain depression has been considered. The present model of depression is the neurotransmitter hypothesis. The neurotransmitter model of depression has led to different classes of antidepressants, including selective serotonin reuptake inhibitors (SSRIs), serotonin and norepinephrine reuptake inhibitors (SNRIs), tricyclic antidepressants (TCAs), monoamine oxidase inhibitors (MAOIs), and others. Most of these medications, except for MAOIs, which inhibit a particular class of enzymes, follow the neurotransmitter model of depression in which the medication is used to keep the neurotransmitter(s) in the synaptic junction for a longer period of time, thus correcting the chemical imbalance thought to cause the depression in the first place. The question that then comes to mind is why is there a chemical imbalance in the first place? A new model of depression has come into play in recent years, challenging the current model and giving us more answers as to what could be the trigger of depression. The other models are the macrophage theory of depression[10] and the cytokine theory of depression.[11]

Those newer theories answer many questions surrounding several associations seen in depression. Depression is more prevalent is women.[12] The role of estrogen in the activation process of macrophages is one explanation in the relationship seen between depression and women.[13] Depression affects cardiac patients more than controls,[14] and rheumatoid arthritis patients are twice as likely to suffer from depression than the general population.[15] There also seems to be a bidirectional link between diabetes and depression in women, meaning that diabetes increases the risk of suffering from depression and vice versa.[16]

In the macrophage theory of depression, Smith emphasizes that when monokines (mostly IL-1) are given to subjects without depression, they can produce the symptoms necessary for the diagnosis of major depressive episodes.[10] Th1 cells can activate macrophages, which may explain why fish oils are an effective treatment for depression. Depressed people have an abnormal metabolism of polyunsaturated fatty acids (PUFAs) and fatty acids alterations.[17] Omega-3 fatty acids have been shown to be effective in the treatment of depression, and the relation between both could be explained via immune as well as inflammatory modulations.[18] Omega-6 fatty acids, on the other hand, can generate a cascade of inflammatory mediators from the eicosanoid class, which, in turn, modulate the immune system. Omega-3 fatty acids and omega-6 fatty acids are thus arachidonic antagonists. It is also thought that the anti-inflammatory effects of omega-3 fatty acids could act by an "eicosanoid-independent mechanism."[19]

In the cytokine theory of depression, cytokines signal the brain and can serve as mediators between the immune system and the central nervous system.[20] Furthermore the severity of depression correlates with the increase of proinflammatory cytokines.[21]

In food allergy, oral tolerance is not attained for certain food items. The body has two distinct ways of protecting the organism from having a food allergy. The first mechanism is the development of the exclusion system performed by the colonization of microorganisms on the surface of the epithelium to inhibit the penetration of harmful agents. The second mechanism is immunosuppression, which leads to oral tolerance.[22] Both systems lead to an inflammatory process. Not only do food allergies induce inflammation, but also this inflammation can lead to depression.

There may also be a link between pollen allergy and depression. Allergen-specific IgE status was associated with a greater increase in depressive scores during exposure to aeroallergens, and the exacerbation of allergic symptoms correlated significantly with a worsening in the depression scores.[23] In 2007, Postolache et al. also concluded that victims of suicide have an increased expression of cytokines in the prefrontal cortex.[24] In 2008, he concluded again that there is a link between the immune function and depression, as he noted that individuals with allergic rhinitis were at greater risk from suffering from depression than the general population.[25]

Also part of a food allergy reaction is histamine. In an allergic reaction, antibodies are released, and they attach to mast cells that, in turn, release histamine. Observations have indicated that cells other than mast cells, namely, macrophages and lymphocytes, can liberate significant amounts of histamine.[26] But as it turns out, histamine also plays a role in regulating the nervous system. Studies have revealed alterations in the histaminergic system in neurological and psychiatric diseases, namely, depression.[27]

Histamine intolerance is defined by a skewed capacity in regulating the histamine load and the ability of the organism to degrade histamine. Histamine is a biogenic amine that occurs to various degrees in many foods. In healthy persons, dietary histamine can be rapidly detoxified by amine oxidases, whereas individuals with low amine oxidase activity are at risk of histamine toxicity. Diamine oxidase (DAO) is the main enzyme for the metabolism of ingested histamine.[28] Although most symptoms of histamine intolerance revolve around the skin and the airway system, some patients describe feeling depressed or anxious after eating foods high in histamine. Histamine is present in aged cheeses, fermented soy products, wine, sauerkraut, and vinegar. Histamine has the potential of downregulating the lymphocytes' activity, and this reaction is worse in atopic individuals when compared to non-atopic individuals.[29]

Since we know that a significant proportion of depressed persons show upregulation of inflammatory factors such as IL-6, C-reactive protein, and TNFα; and inflammatory cytokines can interact with virtually every pathophysiologic domain relevant to depression, including neurotransmitter metabolism, neuroendocrine function, and synaptic plasticity, it is worth taking the time to do a full screen for possible allergies or intolerances and even go to the extent to try an elimination diet or an oligo-antigenic diet where most common allergens are removed from the diet.[30] We have seen a benefit in trying elimination diets in pathologies like irritable bowel syndrome,[31] where, much like in depression, there was neither IgE-mediated food allergies nor any food intolerances. Personalized elimination diets based on IgG, rather than IgE scores, are also an avenue to explore.

NON-IgE FOOD HYPERSENSITIVITIES

THE CASE OF CELIAC DISEASE

Much more research has been published on celiac disease within the past few years, but much remains to be said about this complex autoimmune disease. One of the areas that remains underrecognized is the relationship between depression and celiac disease. When reasoning about depression in celiac disease, one could have the tendency to think the obvious: celiac disease is a pathology that affects the everyday life and thus is difficult to accept and plays on the morale of anyone afflicted by it. Many studies have linked celiac disease with a lowered quality of life.[32,33] The difficulty in assessing whether celiac disease is associated with depression as a feature of the disease or as a result of the burden of having to follow a gluten-free diet for the rest of one's life remains a difficult question to answer. Some patients, even when following a gluten-free diet, still have symptoms of anxiety, fatigue, and a reduced quality of life, but even when changing diet has huge implications, depression is a feature of celiac disease, not merely a consequence.[34]

The Center for Celiac Research at Massachusetts General Hospital, Boston, Massachusetts, defines celiac disease as a genetic disorder affecting children and adults, where gluten sets off an autoimmune reaction that causes the destruction of the villi in the small intestine.[35] People with celiac disease produce antibodies that attack the intestine, causing damage and illness. Symptoms of celiac disease include diarrhea, constipation, weight loss, abdominal pain, chronic fatigue, weakness, malnutrition, and other gastrointestinal problems. In children, the symptoms may include an inability to put on weight, irritability, an inability to concentrate, diarrhea, and bloating.

The immune reaction caused by gluten in celiac disease produces inflammation of the small-intestinal mucosa.[36] Individuals susceptible to developing celiac disease are the ones carrying a particular genetic makeup, carriers of the HLA-DQ2 or HLA-DQ8 genes. However, even if the major genetic risk factor for CD is represented by HLA-DQ genes, which account for approximately 40% of the genetic risk, only a small percentage of carriers develop the disease.[37] If gluten and genes account only for a certain percentage of the problem, one must ask what else?

One of the factors that could give us more answers on the triggers in celiac disease is the intestinal microbiota, the microorganisms, and their genome residing inside a particular microbiome, in this case, the intestinal microbiome.[38] The microbiota in celiac disease patients are in a state of dysbiosis characterized by an increased proportion of *Bacteroides* spp. and a reduction of *Bifidobacterium* spp. as well as *B. Longum*. Once a gluten-free diet is undertaken, those populations tend to normalize.[39] Pozo-Rubio et al. found that intestinal dysbiosis is associated with CD, and that some of the alterations are not only secondary to the inflammatory milieu of the active phase of this disorder, but might play a primary role together with genetics and gluten intake in this disorder.[37]

One of the vectors that could possibly destabilize the intestinal milieu is an infectious agent. Viruses and bacteria have the potential of causing inflammation and tissue damage, thus leading to a lessened tolerance of gluten.[40] A line of communication seems to occur between the intestinal epithelium, the microbiota, the inflammasome, and immunity.

Communication between the gut and the immune system also affects the nervous system and the brain. We now understand why the nervous system and the brain, long considered unattainable, could react. Patients with inflammatory conditions are often afflicted with neuropsychiatric symptoms such as depression, anxiety, and fatigue.[41] Inflammation initiates a number of behavioral adaptations, including depression-like behavior as part of a broader picture called sickness behavior.[42]

If the intestinal epithelium is compromised, problems of malabsorption also tend to occur. At times, even if the gluten-free diet is well installed, patients remain symptomatic. The first issue coming to the clinician's mind must be verifying that the diet really is 100% gluten free. One study involving 12 patients presenting with celiac disease and depression who had been on a gluten-free diet for a year without improvement of the depression, showed that malabsorption not only was an issue but was also inevitable even if the diet was 100% gluten-free.[43] By giving pyridoxine (vitamin B6) to patients already on a gluten-free diet, reversal of the psychopathology was attained. The results indicated a causal relationship between adult celiac disease and concomitant depressive symptoms which seems to implicate metabolic effects from pyridoxine deficiency influencing central mechanisms regulating mood.

Similar observations were made in the pediatric population. In 1991, a team followed 15 untreated celiac children and 12 treated celiac children, and they observed a significantly lower ratio of plasma tryptophan to large neutral amino acids.[44] Impaired brain availability of tryptophan was more pronounced in the untreated group. Decreased tryptophan could indicate decreased central serotonin synthesis and, in turn, would exacerbate behavior disorders in children with celiac disease.

Another area of concern may be vitamin D malabsorption. Vitamin D is a known modulator of inflammation[45] as well as a modulator of the innate immune system as well as the adaptive immune system.[46] A recent study demonstrated that 92% of suicidal patients have low vitamin D levels compared to 59% of nonsuicidal patients.[47] As inflammation is suggested to directly be part of the neural mechanisms underlying depressive and suicidal behavior, it should be of high relevance to detect and cure the vitamin D deficiency in these patients. Bone mineral density (BMD) is also invariably low in patients with untreated celiac disease. Results in treated patients suggest that the gluten-free diet improves but does not normalize BMD. Untreated celiac disease is characterized by high levels of vitamin D and by increased bone turnover, caused by the increase in intact parathyroid hormone level.[48]

Inflammation as a piece of the puzzle might answer the question that was asked by a team of researchers in 2011 when they noticed that individuals with celiac disease have increased risk of depression and death from external causes, but no one had come up with conclusive studies on death from suicide.[49]

On a compromised intestinal milieu, the association between celiac disease and depression, researchers have noticed that adults with untreated celiac disease show signs of reduced central monoamine metabolism.[43]

Celiac disease, long recognized as a gastrointestinal disease, is a more complex disorder than previously thought. Approximately 1% of the population has celiac disease.[50] In a multicenter study of 13,145 patients, 60% of children and 41% of adults diagnosed with celiac disease were asymptomatic, and only 35% of newly diagnosed patients had diarrhea, which has been considered for too long to be required in order to diagnose celiac disease.[51] Even after completing a correct screening, 21% of these patients were denied by their physician for the intestinal biopsy, which is the golden standard for emission of a diagnostic of celiac disease. It comes as no surprise then to learn that the average diagnostic time for a symptomatic person is 4 years.[52] All in all, that translates to 83% of Americans who have celiac disease still being undiagnosed or misdiagnosed with other conditions, and those who are diagnosed and had symptoms before getting their diagnosis have waited an average of 12 years before getting their diagnosis.[53] We know that the longer one waits before having their diagnosis, the more it affects their quality of life.[54]

Although many studies indicate that a gluten-free diet is an effective form of treatment, some individuals may have refractory celiac disease (RCD), although it is quite rare. RCD is defined by persistent or recurrent malabsorptive symptoms and villous atrophy despite strict adherence to a gluten-free diet (GFD) for at least 6 to 12 months in the absence of other causes of nonresponsive treated celiac disease (CD) and overt malignancy.[55] Most studies looking into RCD conclude that what may seem to be RCD may be due to gluten or cross-contamination or a coexisting disease that has not yet been identified.[56]

In 1982, a Swedish team reported that depressive psychopathology may be a feature of adult celiac disease as a result of malabsorption.[43] If the cytokine model of depression is considered, one could hypothesize that not only absorption, but also inflammation, intestinal permeability, and dysbiosis are also possible contributors.

Two studies reported that a third of individuals suffering from celiac disease were also suffering from depression.[57,58] Approximately 31% of the adolescent population with celiac disease also suffer from depression. That is more than four times the rate of depression in the general adolescent population.[59] In a separate study, researchers found that in 10%–15% of celiacs, intolerance could be associated with psychiatric disorders like anxiety, depression, personality disorders, and psychotic symptoms.[60] In 2011, researchers also found elevated levels of IgG antibodies to gliadin, the toxic portion of gluten that triggers the immune reaction in celiac disease, in individuals with bipolar disorder.[61] Further examination is warranted but appears to be in alignment with the cytokine model of depression.

The link between psychiatric disorders and gluten dates further back. In 2002, a team of researchers identified a relationship between celiac disease and depression, behavioral changes, schizophrenia, autism, and disorders of personality. Despite not having a clear understanding of the mechanisms between celiac disease and its psychiatric manifestations, researchers hypothesized that biochemical factors such as a low plasma serotonin level may be a cause.[62]

One research study carried out in Finland studied the link between celiac disease in adolescents and an increased prevalence of depressive and disruptive behavior. Adolescents with untreated celiac disease led to serotonergic dysfunction due to impaired availability of tryptophan.[63] This phenomenon could lead to increased vulnerability to depressive and behavioral disorders. Study participants experienced a significant decrease in psychiatric symptoms following a gluten-free diet for 3 months.

The typical presentation of celiac disease in which gastrointestinal symptoms such as chronic diarrhea, vomiting, abdominal distension, abdominal pain, anorexia, poor weight gain, or weight loss are characteristic, occurs in the 9–24-month-old population. Those symptoms are often accompanied by behavioral changes that include irritability and an introverted attitude. The older the child gets, the less common are the presence of gastrointestinal symptoms.[64]

If the individual stops the gluten-free diet and behavioral symptoms appear, the gluten-free diet should be resumed. Often, when children reach adolescence, either they will no longer see the same pediatrician, or they will relocate. This can lead to a gap in the medical history, which has led researchers to suggest that celiac disease should be taken into consideration in the presence of behavioral or depressive disorders, particularly if they are unresponsive to standard antidepressant therapy.[36]

Double depression is a complication of dysthymia, which is a chronic depressed mood that lasts a minimum of 2 years. In the long run, a fair majority will see their symptoms worsen and lead to a diagnosis of major depression on top of their dysthymia. Adolescents with double depressions tend to have more severe and longer depressive episodes and worse social impairment than adolescents with major depressive disorder or dysthymic disorder alone, and the findings of earlier research suggested that depressed patients with comorbid disruptive behavior disorders have a worse short-term outcome and persisting conduct problems after the depression has remitted.[59]

One study that followed 13,776 individuals with celiac disease investigated the risk of mood disorder in that population. This group was compared to 66,815 individuals. Using the Cox regression model, researchers demonstrated that celiac disease was positively associated with subsequent depression but was not associated with subsequent bipolar disorder.[65] A follow-up study conducted by Addolorato et al. studied a population of 1641 outpatients with gastrointestinal disorders.[66] They showed that depression was associated with IBS, celiac disease, and small intestinal bacterial overgrowth (SIBO).

In 2008, Stein et al. showed a significantly higher prevalence of social phobia in patients with celiac disease compared with the healthy controls. Social anxiety disorder and social phobia in adolescents or young adults with celiac disease may be an important predictor of subsequent depressive disorders.[67]

The link between celiac disease and depression seems even stronger when the person has both celiac disease and type 1 diabetes. It is estimated that 37% of this population suffer from depression.[68] Patients with celiac disease and antithyroid autoantibodies (anti-TPO) are also at greater risk of suffering from panic disorder and major depressive disorder.[69]

Another area of concern in celiac disease is a phenomenon called brain hypoperfusion. Brain hypoperfusion refers to decreased cerebral blood flow in the brain. In 1994, a team of researchers enrolled 15 untreated celiac patients who had no conditions affecting brain perfusion, with no other neurological or psychiatric disorders other than anxiety or depression. They compared those individuals to 15 patients with celiac who had been on the gluten-free diet for one year and 24 healthy volunteers. All individuals went through a cerebral single photon emission computed tomography examination. The results were astonishing; 73% of the untreated celiac patients had at least one hypoperfused brain region compared to only 7% of the celiacs on the gluten-free diet and none in the healthy controls.[70] A possible link between cerebral hypoperfusion, depression, and celiac disease may be due to inflammation.

INFLAMMATION AND SEPSIS

Depression is often associated with a chronic, low-grade inflammatory response and activation of cell-mediated immunity, as well as activation of the compensatory anti-inflammatory reflex system. It is similarly accompanied by increased oxidative and nitrosative stress (O&NS), which contributes to neuroprogression in the disorder.[71] Similarly, the inflammation response observed in sepsis triggers profound changes in the brain, which may lead to sepsis-associated delirium. Observed changes in CBF regulation may be a consequence of inflammation.[72] Functional imaging studies show decreased cerebral metabolism and perfusion in depressed patients relative to normal controls, although the location of the deficits varies.[73]

Depression is thought to start off as an inflammatory process. The inflammatory process sometimes comes from celiac disease. Since celiac disease takes a very long time to be diagnosed, allowing inflammation to continue progressing, the intestinal epithelium and the microbiota are compromised and unable to perform their role of "gate keeping" and containing inflammation within the gut. In a subtype of people, the inflammatory process will further progress to become systemic inflammation. Once this process is initiated, there is an increased risk for developing inflammatory diseases, depression, and many other disorders where low-grade systemic inflammation is an issue.

Recent research suggests a relationship of inflammatory bowel disease (IBD) and depression. Improvement of depressive symptoms with treatment of IBD using immunosuppressive medications was evaluated.[74] Patients who were at risk for moderate to severe depression who were treated with immunosuppressive therapy experienced significant improvement in their depressive symptoms.

THE CASE OF NON-CELIAC GLUTEN SENSITIVITY

Celiac disease may be related to depression in a number of ways. Not only are celiac disease and depression related, gluten seems to be the bridge between depression and gluten-related disorders.[75] As early as 1981, a team of researchers published in *Gastroenterology* what is thought to be the first publication describing non-celiac gluten sensitivity.[76] A few months later, a similar study was done by the same team and led to the same conclusion: patients who presented with diarrhea and were thought to have celiac disease did not. These patients had non-celiac gluten sensitivity.[77]

In relation to wheat, individuals can either be wheat allergic, have celiac disease, have dermatitis herpetiformis, or have non-celiac gluten sensitivity. Non-celiac gluten sensitivity can be described as a "syndrome entity, characterized by intestinal and extra-intestinal symptoms related to the ingestion of gluten-containing food, in subjects that are not affected with either celiac disease (CD) or wheat allergy (WA)."[78]

In non-celiac gluten sensitivity (NCGS), many studies emphasized the relationship between NCGS and neuropsychiatric disorders such as depression. Addolorato et al. postulated that psychiatric symptoms were more or less a personality trait of people with celiac disease and IBD, caused by the burden of having these diseases.[79] They found that anxiety was present as a reactive form, and personality trait anxiety has no effect in celiac and IBD patients. Instead, they identified a possible link between brain function and malabsorption. The result of this particular study could also be associated with NCGS but was not in the study as the new entity was described 15 years later.

In 2007, Bernardo et al. investigated whether gluten was safe for individuals who did not have celiac disease.[80] Biopsy cultures from three individuals with celiac disease on a gluten-free diet and biopsy cultures from three individuals without celiac disease were compared. This pilot study supported the hypothesis that gluten elicits a harmful effect, through an IL15 innate immune response, on all individuals.

The mechanisms behind NCGS remain unclear. However, Brottveit et al. attempted to link a possible somatization of symptoms in people with non-celiac gluten sensitivity.[81] Somatization syndrome is defined as a chronic condition in which a person has physical symptoms that involve more than one part of the body, although no physical cause can be found.[82] Brottveit et al. found that individuals affected by NCGS reported more abdominal and nonabdominal symptoms after an intake of gluten than individuals affected by CD. Mental symptoms were the same in both groups. Symptoms increased after the gluten challenge, and NCGS patients did not exhibit a tendency for general somatization.

In 2014, a double-blind crossover study explored whether gluten provoked symptoms of depression in NCGS individuals.[83] Examiners divided a group of 22 individuals with irritable bowel syndrome where celiac disease was ruled out. These individuals kept on a gluten-free diet to control their symptoms. The participants of the study were assigned to either the group where a gluten challenge was undertaken or a group where whey (dairy) was added to the diet or to a controlled group where the diet was a gluten-free, dairy-free diet. Participants who took the gluten challenge experienced feelings of depression with no effect on emotional disposition. Findings from this study indicate gluten may have the capacity to induce feelings of depression in the celiac population as well as in the non-celiac gluten-sensitive individuals.

Gliadin has the potential of activating zonulin, a protein that modulates the permeability of the intestinal tight junctions.[84-86] Gluten has the potential of inducing gut permeability and has the capacity of inducing depression in a subset of the population. Long considered to only affect individuals with celiac disease, the subset of individuals with NCGS are also affected.

The relationship between carbohydrates and depression may be viewed as a two-way street. Carbohydrates may contribute to depressive symptoms, and depressed individuals exhibit a tendency to consume more carbohydrates.[87] Changes in dietary patterns may be a useful first line of intervention for depression as a way to reduce antidepressant medication use. Antidepressants were the third most common prescription drug taken by Americans of all ages in 2005–2008 and the most frequently used by persons aged 18–44 years. From 1988–1994 through 2005–2008, the rate of antidepressant use in the United States among all ages increased nearly 400%.[88]

EOSINOPHILIC GASTROINTESTINAL DISORDERS

Described only a few years ago, eosinophilic gastrointestinal disorders (EGIDs) are more common in modern times. Primary EGIDs are defined as disorders that selectively affect the gastrointestinal tract with eosinophil-rich inflammation in the absence of known causes for eosinophilia (e.g., drug reactions, parasitic infections, and malignancy). These disorders include eosinophilic esophagitis, eosinophilic gastritis, eosinophilic gastroenteritis, eosinophilic enteritis, and eosinophilic colitis and are occurring with increasing frequency.[89] Many authors have refined the definition of EGIDs, but there is growing evidence to support the role of aeroallergens and food allergens in the pathogenesis of these disorders.[90] EGIDs are also being thought of as being part of a broader continuum. Many children diagnosed with an EGID go on to develop an inflammatory bowel disease.[91] EGIDs are also associated with atopy.[92] An intervention with proven efficacy is the removal of food antigens. Total replacement of foods by an amino acid–based formula resulted in the disappearance of symptoms in 96% of children in one study.[93]

Children affected by an EGID are more anxious and depressed, have social difficulties, have sleep disturbances, and have school problems.[94] Their caretaker also has a reduced quality of life.[95] EGIDs seem to yield a reduction in the quality of life even when compared to obesity and diabetes.[95] The quality of life score for EGIDs as evaluated by the child was comparable with the scores seen in obesity. It has been suggested that routine screening for depression should be incorporated into the clinical care of patients with EGID.[96]

DAIRY

The case of dairy products in relation to depression is much less investigated. One of the reasons behind this lack of evidence is the multiple ways an individual may be sensitive to dairy. Most studies focus on lactose or casein and perceived allergies and intolerances to test "proven" allergies and intolerances. Rarely, food withdrawals for certain periods of time are advised.

Physicians are faced with the problem that there is a huge gap between "perceived allergies" and "real allergies." Previous studies tend to show a 10-fold discrepancy of self-reported food-induced symptoms and physician-diagnosed food hypersensitivity. Through a series of questionnaires, phone surveys, and clinical examinations, study with 13,000 individuals found that roughly 4% of the population surveyed (a pediatric population from 0 to 17 years old) had clinically proven symptoms, and that those symptoms were mainly in relation to the oral allergy syndrome.[98]

For the scope of this text, it is critical to identify the different components of milk. Milk is 87.7% water, 4.9% carbohydrates (lactose), 3.4% fat, 3.3% protein (casein and whey), and 0.7% minerals. There are three types of caseins in cow's milk, alpha, beta, and kappa, and four types of whey, including alpha-lactalbumin, beta-lactoglobulin, bovine serum albumin, and bovine immunoglobulins. The composition of cow's milk varies from species to species. When talking about hypersensitivities related to milk, we focus on beta casein. Most forms of beta casein can be attributed to either beta casein A1 or A2. In short, they are referred to as A1 or A2.

Many people believe that they have an "allergy" to dairy which should be of concern. In the case of irritable bowel syndrome, we notice a majority of people believing they are lactose intolerant. In one recent study, the rate of self-perceived intolerance was 41.1% of the study population. Of these individuals, 47% tested positive on the hydrogen breath test, and 27.4% presented symptoms of lactose intolerance during the test.[99] The fact has been supported in the case of irritable bowel syndrome by the whole FODMAP diet where dairy products are eliminated.[100]

When looking more on the side of dairy allergy, most true milk allergies (IgE mediated) appear early in life, affect mostly children, and tend to resolve around the age of 5 to 6 years old.[101,102] It is surprising that many adults perceive themselves as being allergic to milk. Cow's milk allergy is one of the earliest and most common food allergies. For this reason, cow's milk allergy can be recognized as one of the first indications of an aberrant inflammatory response in early life.[103]

There is a relationship between celiac disease and lactose intolerance, and there seem to be more celiacs in the lactose intolerance population.[104] What is less known is the link between cow's milk proteins and the mucosal reactivity in a subset of patients with celiac disease. In about 50% of celiacs, cow's milk protein induces local inflammation. Once again, the mechanism behind this reaction is probably the increased passage of macromolecules resulting from a damaged epithelium.[105]

Another area of concern is asthma. A food allergy may be a risk factor for increased asthma morbidity in adults.[106] The overlap of depression with several somatic conditions including asthma has been thought of and seen in clinical settings for a very long time.[107] One hypothesis is that the hypersensitivity reactions may prime the hypothalamic-pituitary-adrenal (HPA) axis to respond aberrantly to stressors, resulting in physical and behavioral consequences.[108] As the conditions related to a non-IgE mediated cow's milk hypersensitivity are very broad, one has to question if that could be a reason why there are no clear-cut research studies determining the role of cow's milk allergy in depression. The following symptoms are related to non-IgE-mediated responses: atopic dermatitis, gastroesophageal reflux disease (GERD), crico-pharyngeal spasm, pyloric stenosis, allergic eosinophilic esophagitis (EoE), cow's milk protein-induced enteropathy, constipation, severe irritability (colic), food protein-induced gastroenteritis, proctocolitis, and Heiner's syndrome.[109] Physicians will rarely redirect children in allergology when faced with a problem of constipation. Laxatives using purely mechanical pathways like bulking in the case of fibers or osmosis in the case of lactulose, will work to produce a stool, but they might not address the problem that caused the constipation in the first place. Many children are affected by constipation, which suggests that leaving these children in this state will predispose them to intestinal leakage and eventually systemic inflammation.

Studies often partition the different components of milk or try to identify true IgE-mediated allergy or hydrogen breath test–proven lactose intolerance instead of focusing on the inflammatory cascade produced by milk. Milk is important for proper growth and bone development. A well done research study followed a group of 6500 preadolescent and adolescent girls for a 7-year period.[110] Vitamin D intake was predictive of a lower risk of having a fracture even among the group of girls in the study participating in an intense, high-impact activity. On the other hand, calcium or dairy intake was not protective against the development of fractures. Furthermore, high calcium intake was associated with an elevated risk of developing stress fractures. Dairy products are also under investigation for their possible role in type 1 diabetes, prostate cancer, arthritis, digestive problems, and childhood anemia, among other conditions.[111]

In line with the immune-cytokine model of depression or cytokine-induced depression,[20] inflammation and other immune processes are increasingly linked to psychiatric diseases. Anti-casein IgG reactivity is associated with bipolar I diagnoses and psychotic symptom history. Mania severity scores suggest that casein-related immune activation may relate to the psychosis and mania components of this mood disorder.[112] The link between bipolar disorder and casein was explored recently in 2014, and authors found that immune sensitivity to casein from milk affects a subset of individuals with bipolar disorder.[113] The product of the digestion of casein produces exorphins that have the potential of affecting brain physiology through their action at the site of the opioid receptors. The authors cited that inflammation in the gastrointestinal tract could accelerate an exposure of food antigens to systemic circulation which would explain elevated gluten and casein antibody levels in individuals with bipolar disorder. The same holds true for individuals with schizophrenia.[114]

Another way milk could cause depression is the potential of one of the proteins found in milk, beta-casomorphin-7, to act with an opiate-like activity. Beta-casomorphin is a possible direct histamine liberator in humans. In a study done in 1992, the subjects who were given a dose of H1 antagonist had a decreased reaction from beta-casomorphin-7. Beta-casomorphin-7 can be regarded as a noncytotoxic, direct histamine releaser in humans, although further clinical relevance of these findings warrants further study.[115]

The inflammatory cascade associated with food allergy might also be related to dairy. One study found that exposure to an allergen during early life influenced the development of allergen-specific immune response. The study followed 96 children and measured their IgG antibodies to beta-lactoglobulin levels at 6 months, 18 months, and 8 years. The levels of beta-lactoglobulin, a protein found in cow's milk but not in breast milk, peaked in early childhood before declining until participants were around 8 years of age.[116] A similar kind of assessment was completed in 1999 to determine the effect of giving cow's milk to an infant in the first 3 days of life. The team of researchers divided a group of 129 infants who were exclusively breastfed and gave them either cow's milk, casein hydrolysate formula, or human milk.[117] After the first 3 days of life, infants returned to being breastfed. Researchers found that exposure to cow's milk during the first 3 days of life stimulated IgG antibody production to cow's milk proteins which was still evident at 2 years of age. Infants who were fed with a casein hydrolysate solution developed low levels of IgG antibodies to cow's milk proteins.

This brings up the subject of anti-ganglioside antibodies. In celiac disease, there is an elevated level of these antibodies. Celiacs affected by neurological conditions are the ones most targeted by this elevation.[118] The content of gangliosides in human milk is more elevated than the content of bovine milk.[119] The two main roles of gangliosides are their potential of reducing inflammation in the intestinal epithelium and protecting the intestinal tract by inhibiting infection.[120] In addition to the other problems related to cow's milk, A1 cow's milk is typically used in the process of making cheese, ice cream, and yogurt, and poses a problem similar to gluten.

Gluten is approximately 45% gliadin and 55% glutenins. Glutenins and gliadins are prolamines, and prolamines are rich in proline. Proline is difficult for humans to digest. Gliadin is too large of a molecule to be completely broken down into single amino acids. Thus, when someone consumes gluten, the digestion process will only break the gliadin down into peptides (chains of amino acids). In order to process the gliadin that was ingested, our intestinal cells, tightly standing one beside the other much like the bricks of a wall, will open their tight junctions, via the zonulin system,[51] to let the peptide go through. In the general population, the tight junctions are signaled to open and to close right back up. In celiacs, as long as gluten is consumed, the junctions remain open, and intestinal permeability becomes a day-to-day state. In the celiac population, the gliadin peptides cause an inflammatory reaction as well as an immune reaction. In the general population, the gliadin fragments that are not completely digested are eliminated before the immune system has the chance to recognize this, resulting in gluten elimination without inflammation or immune reactions.

In cow's milk, the structure per se of the milk molecule is also worth mentioning. In A1 beta casein the amino acid present at the 67th position is histidine, whereas in A2 milk, the 67th position is the place of proline—the same proline that causes problems in gluten.

When A1 milk is being consumed, a peptide is formed. This peptide is composed of seven amino acids and is called beta-casomorphin-7. Beta-casomorphin is considered a bioactive peptide with wide-ranging effects on the different functions of one's organism. BCM-7 acts on the nervous, the immune, and the digestive systems through the μ-opioid receptor (MOR). Proline dipeptidyl peptidase IV (DPPIV; EC 3.4.14.5) appears to be the primary degrading enzyme of BCM7. Moreover, DPPIV is known to restrict activity of proinflammatory peptides. BCM7 is considered to modulate an immune response by affecting MOR and DPPIV gene expression.[121] Beta-casomorphin-7 affects gut motility and inflammation and in a recent double-blinded, randomized 8-week crossover study including 47 participants, the team concluded that A1 milk yielded more gastrointestinal complaints than A2 milk.[122]

The protein level of human milk is 1%, whereas bovine milk is about 3%–4%. Furthermore, the protein profile of human milk is mostly whey, whereas in bovines, 80% of the proteins come from casein. Finally, the opioid properties of BC7 from human milk are about 10 times weaker than the bovine form.[123] For several years, many health professionals have been prescribing gluten-free and casein-free diets in autistic populations and in individuals affected by inflammatory conditions. The food-derived peptides (casein from milk and gliadin from gluten) are rich in proline and modulate cysteine uptake in cultured human neuronal and gastrointestinal (GI) epithelial cells via activation of opioid receptors. Decreases in cysteine uptake were associated with changes in the intracellular antioxidant glutathione and the methyl donor S-adenosylmethionine.[124] The disruption in the equilibrium of intracellular glutathione further causes a decrease in the antioxidant magnitude in protecting the organism, on a cellular level, from the prodigious effects of oxidation. When the antioxidant's capacity is reduced, the organism gets put at risk of suffering from the negative effects of inflammation and systemic oxidation, partly explaining the benefits of gluten-free or casein-free diets.[124] A reduction in systemic inflammation and oxidation has been associated with many diseases such as kwashiorkor, seizure, Alzheimer's disease, Parkinson's disease, liver disease, cystic fibrosis, sickle cell anemia, HIV, AIDS, cancer, heart attack, stroke, and diabetes.[125]

The potential of cow's milk–derived products of modulating the cysteine uptake in its effect on SAM-e (S-adenosylmethionine) has huge implications. SAM-e is being increasingly used for its antidepressant effect. The two ways SAM-e positively affects individuals with depression is through its antioxidant potential and its role in neurotransmission.

SAM-e is essential in the production of one of our most potent antioxidants, glutathione.[126] This role is directly linked to the cytokine model of depression, with glutathione being our most potent antioxidant.[127] Additionally, SAM-e has a direct link to neurotransmitters. In an interview given to *Psychiatric Times* in 2001, Richard P. Brown, associate professor of clinical psychiatry at Columbia University College of Physicians and Surgeons, explained that SAM-e is most concentrated in the brain and liver and is crucial to three central pathways of metabolism that stimulate more than 35 different reactions.[128] The three major pathways are transmethylation, transulfuration, and transaminopropylation. Animal studies show that the transmethylation pathway boosts levels of the neurotransmitters serotonin, dopamine, and norepinephrine. This process may contribute to the antidepressant action.

SOY

Understanding the role of soy becomes a more complex problem. Some studies indicate a positive relationship between soy consumption and depression, while others point in the opposite direction.

Methionine in soy products is so low that it needs to be added to infant soy formula.[129] SAM-e is a very effective treatment for depression.[130] When rats are fed soy protein, there is a very-low-density lipoprotein (VLDL) and higher LDL susceptibility to peroxidation in rats compared with casein-fed rats, which could reflect in part the lack of sulfur amino acid availability, since methionine supplementation led to a partial recovery of lipoprotein resistance to peroxidation.[131]

CONCLUSION

In line with the cytokine model of depression, depression could be considered as an immune-mediated inflammatory disease (IMID). Immune-mediated inflammatory disease (IMID) is a concept used to collectively describe a group of ostensibly unrelated conditions that share common inflammatory pathways.[132] Dietary peptides management comes as an organic solution that could manage or aid in the treatment of depression when appropriate.

REFERENCES

1. Logan, A.C. and Jacka, F.N. 2014. Nutritional psychiatry research: An emerging discipline and its intersection with global urbanization, environmental challenges and the evolutionary mismatch. *J Physiol Anthropol* 33: 22.
2. Sathyanarayana Rao, T.S., Asha, M.R., Ramesh, B.N. et al. 2008. Understanding nutrition, depression and mental illnesses. *Indian J Psychiatry* 50(2): 77–82.
3. Baucom, D.H. and Aiken, P.A. 1981. Effect of depressed mood on eating among obese and nonobese dieting and nondieting persons. *J Personality Soc Psychol* 41(3): 577–585.
4. Wurtman, R.J. and Wurtman, J.J. 1995. Brain serotonin, carbohydrate-craving, obesity and depression. *Obesity Res* 3(4): 477S–480S.
5. Randolph, T.G. 1961. Ecologic mental illness—Levels of central nervous system reactions. *Third World Congr Psychiatry* 16: 379–384.
6. Sheinkin, D., Schacter, M., and Hutton, R. 1979. *The Food Connection*. New York, NY: Bobbs-Merrill.
7. Philpott, W.H. 1979. Maladaptive reactions to frequently used foods and commonly met chemicals as precipitating factors in many chronic physical and chronic emotional illnesses. In *A Physician's Handbook on Orthomolecular Medicine*, Ed. Williams, R.J., and Kalita, O.K. New Canaan, CT: Keats.

8. Hoffer, A. 1980. Allergy, depression and tricyclic antidepressants. *Orthomol Psychiatry* 9(3): 164–170.
9. American Academy of Allergy, Asthma, and Immunology (AAAAI). 2014. Oral Allergy Syndrome. http://www.aaaai.org/conditions-and-treatments/conditions-dictionary/oral-allergy-syndrome-(oas).aspx (accessed September 13, 2014).
10. Smith, R.S. 1991. The macrophage theory of depression. *Med Hypotheses* 35(4): 298–306.
11. Loftis, J.M., Huckans, M., and Morasco, B.J. 2010. Neuroimmune mechanisms of cytokine-induced depression: Current theories and novel treatment strategies. *Neurobiol Dis* 37(3): 519–533.
12. Kessler, R.C. 2003. Epidemiology of women and depression. *J Affect Disord* 74(1): 5–1.
13. Hsieh, C.H., Nickel, E.A. Chen, J. et al. 2009. Mechanism of the salutary effects of estrogen on Kupffer cell phagocytic capacity following trauma-hemorrhage: Pivotal role of Akt activation. *J Immunol* 182(7): 4406.
14. Pilote, L., Dasgupta, K., Guru, V. et al. 2007. Comprehensive view of sex-specific issues related to cardiovascular disease. *CMAJ* 176(6): S1–S44.
15. Dickens, C. and Creed, F. 2001. The burden of depression in patients with rheumatoid arthritis. *Rheumatology* 40(12): 1327–1330.
16. Pan, A., Lucas, M., Sun, Q. et al. 2010. Bidirectional association between depression and type 2 diabetes in women. *Arch Intern Med* 170(21): 1884–1891.
17. Maes, M., Christophe, A., Delanghe, J. et al. 1999. Lowered omega-3 polyunsaturated fatty acids in serum phospholipids and cholesteryl esters of depressed patients. *Psychiatry Res* 85(3): 275–291.
18. Grosso, G., Pajak, A. Marventano, S. et al. 2014. Role of omega-3 fatty acids in the treatment of depressive disorders: A comprehensive meta-analysis of randomized clinical trials. *PLoS One* 9(5): e96905.
19. Calder, P.C. and Grimble, R.F. 2002). Polyunsaturated fatty acids, inflammation and immunity. *Eur J Clin Nutr* 56(3): S14–S19.
20. Loftisa, J.M., Huckansa, M., Morascoa, B.J. et al. 2010. Neuroimmune mechanisms of cytokine-induced depression: Current theories and novel treatment strategies. *Neurobiol Dis* 37(3): 519–533.
21. Maes, M., Bosmans, E., De Jongh, R. et al. 1995. Immunoendocrine aspects of major depression. Relationships between plasma interleukin-6 and soluble interleukin-2 receptor, prolactin and cortisol. *Psychiatry Clin Neurosci* 245(3): 172–178.
22. Brandtzaeg, P. 2010. Food allergy: Separating the science from the mythology. *Nature Rev Gastroenterol Hepatol* 7(7): 380–400.
23. Manalai, P., Hamilton, R.G., Langenberg, P. et al. 2012. Pollen-specific immunoglobulin E positivity is associated with worsening of depression scores in bipolar disorder patients during high pollen season. *Bipolar Disord* 14(1): 90–98.
24. Postolache, T.T., Lapidus, M., Sander, E.R. et al. 2007. Changes in allergy symptoms and depression scores are positively correlated in patients with recurrent mood disorders exposed to seasonal peaks in aeroallergens. *Scientific World J* 7: 1968–1977.
25. Postolache, T.T., Komarow, H., and Tonelli, L.H. 2008. Allergy: A risk factor for suicide? *Curr Treat Options Neurol* 10(5): 363–376.
26. Zwadlo-Klarwasser, G., Braam, U., Mühl-Zürbes, P. et al. 1994. Macrophages and lymphocytes: Alternative sources of histamine. *Agents Actions* 41: C99–C100.
27. Kano, M., Fukudo, S., Tashiro, A. et al. 2004. Decreased histamine H1 receptor binding in the brain of depressed patients. *Eur J Neurosci* 20(3): 803–810.
28. Maintz, L. and Novak, N. 2007. Histamine and histamine intolerance. *Am J Clin Nutr* 85(5): 1185–1196.
29. Strannegard, I.L. and Strannegard, O. 1977. Increased sensitivity of lymphocytes from atopic individuals to histamine-induced suppression. *Scand J Immunol* 6(12): 1225–1231.
30. Shelton, R.C. and Miller, A.H. 2010. Eating ourselves to death and despair: The contribution of adiposity and inflammation to depression. *Prog Neurobiol* 91(4): 275–299.
31. Atkinson, W., Sheldon, T.A., Shaath, N. et al. 2004. Food elimination based on IgG antibodies in irritable bowel syndrome: A randomised controlled trial. *Gut* 53(10): 1459–1464.
32. Mustalahti, K. 2002. Gluten-free diet and quality of life in patients with screen-detected celiac disease. *Eff Clin Pract* 5(3): 105–113.
33. Lee, A. and Newman, J.M. 2003. Celiac diet: Its impact on quality of life. *J Am Diet Assoc* 103(11): 1533–1535.
34. Häuser, W., Gold, J., Stein, J. et al. 2006. Health-related quality of life in adult coeliac disease in Germany: Results of a national survey. *Eur J Gastroenterol Hepatol* 18(7): 747–754.
35. Center for Celiac Research, Massachusetts General Hospital for Children. 2014. Center for Celiac Research: Celiac Disease FAQ. http://www.massgeneral.org/children/services/celiac-disease/celiac-disease-faq.aspx (accessed September 13, 2014).

36. Corvaglia, L., Catamo, R., Pepe, G. et al. 1999. Depression in adult untreated celiac subjects: Diagnosis by the pediatrician. *Am J Gastroenterol* 94(3): 839–843.
37. Pozo-Rubio, T., Olivares, M., Nova, E. et al. 2012. Immune development and intestinal microbiota in celiac disease. *Clin Dev Immunol* 2012: I654143. Published online September 11, 2012. doi: 10.1155/2012/654143.
38. Turnbaugh, P.J., Ley, R.E., and Hamady, M. 2007. The human microbiome project. *Nature* 449(7164): 804–810.
39. De Palma, G., Nadal, I., Collado, M.C. et al. 2009. Effects of a gluten-free diet on gut microbiota and immune function in healthy adult human subjects. *Nutr* 102(8): 1154–1160.
40. Bethune, M.T. and Khosla, C. 2008. Parallels between pathogens and gluten peptides in celiac sprue. *PLoS Pathogens* 4(2): e34.
41. Thomson, C.A., McColl, A., Cavanagh, J. et al. 2014. Peripheral inflammation is associated with remote global gene expression changes in the brain. *J Neuroinflammation* 11: 73.
42. Damm, J., Wiegand, F., Harden, L.M. et al. 2011. Fever, sickness behavior, and expression of inflammatory genes in the hypothalamus after systemic and localized subcutaneous stimulation of rats with the toll-like receptor 7 agonist imiquimod. *Neuroscience* 201: 166–183.
43. Hallert, C. 1982. Psychiatric illness, gluten, and celiac disease. *Biol Psychiatry* 17(9): 959–961.
44. Hernanz, A. and Polanco, I. 1991. Plasma precursor amino acids of central nervous system monoamines in children with coeliac disease. *Gut* 32(12): 1478–1481.
45. Miodovnik, M., Koren, R., Ziv, E. et al. 2012. The inflammatory response of keratinocytes and its modulation by vitamin D: The role of MAPK signaling pathways. *J Cell Physiol* 227(5): 2175–2183.
46. Aranow, C. 2011. Vitamin D and the immune system. *J Investig Med* 59(6): 881–886.
47. Grudet, C., Malm, J., Westrin, A. et al. 2014. Suicidal patients are deficient in vitamin D, associated with a pro-inflammatory status in the blood. *Psychoneuroendocrinology* 50: 210–219.
48. Corazza, G.R., Di Sario, A., Cecchetti, L. et al. 1995. Bone mass and metabolism in patients with celiac disease. *Gastroenterology* 109(1): 122–128.
49. Ludvigsson, J.F., Sellgren, C., Runeson, B. et al. 2011. Increased suicide risk in coeliac disease—A Swedish nationwide cohort study. *Dig Liver Dis* 43(8): 616–622.
50. Hoffenberg, E.J., Mackenzie, T., Barriga, K.J. et al. 2003. A prospective study of the incidence of childhood celiac disease. *J Pediatr* 143(3): 308–314.
51. Fasano, A. 2012. Zonulin, regulation of tight junctions, and autoimmune diseases. *Ann N Y Acad Sci* 1258: 25–33.
52. Green, P.H.R., Stavropoulos, S.N., and Panagi, S.G. 2001. Characteristics of adult celiac disease in the USA: Results of a national survey. *Am J Gastroenterol* 96(1): 126–131.
53. Cranney, A., Zarkadas, M., Graham, I.D. et al. 2007. The Canadian celiac health survey. *Digest Dis Sci* 52(4): 1087–1095.
54. Mahadev, S., Simpson, S., Lebwohl, B. et al. 2013. Is dietitian use associated with celiac disease outcomes? *Nutrients* 5(5): 1585–1594.
55. Rubio-Tapia, A. and Murray, J.A. 2010. Classification and management of refractory celiac disease. *Gut* 59(4): 547–557.
56. Abdulkarim, A.S., Burgart, L.J., See, J. et al. 2002. Etiology of nonresponsive celiac disease: Results of a systematic approach. *Am J Gastroenterol* 97(8): 2016–2021.
57. Ciacci, C., Iavarone, A., Mazzacca, G. et al. 1998. Depressive symptoms in adult coeliac disease. *Scand J Gastroenterol* 33(3): 247–250.
58. Arigo, D., Anskis, A.M., and Smyth, J.M. 2012. Psychiatric comorbidities in women with celiac disease. *Chronic Illness* 8(1): 45–55.
59. Pynnönen, P.A., Isometsa, E.T., Aronen, E.T. et al. 2004. Mental disorders in adolescents with celiac disease. *Psychosomatics* 45(4): 325–335.
60. Poloni, N., Vender, S., Bolla, E. et al. 2009. Gluten encephalopathy with psychiatric onset: Case report. *Clin Pract Epidemiol Mental Health* 5: 16.
61. Dickerson, F., Stallings, C., Origoni, A. et al. 2011. Markers of gluten sensitivity and celiac disease in bipolar disorder. *Bipolar Disord* 13(1): 52–58.
62. Martínez-Bermejo, A. and Polanco, I. 2002. Neuropsychological changes in coeliac disease. *Rev Neurol* 34(1): S24–S33.
63. Pynnönen, P.A., Isometsa, E.T., Verkasolo, M.A. et al. 2005. Gluten-free diet may alleviate depressive and behavioural symptoms in adolescents with coeliac disease: A prospective follow-up case-series study. *BMC Psychiatry* 5: 14.

64. Husby S., Koletzko, S., Korponay-Szabo, I.R. et al. 2012. European Society for Pediatric Gastroenterology, Hepatology, and Nutrition guidelines for the diagnosis of coeliac disease. *J Pediatr Gastroenterol Nutr* 54(1): 136–160.

65. Ludvigsson, J.F., Reutfors, J., Osby, U. et al. 2007. Coeliac disease and risk of mood disorders—A general population-based cohort study. *J Affect Dis* 99(1–3): 117–126.

66. Addolorato, G., Mirijello, A., and D'Angelo, C. 2008. State and trait anxiety and depression in patients affected by gastrointestinal diseases: Psychometric evaluation of 1641 patients referred to an internal medicine outpatient setting. *Int J Clin Pract* 62(7): 1063–1069.

67. Stein, M.B., Fuetsch, M., Muller, N. et al. 2001. Social anxiety disorder and the risk of depression a prospective community study of adolescents and young adults. *Arch Gen Psychiatry* 58(3): 251–256.

68. Garud, S., Leffler, D., Dennis, M. et al. 2009. Interaction between psychiatric and autoimmune disorders in coeliac disease patients in the Northeastern United States. *Aliment Pharmacol Ther* 29(8): 898–905.

69. Carta, M.G., Hardoy, M.C., Boi, M.F. et al. 2002. Association between panic disorder, major depressive disorder and celiac disease: A possible role of thyroid autoimmunity. *J Psychosom Res* 53(3): 789–793.

70. Addolorato, G., Di Giuda, D., and De Rossi, G. 2004. Regional cerebral hypoperfusion in patients with celiac disease. *Am J Med* 116(5): 312–317.

71. Berk, M., Williams, L.J., Jacka, F.N. et al. 2013. So depression is an inflammatory disease, but where does the inflammation come from? *BMC Med* 11: 200.

72. Burkhart, C.S., Siegemund, M., and Steiner, L.A. 2010. Cerebral perfusion in sepsis. *Crit Care* 14: 215.

73. Bonne, O., Krausz, Y., Gorfine, M. et al. 1996. Cerebral hypoperfusion in medication resistant, depressed patients assessed by Tc99m HMPAO SPECT. *J Affect Disord* 41(3): 163–171.

74. Horst, S., Chao, A., and Rosen, M. 2014. Treatment with immunosuppressive therapy may improve depressive symptoms in patients with inflammatory bowel disease. *Dig Dis Sci* 60(2): 465–470.

75. Genuis, S.J. and Lobo, R.A. 2014. Gluten sensitivity presenting as a neuropsychiatric disorder. *Gastroenterol Res Pract* 2014: 293206.

76. Cooper, B.T., Holmes, G.K., Ferguson, R. et al. 1980. Gluten-sensitive diarrhea without evidence of celiac disease. *Gastroenterology* 79(5): 801–806.

77. Cooper, B.T., Holmes, G.K., Ferguson, R. et al. 1981. Gluten-sensitive diarrhea without evidence of celiac disease. *Gastroenterology* 81(1): 192–194.

78. Catassi, C., Bai, J.C., Bonaz, B. et al. 2013. Review: Non-celiac gluten sensitivity: The new frontier of gluten related disorders. *Nutrients* 5(10): 3839–3853.

79. Addolorato, G., Stefanini, G.F., Capristo, E. et al. 1996. Anxiety and depression in adult untreated celiac subjects and in patients affected by inflammatory bowel disease: A personality "trait" or a reactive illness? *Hepatogastroenterology* 43(12): 1513–1517.

80. Bernardo, D., Garrote, J.A., Fernandez-Salazar, L. et al. 2007. Is gliadin really safe for non-coeliac individuals? Production of interleukin 15 in biopsy culture from non-coeliac individuals challenged with gliadin peptides. *Gut* 56(6): 889–890.

81. Brottveit, M., Vandvik, P.O., Wojniusz, S. et al. 2012. Absence of somatization in non-coeliac gluten sensitivity. *Scand J Gastroenterol* 47(7): 770–777.

82. Medline Plus. 2014. Somatization disorder. http://www.nlm.nih.gov/medlineplus/ency/article/000955.htm (accessed October 9, 2014).

83. Peters, S.L., Biesiekierski, J.R., Yelland, G.W. et al. 2014. Randomised clinical trial: Gluten may cause depression in subjects with non-coeliac gluten sensitivity—An exploratory clinical study. *Aliment Pharmacol Ther* 39(10): 1104–1112.

84. Clemente, M.G., De Virgiliis, S., Kang, J.S. et al. 2003. Early effects of gliadin on enterocyte intracellular signalling involved in intestinal barrier function. *Gut* 52(2): 218–223.

85. Drago, S., El Asmar, R., Di Pierro, M. et al. 2006. Gliadin, zonulin and gut permeability: Effects on celiac and non-celiac intestinal mucosa and intestinal cell lines. *Scand J Gastroenterol* 41(4): 408–419.

86. Lammers, K.M., Lu, R., Brownley, J. et al. 2008. Gliadin induces an increase in intestinal permeability and zonulin release by binding to the chemokine receptor CXCR3. *Gastroenterology* 135(1): 194–204e.3.

87. Hidaka, B.H. 2012. Depression as a disease of modernity: Explanations for increasing prevalence. *J Affect Disord* 140(3): 205–214.

88. Pratt, L.A., Brody, D.J., Gu, Q. et al. 2011. Antidepressant use in persons aged 12 and over: United States, 2005–2008. CDC: NCHS Data Brief. http://www.cdc.gov/nchs/data/databriefs/db76.htm (accessed September 14, 2014).

89. Rothenberg, M.E. 2004. Eosinophilic gastrointestinal disorders (EGID). *J Allergy Clin Immunol* 113(1): 11–28.

90. DeBrosse, C.W. and Rothenberg, M.E. 2008. Allergy and eosinophil-associated gastrointestinal disorders (EGID). *Curr Opin Immunol* 20(6): 703–708.
91. Mutalib, M., Blackstock, S., Evans, V. et al. 2014. Eosinophilic gastrointestinal disease and inflammatory bowel disease in children: Is it a disease continuum? *Eur J Gastroenterol Hepatol* 27(1): 20–23.
92. Assa'ad, A.H., Putnam, P.E., Collins, M.H. et al. 2007. Pediatric patients with eosinophilic esophagitis: An 8-year follow-up. *J Allergy Clin Immunol* 119(3): 731–738.
93. Liacouras, C.A., Spergel, J.M., Ruchelli, E. et al. 2005. Eosinophilic esophagitis: A 10-year experience in 381 children. *Clin Gastroenterol Hepatol* 3(12): 1198–1206.
94. Ingerski, L.M., Modi, A.C., Hood, K.K. et al. 2010. Health-related quality of life across pediatric chronic. *J Pediatr* 156(4): 639–644.
95. Taft, T.H., Ballou, S., and Keefer, L. 2012. Preliminary evaluation of maternal caregiver stress in pediatric eosinophilic gastrointestinal disorders. *J Pediatr Psychol* 37(5): 523–532.
96. Hommel, K.A., Franciosi, J.P., Gray, W.N. et al. 2012. Behavioral functioning and treatment adherence in pediatric eosinophilic gastrointestinal disorders. *Pediatr Allergy Immunol* 23(5): 494–499.
97. Riehl, M. 2014. *Beyond the Exam Room: How EGIDs Impact Your Social and Emotional Life Experiences*. University of Michigan Health System Division of Gastroenterology—Department of Internal Medicine, Salt Lake City, Utah.
98. Roehr, C.C., Edenharter, G., Riemann, S. et al. 2004. Food allergy and non-allergic food hypersensitivity in children and adolescents. *Clin Exp Allergy* 34(10): 1534–1541.
99. Dainese, R., Casellas, F., Marine-Barjoan, E. et al. 2014. Perception of lactose intolerance in irritable bowel syndrome patients. *Eur J Gastroenterol Hepatol* 26(10): 1167–1175.
100. Shepherd, S.J., Halmos, E., and Glance, S. 2014. The role of FODMAPs in irritable bowel syndrome. *Curr Opin Clin Nutr Metab Care* 17(6): 605–609.
101. Fiocchi, A., Schunemann, H.J., Brozek, J. et al. 2010. Diagnosis and rationale for action against cow's milk allergy (DRACMA): A summary report. *J Allergy Clin Immunol* 126(6): 1119–1128.e12.
102. Suh, J., Lee, H., Lee, J.H. et al. 2011. Natural course of cow's milk allergy in children with atopic dermatitis. *J Korean Med Sci* 26(9): 1152–1158.
103. Jo, J., Garssen, J., Knippels, L. et al. 2014. Review article: Role of cellular immunity in cow's milk allergy: Pathogenesis, tolerance induction, and beyond. *Mediators Inflamm* 2014: 249784.
104. Ojetti, V., Nucera, G., Migneco, A. et al. 2005. High prevalence of celiac disease in patients with lactose intolerance. *Digestion* 71(2): 106–110.
105. Kristjánsson, G., Venge, P., and Hällgren, R. 2007. Mucosal reactivity to cow's milk protein in coeliac disease. *Clin Exp Immunol* 147(3): 449–455.
106. Berns, S.H., Halm, E.A., Sampson, H.A. et al. 2007. Food allergy as a risk factor for asthma morbidity in adults. *J Asthma* 44(5): 377–381.
107. Slavich, G.M. and Irwin, M.R. 2014. From stress to inflammation and major depressive disorder: A social signal transduction theory of depression. *Psychol Bull* 140(3): 774–815.
108. Hurwitz, E.L. and Morgenstern, H. 1999. Cross-sectional associations of asthma, hay fever, and other allergies with major depression and low-back pain among adults aged 20–39 years in the United States. *Am J Epidemiol* 150(10): 1107–1116.
109. Fiocchi, A., Brozek, J., Schunemann, H. et al. 2010. World Allergy Organization (WAO) diagnosis and rationale for action against cow's milk allergy (DRACMA) guidelines. *World Allergy Organ J* 3(4): 57–161.
110. Sonneville, K.R., Gordon, C.M., Kocher, M.S. et al. 2012. Vitamin D, calcium, and dairy intakes and stress fractures among female adolescents. *Arch Pediatr Adolesc Med* 166(7): 595–600.
111. Medicine, Physician's Committee for Responsible. 2012. Got Truth?: The Dairy Industry Junk Science. Good Medicine. Available at: http://www.pcrm.org/sites/default/files/images/gm/autumn2012/Autumn2012GoodMedicine.pdf
112. Severance, E.G., Dupont, D., Dickerson, F.B. et al. 2010. Immune activation by casein dietary antigens in bipolar disorder. *Bipolar Disord* 12(8): 834–842.
113. Severance, E.G., Gressitt, K.L., Yang, S. et al. 2014. Seroreactive marker for inflammatory bowel disease and associations with antibodies to dietary proteins in bipolar disorder. *Bipolar Disord* 16(3): 230–240.
114. Severance, E.G., Lin, J., and Sampson, H.A. 2011. Dietary antigens, epitope recognition, and immune complex formation in recent onset psychosis and long-term schizophrenia. *Schizophr Res* 126(1–3): 43–50.
115. Kurek, M., Przybilla, B., Hermann, K. et al. 1992. A naturally occurring opioid peptide from cow's milk, beta-casomorphine-7, is a direct histamine releaser in man. *Int Arch Allergy Immunol* 97(2): 115–120.

116. Siltanen, M., Kajosaari, M., Savilahti, E.M. et al. 2002. IgG and IgA antibody levels to cow's milk are low at age 10 years in children born preterm. *J Allergy Clin Immunol* 110(4): 658–663.

117. Juvonen, P., Mansson, M., Kjellman, N.I. et al. 1999. Development of immunoglobulin G and immunoglobulin E antibodies to cow's milk proteins and ovalbumin after a temporary neonatal exposure to hydrolyzed and whole cow's milk proteins. *Pediatr Allergy Immunol* 10(3): 191–198.

118. Volta, U., De Giorgio, R., Granito, A. et al. 2006. Anti-ganglioside antibodies in coeliac disease with neurological disorders. *Dig Liver Dis* 38(3): 183–187.

119. Bode, L., Beermann, C., Mank, M. et al. 2004. Human and bovine milk gangliosides differ in their fatty acid composition. *J Nutr* 134(11): 3016–3020.

120. Miklavcic, J.J., Schnabl, K.L., Mazurak, V.C. et al. 2012. Dietary ganglioside reduces proinflammatory signaling in the intestine. *J Nutr Metab* 2012: 280286.

121. Fiedorowicz, E., Kaczmarski, M., Cieslinska, A. et al. 2014. β-Casomorphin-7 alters μ-opioid receptor and dipeptidyl peptidase IV genes expression in children with atopic dermatitis. *Peptides* 62: 144–149.

122. Ho, S., Woodford, K., Kukuljan, S. et al. 2014. Comparative effects of A1 versus A2 beta-casein on gastrointestinal measures: A blinded randomised cross-over pilot study. *Eur J Clin Nutr* 68: 994–1000.

123. Woodford, K. 2009. *Devil in the Milk: Illness, Health and the Politics of A1 and A2 Milk*. New Zealand: Chelsea Green Publishing.

124. Trivedi, M.S., Shah, J.S., Al-Mughairy, S. et al. 2014. Food-derived opioid peptides inhibit cysteine uptake with redox and epigenetic consequences. *J Nutr Biochem* 25(10): 1011–1018.

125. Wu, G., Fang, Y.Z., Yang, S. et al. 2004. Glutathione metabolism and its implications for health. *J. Nut* 134(3): 489–492.

126. Bottiglieri, T. 2002. *S*-Adenosyl-L-methionine (SAMe): From the bench to the bedside—molecular basis of a pleiotrophic molecule. *Am J Clin Nutr* 76(5): 1151S–1157S.

127. Sharma, R., Yang, Y., Sharma, A. et al. 2004. Antioxidant role of glutathione S-transferases: Protection against oxidant toxicity and regulation of stress-mediated apoptosis. *Antioxidant Redox Signal* 6(2): 289–300.

128. *Psychiatric Times*. 2001. Investigating SAM-e for depression. http://www.psychiatrictimes.com/articles/investigating-sam-e-depression (accessed September 13, 2014).

129. Daniel, K.T. 2005. *The Whole Soy Story: The Dark Side of America's Favorite Health Food*. Washington, DC: NewTrends.

130. Mischoulon, D. and Fava, M. 2002. Role of *S*-adenosyl-L-methionine in the treatment of depression: A review of the evidence. *Am J Clin Nutr* 76(5): 1158S–1161S.

131. Moundras, C., Remesy, C., Levrat, M.A. et al. 1995. Methionine deficiency in rats fed soy protein induces hypercholesterolemia and potentiates lipoprotein susceptibility to peroxidation. *Metabolism* 44(9): 1146–1152.

132. Kuek, A., Hazleman, B.L., and Ostor, A.J.K. 2007. Immune-mediated inflammatory diseases (IMIDs) and biologic therapy: A medical revolution. *Postgrad Med J* 83(978): 251–260.

16 Genetic-Based Biomarkers in Psychiatry
An Integrative Approach

Jay Lombard, DO

CONTENTS

INTRODUCTION

Major depression is one of the world's leading causes of morbidity and mortality. It affects approximately 14.8 million American adults, or about 6.7% of the U.S. population age 18 and older, in a given year.[1] Depression can either be chronic or recurrent, and symptoms can be quite heterogeneous with both psychological and physical manifestations. Treatment-resistant depression (TRD), is defined as a failure of two or more medication trials with antidepressants from different pharmacologic classes that fail to produce a significant clinical improvement. TRD is often the norm, not the exception, in the course of treatment for major depression. A multicenter study involving over 2876 patients, referred to as Star-D, revealed that approximately 50% or more of patients with major depression remain refractory to treatment, even after all four treatment levels.[2]

One hypothesis related to the reason for depression being so difficult to treat is that the etiology of depression is heterogenous with distinctive neurobiological underpinnings. There may exist several unique subtypes of depression, and therefore the existing categorical framework of diagnosis and treatment is imprecise and may not address these causal factors. Furthermore, there is a great deal of overlap and comorbidity in depression with systemic disorders, including metabolic and inflammatory conditions.[3] Given the prevalence of depression and its often refractory nature, there is an urgent need for novel paradigms that will potentially improve outcomes.

Currently, the selection of therapy for major depression is purely empirical and based on trial and error. The clinical utility of biomarkers as part of psychiatric practice in depression first requires an understanding of precisely what is being referred to, how these markers have been derived, and how the selection of such markers are potentially able to favorably alter clinical outcomes. Depression is a multifactorial disorder that involves both biological and environmental factors. It is well known that genetic factors play a role in depression vulnerability as family histories reveal a greater than threefold risk of depression in patients in families with first-degree relatives who also have experienced a mood disorder.[4] Our understanding of these genetic biomarkers is critical not only to elucidate the underlying biological mechanisms involved in depression, but also to discover treatments that address the underlying pathophysiological changes as well.

While the focus of this chapter is primarily related to the genetic basis of depression, the reader should also keep in mind the importance of other biological factors related to mood disturbances, including gene transcription and expression, epigenetics, measurements of microRNA, proteomics, brain imaging, and metabolomics. Incorporation of these modalities into the practice of clinical psychiatry will transform our understanding of depression and other diseases of the brain and ultimately allow us to apply a truly integrative systems approach to neuropsychiatric disorders.

GENETICS OF DEPRESSION

Integrative medicine is a relatively new term for alternative approaches in medicine and is ideally suited to approaching complex disorders in conditions of the brain. Integrative medicine is based, on part, in the field of basic science known as systems biology. Systems biology is a framework of investigation that recognizes that biological systems are dynamic and that diseases are fundamentally based on perturbed networks of genes, proteins, and other communication pathways that integrate cellular and higher-order functioning. This integrated approach, based upon a careful analysis of relevant pathways involving altered patterns of gene expression and the downstream changes in protein function, can be detected clinically and will help guide the clinician in choosing a specific treatment or treatments that address the underlying biology of a disorder, rather than treating it only symptomatically.

Much of the available clinical data related to the genetics of depression is derived from genome-wide association studies (GWASs). These studies entail the discovery of variants in a given disorder, such as depression. The diagnosis of depression in these population studies is established through vigorous diagnostic assessments to ensure the accuracy of any potential biological association. Next, certain gene variants are identified which have greater frequency in a particular population compared to unaffected cohorts. Finally, a rigorous statistical analysis of these variants is performed to ensure the veracity of the gene signal within a narrow genomic region. However, the reader needs to keep in mind that the actual causal variant may not be the actual SNP itself but is a currently undetected variant that lies in linkage dysequilibrium.[5]

PHARMACODYNAMIC GENES

This chapter will exclusively emphasize a category of genes referred to as pharmacodynamics genes. In general, there are two broad categories of genes which have been utilized in clinical medicine: pharmacodynamics and pharmacokinetic. The former refers to gene variants that influence how genetically based changes in the genome affect brain metabolism. Some examples of genes in this category include the serotonin transporter, which influences baseline synaptic levels of serotonin in the brain. Pharmacokinetic genes are primarily based upon variants in the hepatic cytochrome p450 system. These enzymes are responsible for drug metabolism and elimination. Variants of the P450 genes, such as an enzyme known as 2D6, can lead to unpredictable blood levels of a given drug with a heightened risk of an adverse drug reaction in some instances. In integrative medicine, the reader should keep in mind some specific examples which impact nonpharmacological therapies in psychiatry. For instance, it is well known that St. John's Wort used for depression has potential interaction with antiviral drugs based upon the cytochrome p450 enzyme.[6]

It is not surprising that many of the pathological genes identified in depression relate to pathways involved in the stress response. For instance, the serotonin transporter gene is one of the first variants discovered in population-based depression studies. The serotonin transporter (5-HTT) is a high-affinity carrier protein that removes serotonin (5-HT) from the synaptic cleft, resulting in serotonin reuptake into the presynaptic terminus. Elevated synaptic serotonin levels are associated with improved mood; thus, the effectiveness of many antidepressant drugs (namely, selective serotonin reuptake inhibitors, SSRIs) is thought to be due to their inhibition of the serotonin transporter, thereby reducing serotonin reuptake into the presynaptic terminus, and increasing serotonin availability in the synaptic cleft.

GENE VARIANTS

Gene variants of the serotonin transporter are characterized as being either long or short. In a prospective study performed by Caspi et al., individuals with one or two copies of the short (S) allele (which results in less expression of the serotonin transporter protein compared to the long [L] form) exhibited more depressive symptoms than individuals who were homozygous for the L allele.[7] Further pharmacogenomics studies have shown that compared to L/L patients, those homozygous for the short allele (S/S) are less likely to respond to antidepressant therapy and more slowly experience and have a greater risk of adverse drug reactions (ADRs) during antidepressant therapy.[8]

A plausible explanation for the association of genetic variants of the serotonin transporter and increased risk of depression relates to enhanced amygdala reactivity in S-allele carriers.[9] Heightened activation of the amygdala in response to stress results in hypothalamic-pituitary-adrenal (HPA)-mediated autonomic arousal and hyperactivity of functional brain circuits involved in the stress response, resulting in elevated cortisol and norepinephrine. Support for this hypothesis includes the observation that 5HTTLPR SS carriers display higher overall cortisol concentrations than L carriers.[10]

In addition to the serotonin transporter, genes that modulate the HPA stress axis with potential downstream dysregulation of cortisol metabolism include FK506-binding protein 5 or FKBP5. FKBP5 is a glucocorticoid receptor-regulating co-chaperone protein that plays a role in the regulation of the HPA system. FKBP5 expression is induced by glucocorticoid receptor activation, which provides a feedback loop for terminating cortisol activity.[11] Polymorphisms of the FKBP5 gene may result in decreased efficiency of the negative feedback of the stress hormone axis, resulting in a prolongation of stress hormone system activation following exposure to stress. This is a potential mechanism as to how glucocorticoid receptor function is impaired in major depression.

THERAPEUTIC MODALITIES

Potential therapeutic modalities which have been speculated to have a genotype specific response include nonpharmacological agents including tryptophan, fish oil, as well as pharmacological agents including lithium and the antidepressant mirtazapine. Lithium has been shown to increase transcription of the serotonin transporter, and the serotonin transporter (5-HTT) gene has been previously implicated in lithium response in bipolar depression. In one study of 122 patients with bipolar I disorder, 49 patients were classified as good responders, 49 as nonresponders, and 24 as partial responders to lithium prophylaxis. A greater response to lithium was correlated with the S allele of 5-HTTLPR.[12]

FISH OIL

The potential anti-stress effects of fish oil may also be based, in part, on the 5HTT genotype. Supplementation with fish oil–rich docosahexaenoic (DHA) and eicosapentaenoic acids (EPA) has been demonstrated to increase serotonergic neurotransmission. Fish oil–supplemented animals display increased hippocampal serotonergic neurotransmission and sensitization of hippocampal 5-HT1A receptors.[13] Animals bred to display a "short variant" of the serotonin transporter, referred to as 5HTT null, were compared to the "wild type" of the serotonin transporter in regard to the potential anti-stress effects of fish oil. 5-HTT$^{-/-}$ and 19 wild-type (5-HTT$^{+/+}$) rats were fed for 3 months on a mixed polyunsaturated fatty acid (PUFA) diet. HTT$^{-/-}$ rats on the control diet displayed increased anxiety-related behavioral responses and impaired fear extinction. These effects were completely offset by the mixed PUFA diet, whereas this diet had no behavioral effect in 5-HTT$^{+/+}$ rats.[14]

Unfortunately, randomized trials of omega-3 polyunsaturated fatty acid (PUFA) treatment for depression are often poorly designed or have widely varied outcome. A recent meta-analyses of the clinical utility of omega-3 fatty acids in depression involving 916 participants revealed that supplements with eicosapentaenoic acid (EPA) $\geq 60\%$ showed benefit on standardized mean depression scores within the range of 200–2200 mg/day of EPA.[14]

TRYPTOPHAN

Tryptophan, an essential amino acid and precursor to serotonin, attenuates the cortisol response to acute social stress depending on the 5-HTTLPR genotype.[15] In a double-blind placebo-controlled parallel design study, 25 S'/S' carriers and 21 L'/L' carriers were randomized to take l-tryptophan (2.8 g/day) or placebo supplements. S'/S' carriers who took l-tryptophan supplements had a significantly lower cortisol response to stress than S'/S' carriers who took placebo.

MIRTAZAPINE

Pharmacologically, lowering the concentrations of free cortisol in depressed patients may be an important prerequisite to prevent glucocorticoid-related sequelae of depression. Pharmacological agents for depression have varying effects on cortisol metabolism, which may explain in part their putative effects. Mirtazapine, an atypical antidepressant that primarily influences noradrenergic rather than serotonergic neurotransmission, has been shown to acutely inhibit cortisol secretion. In one study, for example, the impact of mirtazapine treatment on salivary cortisol secretion was investigated in patients with major depression. A significant reduction in cortisol concentrations was noted after mirtazapine treatment.[16] In a comparative study, mirtazapine significantly lowered afternoon cortisol, whereas venlafaxine did not attenuate saliva cortisol concentrations.[17] In a further study supporting the effects of mirtazapine on cortisol metabolism, mirtazapine significantly reduced elevated cortisol levels, which positively correlated with the percentage reduction in the sum score of the Hamilton Depression Rating Scale.[18]

Neuroactive steroids, such as allopregnanolone, are decreased in the cerebrospinal fluid (CSF) of patients with posttraumatic stress disorder and major depression, and conversely, increased allopregnanolone levels have been detected in CSF and plasma of depressed patients following successful antidepressant treatment.[19] Allopregnanolone is synthesized in the brain from progesterone by the sequential action of 5α-reductase type I (5α-RI), and 3α-hydroxysteroid dehydrogenase (3α-HSD), which converts 5α-dehydroprogesterone into allopregnanolone.[20] Compellingly, levels of 5α-RI mRNA are decreased in depressed patients. In depressed patients, the mRNA expression levels of 5α-RI were strongly decreased compared to those of normal subjects.[21]

Clinically, neurosteroids may have beneficial effects in depression, anxiety, and substance abuse. Adults with bipolar depression were randomized to pregnenolone (titrated to 500 mg/day) or placebo, as add-on therapy, for 12 weeks. Depression remission rates were greater in the pregnenolone group (61%) compared with the placebo group (37%).[22] An additional mechanism related to the neurobiology of stress and depression relates to the brain-derived neurotrophic factor (BDNF) hypothesis of depression. BDNF is a member of the nerve growth factor family, which is essential for neurogenesis and neuronal plasticity. The expression of BDNF may be a downstream target of various antidepressants. The BDNF Val66Met gene variant has been associated with hippocampal dysfunction, anxiety, and depressive traits. Mice bred to express the Met variant of BDNF were found to have atrophy of distal apical dendrites.[23] Lithium, a compound with BDNF-promoting effects, has well-established efficacy as an augmentation strategy of antidepressants, and was one of the first adjunctive strategies used for treatment-resistant depression. A fixed-effects meta-analysis of nine trials that included 237 patients demonstrated that the odds ratio for response to lithium versus placebo in all contrasts combined was 2.89.[24]

GLUTAMATE

Glutamate is the most abundant excitatory neurotransmitter in the brain. Persistent cortisol effects on the brain have been shown to accelerate neurodegenerative processes, and its association with excessive glutamate may be one explanation for higher risk of dementia in untreated depression and PTSD.[25] Altered glutamate neurotransmission in mood disorders may result from genetically based changes in the levels/activity of glutamate transporters which affect termination of the neurotransmitter, N-methyl-D-aspartate (NMDA), α-amino-3-hydroxy-5-methyl-4-isoxazolepropionic acid (AMPA), and kainite receptor activity and calcium ion channels. Regarding the latter, several GWAS studies have confirmed that L-type voltage-gated calcium channel activity has been associated with bipolar depression.[26] The co-occurrence of increased glutamatergic transmission and cortisol hypersecretion raises the possibility that the gray matter volumetric reductions in these depressed subjects is due to interactions between elevated glucocorticoid secretion and (NMDA)-glutamate receptor stimulation.[27] Stress-induced changes in glutamate neurotransmission could potentially be counteracted by increasing the dietary intake of omega-3 polyunsaturated fatty acids (n-3 PUFAs). PUFAs help protect glutamatergic neurotransmission from damage induced by stress and glucocorticoids, possibly preventing the development of stress-related disorders such as depression or anxiety.[28] Additional natural glutamate antagonists which reduce excitotoxicity associated with mood disorders include N-acetylcysteine, magnesium, and cytidine.

N-ACETYLCYSTEINE

N-acetylcysteine (NAC) is a redox-active glutathione precursor that normalizes brain glutamate homeostasis and has putative anti-inflammatory effects, including downregulation of IL-6.[29] In an open-label, randomized, crossover study, proton magnetic resonance spectroscopy (1H-NMR) was used to investigate glutamate changes in the dorsal anterior cingulate cortex (dACC) after a single dose of 2400 mg NAC. In administration of NAC, glutamate levels were reduced in the cocaine-dependent group.[30]

Clinically, NAC has been used both for treatment-resistant depression and for obsessive symptoms, which sometimes are found comorbidly. In a study involving over 250 patients, Berk et al. administered NAC or placebo in patients diagnosed with major depression according to the American Psychiatric Association's DSM-IV-TR criteria. Depressive symptoms were attenuated by week 16, indicating a delayed but significant clinical effect.[31]

GLUTAMATERGIC PATHWAYS

Magnesium deficiency causes NMDA-coupled calcium channels to be biased toward opening, causing neuronal injury and neurological dysfunction. The significance of glutamatergic pathways in depression and the association of this system with the stress pathway and magnesium homeostasis strongly suggests that treatment with NMDA receptor antagonists and magnesium may reverse stress-induced neural changes associated with depression.[32] Cytidine, a pyrimidine, may exert therapeutic effects in the brain of depressed patients by reducing glutamate through a pathway that enhances glial-mediated glutamate reuptake. A study aimed at determining cytidine's efficacy in bipolar depression demonstrated that cytidine supplementation was associated with an earlier improvement in depressive symptoms and also produced a greater reduction in cerebral glutamate/glutamine levels in patients with bipolar depression. Cytidine-related glutamate/glutamine decrements correlated with a reduction in depressive symptoms, an effect not seen in the placebo group.[33]

INFLAMMATORY PATHWAYS

Numerous studies have reported increases in circulating proinflammatory cytokines, interleukin (IL)-1, IL-6, tumor necrosis factor (TNF)-alpha, and C-reactive protein (CRP), in patients with major depression.[34] Furthermore, elevated levels of the inflammatory mediator, prostaglandin E2 (PGE2), have been observed in the saliva, plasma, and CSF of depressed patients.[35] An increased vulnerability for depression related to immune disturbances may be due, in part, to genetically based factors. Findings across the literature suggest that functional allelic variants of genes for IL-1β, TNF-α, and CRP, as well as genetic variations affecting T-cell function, may increase the risk for depression. Moreover, single nucleotide polymorphisms (SNPs) in the IL-1β, IL-6 may be associated with reduced responsiveness to antidepressant therapy.[36]

MITOCHONDRIAL DYSFUNCTION

In addition to inflammatory pathways associated with depression, a growing body of data suggests that mitochondrial dysfunction is involved in the pathophysiology of psychiatric disorders. Targeting mitochondrial function and their role in energy metabolism, synaptic plasticity, and cell survival is an emerging area of interest for the discovery of novel therapeutics for mood and other psychiatric disorders. Mitochondria are crucial for energy production, generated mainly through the electron transport chain, and play an important role in regulating apoptosis and calcium (Ca^{2+}) signaling.[37] Some but not all studies have demonstrated polymorphisms of mitochondria-related genes in bipolar disorder. Most of the antidepressants and mood stabilizers may actually inhibit the activities of respiratory electron transport chain complexes, and complexes I and IV were the most affected. For example, a significant decrease of complex I activity has been observed after administration of valproate and olanzapine.[38] Postmortem studies in bipolar patients revealed decreased electron transport chain activity and expression and increased nitrosative and oxidative stress (OxS) in patient brains.[39] Neuroimaging studies consistently show decreased energy levels in brains of BPD patients.[39] Conversely, dietary supplements that augment mitochondrial function, including creatine, have been observed to have antidepressant effects. For example, 52 women with major depressive disorder were enrolled in an 8-week double-blind placebo-controlled clinical trial and randomly assigned to receive escitalopram in addition to either creatine (5 g/day, $N = 25$) or placebo ($N = 27$). In comparison to the placebo augmentation group, patients receiving creatine augmentation showed significantly greater improvements in HAM-D score, suggesting that creatine augmentation of SSRI treatment may be a promising therapeutic approach that exhibits more rapid and efficacious responses in major depressive disorder.[40]

5,10-METHYLENETETRAHYDROFOLATE REDUCTASE

Many clinicians are aware that certain subtypes of depression are characterized by excessive fatigue, anhedonia, and low motivation. These individuals may respond less favorably to serotonergic-based antidepressants, and preferentially, to agents that augment brain dopamine. Dopamine is a ubiquitous neurotransmitter with diverse function across the neuroaxis. The dopamine-rich emotional valence and reward/executive brain function area (axis) relates to the pain/pleasure response. Dimensionally, individuals with dysfunction in this axis may exhibit abnormalities in motivation, attention, cravings, and addiction. Dysregulation of dopamine neurotransmission in these regions may result from genetic variants involving biogenic amine metabolism. Abnormal biogenic amine biosynthesis has been observed in humans with disturbances in folate metabolism.[41]

A primary role involves the synthesis of dopamine in the brain. Folic acid deficiency results in fatigue, reduced energy, and depression, which may be based, in part, on reduced dopamine synthesis. Specific genetic defects in folate metabolism can result in impaired biogenic amine metabolism. 5,10-Methylenetetrahydrofolate reductase (MTHFR) is a key enzyme for intracellular folate homeostasis and metabolism. Low folate blood levels are correlated with depression, and polymorphisms of the MTHFR gene are closely associated with risk of depression.[42] Individuals with the T/T gene variant of the MTHFR gene experience a reduced capacity for dopamine and serotonin catecholamine synthesis as a result of decreased bioavailability of folate.

In a double-blind, randomized, placebo-controlled trial performed by Papakostas et al., outpatients with SSRI-resistant major depressive disorder received L-methylfolate 15 mg/day for 60 days or placebo followed by L-methylfolate 15 mg/day. Response rates were associated with key biological and genetic markers. Patients with body mass index ≥ 30 kg/m^2, elevated plasma levels of high-sensitivity C-reactive protein or 4-hydroxy-2-nonenal, low S-adenosylmethionine/S-adenosylhomocysteine ratio, and genetic markers associated with folate metabolism had significantly greater changes from baseline on the Hamilton-D rating scale with L-methylfolate versus placebo.[43]

CATECHOL-O-METHYLTRANSFERASE

Catechol-O-methyltransferase (COMT) catabolizes dopamine and is important for regulating dopamine levels in the prefrontal cortex. COMT also inactivates norepinephrine and estrogen catechols, and the levels of dopamine and norepinephrine may be differentially regulated by gene variants of the COMT enzyme. COMT appears to modulate cortical and striatal activation during both reward anticipation and delivery, and to impact reward-related learning and its underlying neural circuitry. In individuals with COMT val/val variation, there is higher enzymatic activity and subsequently greater breakdown of dopamine. Individuals with higher COMT activity and lower prefrontal dopamine display reduced working memory.[44] Potentially using gene variants as a surrogate marker for dopamine neurotransmission may be beneficial in patients who display depressive symptoms associated with these neurotransmitter pathways and may be more responsive to nonpharmacological and/or pharmacological approaches that target elevating brain dopamine levels.

Potential treatment for dopamine hypoexpression genes based on the biomarkers examined may include transcranial magnetic stimulation. Repetitive transcranial magnetic stimulation (rTMS) induces neuronal long-term potentiation or depression. Transcranial magnetic stimulation (TMS) is an effective and FDA-approved modality for the treatment of major depressive disorder (MDD). The relevant mechanisms of action are, however, still unknown. The antidepressant effects of TMS have been speculated to be associated with neurotrophic effects and potential enhancement of dopamine neurotransmission in the prefrontal cortex. The rTMS combined with positron emission tomography (PET) provides evidence of DA modulation following TMS.[45]

CONCLUSION

Biomarkers will enhance the treatment of patients with treatment-resistant depression. Genetic polymorphisms currently used clinically include pharmacokinetic genes and pharmacodynamics genes. Pharmacodynamic genes, the primary focus of this review, include gene variants related to serotonin and cortisol metabolism, dopamine, and glutamate neurotransmission, as well as pathways involving mitochondria and the immune system. The identification of these genes in patients with depression will lead to a more targeted approach to patients with mood disorders, rather than a "one-size-fits-all" approach which is currently used. An integrative medicine approach, based upon identification of specific biological disturbances in the brain associated with depression, will enhance the therapeutic options available for patients. These include alternative medication and/or

augmentation strategies such as omega-3 fish oil, L-tryptophan, methylfolate, lithium, *N* acetylcys-
teine, creatine, and transcranial magnetic stimulation.

REFERENCES

1. Kessler, R.C., Chiu, W.T., Demler, O. et al. 2005. Prevalence, severity, and comorbidity of 12-month DSM-IV disorders in the National Comorbidity Survey Replication. *Arch Gen Psychiatry* 62(6): 617–627.
2. Cain, R.A. 2007. Navigating the sequenced treatment alternatives to relieve depression (STAR*D) study: Practical outcomes and implications for depression treatment in primary care. *Prim Care* 34(3): 505–519.
3. Duivis, H.E., Vogelzangs, N., Kupper, N. et al. 2013. Differential association of somatic and cognitive symptoms of depression and anxiety with inflammation: Findings from the Netherlands Study of Depression and Anxiety (NESDA). *Psychoneuroendocrinology* 38(9): 1573–1585.
4. Weissman, M.M., Wickramaratne, P., Nomura, Y. et al. 2006. Offspring of depressed parents: 20 years later. *Am J Psychiatry* 163(6): 1001–1008.
5. Frazer, K.A., Murray, S.S., Schork, N.J. et al. 2009. Human genetic variation and its contribution to complex traits. *Nat Rev Genetics* 10(4): 241–251.
6. Lee, L.S., Andrade, A.S., and Flexner, C. 2006. Interactions between natural health products and antiretroviral drugs: Pharmacokinetic and pharmacodynamic effects. *Clin Infect Dis* 43(8): 1052–1059.
7. Caspi, A., Sugden, K., Moffitt, T.E. et al. 2003. Influence of life stress on depression: Moderation by the polymorphism in the 5HTT gene. *Science* 301(5631): 386–389.
8. Thomas, K.L. and Ellingrod, V.L. 2009. Pharmacogenetics of selective serotonin reuptake inhibitors and associated adverse drug reactions. *Pharmacotherapy* 29(7): 822–831.
9. Hariri, A.R. and Holmes, A. 2006. Genetics of emotional regulation: The role of the serotonin transporter in neural function. *Trends Cogn Sci* 10(4): 182–191.
10. Wust, S., Kumsta, R., Treutlein, J. et al. 2009. Sex-specific association between the 5-HTT gene-linked polymorphic region and basal cortisol secretion. *Psychoneuroendocrinology* 34(4): 972–982.
11. Buchmann, A.F., Holz, N., Boecker, R. et al. 2014. Moderating role of FKBP5 genotype in the impact of childhood adversity on cortisol stress response during adulthood. *Eur Neuropsychopharmacol* 24(60): 837–845.
12. Tharoor, H., Kotambail, A., Jain, S. et al. 2013. Study of the association of serotonin transporter triallelic 5-HTTLPR and STin2 VNTR polymorphisms with lithium prophylaxis response in bipolar disorder. *Psychiatr Genet* 23(2): 77–81.
13. Carabelli, B., Delattre, A.M., Pudell, C. et al. 2015. The antidepressant-like effect of fish oil: Possible role of ventral hippocampal 5-HT1A post-synaptic receptor. *Mol Neurobiol* 52(1): 206–215.
14. Schipper, P., Kiliaan, A.J., and Homberg, J.R. 2011. A mixed polyunsaturated fatty acid diet normalizes hippocampal neurogenesis and reduces anxiety in serotonin transporter knockout rats. *Behav Pharmacol* 22(4): 324–334.
15. Sublette, M.E., Ellis, S.P., Geant, A.L. et al. 2011. Meta-analysis of the effects of eicosapentaenoic acid (EPA) in clinical trials in depression. *J Clin Psychiatry* 72(12): 1577–1584.
16. Cerit, H., Jans, L.A., and Van der Does, W. 2013. The effect of tryptophan on the cortisol response to social stress is modulated by the 5-HTTLPR genotype. *Psychoneuroendocrinology* 38(2): 201–208.
17. Scharnholz, B., Weber-Hamann, B., Lederbogen, F. et al. 2010. Antidepressant treatment with mirtazapine, but not venlafaxine, lowers cortisol concentrations in saliva: A randomized open trial. *Psychiatry Res* 177(1–2): 109–113.
18. Schule, C., Baghai, T.C., Eser, D. et al. 2009. Effects of mirtazapine on dehydroepiandrosterone-sulfate and cortisol plasma concentrations in depressed patients. *J Psychiatr Res* 43(5): 538–545.
19. Rasmusson, A., Pinna, G., Paliwal, P. et al. 2006. Decreased cerebrospinal fluid allopregnanolone levels in women with posttraumatic stress disorder. *Biol Psychiatry* 60(7): 704–713.
20. Guennoun, R., Labombarda, F., Gonzalez Deniselle, M.C. et al. 2015. Progesterone and allopregnanolone in the central nervous system: Response to injury and implication for neuroprotection. *J Steroid Biochem Mol Biol* 146: 48–61.
21. Agis-Balboa, R.C., Guidotti, A., and Pinna, G. 2014. 5α-Reductase type I expression is downregulated in the prefrontal cortex/Brodmann's area 9 (BA9) of depressed patients. *Psychopharmacology (Berl)* 231(17): 3569–3580.
22. Brown, E.S., Park, J., Marx, C.E. et al. 2014. A randomized, double-blind, placebo-controlled trial of pregnenolone for bipolar depression. *Biol Psychiatry* 39(12): 2867–2873.

23. Liu, R.J., Lee, F.S., Li, X.Y. et al. 2012. Brain-derived neurotrophic factor Val66Met allele impairs basal and ketamine-stimulated synaptogenesis in prefrontal cortex. *Biol Psychiatry* 71(11): 996–1005.

24. Nelson, J.C., Baumann, P., Delucchi, K. et al. 2014. A systematic review and meta-analysis of lithium augmentation of tricyclic and second generation antidepressants in major depression. *J Affect Disord* 168: 269–275.

25. Drevets, W.C. 2004. Neuroplasticity in mood disorders. *Dialogues Clin Neurosci* 6(2): 199–216.

26. Cross-Disorder Group of the Psychiatric Genomics Consortium. 2013. Identification of risk loci with shared effects on five major psychiatric disorders: A genome-wide analysis. *Lancet* 381(9875): 1371–1379.

27. Wolkowitz, O.M., Epel, E.S., Reus, V.I. et al. 2010. Depression gets old fast: Do stress and depression accelerate cell aging? *Depress Anxiety* 27(4): 327–338.

28. Hannebelle, M., Champeil-Potokar, G., Lavialle, M. et al. 2014. Omega-3 polyunsaturated fatty acids and chronic stress-induced modulations of glutamatergic neurotransmission in the hippocampus. *Nutr Rev* 72(2): 99–112.

29. Prakash, A., Kalra, J.K., and Kumar, A. 2014. Neuroprotective effect of *N*-acetyl cysteine against streptozotocin-induced memory dysfunction and oxidative damage in rats. *J Basic Clin Physiol Pharmacol* 26(1): 13–23.

30. Schmaal, L., Veltman, D.J., Nederveen, A. et al. 2012. *N*-Acetylcysteine normalizes glutamate levels in cocaine-dependent patients: A randomized crossover magnetic resonance spectroscopy study. *Neuropsychopharmacology* 37(9): 2143–2152.

31. Berk, M., Dean, O.M., Cotton, S.M. et al. 2014. The efficacy of adjunctive *N*-acetylcysteine in major depressive disorder: A double-blind, randomized, placebo-controlled trial. *J Clin Psychiatry* 75(6): 628–636.

32. Zarate, C., Dumas, R.S., Liu, G. et al. 2013. New paradigms for treatment-resistant depression. *Ann N Y Acad Sci.* 1292: 21–31.

33. Yoon, S.J., Lyoo, I.K., Haws, C. et al. 2009. Decreased glutamate/glutamine levels may mediate cytidine's efficacy in treating bipolar depression: A longitudinal proton magnetic resonance spectroscopy. *Neuropsychopharmacology* 34(7): 1810–1818.

34. Muller, N. 2014. Immunology of major depression. *Neuroimmunomodulation* 21(2–3): 123–130.

35. Ohishi, K., Ueno, R., Nishino, S. et al. 1988. Increased level of salivary prostaglandins in patients with major depression. *Biol Psychiatry* 23(4): 326–334.

36. Cattaneo, A., Gennarelli, M., Uher, R. et al. 2013. Candidate genes expression profile associated with antidepressants response in the GENDEP study: Differentiating between baseline "predictors" and longitudinal "targets." *Neuropsychopharmacology* 38(3): 377–385.

37. Gubert, C., Stertz, L., Pfaffenseller, B. et al. 2013. Mitochondrial activity and oxidative stress markers in peripheral blood mononuclear cells of patients with bipolar disorder, schizophrenia, and healthy subjects. *J Psychiatr Res* 47(10): 1396–1402.

38. Hroudova, J. and Fisar, Z. 2010. Activities of respiratory chain complexes and citrate synthase influenced by pharmacologically different antidepressants and mood stabilizers. *Neuro Endocrinol Lett* 31(3): 336–342.

39. De Sousa, R.T., Machado-Vieira, R., Zarate, C.A. et al. 2014. Targeting mitochondrially mediated plasticity to develop improved therapeutics for bipolar disorder. *Expert Opin Ther Targets* 18(10): 1131–1147.

40. Lyoo, I.K., Yoon, S., Kim, T.S. et al. 2012. A randomized, double-blind placebo-controlled trial of oral creatine monohydrate augmentation for enhanced response to a selective serotonin reuptake inhibitor in women with major depressive disorder. *Am J Psychiatry* 169(9): 937–945.

41. Butler, I.J. and Rothenberg, S.P. 1987. Dietary folate and biogenic amines in the CNS. *J Neurochem* 49(1): 268–271.

42. Bousman, C.A., Potiriadis, M., Everall, I.P. et al. 2014. Methylenetetrahydrofolate reductase (MTHFR) genetic variation and major depressive disorder prognosis: A five-year prospective cohort study of primary care attendees. *Am J Med Genet B Neuropsychiatr Genet* 165B(1): 68–76.

43. Papakostas, G.I., Shelton, R.C., Zajecka, J.M. et al. 2014. Effect of adjunctive L-methylfolate 15 mg among inadequate responders to SSRIs in depressed patients who were stratified by biomarker levels and genotype: Results from a randomized clinical trial. *J Clin Psychiatry* 75(8): 855–863.

44. Tunbridge, E.M., Huber, A., Farrell, S.M. et al. 2012. The role of catechol-*O*-methyltransferase in reward processing and addiction. *CNS Neurol Disord Drug Targets* 11(3): 306–323.

45. Cho, S.S. and Strafella, A.P. 2009. rTMS of the left dorsolateral prefrontal cortex modulates dopamine release in the ipsilateral anterior cingulate cortex and orbitofrontal cortex. *PLoS One* 4(8): e6725.

17 Mood-Related Effects of Medications Prescribed for Non-Psychiatric Indications

Myrto A. Ashe, MD, MPH

CONTENTS

INTRODUCTION

Many medications prescribed for non-psychiatric indications are known to cause depression or to be associated with depression. The mechanisms by which they may cause depression include either a direct effect on neuronal processes related to mood, or an indirect effect of interference with other highly relevant metabolic processes. Medications can also ultimately affect quality of life in ways important enough to be a significant determinant of mood. The use of medication is also a marker for medical conditions or disease processes that may share root causes with depression, such as inflammation, nutrient depletion, or environmental toxicity. Thus the conditions that are comorbid with depression and the specific medications that are a predisposing condition, a trigger, or a perpetuating factor for depression are useful clues that can be used to elucidate the origin of the patient's mood issues.

TIME TREND IN THE USE OF MEDICATIONS IN THE UNITED STATES

Americans are taking more and more medications. According to a 2010 report by the Kaiser Family Foundation,[1] from 1999 to 2009, the number of prescriptions increased 39%, compared to a U.S. population growth of 9%. Throughout 2007–2010, the Centers for Disease Control and Prevention (CDC) surveyed the adult population, and when asked how many prescription medications were taken during the 30 days prior to questioning, 21.7% of all participants stated that they took three or more prescription medications, with 10% taking five or more prescriptions in that time span.[2] The most commonly prescribed classes of medications are analgesics, antihyperlipidemic agents, and antidepressants. Medications belonging to the first two categories can worsen or precipitate depression (Table 17.1).

While the aging of the American population contributes to these increasing numbers, medications account for an increasing proportion of the total health-care expenditures. They are growing much faster than expenditures for hospital care, and doctor- and office-based care. In 20 years, prescription drug expenditures grew 11.4%, compared to 5.2% for hospital care and 6.2% for physicians and clinics.[2,30] Age-adjusted rates for medication use have risen gradually from 1988–1994 to 2007–2010. While in 1988–1994, 61% of Americans used no prescription medications, this number has now decreased to 52%. In 1988–1994, 4% of Americans were using five or more medications: this number has now risen to 10%.

Prescriptions for children are also on the rise, most notably for medications used chronically. In the recent time period 2002–2010, prescriptions to treat attention deficit-hyperactivity disorder (ADHD), asthma, and prescriptions for oral contraceptives increased markedly.[31] This is in contrast to decreasing overall prescriptions, accounted for by fewer antibiotics, medications for allergies, pain, and cough/cold remedies. Once again, two of the categories, hormonal contraceptives and asthma medications, may be related to mood side effects. Prescriptions for depression decreased in that time period, although this apparently came on the heels of a dramatic increase in such prescriptions.[32]

ADVANTAGES AND DISADVANTAGES OF THE USE OF MEDICATIONS

The growth in the use of medications is considered to be responsible in part for the decreasing U.S. age-adjusted mortality rate[33] and increasing life expectancy. The Hoyert article, written for the CDC, attributes gains in the mortality rate to public health efforts and smoking cessation, but other reports attribute it to increasing use of medications. For example, in a 2007 review exploring the causes of the roughly 50% decrease in cardiovascular deaths in the United States (in the 25–84 age group, 1999–2009), the use of medications to improve heart failure, cholesterol, and hypertension accounted for 53% of the total reduction.[34] In the time period 2001–2010, among adults with hypertension, the proportion of patients on antihypertensive medication increased from 63% to 77%.[35] The chance of an individual's hypertension being adequately controlled improved, rising from 40% to 60%. The proportion of patients on multiple antihypertensive drugs increased from 37% to 48%. While they have not been found to exert an overall negative effect on quality of life in the elderly,[36] most classes of antihypertensives are associated with increased risk for depression and death by suicide.[5]

There are some signs that Americans are living longer but not healthier lives. Rates of limitation in complex activities are inching up, especially among 18–64 year olds. However, in general, during 2002 through 2012, there was little change over time, or slight improvement in certain age groups in the limitations in either complex or basic actions. This suggests a sort of trade-off between the gains made from the use of medications and the losses.

Americans suffer very high rates of patient harm resulting from medical care, and in particular, prescription medications. Iatrogenic causes account for at least 100,000 deaths per year, according to a widely quoted 1999 Institute of Medicine report.[37] According to Drug Abuse Warning Network Data, in 2009, 50% of the nearly 4.6 million drug-related emergency room visits nationwide were attributed to adverse reactions to pharmaceuticals taken *as prescribed*.[38] These numbers make it clear that Americans are paying a high price for the ease with which they receive and take prescriptions for medications that seemed justified at one time.

The science of medication side-effects is continuing to evolve. Criteria have been proposed to determine if a medication is the likely cause of an adverse event such as depression.[39] These criteria tend to consider medications "innocent until proven guilty," taking points off, for example, if one can find a reason for the patient's symptoms other than the medication. This is an understandable

TABLE 17.1

List of Medications Associated with Depression

Medication	Type or Condition	Comments	References
Baclofen	Muscle relaxant	GABAergic, but also results in changes in dopamine and serotonin	Oslin[3]
Other muscle relaxers (cyclobenzaprine, carisoprodol, Lioresal, others)	Muscle relaxants for muscle spasm	All affect neuronal transmission and all result in depression in certain individuals; not recommended for patients with a tendency to depression	Oslin[3]
NSAIDs	Pain, inflammation	Association with poorer response to antidepressant therapy, both medical and CBT increases positive impacts of positive events as well as negative impacts of negative events; prostaglandins are involved in affective responses	Gallagher[4]
CCB (amlodipine, Calan®, diltiazem, tizanidine, nifedipine)	Hypertension	Increased risk of depression; lipophilic; affect contractile and secretory functions in many types of cells	Hallas,[5] Lindberg[6]
Accutane®/retinoic acid	Acne	Association; abnormal retinoid levels are thought to have a neurological effect	Bremner[7]
Metoclopramide	GI complaints	Depression, sometimes long-lasting; dopamine antagonist; may increase affective impact of negative events	Oslin[3]
Opiate analgesics	Pain	Associated with depression	Patten[8]
Levofloxacin	Antibiotic	Especially associated with depression; possibly due to interference with receptors	Gunn[9]
Metformin	Diabetes	Appears to exert effects that would appear after years of use through interference with adequate B12 levels	Biemans[10]
Statins	High cholesterol, CV event prevention	May cause depression, may disrupt sleep, cognition, and may cause irritability; decreases likelihood of engaging in regular exercise	Takada,[11] Evans,[12] Golomb,[13] Tuccori,[14] Lee,[15] Golomb[16]
PPI	Reflux, gastritis, esophageal stricture	May be indirect effect due to reduced B12, iron and/or amino acids (due to impaired digestion); increase risk of dementia and Alzheimer's disease	Haenisch[17]
ACEI	Hypertension	Increased risk of depression	Hallas[5]
Methotrexate	Autoimmune disease; cancer	Increased depression rates, possibly through folate depletion	Ribeiro[18]
Tamoxifen, raloxifene	Breast cancer recurrence and prevention	These are associated with rising depression rates in women using them for prevention of breast cancer	Vogel[19]
Vaccinations	Prevention of various illnesses	Depression after vaccination	Glaser[20]
Arava (leflunomide)	Disease-modifying anti-rheumatic drug (DMARD)	Associated with the least depression	Ribeiro[18]
Hydroxychloroquine (Plaquenil)	DMARD	Highest rate of depression and suicidal ideation among drugs used for RA	Ribeiro[18]

(Continued)

TABLE 17.1 (*Continued*)
List of Medications Associated with Depression

Medication	Type or Condition	Comments	References
Finasteride	Androgenic alopecia	Has anti-androgenic properties; more reports of depression when used by younger patients for baldness, fewer when used by older patients for BPH; may reduce GABA activity	Römer[21]
Norplant	Progesterone insert	Side effects include depressive symptoms	Bitzer[22]
Chantix®	Smoking cessation	Suicide risk; though authors argue that quitting smoking can also lead to mood changes	Fagerstrom[23]
Rimonabant	Obesity	Suicide risk (not available in United States, only in Europe)	Moreira[24]
Reserpine	Hypertension	Classical first drug associated with depression, but may not be	Baumeister,[25] Huang[26]
Prednisone	Immune suppressant	Mood swings, irritability, depression	Patten[8]
Topical steroids	Dermatologic	Case report: emotional lability	Malladi[27]
Acyclovir	Antiviral	Case report: depression with psychotic features	Sirota[28]
Ondansetron	Anti-emetic	5-HT3 receptor antagonist; improves depression and fatigue in Hep C patients but can also cause it	Piche[29]

Note: NSAID: non-steroidal anti-inflammatory drug; CBT: cognitive behavioral therapy; CCB: calcium channel blocker; GI: gastrointestinal; CV: cardiovascular; PPI: proton pump inhibitor; BPH: benign prostatic hypertrophy; ACEI: angiotensin converting enzyme inhibitor; RA: rheumatoid arthritis.

attitude in a system that may award court-mandated damages pursuant to a medication side-effect, but it is not consistent with the medical principle of "do no harm."

DEPRESSION: A COMORBIDITY OF MANY CHRONIC MEDICAL CONDITIONS

Patients' underlying medical issues are often correlated (or comorbid) with elevated rates of depression. This can make it difficult to interpret data that find certain medications associated with depression. For example, it has been suggested that patients with rheumatoid arthritis (RA) have high rates of depression at baseline.[40] Authors have suggested that therefore, studies finding a link between specific agents used to treat RA and the development of depression should be discounted. However, one recent study compared RA patients taking different medications for RA and found that some medications are much more highly correlated with depression than others.[18] This finding is consistent with the hypothesis that indeed some medications for RA themselves cause depression, in addition to RA patients' pre-existing tendency to depression. Thus, the fact that a given patient with RA has depression cannot be assumed to be inevitable, if the patient is also taking a medication highly linked to depression. Of course the best research is still a double-blind controlled trial, but that is not always available.

Literature on what happens when patients report side effects to their physicians is not reassuring. It appears that the patient is the one who usually brings up the topic (not the physician) and that the physician usually denies a relationship between the medication and the side effect reported by the patient.[41] Specific criteria for appropriate prescribing have been developed in elderly patients, where this has been most critical, due to both their metabolic characteristics and their likelihood of being on a larger number of medications. Studies show that 20%–25% of elderly patients continue to be on one or more medications recommended as inappropriate using reasonably good scientific evidence.[42] It appears that as a group, physicians strongly believe in the net benefits conferred by medications. Health-care providers may also believe there are few other ways to attain the goals that medications are used for.

MEDICATIONS, SIDE EFFECTS, AND THE REDUCTIONISTIC MODEL OF RESEARCH

Rates of depression in the general population are increasing steadily. Rates have risen from 3.33% to 7.06% from 1991–1992 to 2001–2002 and possibly further to 9% overall in 2005–2008.[43] Use of antidepressant medication has risen nearly 400% in the time period 1988–1994 through 2005–2008.[44]

There is no simple way to prove or disprove a connection between this increase in depression and the increasing use of medications suspected of causing or worsening depression, and at any rate, population-level studies do not always provide information relevant to clinical care of individuals. Where an effort was made to understand the possible contribution of medications prescribed for hypertension, the estimate was that they could account for 1/1000 suicides.[5] This also speaks to the larger issue of the pharmacological treatment of risk factors reducing cardiovascular deaths while increasing deaths from other causes. In the end, overall U.S. age-adjusted mortality is being reduced, and the life expectancy is increasing so far. We seem to be deriving a net benefit from the use of multiple medications.

It may be possible to design an integrative approach that would reduce the need for antidepressant medications, while also reducing the need for the medications prescribed for non-psychiatric indications. For example, regular exercise improves both arthritis (for which a patient might be taking a nonsteroidal anti-inflammatory drug (NSAID), and far too often, a PPI to reduce the side effects of the NSAID), and depression. A diet low in glycemic index and high in plant-based nutrients, with the possible addition of some cold-water fish, is likely to improve hypertension, hypercholesterolemia, obesity, and depression. This is the low-hanging fruit we should not forget about.

INTEGRATIVE APPROACH TO DEPRESSION IN PATIENTS ON PRE-EXISTING MEDICATIONS

From a root-cause orientation to medicine, we find that many diseases have root causes in common with depression. Patients may be on medications that address the manifestations of these root causes, but not the causes themselves. They may even worsen, or add mechanisms that worsen, or cause depression.

Root causes of diseases work through basic pathologic mechanisms and create different diseases depending on the patient's predisposition and other characteristics. The role of the integrative clinician is to understand how the depression developed, and thus what role the patient's pre-existing medications may have played in its development or its exacerbation.

There are underlying processes that may be playing a role in any patient presenting with depression:

1. Inflammation
2. Nutritional deficiencies
3. Inactivity/lack of exercise
4. Poor gut bacterial diversity
5. Inadequate sleep
6. Hormonal dysregulation
7. Long-standing cognitive impairment
8. Inability to engage in previously pleasurable activities

These underlying processes also lead to a number of non-psychiatric diagnoses that could lead a physician to prescribe a depressogenic medication. Inflammation can lead to dyspepsia, leading to a prescription for a PPI. Magnesium or co-enzyme Q10 deficiencies can lead to hypertension, likely related to depression; inflammation is likely involved here as well. A lack of exercise can lead to worsening arthritis and a prescription for a NSAID. Poor gut bacterial diversity can lead to poor intestinal motility and a prescription for metoclopramide. Thus a comprehensive approach that addresses the patient's major issues using a root-cause approach and that is focused on reducing rather than adding medications seems most desirable when approaching a patient on multiple medications. It is a situation where the tools possessed by integrative practitioners help untangle the situation by reducing the total number of prescriptions.

DEPRESSOGENIC MEDICATIONS

Medications used for non-psychiatric purposes can have direct, indirect, and long-term effects on precursors of depression.

Direct effects may include

1. Direct effect on neurons, altering synaptic activity and neuronal communication
2. A general effect of lowering activity in the central nervous system
3. Interference with cytokines, resulting in either improved or worsened depression scores

Indirect effects may include

1. Alteration of nutrient levels over time, depleting vitamin B12 or folate levels, for example
2. Interference with digestion of protein, potentially reducing the quantity of amino acids available to the body to form neurotransmitters
3. Loss of taste and/or loss of appetite, thus reducing nutrient levels
4. Insomnia, thus increasing inflammation and other effects of inadequate sleep
5. Interference with gut bacteria, altering their beneficial effects on mood (we actually have very little research on the direct effect of medications on the gut biome)
6. Worsening insulin sensitivity, and hormone kinetics (altering levels of hormone-binding proteins, for example)

Long-term effects may include

1. Decreased likelihood that a patient will engage in physical exercise, thus reducing the beneficial effects of exercise
2. Cognitive impairment, and thus, interference with quality of life, leading to worsening depression over time
3. Idiosyncratic side effects such as headache, fatigue, nausea, and dizziness that also eventually interfere with quality of life
4. Predictable side effects such as fatigue, loss of libido, weight gain; drug-drug interactions such that a new medication causes the level of an older one to rise, resulting in a new side effect of the old medication

HOW THE INTEGRATIVE APPROACH MAKES USE OF PATIENTS' PRE-EXISTING CONDITIONS AND MEDICATIONS

In clinical practice as in research, the most difficult aspect of understanding the effect of patients' non-psychiatric medications is the question of whether depression is already associated with their diagnosis.

Depression is a comorbidity for many, if not most, non-psychiatric conditions, including cardiovascular disease, cancer, obesity, osteoporosis, hypertension, renal disease, and neurodegenerative conditions. One leading model of depression is "sickness behavior" caused by cytokines that are a part of a normal response to a pathogen: acutely ill people tend to feel dysthymic, discouraged, grumpy, and unmotivated. This can be replicated by injecting certain cytokines into experimental subjects. Chronically ill patients also frequently have dysregulated cytokines and may suffer from depression for the same reason.

While these links introduce complexity in research on the link between certain medications and depression, understanding them can be an advantage to the integrative provider. For example, if a long-standing type 2 diabetic patient on metformin presents with new onset of depression, the conventional approach is to start interpersonal therapy and/or an antidepressant (preferably one that does not cause weight gain). However, from the perspective of an integrative provider looking for the root cause, this patient is more likely to have a B12 deficiency than would a patient who is not on metformin. The diabetic patient also presumably has insulin resistance and frequent variations in glucose levels, perhaps an estrogen imbalance due to insulin-mediated changes in sex-hormone binding globulin, and possibly high levels of cytokines from adipocytes. Thus, when the provider's framework is integrative, both the pre-existing medical condition and the medication used to treat that condition should guide the initial intervention.

ADDITIONAL CONSIDERATIONS FOR SPECIFIC MEDICATIONS

There are convincing case reports of almost any medication causing severe depression, often reversed by discontinuing the medication and sometimes including a positive rechallenge. Thus all new medications should be considered possible candidates in any given patient's depression. This is also true of medications sometimes used to treat depression. For example, while pregabalin (Lyrica®) has been found to be useful at times in the treatment of depressive symptoms,[45] it has also been implicated in causing severe depression.[46]

MEDICATIONS THOUGHT LIKELY TO CAUSE DEPRESSION

DIRECT EFFECTS

Medications are used in general medicine for a variety of conditions involving the function of smooth muscle or skeletal muscle, and these are likely to be targeting the neuromuscular synapse.

This includes the class of medications called muscle relaxers, such as baclofen, cyclobenzaprine, carisoprodol, Lioresal®, and others. These are not recommended for patients with a tendency to depression. The exact mechanism is not known, as they often target more than one neurotransmitter. For example, baclofen is GABAergic but also causes changes in dopamine and serotonin signaling. It is believed that GABA antagonists can relieve depression.

Of the smooth muscle relaxants, only metoclopramide (Reglan®), a gastrointestinal antispasmodic, was directly implicated in predictably causing depression. In one study of normal volunteers, metoclopramide was found to be a dopamine antagonist and appeared to increase the affective impact of negative events on study participants.[3] Other smooth muscle relaxants are strong anticholinergics and will be covered in the section on medications with long-term potential for causing depression.

Prostaglandins are involved in affective responses, though it is generally thought that depression is caused by excessive prostaglandins and that COX inhibitors would be helpful in alleviating it. However, in cohort studies, users of NSAIDs were found less likely to respond to antidepressant or cognitive behavior therapy. It was hypothesized that this was due to the condition causing the inflammation for which the NSAIDs were being taken. However, a further double-blind study involving volunteers who did not have chronic pain showed that NSAIDs increase the positive impact of positive events as well as the negative impact of negative events and thus could in fact interfere with the treatment of depression.[4]

Calcium channel blockers, used for the treatment of hypertension and cardiac arrhythmias, have repeatedly been found to be correlated with higher rates of depression.[5,6] It has been hypothesized that this could be a direct effect of their impact on contractile and secretory functions of many types of cells. Calcium channel blockers include amlodipine, verapamil, diltiazem, tizanidine, nifedipine, and others. They are not normally a first-line treatment for hypertension. It is sometimes said that newer agents (like amlodipine) have fewer reports of adverse effects on mood, but this could be a function of having fewer years of use.

Beta-adrenergic blockers have a controversial association with depression. They were initially associated with fatigue and were believed to also worsen depression.[36] More recent studies have not shown a temporal association between the prescription for a beta-blocker and the subsequent prescription for an antidepressant. However, some population studies do show that patients on beta-blockers are more likely to be depressed than patients on angiotensin-converting enzyme inhibitors (ACEIs).[6]

Reserpine was the original medication thought to be strongly causative of depression. More recent analysis of the historical data refutes this connection. As reserpine is known to alter serotonin signaling, this would be evidence against the serotonin theory of depression.[25,26]

ACEIs may be implicated in preserving cognitive function, and thus there is some theoretical basis to consider at least the centrally acting ones (perindopril, captopril, fosinopril, lisinopril, ramipril, trandolapril) less likely to be harmful in depression as well.[47,48] However, there is at least one study that has found them to be more closely associated with depression than other antihypertensives—though the class includes more the commonly used noncentrally active ACEIs such as benazepril, moexipril, enalapril, and quinapril.

Retinoids such as Accutane® have been strongly associated with depression.[7] It is believed that abnormal retinoid levels have a neurological effect.

Levofloxacin is the antibiotic most commonly found to result in depression. It is believed to have a direct effect on the GABA receptor, though its effect could also be an indirect effect through disruption of gut bacteria.[9]

Opiate analgesics have a generalized depressant effect on the CNS. They are well known to increase rates of depression. They also reduce testosterone levels in the vast majority of male chronic users.

Finasteride is a medication that antagonizes the effects of testosterone. It is normally used in older men for the treatment of symptoms related to benign prostatic hypertrophy, but can also be used to lessen the impact of androgenic alopecia. The connection with depression appears clearer with this latter use.[21]

Indirect Effects

Several medications appear to exert their depressant effect through their disruption of inflammatory mediators. Topical steroids have also been found to lead to emotional lability. It is notable that these are also antimuscarinic anticholinergic agents.

Vaccinations such as the influenza vaccine have been found to result in a mild increase in depression in the weeks after administration, presumably due to transient increase in inflammation.[20]

Disease-modifying anti-rheumatic drugs, though they modulate the immune response in an effort to address certain autoimmune diseases, commonly result in depression. Hydroxychloroquine (Plaquenil®), used for rheumatoid arthritis, for example, has the highest rates of depression and suicidal ideation among drugs used for that condition.[18] Leflunomide (Arava®) is associated with the least depression.

TNF-alpha blockers, which would be expected to help with depression, given that it sometimes involves increased activity of TNF-alpha, actually show only partial effectiveness, and sometimes cause depression.[49]

LONG-TERM EFFECTS

Many medications deplete levels of folate. These include methotrexate, oral contraceptive pills, antacids, steroids, NSAIDs, salicylates, tetracycline, phenytoin, valproic acid, metformin, bile acid sequestrants, niacin, and potassium-sparing diuretics.[50] This can indirectly lead to depression in susceptible individuals, possibly via decreasing synthesis of *S*-adenosyl methionine (SAM-e) an obligatory cofactor in neurotransmitter synthesis.

Many medications may interfere with absorption of vitamin B12. These include metformin and antacids, including alkalinized water, calcium carbonate tablets, Carafate, H2 blockers like cimetidine and ranitidine, and most powerfully, the proton-pump inhibitors such as omeprazole, pantoprazole, and more.

Estrogens and progestins can result in depression in susceptible individuals. This is true of oral contraceptives, as well as hormone therapy, including bioidentical hormone therapy. Individuals may report that they can tolerate estrogen only, without progesterone, or neither. The strongest effect found for a specific indication seems to be that of the contraceptive implant Norplant®, which was the subject of a successful class action suit.[22]

Another way that medications can lead to depression in the long term is through their impact on cognitive function, especially in the elderly, but also other susceptible patients. Some studies show that cognitive dysfunction precedes the development of depression and could be causative.[51] Anticholinergic medications have been shown to cause cognitive decline over time. For this reason, they are not recommended for elderly patients, but a majority of older patients are nevertheless taking one or more of these medications.

A large number of medications have an effect on the muscarinic cholinergic receptor. These include powerful inhibitors such as certain urinary antispasmodics (oxybutynin), digoxin, furosemide, disopyramide, H1 and H2 blockers, meclizine, antiparkinson drugs, muscle relaxers, antiemetics, asthma medications such as atropine and Spiriva® and antispasmodics such as dicyclomine, and antiepileptics such as carbamazepine and trileptal. In addition, a large number of medications have weak anticholinergic activity, including many antibiotics (ampicillin, cefoxitin, clindamycin, piperacillin, vancomycin), valproic acid, asthma medication Advair®, and beta-blockers.

UNKNOWN RELATIONSHIP

Several medications have shown research associations over time that are not well-understood. These include raloxifene and tamoxifen, when prescribed for the prevention of breast cancer in patients at high risk but without a history of breast cancer.[19]

Statins are a special case due to the number of different ways they could potentially disrupt cognition, mitochondrial function, decrease in levels of coenzyme Q10, building blocks for major hormones (vitamin D, sex steroids, thyroid hormone, cortisol), myelination of brain pathways and also liver function, chronic pain through myalgias and muscle damage, and finally, decreased likelihood of engaging in exercise. On the other hand, in certain patients, they may exert a positive effect on depression and on cognition by their impact on inflammation. A quarter of American adults are presently being prescribed a statin drug, often for primary prevention of adverse cardiovascular outcomes.

It is never appropriate to assume that because most people have no adverse effects, that any given patient must have another cause for his or her symptoms.

CONCLUSION

The integrative approach offers a significant advantage in that it may address root causes of disease instead of adding to the mix a medication that lowers effectiveness or has side effects of its own. Thus integrative practitioners should carefully examine a patient's pre-existing medications and conditions and take them into account when designing a treatment for depression.

Side effect profiles of most medications frequently include depression. In the comprehensive evaluation of the patient, medications should be included as possible contributors to the patient's symptoms. Moreover, medications can be the clue to underlying causes of mood issues, either by their direct or indirect actions, or because they were started to address a condition that offers clues to the patient's genetic, nutritional, and inflammation status.

REFERENCES

1. Kaiser Family Foundation. 2010. Prescription Drug Trends. Available at: http://kaiserfamilyfoundation. files.wordpress.com/2013/01/3057-08.pdf
2. Centers for Disease Control and Prevention (CDC). 2013. Health, United States. Available at: http://www.cdc.gov/nchs/data/hus/hus13.pdf
3. Oslin, D.W. and Thomas, R.T. 1999. Exploring the affective toxicity of commonly prescribed medications in the elderly. *Dialogues Clin Neurosci* 1(2): 125–128.
4. Gallager, P.J., Castro, V., Fava, M. et al. 2012. Antidepressant response in patients with major depression exposed to NSAIDs: A pharmacovigilance study. *Am J Psychiatry* 169(10): 1065–1072.
5. Hallas, J. 1996. Evidence of depression provoked by cardiovascular medication: A prescription sequence symmetry analysis. *Epidemiology* 7(5): 478–484.
6. Lindberg, G., Bingefors, K., Ranstam, J. et al. 1998. Use of calcium channel blockers and risk of suicide: Ecological findings confirmed in population based cohort study. *BMJ* 3167133: 741–745.
7. Bremner, J.D., Shearer, K., and McCaffery, P. 2012. Retinoic acid and affective disorders: The evidence for an association. *J Clin Psychiatry* 73(1): 37–50.
8. Patten, S.B. and Lavorato, D.H. 2001. Medication use and major depressive symptoms in a community population. *Compr Psychiatry* 42(2): 124–131.
9. Gunn, B.G., Brown, A.R., Lambert, J.J. et al. 2011. Neurosteroids and GABA(A) receptor interactions: A focus on stress. *Front Neurosci* 5: 131.
10. Biemans, E., Hart, H.E., Rutten, G.E. et al. 2015. Cobalamin status and its relationship with depression, cognition, and neuropathy in patients with type 2 diabetes mellitus using metformin. *Acta Diabetol* 52(2): 383–393.
11. Takada, M., Fujimoto, M., Yamazaki, K. et al. 2014. Association of statin use with sleep disturbances: Data mining of a spontaneous reporting database and a prescription database. *Drug Saf* 37(6): 421–431.
12. Evans, M.A. and Golomb, B.A. 2009. Statin-associated adverse cognitive effects: Survey results from 171 patients. *Pharmacotherapy* 29(7): 800–811.
13. Golomb, B.A., Kane, T., and Dimsdale, J.E. 2004. Severe irritability associated with statin cholesterol-lowering drugs. *QJM* 97(4): 229–235.
14. Tuccori, M., Montagnani, S., Mantarro, S. et al. 2014. Neuropsychiatric adverse events associated with statins: Epidemiology, pathophysiology, prevention and management. *CNS Drugs* 28(3): 249–272.
15. Lee, D.S.H., Markwardt, S., Goeres, L. et al. 2014. Statins and physical activity in older men: The Osteoporotic Fractures in Men Study. *JAMA Intern Med* 174(8):1263–1270.
16. Golomb, B.A. 2014. Statins and activity: Proceed with caution. *JAMA Intern Med* 174(8): 1270–1272.
17. Haenisch, B., von Holt, K., Wiese, B. et al. 2014. Risk of dementia in elderly patients with the use of proton pump inhibitors. *Eur Arch Psychiatry Clin Neurosci* 265(5): 419–428.
18. Pinho de Oliveira Ribeiro, N., Rafael de Mello Shier, A., Ornelas, A.C. et al. 2013. Anxiety, depression and suicidal ideation in patients with rheumatoid arthritis in use of methotrexate, hydroxychloroquine, leflunomide and biological drugs. *Compr. Psychiatry* 54(8): 1185–1189.
19. Vogel, V.G. 2009. The NSABP Study of Tamoxifen and Raloxifene (STAR) trial. *Expert Rev Anticancer Ther* 9(1): 51–60.
20. Glaser, R., Robles, T.F., Sheridan, J. et al. 2003. Mild depressive symptoms are associated with amplified and prolonged inflammatory responses after influenza virus vaccination in older adults. *Arch Gen Psychiatry* 60(10): 1009–1014.
21. Römer, B. and Gass, P. 2010. Finasteride-induced depression: New insights into possible pathomechanisms. *J Cosmet Dermatol* 9(4): 331–332.
22. Bitzer, J., Tschudin, S., and Alder, J. 2004. Acceptability and side-effects of Implanon in Switzerland: A retrospective study by the Implanon Swiss Study Group. *Eur J Contracept Reprod Health Care* 9:278–284.
23. Fagerström, K. and Hughes, J. 2008. Varenicline in the treatment of tobacco dependence. *Neuropsychiatr Dis Treat* 4(2): 353–363.

24. Moreira, F.A. and Crippa, J.A. 2009. The psychiatric side-effects of rimonabant. *Rev Bras Psiquiatr* 31(2): 145–153.
25. Baumeister, A.A., Hawkins, M.F., and Uzelac, S.M. 2003. The myth of reserpine-induced depression: Role in the historical development of the monoamine hypothesis. *J Hist Neurosci* 12(2): 207–220.
26. Huang, Q.J., Jiang, H., Hao, X.L. et al. 2004. Brain IL-1 beta was involved in reserpine-induced behavioral depression in rats. *Acta Pharmacol Sin* 25(3): 293–296.
27. Malladi, S.S. 2009. Emotional lability secondary to the application of a very potent topical corticosteroid. *Indian J Psychiatry* 51(3): 212–213.
28. Sirota, P., Stoler, M., and Meshulam, B. 1988. Major depression with psychotic features associated with acyclovir therapy. *Drug Intell Clin Pharm* 22(4): 306–308.
29. Piche, T., Vanbiervliet, G., Cherikh, F. et al. 2005. Effect of ondansetron, a 5-HT3 receptor antagonist, on fatigue in chronic hepatitis C: A randomised, double blind, placebo controlled study. *Gut* 54(8): 1169–1173.
30. CDC Faststats. 2012. Therapeutic Drug Use. Available at: http://www.cdc.gov/nchs/fastats/drug-use-therapeutic.htm
31. Chai, G., Governale, L., McMahon, A.W. et al. 2012. Trends of outpatient prescription drug utilization in US children, 2002–2010. *Pediatrics* 130(1): 23–31.
32. Olfson, M., Marcus, S.C., Weissman, M.M. et al. 2002. National trends in the use of psychotropic medications by children. *J Am Acad Child Adolesc Psychiatry* 41(5): 514–521.
33. Hoyert, D.L. 2012. *75 Years of Mortality in the United States, 1935–2010.* NCHS Data Brief, no 88. Hyattsville, MD: National Center for Health Statistics.
34. Ford, E.S., Ajani, U.A., Croft, J.B. et al. 2007. Explaining the decrease in U.S. deaths from coronary disease, 1980–2000. *N Engl J Med* 356(23): 2388–2398.
35. Gu, Q., Burt, V.L., Dillon, C.F. et al. 2012. Trends in antihypertensive medication use and blood pressure control among United States adults with hypertension: The National Health and Nutrition Examination Survey, 2001 to 2010. *Circulation* 126(17): 2105–2114.
36. Fogari, R. and Zoppi, A. 2004. Effect of antihypertensive agents on quality of life in the elderly. *Drugs Aging* 21(6): 377–393.
37. Kohn, L.T., Corrigan, J.M., and Donaldson, M.S. 1999. *To Err Is Human: Building a Safer Health System.* Institute of Medicine. Washington, DC: National Academy Press.
38. National Institute on Drug Abuse. 2014. Drug-Related Hospital Emergency Room Visits. http://www.drugabuse.gov/publications/drugfacts/drug-related-hospital-emergency-room-visits
39. Rogers, D. and Pies, R. 2008. General medical drugs associated with depression. *Psychiatry* 5(12): 28–41.
40. Hyrich, K., Symmons, D., Watson, K. et al. 2006. Baseline comorbidity levels in biologic and standard DMARD treated patients with rheumatoid arthritis: Results from a national patient register. *Ann Rheum Dis* 65(7): 895–898.
41. Golomb, B.A., McGraw, J.J., Evans, M.A. et al. 2007. Physician response to patient reports of adverse drug effects: Implications for patient-targeted adverse effect surveillance. *Drug Saf* 30(8): 669–675.
42. Pugh, M.J., Hanlon, J.T., Zeber, J.E. et al. Assessing potentially inappropriate prescribing in the elderly Veterans Affairs population using the HEDIS 2006 quality measure. *J Manag Care Pharm* 12(7): 537–545.
43. Compton, W.M., Conway, K.P., Stinson, F.S. et al. 2006. Changes in the prevalence of major depression and comorbid substance use disorders in the United States between 1991–1992 and 2001–2002. *Am J Psychiatry* 163(12): 2141–2147.
44. Pratt, L.A., Brody, D.J., and Gu, Q. 2011. *Antidepressant Use in Persons Aged 12 and Over: United States, 2005–2008.* NCHS data brief, no 76. Hyattsville, MD: National Center for Health Statistics.
45. Stein, D.J., Baldwin, D.S., Baldinetti, F. et al. 2008. Efficacy of pregabalin in depressive symptoms associated with generalized anxiety disorder: A pooled analysis of 6 studies. *Eur Neuropsychopharmacol* 18(6): 422–430.
46. Hall, T.D., Shah, S., Ng, B. et al. 2014. Changes in mood, depression and suicidal ideation after commencing pregabalin for neuropathic pain. *Aust Fam Phys* 43(10): 705–708.
47. Mogi, M., Iwanami, J., and Horiuchi, M. 2012. Roles of brain angiotensin II in cognitive function and dementia. *Int J Hypertens* 2012(169649): 1–7.
48. O'Caoimh, R., Healy, L., Gao, Y. et al. 2014. Effects of centrally acting angiotensin converting enzyme inhibitors on functional decline in patients with Alzheimer's disease. *J Alzheimers Dis* 40(3): 595–603.
49. Finn, D.A., Beadles-Bohling, A.S., Beckley, E.H. et al. 2006. A new look at the 5α-reductase inhibitor finasteride. *CNS Drug Rev* 12(1): 53–76.

50. UMMC. 2015. Drugs that deplete: Vitamin B9 (folic acid). Available at: http://umm.edu/health/medical/altmed/supplement-depletion-links/drugs-that-deplete-vitamin-b9-folic-acid

51. Katz, I.R. 1999. Depression in late life: Psychiatric-medical comorbidity. *Dialogues Clin Neurosci* 1(2): 81–94.

52. van Melle, J.P., Verbeek, D.E.P, van den Berg, M.P. et al. 2006. Beta-blockers and depression after myocardial infarction: A multicenter prospective study. *J Am Coll Cardiol* 48(11): 2209–2214.

18 The Rationale for Treating with a Broad Spectrum of Minerals and Vitamins

Julia J. Rucklidge, PhD and Bonnie J. Kaplan, PhD

CONTENTS

INTRODUCTION

There are some very simple facts about the brain that are well-known to all neuroscientists, yet have thus far not attracted the attention of many clinicians and clinical researchers. For instance, the brain is the most metabolically active organ in the body, which means that it requires the most energy in the form of ATP to function optimally. What do our mitochondria need to produce more ATP? They need many nutrients, including glucose. Here is an indication of how demanding the brain is: a liter of blood flows through our brains every minute that our hearts are beating. What is that blood doing? Of course it delivers oxygen and carries away waste products; however, it also delivers the nutrients needed to feed our mitochondria and sustain brain function.

Here is a second basic fact: nutrients are cofactors in virtually every enzymatic function in every pathway of the brain. With insufficient nutrients, those metabolic steps (including synthesis of neurotransmitters) cannot function at their optimal level. Interestingly, at least 50 genetic mutations have been defined that result in people needing an unusually large amount of nutrients for those metabolic steps to work well; in every one of those known inborn errors of metabolism (all of which are associated with primarily physical symptoms), treatment of the patients consists of providing them with additional nutrients to restore normal function, presumably by saturating the enzymes with sufficient cofactors.[1] The RDA levels of nutrients found in ordinary multivitamin tablets are not sufficient for people with these inborn errors of metabolism. As discussed below, this framework can be helpful in understanding some mental disorders: some people eating very healthy diets still improve emotionally when they take broad-spectrum micronutrient formulas, which suggests that they may have inborn errors of metabolism resulting in this need for unusually large amounts of nutrients for optimal function.

And here is a third and final basic fact that is often overlooked: humans have evolved to need around 50 essential nutrients that we know of (and maybe more, whose roles are not yet defined), and these need to be consumed *together, in balance*. Consuming large amounts of just one or a few can actually be harmful. The brilliant feature of many food sources is that they have also evolved to provide most of those nutrients in optimal proportions (if they have not been genetically modified). So, for instance, plants that provide calcium tend to also provide nutrients such as magnesium which facilitate absorption of calcium, and foods rich in copper (e.g., oysters) also provide zinc in the perfectly balanced, healthy ratio to benefit human needs.

The purpose of this chapter is to demonstrate why it makes perfect sense to treat mental disorders with nutrients, and why treating with broad-spectrum nutrients is effective. The evidence will be reviewed, demonstrating the overall clinical benefit from broad-spectrum nutrients, followed with a discussion of where further research is urgently needed.

NUTRITION CONCEPTS

Every field has its technical terms and jargon, and nutrition is no exception. As two psychologists who study nutrition, a few basic terms have been especially useful.

Food is usually described in terms of its *macronutrients*: grams of protein, carbohydrates (including sugars), and fats. In contrast, supplements (nutrients that we take in pill form) usually contain *micronutrients:* milligrams and micrograms of dietary minerals and vitamins, perhaps amino acids, and essential fatty acids (such as omega 3s). Millions of people consume other supplements (e.g., botanicals), but this chapter is restricted to the most commonly consumed and most frequently studied nutrients: *micronutrients*.

When North Americans want to know whether they are getting "enough" or "too much" of a nutrient, the primary source of information is the Dietary Reference Intakes (DRI), a series of volumes developed in the United States and Canada, principally by the Institute of Medicine, which is part of the U.S. National Academy of Sciences, and published over several years in the early part of this century.[2] The DRIs are freely available on the Internet and can vary from country to country. An important point to know is that for many nutrients the optimal amounts are not yet known. For instance, there are more than 600 naturally occurring carotenoids in our plants (lutein and lycopene are examples), and people who consume a lot of plants with carotenoids are generally healthier than those who do not.[3] Yet, the functions of many of those carotenoids have not yet been defined, and very little information about them is included in the DRIs. But the primary minerals and vitamins are in the DRIs, and three types of reference values are particularly useful to know when questioning safe and adequate amounts to be consumed: Estimated Average Requirement (EAR), Recommended Dietary Allowance (RDA), and tolerable Upper intake Levels (ULs).

The EAR is defined as a nutrient intake value that is estimated to meet the requirements of half of the healthy individuals in a group. The EAR is used to assess adequacy of intake of population groups and, along with knowledge of the distribution of requirements, to develop the RDAs. The RDA is defined as the average daily dietary intake level that is sufficient to meet the nutrient requirements of nearly all (98%) healthy individuals in a group. It is a target for individuals, to ensure enough intake. The UL is defined as a recommended daily nutrient intake that is likely to pose no risks of adverse health effects to almost all individuals in the general population. As intake increases above the UL, the risk of adverse effects increases.

These three types of reference values have to be used carefully. For instance, notice that the EAR and RDA are defined for healthy people. The third type of reference value also requires caution. Notice that the UL is defined for an individual ingredient, and so application of ULs to broad-spectrum formulas requires thought. One well-known example illustrates why ULs cannot be accepted uncritically. It has been understood for about 150 years that vitamin B12 deficiency can cause depression, psychosis, and other mental symptoms. And it is also known that taking large doses of another B vitamin, folate, can mask that deficiency. Hence, the UL for folate is kept low to avoid the problem of inadvertently masking a B12 deficiency, and putting a patient at risk of ill physical and mental health. But good quality multinutrient formulas always provide enough B12 that the consumer will not experience a B12 deficiency, so the entire basis of the UL for folate would not apply to such formulas.

ORTHOMOLECULAR PSYCHIATRY

The goal of the orthomolecular approach, as proposed by Nobel Laureate Linus Pauling in 1968, is to restore health by treating people with natural substances. But even more than Pauling, it is the name Hoffer that is most closely associated with the term. Abram Hoffer (1917–2009) was a Canadian psychiatrist with a PhD in biochemistry. He was highly respected for his clinical work, and for helping to develop the International Society of Orthomolecular Medicine. Hoffer demonstrated that some psychiatric patients improved if treated with large doses of vitamins, and his primary focus was on one: niacin.[4] Although Hoffer was widely respected as a brilliant clinician and a pioneer in this field, the orthomolecular approach is difficult to study because it is individualized for each patient. Hence, there have been few well-conducted trials done on orthomolecular methods, making it difficult for the field to gain credibility.

DISAPPOINTING RESEARCH OF THE TWENTIETH CENTURY

There is a massive amount of research on the importance of various nutrients for brain cells, and the application of that knowledge to brain dysfunction has also been explored for at least a century. Some readers may be surprised to learn that as early as 1929, psychiatrists were publishing reports of improved mental health in patients given extra nutrients. But the key feature that discriminated most of the reports from 1929 to 2000 from nutrient treatment studies published in the current century is this: the early research studied one nutrient at a time, whereas now the best scientific data are primarily emanating from studies of multinutrient formulas. The importance of the early work should not be dismissed; however, as those studies showed modest improvements in mental health with nutrient supplementation, especially vitamins A, B, C, and E, as well as choline, calcium, chromium, iron, magnesium, zinc, and selenium and also provide useful insights into mechanisms of action of individual nutrients.[5]

The broad-spectrum research is discussed in the section "Scientific Basis of Treating Mental Illness Nutritionally" in this chapter. In the following section, the single-nutrient approach employed in twentieth century research is described, along with how it created an obstacle to progress and, in fact, directly contributed to the current widespread attitude that nutrient treatment is of trivial importance.

SEARCHING FOR MAGIC BULLETS

Scientists have raised public awareness of the benefit to mental health of many individual nutrients: omega-3 fatty acids and vitamin D are particularly salient and recent examples. Ongoing studies of vitamin D, S-adenosylmethionine (SAMe), co-enzyme Q10, and so on, contribute to our understanding of the potential therapeutic role that individual nutrients can play in treating people with emotional instability. However, given that there are over 50 micronutrients (vitamins, minerals, amino acids, and essential fatty acids) that are critical for good health, plus others (e.g., the conditionally essential nutrient α-lipoic acid, as well as SAMe and others) that may also influence mental health, doing extensive clinical trials of each one individually would require many decades of work and extensive funding. For each nutrient, multiple studies would be needed that varied the formulation (e.g., different chelates for minerals), the dose, the target symptom/disorder, and duration of intervention.

As mentioned above, recent reviews have shown that over a century of investigations of single nutrients has resulted in only modest treatment benefits. Although even in the current century there are sporadic suggestions that there is an urgent need to mount clinical trials on individual micronutrients (e.g., vitamin D[6,7]), perhaps it is time to question whether this tactic makes sense. Presented below is the argument that studying a single nutrient may be a reasonable methodology when the purpose is to target a specific physiological pathway, but that a more sensible approach both financially and physiologically is to address broad questions of clinical benefit with complex, multinutrient formulas.

SINGLE CAUSE FALLACY AND SCIENTIFIC METHOD

Historically, the single-nutrient strategy yielded significant progress in mental health, such as the discovery that myxedema madness could be reversed with iodine, that the mental symptoms of pellagra were due to insufficient niacin (nicotinic acid, vitamin B3), that psychosis was sometimes a sign of pernicious anemia (insufficient cobalamin, vitamin B12), and that Wernicke's encephalopathy should be treated with thiamine (vitamin B1), but no new single-nutrient causes have been identified in recent years. Consequently, continuation of this single-nutrient strategy has yielded only small benefits, in particular from other B vitamins, iron, zinc, copper, and vitamins D (cholecalciferol) and E (tocopherols and tocotrienols). Years ago the eminent nutrition researcher Walter Mertz pointed out that the concept of "one-disease, one-nutrient" had become outdated, because most nutrient risk factors are now understood to be multifactorial.[8]

The single cause fallacy continues to influence research on nutritional interventions for various reasons. One reason is that it fits comfortably with the paradigm called the scientific method, which requires the manipulation of only one independent variable (such as a nutrient) at a time. The definition of a single independent variable has relaxed a bit in the nonbiological world (consider the complexity of a cognitive behavioral intervention), but of course has changed little in the realm of physiological research. A second reason the single cause fallacy continues to be influential is that it fits comfortably with the pharmaceutical paradigm, in which the vast majority of medications are single-ingredient drugs. Combination drugs are rare, in part because they require extraordinary testing to obtain government approval for marketing. Consequently, clinical research for both physical and mental health problems is dominated by single-ingredient approaches. Finally, a third reason that the single cause fallacy continues to be influential is because it fits into a particularly Western way of viewing the world commonly referred to as magic or silver bullet thinking: when there is a problem, the optimal solution is expected to be a single remedy.

Though single nutrients were historically suitable for certain frank deficiency syndromes (e.g., using ascorbic acid, vitamin C, to treat scurvy), a multifactorial approach (as suggested by Mertz[8]) is more consistent with the evolutionary process that favors variability. Equifinality, a term used to describe the fact that different genetic and environmental factors can lead to a similar outcome, could apply to nutrients (one of the most significant of all environmental factors, as exposure is pervasive and continues throughout life). For instance, various genetic mutations affecting different pathways involving micronutrients could result in the same mental symptoms. The search for one causal nutrient deficiency to explain the etiology of one disorder ignores the wealth of data showing that the success of an organism evolving over time is not through identical changes affecting one system but via constant reshuffling of genes as well as infinite mutations occurring over time.

The elegant Lenski experiments on *Escherichia coli* illustrated this process over 45,000 generations of *E. coli* in which one population was used to infect 12 identical flasks, all containing a finite supply of the same nutrient broth.[9] These 12 flasks founded 12 different lines of evolution tracked for over two decades; nonetheless, the varied genetic changes occurring across the 12 lineages often resulted in similar improved fitness and, hence, survival, showing that different mutations in genes can result in similar outcomes. However, there was one interesting exception. After about 33,000 generations, one lineage suddenly showed a dramatic rise in population density after a genetic mutation resulted in the bacteria acquiring the ability to use another nutrient in the broth (citrate) in addition to glucose. What this change showed was that in the bacterial world, a mutation enabling the bacteria to use more than one nutrient resulted in a dramatic evolutionary advantage.

In human health research, there is reemergence of understanding that human physiology requires many nutrients, and so a few scientists have begun to study complex micronutrient formulas in both physical and mental health.

LOGIC OF TREATING MENTAL ILLNESS WITH NUTRIENTS

NEUROTRANSMITTER PATHWAYS AND METABOLISM

Earlier, when discussing the role of nutrients in brain function, inborn errors of metabolism were discussed. The word *metabolism* refers to the fact that chemicals that enter our body need to go through various transformations in order to be available to serve our cells in the manner needed. Every step of metabolism is catalyzed by enzymes, which are dependent on the availability of cofactors (sometimes called coenzymes). When there are sufficient amounts of the requisite cofactors present, our enzymes can function optimally, and our metabolism occurs at its maximum pace. To optimize health, we want to optimize metabolic activity so that it approaches its maximum, and for that, we need sufficient cofactors.

The role of nutrients in metabolic pathways is the important point to remember: cofactors are often nutrients, especially vitamins, and the metal ions that are dietary minerals (e.g. iron, magnesium, copper, zinc). So if we want to ensure that our brains are synthesizing sufficient chemicals such as neurotransmitters, and if we also want to ensure that all the neurotransmitter precursors are present when needed and that they are all broken down (metabolized) when not needed, then every step must be supported by the nutrients that make up the precursors as well as the cofactors that facilitate the critical enzymatic reactions.

To think of the relationship between nutrition and neurotransmitters another way, consider this: there are medications that increase availability of serotonin in the synaptic cleft. But perhaps the better way to increase serotonin availability is the natural way, by providing sufficient cofactors (nutrients) to the enzymes to maximize metabolic speed in pathways involved in synthesis.

DYSBIOSIS, INFLAMMATION, AND MENTAL HEALTH

The *immunity hypothesis* of depression has been strongly supported for almost three decades: depression is associated with activation of inflammatory responses.[10,11] For instance, the Cooper Center Study of almost 12,000 adults found that elevated homocysteine levels (biomarker of systemic inflammation) were associated with 26% increased odds of scoring in the depression range on the Center for Epidemiologic Studies Depression Scale, even after controlling for many variables likely to influence both inflammation and depression (e.g., age, sex, body mass index, and exercise).[12,13] Although some of the reports are inconsistent, the association of other biomarkers of inflammation (e.g., TNF-alpha and IL-6) with diagnosed depression has been strongly supported.[10]

Bipolar disorder has also been associated with elevated biomarkers of inflammation,[14] although the relationships being studied can be complicated. Sometimes inflammatory biomarkers have shown the elevated levels expected in association with symptom severity, but other inflammatory markers have been low, resulting in the hypothesis that lower markers of inflammation may actually indicate the body's attempt to limit pro-inflammatory processes. A meta-analysis of clinical trials of nonsteroidal anti-inflammatory drugs (NSAIDs) used as adjuncts in treatment for schizophrenia found a mean effect size of 0.43, indicating that the NSAIDs (celecoxib in four studies, and aspirin in the fifth) had a moderately beneficial impact on symptoms.[15] The question is, what causes systemic, chronic inflammation?

It is often said that at least 90% of the cells in and on our bodies are not human: they are the microbial cells (especially bacteria) that constitute our microbiome. Most of these microbial cells live in the gastrointestinal (GI) system, where they serve many functions: they protect the intestinal barrier defense system, digest our food, extract the nutrients that we need, and in some cases synthesize those nutrients for us.[16] There is bidirectional communication between the gut and the brain, termed the *gut-brain axis*, which is dependent on the health of the community of organisms. An imbalance in gut bacteria is called dysbiosis, which can lead to problems such as overgrowth of already-present opportunistic micro-organisms such as *Clostridium difficile*.[17] Insufficient quantities of the "good" bacteria can lead to the induction of inflammatory responses,[10] which are associated with many chronic inflammatory disorders, including inflammatory bowel disease and rheumatoid arthritis.[18] In addition, these same inflammatory responses caused by dysbiosis can lead to some mental disorders such as depression.

Gut dysbiosis can be caused by many things: use of broad-spectrum antibiotics, poor diet, and an excessively clean modern environment (the hygiene, or "Old Friends," hypothesis).[19,20] Psychological stress is another causal factor, as shown in animal models prenatally,[21] in early life,[22] and in adulthood.[17] These effects can be long-lasting: when baby rats were removed from their mothers for 3 hours per day, only during the 10 days after birth, the induced dysbiosis was maintained all the way into adulthood.[23] This effect of psychological stress on the microbiota has also been demonstrated in humans.[24]

Some effects of probiotics on mood and anxiety have been found in recent trials,[25,26] but the data are quite preliminary and require replication and expansion. There are several mechanisms that explain how gut health can influence inflammation, which can then affect mental health. Though slightly oversimplified, these processes can be conceptualized as three steps: (1) broad-spectrum antibiotics, psychological stress, excessively clean environments, or a chronically poor diet cause dysbiosis; (2) dysbiosis causes inflammation by increasing susceptibility to intestinal pathogens, impairing the development of a healthy immune system (which requires sufficient supply of "good" bacteria); and (3) inflammation results in a breakdown of the gut's mucosal barrier, permitting migration of bacteria to areas outside the intestinal tract, thereby affecting brain function.

The association between dysbiosis and inflammatory activation is a robust one, but there are many other potential causative agents for chronic inflammation, including psychological factors (e.g., childhood adversity and environmental toxins).[27]

One might ask, how does the human body deal with dysbiosis and inflammation under normal circumstances? The mitochondria in our cells are our first line of defense. Given adequate quantities of the nutrients that they need to function, our mitochondria efficiently produce adenosine triphosphate (ATP) which combats inflammation and its harmful effects.[28] As we see below, it is the adequacy of nutrients that is the target of micronutrient treatment for mental disorders.

MITOCHONDRIA AND MENTAL HEALTH

Mitochondria are the cellular structures that have evolved in humans to manage inflammation and oxidative stress. During our education we all learned about their role as the "powerhouse" of the cell, generating energy in the form of a molecule called ATP. Billions of years ago eukaryotic cells (those with membrane-bound nuclei) engulfed primitive mitochondria-like bacteria, resulting in a "composite" organism with an energy-producing advantage.[29] Through millions of years of evolution, these composite cells became complex organisms. All of our cells contain multiple mitochondria, which produce ATP. The production of ATP via (a) the Krebs cycle (also known as the citric acid cycle) and the (b) electron transport chain (also known as oxidative phosphorylation) is well defined. The Krebs cycle sequentially oxidizes (i.e., removes electrons from) acetyl coenzyme-A (acetyl-CoA), produced from the breakdown of carbohydrates, fats, and proteins. The important products of the Krebs cycle are two high-energy molecules, nicotinamide adenine dinucleotide and flavin adenine dinucleotide (known as NADH and $FADH_2$, respectively), which receive the electrons from acetyl-CoA.

The second step is being studied particularly in relationship to mental disorders: the electron transport chain (ETC). The ETC is composed of five enzyme complexes.[29] NADH and $FADH_2$, generated previously in the Krebs cycle, donate their electrons to the ETC. These electrons are transferred through a cascade of chemical reactions that create a chemical environment suitable for the generation of ATP. Many cofactors (coenzymes) required for proper enzymatic function in the Krebs cycle and ETC are dependent on the availability of dietary nutrients.

When genes are discussed, it is generally in reference to the DNA contained in the nuclei of cells, called *nuclear DNA* (nDNA). But mitochondria are not inside the nucleus, and yet they possess their own DNA, mitochondrial DNA (mtDNA). The mtDNA is so small it accounts for only 0.3% of total cellular DNA; the other 99.7% is the nDNA. Relevant to our description of the ETC, it is interesting to note that mtDNA encodes 13 enzymes involved in the ETC. Ninety-five percent of enzymes present in the ETC, however, are expressed in the nucleus and are shuttled to the mitochondria. Therefore, to summarize this simple description of mitochondria in a different way, they are semi-autonomous organelles that are responsible for energy production in the form of ATP, and they have a small (but important) number of coding genes that are distinct from nuclear DNA.

The ETC is efficient at generating energy, but oxygen is required for this process. Errors in the reactions involving oxygen are capable of generating reactive oxygen species (ROS) such as super-oxide and peroxide. Importantly, these ROS can damage mitochondria and cause DNA mutations, and mtDNA is particularly susceptible to ROS-induced damage because of its proximity to the ETC. Furthermore, mtDNA has less efficient DNA repair mechanisms and protective measures than nDNA, resulting in mutations accumulating 10–16 times faster than in nDNA.[29] Accumulated mtDNA mutations affect enzyme function in ways that can decrease energy production, causing mitochondrial disease. Consequently, it seems that most, if not all, mitochondrial diseases are the result of mtDNA mutations causing a reduction of ATP production. This topic is relevant to mental health, requiring a bit of background about mitochondrial illness.

The term *mitochondrial medicine* was coined by Luft in 1994; even at that time, he reported that mitochondrial dysfunction was relevant in more than 100 diseases.[30] Mitochondrial dysfunction can affect every organ and system in our bodies, because all tissues are dependent upon the ETC process, and mitochondria are in all of our cells. In their article on "mitochondrial psychiatry," Gardner and Boles explained that the tissues most commonly affected by mitochondrial dysfunction are in the brain, ears, eyes, muscle, heart, nerves, endocrine system, gastrointestinal system, skin, and autonomic nervous system.[31] In other words, almost everywhere. Given the high-energy demands of the brain and the susceptibility of mtDNA to oxidative stress and mutation, it is not surprising that investigators have proposed mitochondrial dysfunction as a "new" causal pathway to consider in some mental disorders.

Estimates vary, but it is generally thought that our brains account for only ~2% of our body in terms of cellular mass, but they consume at least 20% of the energy our mitochondria generate.[32] As the biggest energy consumer in our body, the brain makes huge demands on mitochondrial function. The primary energy demand is for excitatory neurotransmission in the cortex, most of which is mediated by the amino acid glutamate, the most common excitatory neurotransmitter in the human brain.

Overall then, when our mitochondria work well, they provide the energy our cells use to generate glutathione and other antioxidants to minimize the oxidative damage that would otherwise harm our brains. Some believe that when they do not work well, psychiatric symptoms may emerge.

SOME MENTAL DISORDERS MAY BE MITOCHONDRIAL DISORDERS

Gardner and Boles proposed a mitochondrial psychiatry model based on defective mitochondrial energy metabolism as a predisposing factor in the development of psychiatric disorders.[31] Two years later the title of a provocative editorial asked, "Is bipolar disorder a mitochondrial disease?"[33] And now, for the last 5 years, the evidence of mitochondrial dysfunction in association with mental disorders has been increasing.[28]

For example, in a sample of Italian adults with well-characterized mitochondrial disease, the prevalence of psychiatric symptoms was found to be very high (~60%) relative to population rates (20%–25%).[34] A neurological comparison group was examined in a report from Hungary, which evaluated mental disorders in a group of patients whose mitochondrial mutations had been identified; they were then compared to people with hereditary sensorimotor neuropathy.[35] The groups were well-matched in terms of sociodemographic variables and overall level of disability, and also on the somatization subscale of the Symptom Check List-90-Revised. What this group found was that the patients with identified mitochondrial disorders had significantly more depression and anxiety, based on structured interviews. Of the mitochondrial patients, 47% met criteria for lifetime prevalence of psychiatric disorders, compared to 30% of the neuropathy group. The results from these two studies suggest that psychiatric symptoms may be a direct manifestation of mitochondrial dysfunction, and not just a secondary development associated with the distress of illness.

The field of psychiatry has acknowledged the presence of somatic symptoms in mental disorders for decades, but the coexistence of physical and mental problems has rarely been interpreted as a clue regarding etiology. How many clinical psychologists and psychiatrists have been confronted with unanswerable questions from patients such as, "Why do my legs hurt when I am sad?" It is perhaps of great relevance, then, that higher ATP production in 21 patients with chronic depression and somatic symptoms was correlated with lower severity of their somatic complaints.[36] In other words, severity of somatic complaints may be a marker of low ATP production and perhaps also the severity of mental symptoms.

Describing the role of various nutrients in optimizing mitochondrial function is difficult, because some have direct functions (e.g., both niacin and riboflavin are structural components of cofactors that are critical for ATP production) and others have an indirect impact (e.g., heme deficiency causes mitochondrial decay and oxidative stress, and the production of this form of iron is dependent on several nutrients such as vitamin B6, copper, and zinc). When all the steps of cellular metabolism and energy production are combined for consideration, it appears as if virtually all the known minerals, vitamins, amino acids, and essential fatty acids are involved. For that reason, it is logical to consider the topic of using multiple nutrients to optimize mitochondrial function.

SCIENTIFIC BASIS OF TREATING MENTAL ILLNESS NUTRITIONALLY

DATA FROM NUTRITIONAL EPIDEMIOLOGY

Large population cohorts have been studied in several countries, particularly Spain, Australia, Japan, and the United Kingdom. Typically, groups who eat lots of fruits and vegetables, whole foods, and very few fast foods (whole food or Mediterranean diets) are compared with groups eating more typical Western diets that are high in processed foods. The studies have consistently shown that a dietary pattern of fast food, or processed food, with low intake of fruits and vegetables, is associated with increased rates of anxiety and depression.

In Spain, the SUN (Seguimiento University of Navarra) cohort was established in 2000 to study the effect of diet on a host of physical diseases. The almost 20,000 participants, most of whom are graduates of the University of Navarra, are asked to complete a variety of questionnaires every 2 years. Various diet-health relationships have been reported over the years, particularly showing an association between a Mediterranean diet and better control of diabetes, cardiovascular health, and glaucoma. With respect to mental health, amounts of fast food and commercial baked goods consumed have been shown to be correlated with the chances of being diagnosed with depression.[37] A subgroup of 9000 participants were asked to report on how much fast food (defined as sausages, hamburgers, and pizza) and how many processed pastries (defined as doughnuts, store-bought muffins, and croissants) they ate. During the 6 years they were followed up, 493 cases of newly diagnosed depression were reported. The researchers compared those consuming the least amount of processed foods with those consuming the most and found that those in the higher consumption groups had a 36%–38% greater risk of becoming depressed.

Research conducted in Australia established a positive correlation between the amount of processed food eaten and women's mood and anxiety symptoms.[38] Consequently, researchers explored whether poor dietary patterns preceded mental health issues in children. They assessed approximately 3000 children (11–18 years of age) over a 2-year period.[39] Mental health was measured with the Pediatric Quality of Life Inventory, and dietary patterns were evaluated with a food frequency questionnaire. The study established that changes in the quality of their diet predicted changes in mental health in the expected direction. This finding is of particular importance because it involved teenagers, a time of life when their parents are losing influence over their dietary intake. Adolescents are at high risk for developing mood disorders when consumption of carry-out and junk food is common. Dietary interventions could be especially important at this vulnerable stage of development.

A study was conducted with 97 adults diagnosed with mood disorders.[40] They were asked to keep detailed food records of what they consumed (weighed and measured) for 3 days, and these records were then evaluated for actual mineral and vitamin content. Seven minerals and seven vitamins were targeted, and 13 out of 14 of these nutrients were significantly correlated with mental health (sodium was the exception). This appears to be the first study in which actual nutrient intake (as opposed to dietary pattern) was shown to be related to quality of mental health in a dynamic way, over a short time period. The results strongly supported the importance of a healthy diet, especially among those diagnosed with a mental illness. All of these studies certainly suggest that adequate nutrient intake is relevant to the prevention of mental illness.

DATA FROM TREATMENT RESEARCH IN NONCLINICAL SAMPLES

Many randomized controlled trials (RCTs) have been conducted to look at the impact of micronutrients on anxiety and mood symptoms in nonclinical samples, with mixed results. For example, Schlebusch and colleagues found that adults randomized to consume a broad-spectrum micronutrient formula improved on all measures of stress during a 30-day RCT, compared with participants randomized to receive a placebo.[41] In a 16-week RCT of 114 adults, those randomized to receive a multivitamin (Swisse Men's Ultivite™ or Swisse Women's Ultivite™) reported significantly better energy levels and mood than those randomized to placebo.[42] Other research has replicated these findings, showing that healthy volunteers who received a complex nutrient formula (e.g., Berocca™, Blackmores™ Executive B Active, or Centrum™ Advanced 50+) reported greater improvement in mood, anxiety, or perceived stress as compared to placebo control groups,[43–45] although not all trials have documented benefit in nonclinical samples on ratings of mood.[46–49] Within elderly populations known for comorbid physical health problems, some trials show additional benefit of nutrients on psychological symptoms, although not all.[50] For example, in an RCT with 73 nursing home residents, micronutrients (Recip AB™) were found to assist with mood in those residents with low levels of selenium.[51] In an RCT of a complex micronutrient formula in 225 hospitalized elderly patients suffering from a variety of acute illnesses, those receiving the micronutrients showed greater change in measures of depression as compared with those receiving placebo, even if they had not been clinically depressed.[52] There was evidence of improved mood in everyone receiving the micronutrients, from those with severe or mild depression to those not previously reporting low mood.

Long and Benton conducted a meta-analysis of all RCTs examining mood in healthy adults and showed no overall effect of nutrients on general mood, although they did note small but significant effects of the nutrients on perceived stress, anxiety, mental fatigue, fog, and hostile mood.[45] Nevertheless, the meta-analysis also showed that micronutrient formulations with higher doses of B vitamins had more effect on mood ratings, especially when the doses were well above RDA levels. These findings challenge our overreliance on RDA levels to direct the use of vitamins for the regulation of psychological symptoms. Although these studies show a modest effect of micronutrient supplementation in a nonclinical sample, it is important that they be interpreted within the context in which they were conducted. These studies have a limited opportunity to show large effects on psychological variables given that most people begin the studies already falling in the normal, nonclinical range of functioning. It is important that these results not be extrapolated to clinical populations; one cannot assume that the effects would be equally modest.

Nevertheless, there is compelling reason to consider the public health implications of supplementation with broad-spectrum formulas that include both minerals and vitamins based on research conducted during and after a natural disaster. One case-control study showed that people who happened to be taking nutrients (EMPowerplus™) at the time of a large earthquake recovered more quickly from the associated stress as compared with people who happened to not be taking nutrients at the time of an earthquake.[53] Those taking the nutrients also exhibited large changes in measures of depressed mood. An RCT conducted after a 6.3 earthquake using different doses of micronutrients demonstrated that supplementation improved resistance to stress and reduced rates of post-traumatic stress symptoms, changes that were maintained one year later.[54,55] The message is clear: providing adequate levels of micronutrients following an environmental catastrophe is an effective way to improve the mental health of a population. Micronutrients support the energy output of mitochondria and also provide protection from oxidative stress in the form of antioxidants. Therefore it is plausible that the micronutrients help people cope with the harmful effects of stressors, indicating the value to public health of having a well-nourished populace. A very inexpensive public health initiative would be to incorporate micronutrient supplements into every disaster relief effort.

DATA FROM TREATMENT RESEARCH IN CLINICAL SAMPLES

Over the last decade, there has been a slow increase in the number of publications on multi-ingredient micronutrient formulas for the treatment of mental illness across the life span with far more positive effects being observed than in nonclinical samples. With the exception of a few studies conducted with inappropriately high megadoses of vitamins in the 1970s and 1980s,[56,57] all the studies using broad-spectrum micronutrient supplementation have been conducted within the last 20 years. The clinical trials conducted on depression were recently reviewed extensively by Popper.[58]

Antisocial Behaviors and Other Associated Behavioral Disturbances

The idea that nutrients can affect problem behaviors may date back to World War II when most children were supplemented with orange juice and cod-liver oil to reduce antisocial behavior.[59] In the 1980s, Schoenthaler and colleagues started publishing research trials investigating the role that sugar and other refined foods lacking micronutrients played in the expression of antisocial behaviors in children and adolescents.[60,61]

In 1997, these researchers published the results of an RCT with 62 incarcerated juveniles.[62] They found that giving these children a broad array of minerals such as magnesium, calcium, and zinc alongside vitamins such as riboflavin, thiamine, and folate in doses at least equivalent to, if not higher than, the RDA resulted in a 28% greater decrease in rule violations compared with those children receiving the placebo. Another RCT conducted by these same researchers showed that giving delinquent children (aged 6–12 years of age) a broad spectrum of nutrients yielded even better results.[63] The 40 children in the experimental group who were randomized to a broad spectrum of nutrients (most provided at about 50% RDA) exhibited 47% fewer antisocial behaviors requiring discipline than the 40 children randomized to receive a placebo. Other studies have been conducted with adult incarcerated populations with similar effects on violent behaviors within prisons.[58,64]

These studies compel us to appreciate that a simple intervention involving nutritional supplements could have wide-reaching effects on our communities at large, whereas conventional behavioral programs with young offenders have generally had very modest success. It is disheartening that this research has been around for over a decade and has not influenced how we address aggressive and violent behavior in children and adults. Further, although not directly targeted, the results may also have implications for management of mood disorders, given that antisocial behaviors can often be driven by an inability to regulate emotions.

There have been a number of trials using a micronutrient formula called EMPowerplus for the treatment of various symptoms in children and adults with complex behavioral and neurodevelopmental disorders that again, may have implications for management of mood disorders. This formula consists of 14 vitamins, 16 minerals, 3 antioxidants, and 3 amino acids in doses higher than the RDA but not approaching toxic levels. For example, in 2004, Kaplan and colleagues conducted an open-label trial with children with a variety of psychiatric disorders, including bipolar disorder, anxiety, oppositional behaviors, ADHD, and Asperger's disorder.[65] After 16 weeks of taking EMPowerplus, parent ratings on standardized tests such as the Child Behavior Checklist revealed significant improvements in delinquency, anxiety, aggression, attention, and mood. Few adverse effects were reported, and those that did occur were mild for all except two who were concurrently taking psychiatric medications. Indeed, Popper has warned against taking such supplements concurrently with medications due to the hypothesized potentiating effect these combination formulas can have on the medication, and he has cautioned about the need to lower the dose of medications very carefully.[58,66]

Depression and Bipolar Disorder

There is a long history of using single nutrients for the treatment of mood disorders, reviewed by Kaplan et al.[5] and Popper.[58] Research on multinutrient treatments is in its infancy, especially in clinical samples. There are almost 20 studies of broad-spectrum micronutrient treatments conducted on individuals with mood disorders; however, only two of these have been blinded RCTs. The rest have been open-label, database analyses and case studies.

In all five published reports of open-label trials of EMPowerplus for the treatment of children and adults with bipolar disorder or bipolar symptoms, the effects of this formula have been positive, sometimes within a few days of commencing treatment. All five trials showed significant change sustained over at least a 6-month period, with about 70%–80% of participants showing much or very much improved bipolar symptoms and a reduction in the amount of medications required to maintain symptom control.[67] In a database analysis of a large sample of 358 adults with bipolar disorder, more than half were identified as positive responders (defined as >50% decrease in symptom severity) after 3 months of consuming the micronutrients.[68] Importantly, their symptom improvement was sustained at 6 months, making it unlikely that placebo or expectancy effects accounted for the reported changes. These findings were replicated in a similar database analysis of 120 children and adolescents with bipolar disorder with parent-reported mood symptoms decreasing by 46% with a simultaneous decrease in the number of patients using medications from 79% to 38%.[69] Both of these database analyses showed a large effect size from baseline to end of 6 months (ES 0.8). Case studies have been consistent with group data, showing on-off control of symptoms depending on the presence or absence of the nutrient formula, and long-term maintenance of benefit.[70,71] Part of the value of the case studies is that they provided empirical evidence of symptom remission that was sustained for at least 4 years and could be compared to a clinically documented history of 6 years of extensive conventional treatment. [70,72,73]

The two RCTs conducted on people with a mood disorder have both been positive, albeit one was a post hoc analysis of a subsample with mood disorders. A trial of 60 adults with depressive disorder showed greater reductions on the Beck Depression Inventory for those who were randomized to receive a B-Complex formula (Max Stress B™) compared with those receiving a placebo.[74]

The other RCT was conducted by Rucklidge and colleagues who studied 80 adults diagnosed with ADHD, half of whom were given EMPowerplus, and the other half, a placebo.[75] Those who received the micronutrient treatment reported greater change in attention, hyperactivity, and impulsivity than those who received the placebo. Of note, better functioning and greater improvement in overall psychiatric symptoms in the micronutrient group compared with the placebo group was also observed by clinicians, who saw participants only once a fortnight. Importantly, participants (about one fifth of the sample) who were also struggling with depression (identified as being in the moderate to severe range of depression) showed greater benefit from the nutrients compared to placebo (ES 0.64), an effect comparable to antidepressant effects.[58] It is especially noteworthy that the significant effects of the micronutrients on mood were maintained one year later for those who stayed on the micronutrients.[76] Replication of these results in participants specifically recruited for mood disorders is now warranted.

The improvements in depression, anxiety, and mood regulation that are described above have also been noted in samples of people with other diagnoses. Adams and his colleagues used a formulation of micronutrients (Syndion™) and found positive results compared with placebo in reducing tantrums and hyperactivity as well as improving receptive language and overall functioning in children with autism spectrum disorder (ASD).[77] In another illustration of such results, a psychiatrist in private practice followed 44 children in his clinic diagnosed with ASD whose parents agreed to treat them with EMPowerplus. He matched these 44 children to another 44 children from his clinic whose parents elected to follow a more conventional course of treatment involving psychiatric medication. His research showed that not only was this micronutrient formula superior in reducing symptoms such as irritability and mood dysregulation as compared with medication, it also reduced self-injurious behaviors, changes that did not occur in the medication group.[78]

The consistency of findings across universities and countries suggests that broad-spectrum micronutrient treatments are worthy of further study using more rigorous designs. Unlike the medications typically prescribed to people with bipolar disorder—antipsychotics and mood stabilizers—whose adverse effects are well documented, micronutrient supplements *at worst* will confer general health benefits with no benefit for mental health and with no adverse effects.[79] The research thus far certainly suggests that trial supplementation with people diagnosed with bipolar disorder may be helpful and is certainly unlikely to do any harm.

CONCLUSION

Several key messages are presented in this chapter. There are at least 50 essential nutrients that function as cofactors for our very metabolically demanding brains. Until about 20 years ago, researchers looked for magic bullets to treat brain dysfunction, but the single cause fallacy neglects the fact that we have evolved to need a broad spectrum of minerals, vitamins, amino acids, and essential fatty acids consumed in balance.

Nutrient treatment was discussed as "logical" because of the known role of nutrients in brain metabolism, and also their role in combatting inflammatory activity often triggered by gut dysbiosis. Also, the review explained why optimizing nutrient availability for mitochondrial function is a pathway relevant for brain (mental) health.

Finally, research was reviewed that showed that nutrients are a viable treatment for mood and anxiety symptoms, regardless of the complexity of diagnoses in the patients being treated. There are excellent clinical trials showing that broad-spectrum micronutrient treatment ameliorates antisocial behavior, depression, anxiety, mood dysregulation, and so on. And these results have emanated from multiple countries and laboratories, based on both child and adult research, and using multiple formulas. Of perhaps most importance is the fact that broad-spectrum micronutrient treatments appear to be quite safe, causing no significant adverse events.

Much more research is needed in this area, because many questions remain about the use of multiple nutrients for both prevention and treatment of mental disorders. In the area of prevention, there is only one solid RCT showing that a particular nutrient (omega 3 fatty acids) can prevent episodes of psychosis in adolescents at high risk.[80] But what about dietary interventions? Could a change in dietary patterns (e.g., moving toward a Mediterranean diet) in a targeted group of high-risk young-sters prevent onset of symptoms? Similarly, could broad-spectrum micronutrients? Would combin-ing micronutrients with probiotics improve efficacy?

In the area of treatment, many more RCTs are needed to determine whether broad-spectrum micronutrient formulas are superior to placebo in people with major depressive disorder, bipolar disorder, and various anxiety syndromes. Similar to the questions above, studies should be mounted to determine whether comparable improvements could be achieved with changed dietary patterns, and whether adding probiotics might improve efficacy.

Further into the future, there should be studies to determine whether it is possible to use genetic methodologies to determine who might have inherited a need for unusually large amounts of nutrients (and which ones) so that they can be supplemented from an early age to optimize brain function.

REFERENCES

1. Ames, B.N., Elson-Schwab, I., and Silver, E.A. 2002. High-dose vitamin therapy stimulates variant enzymes with decreased coenzyme binding affinity (increased Km): Relevance to genetic disease and polymorphisms. *Am J Clin Nutr* 75(4): 616–658.
2. Institute of Medicine. 2000. *Dietary Reference Intakes: Applications in Dietary Assessment.* Washington, DC: National Academies Press.
3. Diplock, A.T., Charleux, J.L., Crozier-Willi, G. et al. 1998. Functional food science and defence against reactive oxidative species. *Br J Nutr* 80(Suppl 1): S77–S112.
4. Hoffer, A. and Saul, A.W. 2008. *Orthomolecular Medicine for Everyone: Megavitamin Therapeutics for Families and Physicians.* Laguna Beach, CA: Basic Health.
5. Kaplan, B.J., Crawford S.G., Field, C.J. et al. 2007. Vitamins, minerals, and mood. *Psychol Bull* 133(5): 747–760.
6. McGrath, J. 2010. Is it time to trial vitamin D supplements for the prevention of schizophrenia? *Acta Psychiatrica Scand* 121: 321–324.
7. Young, S.N. 2009. Has the time come for clinical trials on the antidepressant effect of vitamin D? *J Psychiatry Neurosci* 34: 3.
8. Mertz, W. 1994. A balanced approach to nutrition for health: The need for biologically essential miner-als and vitamins. *J Am Dietetic Assoc* 94: 1259–1262.
9. Blount, Z.D., Borland, C.Z., and Lenski, R.E. 2008. Historical contingency and the evolution of a key innovation in an experimental population of *Escherichia coli. Proc Natl Acad Sci USA* 105(23): 7899–7906.
10. Berk, M., Williams, L.J., Jacka, F.N. et al. 2013. So depression is an inflammatory disease, but where does the inflammation come from? *BMC Med* 11(1): 200.
11. Dowlati, Y., Herrmann, N., Swardfager, W. et al. 2010. A meta-analysis of cytokines in major depres-sion. *Biol Psychiatry* 67(5): 446–457.
12. Gu, P., DeFina, L.F., Leonard, D. et al. 2012. Relationship between serum homocysteine levels and depressive symptoms: The Cooper Center Longitudinal Study. *J Clin Psychiatry* 73(5): 691–695.
13. Reber, S.O. 2012. Stress and animal models of inflammatory bowel disease—An update on the role of the hypothalamo-pituitary-adrenal axis. *Psychoneuroendocrinology* 37 (1): 1–19.
14. Hamdani, N., Tamouza, R., and Leboyer, M. 2012. Immuno-inflammatory markers of bipolar disorder: A review of evidence. *Front Biosci* 4: 2170–2182.
15. Sommer, I.E., de Witte, L., Begemann, M. et al. 2012. Nonsteroidal anti-inflammatory drugs in schizo-phrenia: Ready for practice or a good start? A meta-analysis. *J Clin Psychiatry* 73(4): 414–419.
16. Carpenter, S. 2012. That gut feeling: Exploring the mind-belly-bacteria connection. *Monitor Psychol* 43(8): 51–55.
17. Bailey, M.T., Dowd, S.E., Galley, J.D. et al. 2011. Exposure to a social stressor alters the structure of the intestinal microbiota: Implications for stressor-induced immunomodulation. *Brain Behav Immun* 25(3): 397–407.
18. Round, J.L. and Mazmanian, S.K. 2009. The gut microbiota shapes intestinal immune responses during health and disease. *Nature Rev Immunol* 9(5): 313–323.
19. Rook, G.A.W., Raison, C.L., and Lowry, C.A. 2012. Can we vaccinate against depression? *Drug Discov Today* 17(9): 451–458.

20. Hawrelak, J.A. and Myers, S.P. 2004. The causes of intestinal dysbiosis: A review. *Altern Med Rev* 9(2): 180–197.
21. Bailey, M.T., Lubach, G.R., and Coe, C.L. 2004. Prenatal stress alters bacterial colonization of the gut in infant monkeys. *J Pediatr Gastroenterol Nutr* 38(4): 414–421.
22. Bailey, M.T. and Coe, C.L. 1999. Maternal separation disrupts the integrity of the intestinal microflora in infant rhesus monkeys. *Dev Psychobiol* 35(2): 146–155.
23. O'Mahony, S.M., Marchesi, J.R., Scully, P. et al. 2009. Early life stress alters behavior, immunity, and microbiota in rats: Implications for irritable bowel syndrome and psychiatric illnesses. *Biol Psychiatry* 65(3): 263–267.
24. Knowles, S.R., Nelson, E.A., and Palombo, E.A. 2008. Investigating the role of perceived stress on bacterial flora activity and salivary cortisol secretion: A possible mechanism underlying susceptibility to illness. *Biol Psychol* 77(2): 132–137.
25. Messaoudi, M., Lalonde, R., Violle, N. et al. 2010. Assessment of psychotropic-like properties of a probiotic formulation (*Lactobacillus helveticus* R0052 and *Bifidobacterium longum* R0175) in rats and human subjects. *Br J Nutr* 105(5): 755–764.
26. Rao, A.V., Bested, A.C., Beaulne, T.M. et al. 2009. A randomized, double-blind, placebo-controlled pilot study of a probiotic in emotional symptoms of chronic fatigue syndrome. *Gut Pathogens* 1(1): 6.
27. Miller, G.E. and Cole, G.W. 2012. Clustering of depression and inflammation in adolescents previously exposed to childhood adversity. *Biol Psychiatry* 72(1): 34–40.
28. Kaplan, B., Rucklidge, J.J., McLeod, K. et al. 2015. The emerging field of nutritional mental health: Inflammation, the microbiome, oxidative stress, and mitochondrial function. *Clin Psychol Sci* 1–17.
29. Karp, G. 2012. *Cell and Molecular Biology: Concepts and Experiments*. New York, NY: Wiley.
30. Luft, R. 1994. The development of mitochondrial medicine. *Proc Natl Acad Sci USA* 91(19): 8731–8738.
31. Gardner, A. and Boles, R.G. 2005. Is a "Mitochondrial Psychiatry" in the future? A review. *Curr Psychiatry Rev* 1: 255–271.
32. Belanger, M., Allaman, I., and Magistretti, P.J. 2011. Brain energy metabolism: Focus on astrocyte-neuron metabolic cooperation. *Cell Metab* 14(6): 724–738.
33. Young, L.T. 2007. Is bipolar disorder a mitochondrial disease? *J Psychiatry Neurosci* 32(3): 160–161.
34. Mancuso, M., Orsucci, D., Ienco, E.C. et al. 2011. Psychiatric involvement in adult patients with mitochondrial disease. *Neurol Sci* 34(1): 71–74.
35. Inczedy-Farkas, G., Remenyi, V., Gal, A. et al. 2012. Psychiatric symptoms of patients with primary mitochondrial DNA disorders. *Behav Brain Funct* 8: 9081–9089.
36. Gardner, A. and Boles, R.G. 2008. Mitochondrial energy depletion in depression with somatization. *Psychother Psychosom* 77(2): 127–129.
37. Sánchez-Villegas, A., Toledo, A., Irala, J. et al. 2012. Fast-food and commercial baked goods consumption and the risk of depression. *Public Health Nutr* 15(03): 424–432.
38. Jacka, F.N., Pasco, J.N., Mykletun, A. et al. 2010. Association of Western and traditional diets with depression and anxiety in women. *Am J Psychiatry* 167: 305–311.
39. Jacka, F.N., Kremer, P.J., Leslie, E.R. et al. 2010. Associations between diet quality and depressed mood in adolescents: Results from the Australian healthy neighbourhoods study. *ANZ J Psychiatry* 44(5): 435–442.
40. Davison, K.M. and Kaplan, B.J. 2012. Nutrient intakes are correlated with overall psychiatric functioning in adults with mood disorders. *Canadian J Psychiatry* 57(2): 85–92.
41. Schlebusch, L., Bosch, B.A., Polglase, G. et al. 2000. A double-blind, placebo-controlled, double-centre study of the effects of an oral multivitamin-mineral combination on stress. *S Afr Med J* 90: 1216–1223.
42. Sarris, J., Cox, K.H., Camfield, D.A. et al. 2012. Participant experiences from chronic administration of a multivitamin versus placebo on subjective health and wellbeing: A double-blind qualitative analysis of a randomised controlled trial. *Nutr J* 11 (1): 110.
43. Kennedy, D.O., Veasey, R., Watson, A. et al. 2010. Effects of high-dose B vitamin complex with vitamin C and minerals on subjective mood and performance in healthy males. *Psychopharmacology* 211: 55–68.
44. Stough, C., Scholey, A., Lloyd, J. et al. 2011. The effect of 90 day administration of a high dose vitamin B-complex on work stress. *Human Psychopharmacol* 26(7): 470–476.
45. Long, S.J. and Benton, D. 2013. Effects of vitamin and mineral supplementation on stress, mild psychiatric symptoms, and mood in nonclinical samples: A meta-analysis. *Psychosom Med* 75(2): 144–153.
46. Cockle, S.M., Haller, J., Kimber, S. et al. 2000. The influence of multivitamins on cognitive function and mood in the elderly. *Aging Ment Health* 4(4): 339–353.

47. Haskell, C.F., Scholey, A., Jackson, A. et al. 2008. Cognitive and mood effects in healthy children during 12 weeks' supplementation with multi-vitamin/minerals. *Br J Nutr* 100(5): 1086–1096.
48. Neri, M., Andermarcher, E., Pradelli, J.M. et al. 1995. Influence of a double blind pharmacological trial on two domains of well-being in subjects with age associated memory impairment. *Arch Gerontol Geriatr* 21(3): 241–252.
49. Pipingas, A., Camfield, D.A., Stough, C. et al. 2013. The effects of multivitamin supplementation on mood and general well-being in healthy young adults. A laboratory and at-home mobile phone assessment. *Appetite* 69: 123–136.
50. Manders, M., De Groot, L.C., Hoefnagels, W.H. et al. 2009. The effect of a nutrient dense drink on mental and physical function in institutionalized elderly people. *J Nutr Health Aging* 13(9): 760–767.
51. Gosney, M.A., Hammond, M.F., Shenkin, A. et al. 2008. Effect of micronutrient supplementation on mood in nursing home residents. *Gerontology* 54(5): 292–299.
52. Gariballa, S. and Forster, S. 2007. Effects of dietary supplements on depressive symptoms in older patients: A randomised double-blind placebo-controlled trial. *Clin Nutr* 26(5): 545–551.
53. Rucklidge, J.J., Johnstone, J., Harrison, R. et al. 2011. Micronutrients reduce stress and anxiety following a 7.1 earthquake in adults with attention-deficit/hyperactivity disorder. *Psychiatry Res* 189: 281–287.
54. Rucklidge, J.J., Andridge, R., Gorman, B. et al. 2012. Shaken but unstirred? Effects of micronutrients on stress and trauma after an earthquake: RCT evidence comparing formulas and doses. *Human Psychopharmacol Clin Experimental* 27(5): 440–454.
55. Rucklidge, J.J., Blampied, N., Gorman, B. et al. 2014. Psychological functioning one year after a brief intervention using micronutrients to treat stress and anxiety related to the 2011 Christchurch earthquakes: A naturalistic follow-up. *Human Psychopharmacol Clin Exp* 29(3): 230–243.
56. Arnold, L.E., Christopher, J., Huestis, R.D. et al. 1978. Megavitamins for minimal brain dysfunction: A placebo-controlled study. *JAMA* 240(24): 2642–2643.
57. Haslam, R.H.A., Dalby, J.T., and Rademaker, A.W. 1984. Effects of megavitamin therapy on children with attention deficit disorders. *Pediatrics* 74(1): 103–111.
58. Popper, C.W. 2014. Single-micronutrient and broad-spectrum micronutrient approaches for treating mood disorders in youth and adults. *Child Adolesc Psychiatr Clin N Am* 23(3): 591–672.
59. Gesch, B., Hammond, S., Hampson, S. et al. 2002. Influence of supplementary vitamins, minerals and essential fatty acids on the antisocial behaviour of young adult prisoners. *Br J Psychiatry* 181: 22–28.
60. Schoenthaler, S. J. 1982. The effect of sugar on the treatment and control of antisocial behavior: A double-blind study of an incarcerated juvenile population. *Int J Biosoc Res* 3(1): 1–9.
61. Schoenthaler, S.J. 1983. Diet and crime: An empirical examination of the value of nutrition in the control and treatment of incarcerated juvenile offenders. *Int J Biosoc Res* 4(1): 25–39.
62. Schoenthaler, S.J., Amos, S.P., Doraz, W.E. et al. 1997. The effect of randomized vitamin-mineral supplementation on violent and non-violent antisocial behavior among incarcerated juveniles. *J Nutr Env Med* 7: 343–352.
63. Schoenthaler, S.J. and Bier, I.D. 2000. The effect of vitamin-mineral supplementation on juvenile delinquency among American schoolchildren: A randomized, double-blind placebo-controlled trial. *J Altern Complement Med* 6(1): 7–17.
64. Zaalberg, A., Nijman, H., Bulten, E. et al. 2010. Effects of nutritional supplements on aggression, rule-breaking, and psychopathology among young adult prisoners. *Aggress Behav* 36(2): 117–126.
65. Kaplan, B.J., Fisher, J.E., Crawford, S.G. et al. 2004. Improved mood and behavior during treatment with a mineral-vitamin supplement: An open-label case series of children. *J Child Adolesc Psychopharmacol* 14(1): 115–122.
66. Popper, C.W. 2001. Do vitamins or minerals (apart from lithium) have mood-stabilising effects? *J Clin Psychiatry* 62(12): 933–935.
67. Rucklidge, J.J. and Kaplan, B.J. 2013. Broad-spectrum micronutrient formulas for the treatment of psychiatric symptoms: A systematic review. *Expert Rev Neurother* 13(1): 49–73.
68. Gately, D. and Kaplan, B.J. 2009. Database analysis of adults with bipolar disorder consuming a multinutrient formula. *Clin Med Psychiatry* 4: 3–16.
69. Rucklidge, J.J., Gately, D., and Kaplan, B.J. 2010. Database analysis of children and adolescents with bipolar disorder consuming a multinutrient formula. *BMC Psychiatry* 10: 74. doi:10.1186/1471-244X-10-74.
70. Kaplan, B.J., Crawford, S.G., Gardner, B. et al. 2002. Treatment of mood lability and explosive rage with minerals and vitamins: Two case studies in children. *J Child Adolesc Psychopharmacol* 12(3): 205–219.
71. Rucklidge, J.J. and Harrison, R. 2010. Successful treatment of Bipolar Disorder II and ADHD with a micronutrient formula: A case study. *CNS Spectrums* 15(5): 289–295.

72. Rodway, M., Vance, A., Watters, A. et al. 2012. Efficacy and cost of micronutrient treatment of childhood psychosis. *BMJ Case Rep* 2012.

73. Frazier, E., Fristad, M.A., and Arnold, L.E. 2009. Multinutrient supplement as treatment: Literature review and case report of a 12-year-old boy with bipolar disorder. *J Child Adolesc Psychopharmacol* 19(4): 453–460.

74. Lewis, J.E., Tiozzo, E., Melillo, A.B. et al. 2013. The effect of methylated vitamin B complex on depressive and anxiety symptoms and quality of life in adults with depression. *ISRN Psychiatry* 2013: 621453.

75. Rucklidge, J.J., Frampton, C.M., Gorman, B. et al. 2014a. Vitamin-mineral treatment of ADHD in adults: A double-blind, randomized, placebo controlled trial. *Br J Psychiatry* 204: 306–315.

76. Rucklidge, J.J., Frampton, C.M., Gorman, B. et al. 2014b. Vitamin-mineral treatment of ADHD in adults: A 1-year naturalistic follow-up of a randomized controlled trial. *J Atten Disord.* [Epub ahead of print].

77. Adams, J.B., Audhya, T., McDonough-Means, S. et al. 2011. Effect of a vitamin/mineral supplement on children and adults with autism. *BMC Pediatr* 11: 111.

78. Mehl-Madrona, L., Leung, B., Kennedy, C. et al. 2010. A naturalistic case-control study of micronutrients versus standard medication management in autism. *J Child Adolesc Psychopharmacol* 20(2): 95–103.

79. Simpson, J.S.A., Crawford, S.G., Goldstein, E.T. et al. 2011. Systematic review of safety and tolerability of a complex micronutrient formula used in mental health. *BMC Psychiatry* 11(62). [online].

80. Amminger, G.P., Schäfer, M.R., Papageorgiou, K. et al. 2010. Long-chain omega-3 fatty acids for indicated prevention of psychotic disorders: A randomized, placebo-controlled trial. *Arch Gen Psychiatry* 67(2): 146–154.

19 Amino Acids and Other Nutrients That Enhance the Synthesis and Regulation of Neurotransmitters

Richard M. Carlton, MD

CONTENTS

INTRODUCTION

Supplementation of specific nutrients can be effective in supporting the treatment of a wide variety of psychiatric disorders, including depression, anxiety, and attention deficit-hyperactivity disorder (ADHD). Nutrients work in part by increasing the rate of synthesis of neurotransmitters that modulate mood and cognition. This increase results from saturation of enzymes with supratherapeutic dosages of the essential nutrients that serve either as the precursor molecule (amino acids) or as cofactors (e.g., vitamin B6, vitamin C, folate, SAMe, zinc, iron, and copper) required for those enzymes. Saturation with these essential nutrients can drive enzymatic production of far greater amounts of neurotransmitters than is possible with the physiologically low levels of nutrients found in many current dietary patterns. A common feature found in the diets from individuals suffering from mental illness is the lack of adequate essential vitamins, minerals, and amino acids. Studies show that daily supplementation of essential nutrients is often effective in reducing patients' symptoms, particularly supplements containing amino acids.[1] The literature suggests that amino acid supplementation may reduce symptoms by converting to neurotransmitters which subsequently ameliorate symptoms of depression.

This chapter summarizes the neuroscience that underlies the phenomena described above; provides documentation from clinical studies demonstrating efficacy; shows how to logically predict which nutrients may help a given disorder; and explains the inherent limitations, side effects, and contraindications of this approach.

BASIC PRINCIPLES

The late biochemist Roger Williams documented the existence of medical conditions where individuals require specific nutrients in dosages many times higher than minimum daily requirement (MDR) levels needed to prevent a deficiency state.[2] The individual's health is derailed if high levels of the specific nutrients are not obtained. In these cases a pharmacological, or supraphysiologic, dose is appropriate. Nevertheless, these individuals may often have blood levels of the nutrients in question that are considered within normal limits.

Antidepressants act in part by increasing the concentration of neurotransmitters in the synapse. Disorders of mood or cognition are often treated with prescription medications that work, in part, by achieving net increases in the amounts of a given neurotransmitter in the synaptic cleft. There are three primary medication categories for achieving such an effect. First some stimulant medications induce the release of neurotransmitter molecules stored within synaptic vesicles. Second, medications inhibiting monoamine oxidase enzymes can inhibit the enzymatic breakdown of certain neurotransmitters. Finally, a group of medications such as selective serotonin reuptake inhibitors (SSRIs) and selective norepinephrine reuptake inhibitors (SNRIs) function by inhibiting the reuptake of neurotransmitters once they are released within the synapse.

This process can be further augmented by nutritional supplementation of amino acids and minerals to further enhance neurotransmitter levels within the synapse. If one of the goals of treatment is to increase the net concentration of neurotransmitters in the synapse, we can take advantage of the capacity for nutrients to facilitate this process. Most of the neurotransmitters that control mood and cognition are synthesized through a process wherein an essential amino acid is converted to the neurotransmitter with the help of one or more enzymes. Vitamins and minerals are also required for the enzyme to become properly arrayed in the functional three-dimensional configuration necessary for activation. These nutrients are referred to as co-catalysts, co-enzymes, and/or cofactors.

The enzymes involved in neurotransmitter synthesis can be galvanized to producing higher-than-normal amounts of the neurotransmitter by being saturated with pharmacological dosages of these essential nutrients that serve as precursors and cofactors to neurotransmitter synthesis.[3,4]

Many double-blind clinical studies support nutrition supplementation. In one study, 19 learning-disabled schoolchildren showed significant academic and behavioral improvements within months from treatment with nutritional supplements.[5] Twelve children completed the full one-year double-blind phase, and those who remained on the nutrients showed continual upward improvement. The children who discontinued nutrient therapy experienced declines in their academic performance one year after discontinuing nutrient therapy. At the end of the fourth year, the rates of decline between the two groups were statistically significant ($P < .01$).

Unfortunately, a typical diet at best provides only the physiologic amounts of nutrients needed to prevent deficiency states (such as *scurvy* and *beri-beri*). However, dietary intake cannot provide the pharmacological dosages of nutrients needed to support increased production or to overcome inborn or epigenetic variants interfering with optimal physiology. As an analogy, for the typical water needs of a household, a garden hose will suffice. But if a fire is raging, a fire hose is needed to deliver the sheer volume of water required. In enzymology, this bolus of nutrients produces what is called the *mass effect*.

NUTRITION RESPONSIVE CONDITIONS

A patient does not have to have a vitamin "deficiency" to benefit from pharmacological dosages of nutrients. Because of biochemical individuality, a patient may fail to thrive (and even die) if pharmacological dosages of a particular nutrient are not given even though the patient shows no evidence (in terms of laboratory results or clinical symptoms) of a nutrient deficiency state. The seminal example of this phenomenon is a condition called pyridoxine-responsive neonatal seizures (West syndrome).[6] In the 1950s, a neonatologist named West was treating a neonate hospitalized for intractable generalized seizures, refractory to all anticonvulsants. At one point the little girl became febrile, stopped nursing, and went into status epilepticus. Intravenous (IV) fluids were initiated. Unexpectedly, the seizures stopped—completely. When the fever abated and she resumed nursing, the IV fluids were discontinued—at which point the seizures promptly recurred. West discovered that it was the vitamin B6 (pyridoxine) in the IV solution that was controlling the seizures. This child's baseline blood levels of pyridoxine were entirely within normal limits. In the decades following West's discovery, investigators determined the mechanisms of action whereby vitamin B6 controlled the seizures. Some neonates with intractable seizures have an inborn error of metabolism in which the enzyme glutamic acid decarboxylase (GAD) is profoundly inefficient. GAD converts the essential amino acid glutamine into the inhibitory neurotransmitter GABA.

When synaptic levels of GABA are abnormally low, abnormal bursts of firing go unquenched and are able to spread unopposed. It so happens that pyridoxine and magnesium are the cofactors for GAD, and that when this enzyme is highly inefficient, saturating it with pharmacological amounts of pyridoxine can galvanize it to producing at least enough GABA to stop the ictal activity from spreading. Other neonates with seizures responsive to vitamin B6 may have a deficiency of alpha-aminoadipic semialdehyde dehydrogenase (antiquitin), which is encoded by ALDH7A1. Here, too, pharmacologic dosages of B6 decrease the seizures. For neonatologists it is axiomatic that, in treating nutrient-responsive inborn errors of metabolism, therapy with the nutrient in question must *not* be withheld simply because blood levels of that nutrient are "within normal limits."

SPECIFIC NUTRIENTS THAT DRIVE ENZYMES THAT SYNTHESIZE MOOD-MODULATING NEUROTRANSMITTERS

SYNTHESIS OF THE MONOAMINE NEUROTRANSMITTERS AND GABA

Figure 19.1 shows that there are two different one-step processes required for the synthesis of phenylethylamine and of GABA; two steps needed for the synthesis of dopamine and serotonin; and three steps for the synthesis of norepinephrine. Recurring patterns are also apparent, such as the participation of hydroxylase enzymes that use vitamin C, iron, and tetrahydrobiopterin [BH4] as cofactors. The decarboxylase enzymes use vitamin B6 and magnesium as cofactors.

SYNTHESIS OF ACETYLCHOLINE

Figure 19.2 shows that choline (an essential nutrient) is converted into acetylcholine under the action of the enzyme choline acetyltransferase, for which acetyl-coenzyme A is the cofactor.

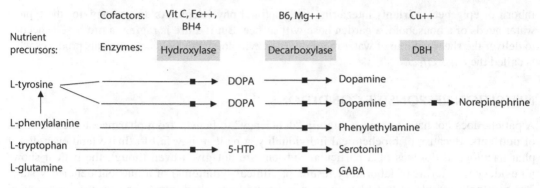

Key: DBH = Dopamine beta-hydroxylase; BH4 = Tetrahydrobiopterin

FIGURE 19.1 In order for the major neurotransmitters shown above to be synthesized, there is an absolute requirement for the participation of *essential* nutrients. For example, essential amino acids serve as the precursors, and vitamin and mineral cofactors (co-enzymes) are required to drive the respective enzymes of synthesis.

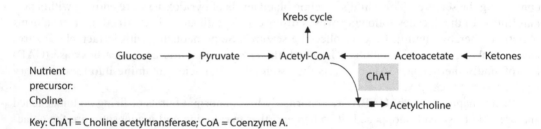

Key: ChAT = Choline acetyltransferase; CoA = Coenzyme A.

FIGURE 19.2 The essential nutrient choline is the precursor for the synthesis of acetylcholine (ACh). The co-factor for this synthetic pathway is acetyl-coenzyme A (ACoA), normally produced from metabolism of glucose. In diseases with poor entry of glucose due to defects in neuronal insulin receptor signaling such as Alzheimer's disease, the brain is a hybrid engine that can use ketone bodies as an alternative fuel: the ketones are metabolized to produce the ACoA needed to drive ACh synthesis and to generate ATP through the Krebs cycle.

NUTRIENTS, NUTRACEUTICALS, AND HERBS USEFUL "UPSTREAM" AND "DOWNSTREAM" FROM THE ENZYMES OF NEUROTRANSMITTERS

Hydroxylase enzymes are the first step in converting the precursor molecules (tyrosine and tryptophan) into their respective neurotransmitters (dopamine and norepinephrine, and serotonin, respectively). Those enzymes—tyrosine hydroxylase and tryptophan hydroxylase—are the rate-limiting enzymes in the synthetic pathways. They both utilize iron, ascorbic acid, and tetrahydrobiopterin (BH4) as cofactors. Saturating these hydroxylases with higher amounts of BH4 can increase their throughput, which is important because the body's ability to produce BH4 declines with age and with certain single nucleotide polymorphisms such as the MTHFR 1298 mutation. This decline in BH4 production can be corrected, and production of dopamine and serotonin increased, by administering S-adenosylmethionine (SAMe) and L-methylfolate.

S-Adenosylmethionine

SAMe is a naturally occurring high-energy intermediate formed in most of our cells when the sulfur-bearing amino acid methionine condenses with ATP in a reaction catalyzed by methionine adenosyltransferase (MAT). SAMe contributes two molecules of great importance in a wide range of metabolic functions: methyl groups (CH_3) and sulfate groups (SO_4).

The methyl groups contributed by SAMe are used in the production of neurotransmitters, DNA, proteins, and phospholipids. The sulfate groups that SAMe contributes are used in the production of a number of important molecules, including the potent neuroprotective molecule glutathione. There have been over 40 clinical trials published within the last two decades confirming the efficacy of SAMe in the treatment of depressive disorders.[7] In one meta-analysis involving the outcomes from 25 controlled trials and 791 patients, SAMe had a significantly greater response rate than placebo and was comparable to tricyclic antidepressants, including escitalopram.[8,9] In 18 controlled trials, SAMe was as effective as impramine, chlorimipramine, nomifensine, and minaprine; however, it is important to note that those receiving SAMe supplementation experienced fewer and milder side effects compared to those on medications.[10] SAMe's comparable efficacy to antidepressants without the undesirable side effects makes it a desirable alternative to standard antidepressant therapy.

In one placebo-controlled trial, SAMe concentrations in cerebrospinal fluid (CSF) were measured before and after treatment in patients with severe depression who scored 20 or more points on the Hamilton Rating Scale.[11] Thirty participants received either 200 mg daily of intravenous SAMe ($n = 16$) or placebo ($n = 14$) for 14 days. A significant increase in CSF SAMe concentrations was observed in patients receiving intravenous SAMe compared to the placebo.

A later study evaluated the effectiveness of SAMe compared to placebo in patients who had not responded to antidepressant treatment with SSRIs.[12] A total of 73 patients participated in this 6-week randomized controlled trial. Those taking SAMe had lower scores on the Hamilton depression scale (25% versus 36%) and higher remission rates (17.6% versus 11.7%) than those study participants taking placebo. These preliminary results suggest that SAMe is safe, effective, and well tolerated.

Published clinical studies also report that the average depressed patient will require dosages of SAMe in the range of 600 to 1200 mg per day, while some patients may need to go as high as 2000 mg per day to get a response. There are some limitations of treatment with SAMe, and patients have reported several possible side effects, which include gastrointestinal discomfort and agitation. Gastrointestinal discomfort is fairly common once the patient approaches the higher end of the therapeutic dosage range. SAMe supplementation is not recommended for patients with bipolar depression, as it has been reported to activate hypomania. It is recommended that patients take SAMe before or after meals so it does not compete with other amino acids for absorption. However, if SAMe causes gastrointestinal upset, it can be taken with a meal. SAMe should not be taken late in the day or before bedtime due to its tendency to be activating.

L-Methylfolate

Numerous studies show that blood levels of folate tend to be low in depressed patients, that supplements with folate produce clinically meaningful relief of the depression, and that folate supplements can augment the effects of conventional antidepressants in patients whose depression had been refractory.[13]

However, some patients suffer depression not only with normal blood levels of folate but even when taking supplemental folate. This poor response appears to result from a commonplace genetic defect that blocks the reduction of folate to its "activated" form, L-methylfolate (also referred to as 5-methyltetrahydrofolate, 5-MTHF). The enzyme in question is methylenetetrahydrofolate reductase (MTHFR). Once it became feasible to do genome-wide analyses on large swaths of the population, it became apparent that mutations in the MTHFR gene are among the most commonplace mutations in the human population—with approximately 12% of Caucasians and 22% of the Latino population having such mutations.[14] These high rates of mutation have serious repercussions, because mutations in the MTHFR gene slow down the enzymatic conversion of homocysteine to methionine. With less methionine available to generate SAMe, methylation steps needed "upstream" to synthesize serotonin, dopamine, and norepinephrine are impaired.

A clinical study in which patients with SSRI-resistant depression were treated with large dosages of L-methylfolate (15 mg per day) revealed statistically significant improvements in measures of mood (CGI-SI and HDRS-28). The authors concluded that biomarkers associated with inflammation or metabolism or genomic markers associated with L-methylfolate synthesis and metabolism may help identify patients with treatment-resistant depression who may benefit from adjunctive therapy with L-methylfolate 15 mg, although more confirmatory studies are warranted.[15]

The clinical trials with L-methylfolate and/or SAMe demonstrate significant improvements in depression and provide strong validation for the strategy in the treatment of depression by utilizing cofactors required for optimal neurotransmitter synthesis.

"DOWNSTREAM" ISSUES

Once a neuron has synthesized neurotransmitter molecules and has released them into the synapse, there are still several factors to overcome before neurons are fired adequately. For instance, the receptor may be defective, and therefore relatively unresponsive to even supranormal levels of the neurotransmitter.[16] Also, the membrane in which the receptor protein is anchored may be too rigid. Then, when the neurotransmitter has bound to the receptor site, the receptor protein may not be able to diffuse laterally in the membrane to ensure receptor activation and signal transduction.[17] Furthermore, the signal transduction pathways downstream from the receptor may be defective.[18]

There are several nutrients that are critical for optimal composition and fluidity of neuronal membranes. The list includes cholesterol, inositol, phosphatidylserine, phosphatidylcholine, omega-3s, essential fatty acids, and vitamin D3. There are nutrients that also improve signal transduction; key among them is the sugar inositol.[19]

NUTRIENTS THAT INHIBIT ENZYMES

D,L-PHENYLALANINE

D,L-Phenylalanine (DLPA) can increase the net level of enkephalins (one of the classes of endogenous opiates). It is the racemic mixture of the D- and L- forms of this amino acid; the L- isomer of phenylalanine is the one normally found in nature. DLPA serves as the direct precursor to phenylethylamine (PEA), and it can be converted to L-tyrosine, which will thereby increase production of dopamine and/or norepinephrine. The D- isomer of phenylalanine happens to inhibit enkephalinase, the enzyme that breaks down the enkaphalins.[20] Inhibiting an enzyme that breaks down a neurotransmitter will bring about a net increase in the level of that neurotransmitter in the synapse. Clinical studies have shown that DLPA is useful in treating depression, certain addictions, and pain.[21] However, both the DL- form and the L- form of phenylalanine can induce activation, agitation, and irritability, requiring a reduction in dosage or discontinuation.

RHODIOLA ROSAE

Rhodiola rosae is an adaptogenic herb that has been shown to be helpful in treating those depressive disorders where anergy and/or anhedonia are prominent.[22,23] The putative mechanisms by which Rhodiola functions as an antidepressant include (a) facilitating the entry of tryptophan across the blood-brain barrier; and (b) inhibiting the enzyme catechol-*O*-methyl transferase (COMT),[24] decreasing inactivation of dopamine in the synapse.

An extract of *Rhodiola rosae* rhizomes was studied in a 6-week randomized, double-blind phase III clinical trial in patients with mild to moderate depression. Patients receiving the lower dose (340 mg/day) as well as those receiving the higher dose (680 mg/day) had a statistically significant (approximately eight-point) drop in HAM-D scores, whereas those randomized to placebo had a nonsignificant half-point drop.[25] Patients randomized to receive the herb reported significant improvement with overall depression, insomnia, emotional stabilization, and somatization.

There is a great deal of variability among the Rhodiola products available on the market. Efficacy is determined by factors such as the climate and soil in which the plants were grown, the methods of extraction, and the presence or absence of specific fractions. At a minimum, the product should be standardized to at least 3% rosavins and 1% salidrosides. Extensive discussion on the uses of this highly effective adaptogenic herb may be found in *The Rhodiola Revolution*.[26]

TRACE MINERALS

Of the micronutrient groups, deficiencies of minerals are of particular concern. As the human body cannot create enough of these minerals for effective metabolism, a balanced diet with ample drinking water is critical. A 2004 study sponsored by the American College of Nutrition cited growing pollution, rampant pesticide use, over-mining, and exploitive agricultural practices as factors leaching minerals out of the oceans, soils, and consequently, out of our food supply.[27]

The trace minerals calcium, zinc, magnesium, chromium, and iron may be implicated in the pathophysiology of depression. Numerous studies have linked hyperactivation of *N*-methyl-D-aspartate (NMDA) receptors and depression.[28,29] NMDA receptors respond to glutamate by increasing their permeability to calcium. This can lead to overstimulation and excitotoxic damage, a cause of neuro-degeneration associated with depression.[30] Zinc and magnesium prevent depressive symptoms by inhibiting NMDA receptors.[31] These minerals reduce the harmful effects of NMDA receptor overactivation by decelerating calcium reception.[32,33]

Chromium is involved in monoamine function. In animal trials chromium administration has been associated with increased tryptophan, serotonin, and noradrenaline.[34] Chromium is therefore predicted to increase selective amino acid transport to the brain, enhancing the function of neurotransmitters involved in depression.

Several studies have investigated the relationship between iron and neurotransmitter receptors, suggesting a possible pathway through which iron affects mood. Iron is required for binding of nitric oxide, NMDA receptor functioning, glutamate activity, GABA homeostasis, and adequate energy metabolism.[35,36] Brain function and mood are therefore sensitive to changes in iron status. Supplementation as needed with trace minerals in addition to amino acid precursors is part of an integrative treatment for depression.

TARGETING NUTRIENT SUPPLEMENTATION FOR PSYCHIATRIC CONDITIONS

DEPRESSION

Figure 19.1 shows that the catecholamine neurotransmitters are synthesized from the precursor amino acids L-tyrosine, precursor to dopamine and norepinephrine; and L-phenylalanine, a precursor to the neuromodulator phenylethylamine. Phenylalanine can also be converted to tyrosine (and then to dopamine and norepinephrine). L-Tryptophan is the precursor to serotonin.

The documentation that these precursor amino acids regulate mood in clinically significant ways comes from two lines of clinical evidence: studies in which the amino acids are intentionally depleted, and studies in which the amino acids are supplemented. A number of placebo-controlled clinical studies on humans have shown that diets depleted in tryptophan as well as diets depleted in tyrosine and phenylalanine can cause clinically significant worsening of mood and anxiety. For example, Smith et al. studied 15 women (age 21–45 years) with clinical depression.[37] Ten of the women who received a tryptophan-free mixture (75% reduction in plasma tryptophan concentration) experienced temporary but clinically significant depressive symptoms and higher mean HAM-D scores after 7 hours than those who received a tryptophan-rich mixture (7.3 versus 0.15 [95% CI 4.5–9.9]; $p < 0.001$). In a more recent study, Robinson et al. demonstrated that women who have a history of depressed mood with subsequent acute tryptophan depletion (ATD) have a higher risk for recurrent negative mood than healthy females.[38] However, previous findings indicate that serotonergic vulnerability also exists in healthy individuals with a positive family history (FH+) for depression (first-degree relatives).[39] Tryptophan depletion in these individuals induced depression (increased score on the POMS depression scale) in 50% of FH+ females ($N = 5$) compared to 9% in FH- individuals. Although this study only enrolled female participants, the findings are consistent with other studies conducted with male subjects.

Similar to the synthesis of serotonin from tryptophan, tyrosine and phenylalanine are precursor amino acids responsible for the formation of the catecholamine neurotransmitters dopamine, norepinephrine, and phenylethylamine. One study involved 12 healthy male individuals who were randomized to receive either a nutritionally balanced mixture or one devoid of phenylalanine and tyrosine (PT-).[40] After 5 hours of ingesting the mixture, patients in the PT- group showed lower alertness scores (VAMS factor I) and increased anxiety scores (Profiles of Mental State composed-anxious dimension, $p = 0.022$). In a similar study, 12 healthy women subjected to acute phenylalanine/tyrosine depletion (APTD) experienced lower moods, especially after aversive physiologic challenge, compared to their counterparts.[41]

The results of several placebo-controlled clinical studies show that major depressive disorder can be significantly alleviated by supplements of tryptophan (and/or 5-OH tryptophan), and/or by supplements of phenylalanine. For example, a clinical trial on tryptophan supplementation in eight patients demonstrated that a combination supplementation [tryptophan plus 5-OH tryptophan] was superior to monotherapy with tryptophan or nomifensine administration.[42] Another clinical trial, using phenylalanine supplementation, studied the effects of 2-phenylethylamine in healthy and depressed individuals.[43] Phenylacetic acid (PAA), a metabolite of 2-phenylethylamine, was measured via plasma and urine samples. Mean plasma PAA concentration was higher (491.83 ± 232.84 ng/mL; $N = 12$) in healthy individuals than in those with depression (300.33 ± 197.44 ng/mL; $N = 23$). Twenty-four-hour urine PAA in healthy individuals (141.1 ± 10.2 mg; $N = 48$) was also higher than in the depressed group (78.2 ± 41.0 mg; $N = 144$). These metabolites have a potential use as biomarkers for depression. Additionally, the study supplemented 40 depressed participants with 2-phenylethylamine's precursor, L-phenylalanine, and the results showed elevated mood in 77.5% (31) of the group.

Nutrient augmentation of traditional pharmacologic therapy has also been studied. Levitan et al. suggested augmenting fluoxetine with tryptophan to overcome the delayed onset of action of antidepressants and/or the associated insomnia.[44] Thirty individuals with major depressive disorder were given 20 mg daily of fluoxetine and either 2 to 4 g of tryptophan or placebo over the course of 8 weeks. Results were tracked via the Hamilton Depression Rating Scale (HDRS-29) and Beck Depression Inventory (BDI). During the first week, scores were significantly lower on both scales in the fluoxetine/tryptophan group compared to the fluoxetine/placebo group. No significant difference was present after the first week. Also, slow-wave sleep was significantly decreased in the fluoxetine/placebo group at 4 weeks but not in the fluoxetine/tryptophan group. Augmentation protocol may provide early relief of symptoms of low mood and insomnia in depressed patients.

In treating depression, many practitioners recommend L-phenylalanine (500 mg 1 hour before breakfast and sometimes another 500 mg 1 hour before lunch), along with the cofactors vitamin B6 (50 mg once per day) and magnesium (100 mg at night). For tryptophan supplementation, similar dosing and augmentation with cofactors would be used, but the dose should be taken in the evening, as tryptophan can induce drowsiness. These precursor amino acids should not be taken with food in order to avoid competition with the other large neutral amino acids (LNAAs), present in the food, for receptor-mediated entry across the blood-brain barrier. To further enhance the antidepressant effect, many practitioners add SAMe. In addition, if the patient is lethargic and/or anhedonic, practitioners further augment with the adaptogenic herb *Rhodiola rosae*, at minimal doses of 100 mg once per day in the morning.

In contrast to the clinical benefits seen for supplementation with tryptophan and phenylalanine, results of clinical studies using supplements of tyrosine to treat depression have been equivocal.[45,46] The failure of tyrosine to significantly relieve depression may result from the fact that the investigators were using that precursor amino acid alone, as a "silver bullet." In clinical practice, most integrative practitioners eschew the "silver bullet" approach and, instead, recommend a combination of nutrients, such as augmenting the precursor amino acid with supplements of the vitamin and mineral cofactors that are required to convert the precursor to the finished product.[47,48]

BIPOLAR DEPRESSION

Nutrients can downmodulate mood swings by counterbalancing catecholaminergic versus cholinergic tone (see Table 19.1). A see-saw–like relationship exists between catecholaminergic and cholinergic inputs into the regions of the brain (e.g., the basal ganglia, and the striatum in particular) that modulate mood.[49,50] Increasing catecholaminergic tone can elevate low mood, but too great an increase in this tone can drive the patient past euthymia and into mania. Conversely, increasing cholinergic tone can dampen a manic mood, but too great an increase in this tone can drive the patient past euthymia and into depression.

A nutrient approach is particularly valuable with bipolar patients who have suffered severe adverse events from the mood stabilizers and/or the neuroleptics that had previously been tried. For lecithin, a generally recommended dose is 1200 mg per day, preferably in a chewable formulation so that the patient can gradually decrease the dose as the mania subsides. In a double-blind, placebo-controlled trial studying the efficacy of lecithin in controlling mania, five of six patients experienced significantly greater improvement compared to placebo.[51]

Branched-chain amino acid (BCAA) supplements[52] decrease catecholaminergic tone by competing with the precursor amino acids tyrosine and tryptophan for receptor-mediated entry across the blood-brain barrier. BCAAs should only be administered under medical supervision. Another approach is a tyrosine-depleted diet. Prescribing high-dose ascorbate as an adjunctive therapy for psychosis or mania has also shown promise. In one study, 10 out of 13 patients on neuroleptics improved symptomatically on high-dose vitamin C.[53] Remission of psychosis (whether from hypermania or schizophrenia) can be promoted by adding ascorbic acid (vitamin C) to the regimen of nutrients and/or neuroleptics. Dosages of about 2000 mg (2 g) per day are needed. The effect may be due to the achievement of ascorbate-induced D2 receptor blockade.

TABLE 19.1
Nutrients That Can Increase Catecholaminergic versus Cholinergic Tone

Nutrients to Treat Depression by Increasing *Catecholaminergic Tone* in the Basal Ganglia	Nutrients to Treat Mania by Increasing *Cholinergic Tone* in the Basal Ganglia
Nutrients such as tyrosine, phenyl-alanine, and SAMe increase the synthesis of dopamine, norepinephrine, and/or phenylethylamine (collectively, the catecholamines).	Nutrients such as lecithin (a source of choline) increase the synthesis of acetylcholine.[50]

SIDE EFFECTS AND CONTRAINDICATIONS

Pharmacologists like to point out: "If it's strong enough to help, it's strong enough to harm." This principle applies to nutrients and herbs as well as to prescription medications. This is important, because many people (and even a few integrative physicians) labor under the misconception that nutrients cannot possibly cause side effects. Granted, the side effects of nutrients tend to be mild compared to the devastating adverse effects that many psychotropics can induce, such as liver failure, bone marrow dysplasia, Stevens-Johnson syndrome, and successful suicide. Nevertheless, nutrients can induce side effects. Some of the more common ones are headache, irritability, heartburn, mild sedation, and (for the more stimulating compounds) a "wired" feeling like drinking too much coffee. Patients need to be routinely advised that there *can* be side effects, so that they do not second-guess themselves.

Table 19.2 lists some of the contraindications for certain nutrients. Glutamine is contraindicated with cirrhosis of the liver as glutamine contains two amino acid residues.[54] The cirrhotic liver is said to be overly burdened by the extra ammonia that can result. Contraindications for L-tryptophan (LTP) and 5-HTP involve potential toxicity to patients with certain conditions or taking certain drugs. While some part of a dose of LTP is converted to serotonin, a large proportion is cleaved by the enzyme indoleamine dioxygenase (IDO) and shuttled down the kynurenine pathway, becoming converted into neurotoxic metabolites such as 6-OH kynurenine, a compound commonly used for inducing symptoms of Parkinson's disease in animal models of this condition. Given that the end-product of the kynurenine pathway is niacinamide (NAA), supplements of this vitamin can induce end-product inhibition and thereby block the kynurenine pathway, allowing more of the tryptophan to be converted to serotonin (while minimizing the risk of the kynurenine neurotoxins being formed).

The reason for caution in recommending 5-hydroxytryptophan (5-HTP) is that it is analogous to L-DOPA, in terms of its position in the biosynthetic pathways. In Figure 19.1, which shows the pathways for synthesizing the monoamine neurotransmitters, we see that there is a hydroxylase enzyme that converts tyrosine to DOPA, and that an analogous hydroxylase enzyme converts tryptophan to 5-HTP. Given that L-DOPA can cause such a wide array of serious side effects, it is logical to assume that 5- HTP would, theoretically, be likely to cause its own array of serious side effects. Strictly speaking, 5-HTP is not a "nutrient." Rather, it is a derivative of a nutrient (tryptophan), just as L-DOPA is a derivative of a nutrient (tyrosine). More research is needed to evaluate the efficacy and safety of 5-HTP and tryptophan before widespread use may be recommended.

SUMMARY OF INDICATIONS, DOSES, AND TIMING OF KEY NUTRIENTS

Table 19.3 provides a summary of the indications, dosages, timing, and other issues for several nutrients and herbs used in psychiatry.

TABLE 19.2

Relative and/or Absolute Contraindications for Certain Nutrients

Nutrient or herb	Contraindication
L-glutamine	Presence of cirrhosis of the liver
St. John's wort (SJW)	Increases the metabolism of (and thereby counteracts) a wide range of medications, including birth control pills and anticoagulants; induces photo-sensitivity
SAMe, SJW, tyrosine, LTP	Recent or past history of switches to mania
L-tryptophan (LTP)	Its breakdown products can be toxic to Parkinson's and Alzheimer patients
5-OH tryptophan (5-HTP)	Absolute: Use of MAOIs
SAMe, tryptophan, SJW	Relative contraindication for concurrent use of serotonergic agents, because of risk for serotonin syndrome

TABLE 19.3

Some Commonly Used Nutrients: Indications, Dosages, Timing, and Other Issues

Supplement	Indications	Initial Dose/Final Dose	Timing; Relationship to Meals	Comments (If Any)
L-Tyrosine or L-Phenylalanine	Depression; bipolar depression (cautiously)	500 mg 1 qd for starters; 1500 mg/d max	Take 1 h before breakfast +/ or lunch	Do not take in evening, because it is activating. As depression subsides, doses have to be progressively tapered so as not to provoke a new round of mania.
Vitamin B6	Depression; bipolar depression; PMS	50 mg per day	N/A	Add magnesium (at bedtime), because B6 supplements deplete magnesium stores, causing hyperacusis.
Magnesium	Anxiety; migraines; insomnia; PMS	100 mg hs	N/A	Amino acid chelates are preferred. Weight shown is elemental, not the gross weight of the salt.
Lecithin	Dementia and mild cognitive impairment; Psychosis (manic or schizophrenic)	Dementia: 1200 mg/d Mania: 1200 mg/d, but decrease dose progressively as mania subsides	N/A	As mania subsides, doses of choline sources have to be progressively tapered so as not to provoke a new round of depression.
Vitamin C (ascorbic acid)	Psychosis (manic or schizophrenic)	2000 mg/day, in two to three divided doses	N/A	Buffered formulations of vitamin C reduce the likelihood of gastritis.
L-glutamine	Alcohol abuse, GAD, panic attacks	500 mg one to two times per day	N/A	If slightly sedating, bias the dose towards hs.
Rhodiola rosae	Anergic depression, suicidality	Approximately 100 mg one to two times per day	1 h before breakfast	Can be activating, might have to decrease intake of caffeine.
Lemon balm	Anxiety disorders	300 mg one to two times per day	N/A	Slows enzymatic breakdown of GABA
SAMe	Depression, especially with suicidal ideation	Start with 200 mg/day, work up slowly to 2000 mg/day if needed	1 h before breakfast and/or lunch	Can activate hypomania, thus relatively contraindicated in bipolar patients.

Note: AD, antidepressants; LNAAs, large neutral amino acids (e.g., tryptophan and tyrosine).

CONCLUSION

Although much research is still to be done, a small research base currently exists to support the use of amino acids, vitamins, herbs, and trace minerals as treatment for depression and other psychiatric disorders. These therapies have the advantage of being safe and well tolerated in addition to being effective. Following the dosage recommendations in this chapter, the clinician can target nutrient therapy—either as a single nutrient or in combinations—to the individual biochemistry of his/her patients. Pharmacologic doses of selected nutrients restore balance in neurotransmitter levels, thereby helping to resolve the ravages of depression.

REFERENCES

1. Shaheen, S.E. and Vieira, K.F. 2008. Nutritional therapies for mental disorders. *Nutr Jr* 7: 2.
2. Williams, R.J. 1998. *Biochemical Individuality: The Basis for the Genetotrophic Concept.* New Canaan, CT: Keats.

3. Lehnert, H. and Wurtman, R.J. 1993. Amino acid control of neurotransmitter synthesis and release: Physiological and clinical implications. *Psychother Psychosom* 60(1): 18–32.

4. Wurtman, R.J. 2011. Non-nutritional uses of nutrients. *Eur J Pharmacol* 668(1): S10–S15.

5. Carlton, R.M., Ente, G., Blum, L. et al. 2000. Rational dosages of nutrients have a prolonged effect on learning disabilities. *Altern Ther* 6(3): 85–91.

6. Basura, G.J., Hagland, S.P., Wiltse, A.M. et al. 2009. Clinical features and the management of pyridox-ine-dependent and pyridoxine-responsive seizures: Review of 63 North American cases submitted to a patient registry. *Eur J Pediatr* 168(6): 697–704.

7. Brown, R., Gerberg, P., and Bottiglieri, T. 2000. S-Adenosylmethionine in the clinical practice of psychiatry, neurology and internal medicine. *Clin Pract Intern Med* 1: 230–241.

8. Bressa, G.M. 1994. S-Adenosyl-L-methionine (SAMe) as antidepressant: Meta-analysis of clinical studies. *Acta Neurol Scand* 154: 7–14.

9. Papakostas, G.I. 2009. Evidence for S-adenosyl-L-methionine (SAM-e) for the treatment of major depressive disorder. *Clin Psychiatry* 70 Suppl 5: 18–22.

10. Sarris, J., Papakostas, G.I., Vitolo, O. et al. 2014. S-adenosyl methionine (SAMe) versus escitalopram and placebo in major depression RCT: Efficacy and effects of histamine and carnitine as moderators of response. *J Affect Disord* 164: 76–81.

11. Bottiglieri, T., Godfrey, P., Flynn, T. et al. 1990. Cerebrospinal fluid S-adenosylmethionine in depression and dementia: Effects of treatment with parenteral and oral S-adenosylmethionine. *J Neurol Neurosurg Psychiatry* 53: 1096–1098.

12. Papakostas, G.K., Mischoulon, D., Shyu, I. et al. 2010. SAMe augmentation of SSRIs for antidepressant nonresponders with major depressive disorder: A double blind, randomized clinical trial. *Am J Psychiatry* 167(8): 942–948.

13. Morris, D.W. 2008. Folate and unipolar depression. *J Altern Complement Med* 14(3): 277–285.

14. Liew, S.C. et al. 2015. Methylenetetrahydrofolate reductase (MTHFR) C677T polymorphism: Epidemiology, metabolism and the associated diseases. *Eur J Med Genet* 58(1): 1–10.

15. Papakostas, G.I., Shelton, R.C., Zajecka, J.M. et al. 2014. Effect of adjunctive L-methylfolate 15 mg among inadequate responders to SSRIs in depressed patients who were stratified by biomarker levels and genotype: Results from a randomized clinical trial. *J Clin Psychiatry* 75(8): 855–863.

16. Van Ijzendoorn, M.H. et al. 2015. Genetic differential susceptibility on trial: Meta-analytic support from randomized controlled experiments. *Dev Psychopathol* 27(1): 151–162.

17. Czysz, A.H. et al. 2015. Lateral diffusion of Gαs in the plasma membrane is decreased after chronic but not acute antidepressant treatment: Role of lipid raft and non-raft membrane microdomains. *Neuropsychopharmacology* 40(3): 766–773.

18. Kim, H. et al. 2005. A review of the possible relevance of inositol and the phosphatidylinositol second messenger system (PI-cycle) to psychiatric disorders—Focus on magnetic resonance spectroscopy (MRS) studies. *Hum Psychopharmacol* 20(5): 309–326.

19. Shears, S.B., Ganapathi, S.B., Gokhale, N.A. et al. 2012. Defining signal transduction by inositol phosphates. *Subcell Biochem* 59: 389–412.

20. Von Knorring, L., Almay, B.G., Johansson, F. et al. 1979. Endorphins in CSF of chronic pain patients, in relation to augmenting-reducing response in visual averaged evoked response. *Neuropsychobiology* 5: 322–326.

21. Russell, A.L. and McCarty, M.F. 2000. DL-phenylalanine markedly potentiates opiate analgesia—An example of nutrient/pharmaceutical up-regulation of the endogenous analgesia system. *Med Hypotheses* 55(4): 283–288.

22. Quereshi, N.A. and Al-Bedah, A.M. 2013. Mood disorders and complementary and alternative medicine: A literature review. *Neuropsychiatr Dis Treat* 9: 639–658.

23. Iovieno, N., Dalton, E.D., Fava, M. et al. 2011. Second-tier natural antidepressants: Review and critique. *J Affect Disord* 130(3): 343–357.

24. Blum, K., Chen, T.J., Meshkin, B. et al. 2007. Manipulation of catechol-*O*-methyl-transferase (COMT) activity to influence the attenuation of substance seeking behavior, a subtype of Reward Deficiency Syndrome (RDS), is dependent upon gene polymorphisms: A hypothesis. *Med Hypotheses* 69(5): 1054–1060.

25. Darbinyan, V., Aslanyan, G., Amroyan, E. et al. 2007. Clinical trial of *Rhodiola rosea* L. extract SHR-5 in the treatment of mild to moderate depression. *Nord J Psychiatry* 61(5): 343–348.

26. Brown, R.P., Gerberg, P.L., and Graham, B. 2004. *The Rhodiola Revolution: Transform Your Health with the Herbal Breakthrough of the 21st Century.* Emmaus, PA: Rodale Press.

27. Davis, D.R., Epp, M.D., and Riordan, H.D. 2004. Changes in USDA food composition data for 43 Garden Crops, 1950 to 1999. *J Am Coll Nutr* 23(6): 669–682.

28. Costa, B.M., Irvine, M.W., Fang, G. et al. 2010. A novel family of negative and positive allosteric modulators of NMDA receptors. *J Pharmacol Exp Ther* 335(2): 614–621.

29. Szewczyk, B., Poleszak, E., Sowa-Kucma, M. et al. 2010. The involvement of NMDA and AMPA receptors in the mechanism of antidepressant-like action of zinc in the forced swim test. *Amino Acids* 39: 205–217.

30. Salimi, S., Kianpoor, M., Abassi, M.R. et al. 2008. Lower total serum protein, albumin and zinc in depression in an Iranian population. *J Med Sci* 8: 587–590.

31. Swardfager, W., Herrmann, N., Mazereeuw, G. et al. 2013. Zinc in depression: A meta-analysis. *Biol Psychiatry* 74: 872–878.

32. Videbech, P. and Ravnkilde, B. 2004. Hippocampal volume and depression: A meta-analysis of MRI studies. *Am J Psychiatry* 161(1): 1957–1966.

33. Lee, A.L., Ogle, W.O., and Sapolsky, R.M. 2002. Stress and depression: Possible links to neuron death in the hippocampus. *Bipolar Disord* 4(2): 117–128.

34. Franklin, M. and Odontiadis, J. 2003. Effects of treatment with chromium picolinate on peripheral amino acid availability and brain monoamine function in the rat. *Pharmacopsychiatry* 36(5): 176–180.

35. Jaffrey, S.R., Cohen, N.A., Rouault, T.A., Klausner, R.D., and Snyder, S.H. 1994. The iron-responsive element binding protein: A target for synaptic actions of nitric oxide. *Proc Natl Acad Sci USA.* 91(26): 12994–12998.

36. Ward, K.L., Tkac, I., and Jing, Y. 2007. Gestational and lactational iron deficiency alters the developing striatal metabolome and associated behaviors in young rats. *J Nutr* 137(4): 1043–1049.

37. Smith, K.A. 1997. Relapse of depression after rapid depletion of tryptophan. *Lancet* 349(9056): 915–919.

38. Robinson, O.J. 2009. Acute tryptophan depletion evokes negative mood in healthy females who have previously experienced concurrent negative mood and tryptophan depletion. *Psychopharmacology (Berl)* 205(2): 227–235.

39. Riedel, W.J. 2002. Tryptophan, mood, and cognitive function. *Brain Behav Immun* 16(5): 581–589.

40. Grevet, E.H. 2002. Behavioural effects of acute phenylalanine and tyrosine depletion in healthy male volunteers. *J Psychopharmacol* 16(1): 51–55.

41. Leyton, M. 2000. Effects on mood of acute phenylalanine/tyrosine depletion in healthy women. *Neuropsychopharmacology* 22: 52–63.

42. Quadbeck, H. 1984. Comparison of the antidepressant action of tryptophan, tryptophan/5-hydroxytryptophan combination and nomifensine. *Neuropsychobiology* 11(2): 111–115.

43. Sabelli, H.C. 1986. Clinical studies on the phenylethylamine hypothesis of affective disorder: Urine and blood phenylacetic acid and phenylalanine dietary supplements. *J Clin Psychiatry* 47(2): 66–70.

44. Levitan, R.D., Shen, J.H., Jindal, R. et al. 2000. Preliminary randomized double-blind placebo-controlled trial of tryptophan combination with fluoxetine to treat major depressive disorder: Antidepressant and hypnotic effects. *J Psychiatry Neurosci* 25(4): 337–346.

45. Gelenberg, A.J., Wojcik, J.D., Falk, W.E. et al. 1984. Tyrosine for depression: A double-blind trial. *Nutr Health* 3(3): 163–173.

46. Parker, G. and Brotchie, H. 2011. Mood effects of the amino acids tryptophan and tyrosine: "Food for Thought" III. *Acta Psychiatr Scand* 124(6): 417–426.

47. Doll, H., Brown, S., Thurston, A. et al. 1989. Pyridoxine (vitamin B6) and the premenstrual syndrome: A randomized crossover trial. *J R Coll Gen Pract* 39(326): 364–368.

48. De Souza, M.C. 2000. A synergistic effect of a daily supplement for 1 month of 200 mg magnesium plus 50 mg vitamin B6 for the relief of anxiety-related premenstrual symptoms: A randomized, double-blind, crossover study. *J Womens Health Gend Based Med* 9(2): 131–139.

49. van Enkhuizen, J., Janowsky, D.S., Olivier, B. et al. 2014. The catecholaminergic-cholinergic balance hypothesis of bipolar disorder revisited. *Eur J Pharmacol* 753: 114–126. pii:S0014–2999(14)00585–8.

50. Cohen, E.L. et al. 1976. Brain acetylcholine: Control by dietary choline. *Science* 191(4227): 561–562.

51. Cohen, B.M. et al. 1982. Lecithin in the treatment of mania: Double-blind, placebo-controlled trials. *Am J Psychiatry* 139(9): 1162–1164.

52. Scarna, A. et al. 2003. Effects of a branched-chain amino acid drink in mania. *Br J Psychiatry* 182: 210–213.

53. Beauclair, L., Vinogradov, S., Riney, S.J. et al. 1987. An adjunctive role for ascorbic acid in the treatment of schizophrenia? *J Clin Psychopharmacol* 7(4): 282–283.

54. Oppong, K.N., Al-Mardini, H., Thick, M., and Record, CO. Oral glutamine challenge in cirrhotics pre- and post-liver transplantation: A psychometric and analyzed EEG study. *Hepatology* 26(4): 870–876.

20 Botanicals for Depression
Rhodiola, St. John's Wort, Curcumin, and Saffron

Judith E. Pentz, MD

CONTENTS

INTRODUCTION

Botanicals, also known as herbs, have been part of the healing traditions of human cultures from ancient times. We usually think of their ability to heal the body but often overlook their potent effect on the mind. Their effect on both body and mind is what makes them quite remarkable and unique. Researchers have found ample evidence to support utilizing botanicals as interventions for mental health, particularly depression. Using herbs for depression has become increasingly common in the population at large. A study from 2001 reported that 54% of individuals interviewed, or more than 2000 people, had taken an herbal remedy to alter their mood.[1]

Given the rising costs of modern research and health care, medicinal herbs are a promising alternative therapeutic strategy, one that may be as effective as and possibly safer than pharmaceutical treatment. Approaching herbal medicine using the scientific method is a discipline known as *phytotherapy*. Botanicals can be part of an integrative approach, in which the clinician addresses the patient's nutrition, genetics, social/community connections, culture, spiritual/religious traditions, baseline health/physiology, work, and environment. As each herb has distinctive properties and leads to a slightly different reaction in each individual, an integrative approach provides the greatest potential for success by customizing the treatment plan to the patients' needs.

It is important to note that herbal medicine is not as rigorously defined as traditional medicine, and many factors affect the botanicals themselves. Therefore, the clinician must be vigilant in adapting dosages and combinations in order to achieve the best results. The concentration of bioactive ingredients within a plant is affected by growth conditions, time to harvest, preparation, and method of extraction. Seeking reputable and knowledgeable practitioners should ensure the highest quality and consistency of bioactive compounds to maximize herbal impact. We are in the early stages of understanding the active ingredient(s) in herbs. For example, the recent clinical research of St. John's wort reveals the presence of two active ingredients, hypericin and hyperforin, even though previously only one active ingredient was thought to be present. It is still not known which of the two is more active or if they act synergistically in reducing depression. Studies are underway to explore further the activity of both ingredients.

GENERAL CONSIDERATIONS

Many models are available to help the clinician identify the best herbal treatment and dosage for the individual patient. One model, as described by David Hoffman in *Medical Herbalism*, suggests the importance of several factors.

It is important to consider the potential impact of the herb on the mind and body. According to herbal nomenclature, some compounds are referred to as *adaptogens,* including Rhodiola. These herbs provide greater balance and homeostasis, normalizing the body-mind dynamic.[2] In 1968, Brekman and Dardymov reported that these gentle and nourishing herbs yield a nontoxic, nonspecific response that confers resilience and adaptability under stress.[3] Other herbs are classified as *effectors,* due to their observable impact on the body. Thus, these herbs, such as St. John's wort, are more suited for treating specific conditions.

Factors in compliance, ecological concerns, and financial considerations should be addressed. A combination of herbs that are pleasant to both taste and smell can help ensure compliance with herbal treatment. A cup of herbal tea can be both pleasant and a therapeutic remedy. Environmentally, herbal medicine is much less resource-draining than pharmacotherapy and causes less pollution than the pharmaceutical production of its counterpart. Those involved in medicinal herb production are generally aware of the need for responsible harvesting in ensuring sustainable production. In addition, herbs provide a financial benefit to the patient as they are often significantly less costly than their pharmaceutical alternative, with a lower risk profile.

Existing research data should be carefully considered. Sarris et al., in exploring herbal medicine for the treatment of depression, anxiety, and insomnia, noted some areas of concern about the use of herbal treatment.[4] Despite the common misperception that herbs are natural and thus cause no adverse effects, some case reports suggest the contrary. For instance, in patients with bipolar disorder, St. John's wort can possibly induce mania.[5,6] The "polyvalence" concept, defined as the "range of biological activities that a herbal extract may exhibit, can prove useful in determining a herbs overall clinical effect."[7]

Studies need to be constructed rigorously to address consistency and reliability, concerns not stressed in traditional herbal medicine. Research should attempt to identify the effects of the active ingredients as well as the effects of other chemicals in the treatment's composition. Each batch of the herb is unique and influenced by its own environmental factors.

A new area of research that promises expanded knowledge about herbs is the field of genetic technologies. One exciting area is the study of the role of herbal medicine on epigenetics utilizing proteomic assays. An 8-week animal study treated animals with either St. John's wort or imipramine and assessed alteration in hypothalamic genes with therapies targeted for depression.[8] Results indicated that 66 genes were altered in those animals that received St. John's wort compared to 74 genes in those that received imipramine.[8]

Careful exploration of the properties and uses of botanicals will reward the effort. Given the heterogeneous nature of depression, the synergistic and polyvalence of herbs can address its inherent complexities. Herbal medicines possess a range of therapeutic actions beyond being simply antidepressants. They can also have anxiolytic, sedative/hypnotic, and analgesic properties, and can enhance cognitive function.

Much of the research on botanicals has focused on single herbs as primary interventions.

RHODIOLA ROSEA

Historically, *Rhodiola rosea* was mentioned as long ago as 77 AD in the *De Materia Medica* of Dioscorides. In an excellent monograph about herbs, Brown and Gerbarg review the history of this unique herb, noting that the majority of the literature on the subject has been written in Russian, Slavic, or the Scandinavian languages.[9] Over time *Rhodiola rosea* has been used in Eastern Asia, Siberian, Eastern Europe, and Scandinavia for relieving mental and physical fatigue, increasing endurance, enhancing fertility, and providing a sexual tonic.[9] Currently, *Rhodiola rosea* is recognized by the Russian Ministry of Health as both a medicine and an herbal tonic to reinvigorate general well-being. Similarly, in Sweden, it is popular for its unique anti-fatigue properties.

Today *Rhodiola rosea* is commonly referred to as golden root, arctic root, or rose root. In taste it is sweet, slightly bitter, and spicy, and possesses a texture that feels dry and cool. The root is the most commonly used part of the plant for medicinal purposes. It is native to higher elevations in Siberia, Scandinavia, and Canada. It has also been found in the Alps, Pyrenees, and Carpathian Mountains and in the western mountains of the United States. Growing up to 30 inches, *Rhodiola rosea* produces a yellow perennial flower with a life span of above 2 years. The root when cut has a fragrance similar to that of a rose. It is also both cardio- and neuroprotective. However, its main feature is its ability as an adaptogen to alter hormones and neurotransmitters for maintaining homeostatic balance. Although other Rhodiola plants exist, they do not have the same properties as *Rhodiola rosea*, with its unique phytochemistry and pharmacology.

Rhodiola rosea is composed of many different molecules including rosin, rosarin, rosavin, salidrosides, and flavonoids such as rodiolin and rodionin.[2] Chief among these are the molecules rosavins and salidrosides, as they are believed to be the bioactive ingredients. The standardized extract from *Rhodiola rosea* is the SHR-5 compound from the artic root, a proprietary compound of the Swedish Health Council. Despite significant research into the biochemistry of *Rhodiola rosea*, the mechanism of action is still not fully understood, though several working models and hypotheses exist.

In its capacity as an adaptogen, *Rhodiola rosea* assists in normalizing the stress response in the body. It impacts both the sympatho-adrenal system and the hypothalamic axis. Therefore, it leads to increased resilience, with rapid response to stress along with improved capacity for long-term adaptation.[9] It is an excellent choice for providing cognitive stimulation while maintaining emotional stability. The stimulating effect of *Rhodiola rosea* differs from the effects of typical stimulants, which can result in subsequent drainage of energy from the body and mind, leading to symptoms of withdrawal. No withdrawal syndrome is associated with *Rhodiola rosea*, as shown by Breckman and Dardimov in 1968.[3] Additionally, the stimulating effect is best during fatigue and stress as it increases the individual's physical capacity for work while also enhancing cognitive performance.

More recently, an overview by Panossian et al. in 2005 also shows that *Rhodiola rosea* contains high antioxidant levels.[10] Rhodiola has been shown to have an impact on the monoamine neurotransmitters, dopamine, serotonin, and norepinephrine. In a 2009 study by Van Dierman et al., *Rhodiola rosea* was found to inhibit monamine oxidases (MAO A and B), providing both antidepressant activity and potential applicability for treating senile dementia.[11] Monoamine oxidase is an enzyme that catalyzes the breakdown of certain monoamine neurotransmitters within the nervous system.

Thus, the herb is able to act as a MAO inhibitor without the side effects seen in pharmaceuticals known as MAOIs.[11]

Animal research has further demonstrated that *R. rosea* also impacts brain function, reduces fatigue, improves long-term memory, and enhances learning behavior as well as reducing corticotropin-releasing factor, often higher during times of stress. In fact, studies show that compared to other nootropics, or substances that enhance cognition, Rhodiola resulted in increased levels of frontal lobe 5-HT in animals.[12,13] In studying its stimulative properties, Saratikov et al. showed that it also boosts adenosine triphosphate (ATP) and creatine phosphate (CP) in animal brain and muscle cells, thereby increasing cellular energy.[14]

CLINICAL RESEARCH

Rhodiola's ability to directly stimulate nicotinic, noradrenergic, dopamine, cholinergic, and 5-hydroxytryptaminic actions in certain parts of the brain is well documented.[15] A study from 1986 by Brichenko et al. evaluated the efficacy of *Rhodiola rosea* compared to placebo for treating depression. The patients receiving Rhodiola showed a significant improvement in symptoms, while patients on placebo did not.[15] Subsequently, in 1987, Brichenko et al. conducted an augmentation trial with *Rhodiola rosea* and tricyclic antidepressants in hospitalized patients, reporting positive results.[16]

Other studies have confirmed positive effects for *R. rosea* in treating mild to moderate depression. A 6-week Phase III randomized double-blind placebo-controlled study with parallel groups was conducted with patients ranging from 18–70 years, utilizing the Beck Depression Inventory and Hamilton Rating Scale for Depression (HAM-D) for identifying patients with depression.[17] The patients were randomized to three groups. Of the patients with initial HAM-D from 21 to 31, the first group ($N = 31$) received 340 mg of SHR-5 in divided doses, the second group received 680 mg of SHR-5 in divided doses ($N = 29$), and the third group received two placebo pills ($N = 29$).[17] After 42 days, individuals in both treatment arms were experiencing less depression, improved emotional stability, and less somatization compared to those taking placebo.[17] No difference in self-esteem was evident except in those on the higher dose (680 mg) of Rhodiola, which does suggest a possible dose response.[17] No serious side effects were noted in any of the groups.[17] The researchers concluded that SHR-5, standardized extract of *Rhodiola rosea,* has antidepressive effects in individuals diagnosed with mild to moderate depression.

In 2007, Fintelmann and Gruenwald conducted a 12-week monitoring study that tested the efficacy of SHR-5 extract along with vitamins and minerals.[18] Patients' age range was from 50–89 years old.[18] Significant improvements were noted in physical and cognitive deficiencies.[18] The overall global assessment of efficacy was between either "good" or "very good" for 81% of the patients.[18] Another double-blind, randomized, placebo-controlled study evaluated the effects of SHR-5 at 576 mg/day in 60 patients over 4 weeks.[19] Stress-related fatigue was the focus of this study.[19] Decreased cortisol response was noted as well as improvement in fatigue and concentration.[19] Previous clinical trials had focused on concomitant dosing of Rhodiola with tricyclic antidepressants but never as a single agent to treat depression. The results of these studies indicated that treatment with *Rhodiola rosea* resulted in both improvement of depression and fewer side effects than treatment with tricyclic antidepressants.

DOSAGE AND ADMINISTRATION

Due to the stimulating characteristics of *Rhodiola rosea,* it is best to take it earlier in the day, before breakfast and lunch. This provides for more effective absorption. The recommended starting dose for *Rhodiola rosea* is a standardized 100 mg. Titration can commence from as early as 3 days to 14 days and depends on the capacity of the person's individual capacity to tolerate stimulation. Diluting the 100-mg capsule in water or taking a smaller portion of the dose is also recommended for those more sensitive to stimulation, before gradually increasing the dose to the recommended level.

The maximum daily dose of Rhodiola is determined by overall health. Healthy individuals can take as much as 450 mg/day. In elderly individuals along with children and those with medical comorbidities, a lower starting dose of 25–50 mg is recommended, with slow up-titration. Clinical response after starting therapy varies from 2 weeks to 2 months.

SIDE EFFECTS AND TOXICITY

Side effects of *Rhodiola rosea* include overstimulation, vivid dreams, and occasional nausea. Although it is not contraindicated in individuals diagnosed with bipolar disorder, caution is recommended, as *Rhodiola rosea* has the potential to induce mania in these individuals. Saratikov et al., in a 1987 study, also advised caution.[14] Although the patients these researchers referred to as schizophrenic would now be considered to have bipolar disorder, their results suggest that *R. rosea* can exacerbate irritation and excitability.[20] Substances that are stimulating like Rhodiola require great caution in patients with bipolar tendencies.

Other side effects have been reported. There have been rare reports of hypersexuality and agitation with increased blood pressure in postmyocardial infarction patients.[2] *Rhodiola rosea* is absolutely contraindicated in individuals taking MAOIs because of the herb's action to inhibit monoamine oxidases. Current research does not show significant in vivo alteration in the functioning of cytochrome P450 enzymes (CYP3A4).[21] To this point, in vitro studies on cytochrome enzymes are not reliable predictors of in vivo activity of the enzymes for metabolism of drugs. The latter is complicated by a number of factors, including digestive bioavailability, intermediate metabolites, presence of multiple constituents, and different binding capacities.

Currently, there is Level 2 evidence of the efficacy of *Rhodiola rosea* for the treatment of depression, and therefore there is great need for replication of larger clinical studies. Overall, *Rhodiola rosea* appears to be a safe, effective option for the treatment of mild to moderate depression. Its onset of action is slightly faster than pharmaceutical medications, and it appears to have fewer side effects. Added benefits include the ability of *R. rosea* to boost cognition and immunity and to stabilize the HPA axis, leading to a positive impact on the sympathetic nervous system.

Although much of the research of the effects of *R. rosea* is aimed at the treatment of depression, clinical evidence supports the treatment of other medical conditions with *R. rosea*. The herb has provided demonstrated cognitive and physical support in the following conditions: attention deficit-hyperactivity disorder, fatigue (including during and after cancer treatment), stress, menopause, immunity issues, fibromyalgia, and Parkinson's disease.[22] *Rhodiola rosea* has also been able to reverse the sexual side effects of selective serotonin reuptake inhibitor (SSRI)-induced dysfunction.[22]

ST. JOHN'S WORT

The scientific name for St. John's wort (SJW) is *Hypericum perforatum*. The literal translation is "above a ghost," as the herb was initially gathered to ward off evil spirits. SJW is also referred to as klamath weed or goatweed. The most commonly used part of the plant is the "aerial portions" or the part above ground. *Hypericum perforatum* is native to Europe and Asia but has over time come to be found also in North America. It is a tall, erect perennial herb with yellow flowers containing oblong-oval leaves surrounded by black dots at the margins. It blooms primarily in the summer.

The constituents of SWJ are essential oil, hypericin (glycoside-red pigment), hyperforin, and polyphenol flavonoid derivatives. Its fame is attributed to its ability to elevate mild to moderate depression. It is heavily utilized as an alternative natural therapy for low mood in place of traditional pharmaceutical drugs. In Europe, SJW is often the first-line treatment for mild to moderate depression. SJW also possesses antispasmodic and anti-inflammatory properties and is utilized as a pain-relieving sedative for the treatment of neuralgia and anxiety. Therefore, SJW is believed to have multiple properties culminating in a global calming effect within the body and brain for treatment of depression and anxiety.

BIOCHEMISTRY

Research studies evaluating the effectiveness of SJW for the treatment of depression have focused on two active ingredients: hypericin and hyperforin. A growing body of evidence suggests that these two active ingredients are responsible for SJW's utility in treating mild to moderate depression, though the actual mechanism of action for SJW is still unknown. However, animal studies have indicated the presence of weak MAO-A and MAO-B inhibition.[23] It is possible that this prolongation in breakdown of essential neurotransmitters, such as serotonin, dopamine, and norepinephrine, is what makes SJW lead to results similar to those of SSRIs.[23] Additionally, SJW has also been shown to modulate both the gamma-amino butyric (GABA) and N-methyl-D-aspartate (NMDA) receptors.[24]

CLINICAL RESEARCH

SJW is one of the most heavily studied herbs of all time and has therefore been extensively compared to standard pharmaceutical therapy for the treatment of mild to moderate depression. A randomized, controlled, double-blind (RCT) study found SJW as effective as treatment with imipramine 150 mg.[25] Similar findings were also noted in another study that compared SJW to fluoxetine 20 mg in patients with mild to moderate depression.[26] A 42-day RCT conducted by Kasper et al. in 2006 demonstrated positive results with SJW (WS-5570 extract) in outpatient adults recovering from an acute episode of moderate depression.[27] Symptom resolution and overall improvement were greater in patients who took SJW than in patients who received placebo.[27] SJW (WS-5570 extract) was also found to be effective in preventing relapse of depression.[27] SJW was also shown to be effective for the treatment of seasonal affective disorder in one study utilizing Kira [LI-160] extract along with light therapy.

St. John's wort has not shown effectiveness in treating severe depression. Short-term RCT studies in severely depressed patients have been conducted. Patients were given SJW (Kira [Li-160 extract]) 900–1500 mg, sertraline 50–100 mg or placebo. Results indicated that neither sertraline nor Kira were more effective than placebo.[28] This finding has since been replicated in subsequent studies. Therefore, SJW is not recommended for the treatment of severely depressed patients.

St. John's wort is seen as a second-line agent in the United States. An exception to this would be women who have responded to low-dose SSRIs. From a clinical perspective, Gerbarg and Brown have noted this particular finding in their work with patients over the past 20 years. Although there are no published studies regarding combining of SJW with other antidepressants therapies such as bupropion, venlafaxine, or SAMe, the concept of augmenting with SJW has occurred in clinical practice for many years with good response.

SJW is a therapy with Level 1 evidence due to the multitude of replicated effectiveness studies and its established safety profile. It is a substantiated herbal treatment recommended for treatment for mild to moderate depression, including seasonal affective disorder for adults. It has been shown to be comparable if not superior to conventional antidepressants.[29]

DOSAGE AND ADMINISTRATION

The dosing for St. John's wort is typically from 900 to 1500 mg/day taken orally, though up to 1800 mg has benefitted some patients. In recommending quality sources with standardized dosing, it is best to look for a brand name with 0.3%–5% hypericin or hyperforin available in each capsule. Brands used in clinical trials are available. Brand names to consider include Kira (LI-160), Perika. Manufacturers with good manufacturing practices and that have independent testing done on their products includes Nature's Way, Healthcare, and Alokit. Relief from depression can take up to 1 month.

SIDE EFFECTS AND TOXICITY, RECOMMENDATIONS

Though generally safe, SJW does have a few dose-dependent side effects, which are similar to those from tricyclic antidepressants and less than those from SSRIs. These symptoms include nausea, heartburn, insomnia, fatigue, and loose stools. Stopping SJW 10 days before surgery is recommended due to the effect of the herb on heart rate and blood pressure with anesthesia. Adverse effects can include serotonin syndrome, photosensitivity, and induced mania similar to effects observed with SSRIs.[29] Induced mania occurs in individuals who have a bipolar history but is less likely to happen if the patient is on a mood stabilizer. Photosensitivity has been associated with a rash at the higher doses of a synthetic form of hypericin with HIV-positive patients.

Drug interactions are of concern, as SJW can induce the hepatic cytochrome P450 (CYP) 3A4 and CYP 1A2 enzymes. This can reduce the amount of active drug in the bloodstream of medications such as warfarin, digoxin, theophylline, cyclosporine, dextromethorphan, alprazolam, simvastatin, and oral contraceptives. Informing patients of the risk that SJW can reduce the concentration of other drugs is important. For example, the risk of pregnancy is higher if a young woman is on both birth control pills and SJW. Due to the complex chemistry of SJW, informing patients to *not* take SJW with MAOI antidepressants is recommended.

It is best to stop taking SJW during pregnancy, as safety data are limited about its potential impact on the growing fetus. SJW is currently classified as a Category C drug during pregnancy. Two case reports of SJW during pregnancy documented no observable adverse events. One case report noted that only hyperforin was excreted in human milk upon repeated testing. Neither hypericin nor hyperforin were found in the infant's plasma.[30] A cohort of 33 breastfeeding women on SJW in an observational study were followed for 2 years along with a group of 33 age-matched and parity-matched controls.[31] There were no significant differences in adverse events with the babies.[31] One case of colic was present in the control group.[31] The treatment group reported two cases of colic, one case of lethargy, and two cases of drowsiness.[31] None of the babies required medical treatment.[31]

CURCUMIN

The scientific name for curcumin is *Curcuma longa*, Zingiberaceae (ginger family). It is also referred to by other common names such as turmeric and Asian yellow spice, due to its orange-yellow color. It has a spicy, bitter taste. The active ingredients of curcumin are essential oil, valepotriates, and alkaloids. Clinically, curcumin stimulates blood flow, acts as an aromatic stimulant, regulates bile flow, relieves pain, and possesses antimicrobial properties.[32] The most commonly used part of the plant is the rhizome (underground stem), which is processed by grinding after drying. Turmeric can grow up to 5 feet with leaves resembling a lily. It has yellow flowers with a funnel shape in pairs near the leaf axils. Curcumin is the primary active curcuminoid ingredient present within turmeric, comprising 2%–8% of most turmeric preparations. It is a low molecular weight polyphenol.

Turmeric is primarily grown in China and India, where it is a common herb used daily in East Indian curries. It is often cooked with ghee or pepper, which aids in the absorption of the curcumin. In research trials, this preparation has been utilized to ensure the absorption of the herb. Curcumin has been part of the Ayurvedic and Chinese *Materia Medica* for thousands of years. In Chinese herbal therapy, turmeric has been specifically used to treat stress and depression as a major herb in Xiaoyao-san and Jieyu-wan.

BIOCHEMISTRY

The mechanism of action for curcumin appears to affect monoaminergic activity, oxidative pathways, the hypothalamic-pituitary-adrenal (HPA) axis, and immune/inflammatory pathways. In addition, it has a neuroprotective effect.[33] All these pathways have been the focus of recent research on depressive disorders. As curcumin influences all these pathways, interest has increased in this herb for the treatment of depression.

Several animal studies have shown that curcumin is a powerful antioxidant that lowers markers of oxidative stress.[34] In a study by Rinwa et al., rats with depression induced by olfactory bulbectomy and subsequent 2 weeks of curcumin and Piperin therapy exhibited neuroprotection through a possible curbing of oxidative-nitrosative stress induced neuroinflammation and apoptosis.[35] Modulation of inflammation as a COX-2 inhibitor has also been noted.[36] Neuroprotection and modulation of the HPA axis were findings from a study conducted by Huang et al. in 2011.[37] The investigators showed that curcumin significantly reduced depression-like behavior and brain-derived neurotrophic factor (BDNF) levels in rats with corticosterone-induced depression.[37] Also, curcumin has been demonstrated to have an increased effect on serotoninergic[38] and/or dopaminergic activity in several animal studies.[39] When serotonin receptors are pharmacologically blocked prior to curcumin administration, rats seem to lose the anti-immobility effect of curcumin on the forced swim test (FST).[40]

Additionally, curcumin appears to restore levels of serotonin and dopamine depleted in chronic stress situations.[41] Jiang et al. studied rats subjected to chronic mild stress for 21 days for induction of depression-like behavior.[42] Curcumin effectively inhibited cytokine gene expression with lower mRNA and protein expression and reduced activation of NF-kB, further showing its antidepressant effect.[42] Similarly, Bhutani et al. reported that curcumin significantly reversed chronic unpredictable stress-induced behavioral, biochemical, and neurochemical alterations.[43] Moreover, adult male Wistar Kyoto (WKY) rats were both acutely and chronically injected with curcumin by Hurley et al. in a 2013 study.[44] Helplessness was measured via open field locomotor activity and FST at 1 hour after the acute injection and 18–20 hours after the last chronic injection.[44] Results showed a dose-dependent reduction in immobility in FSTs both acutely and chronically.[44]

Most interestingly, animal models also provide evidence of neurogenesis in the frontal cortex and hippocampus.[41] This exciting research and its potential impact reach beyond treatment for depression. Patients with other disorders of the brain could potentially benefit from curcumin as well, including those with Alzheimer's disease, stroke, schizophrenia, epilepsy, Parkinson's disease, drug addiction, and aluminum toxicity.[41]

CLINICAL RESEARCH

Research studies have evaluated the benefits of curcumin in treating humans with depression. In one study, curcumin was used as an antidepressant augmentation with no treatment enhancement evident.[45] In another study by Sanmukhni et al., which utilized highly absorbed BCM-95, the effects of curcumin equaled the effects of fluoxetine without adverse effects.[46] A 6-week study divided 60 patients diagnosed with major depression into three groups. The first group was placed on fluoxetine 20 mg, the second group on BCM-95 curcumin 500 mg twice daily, and the third group received a combination of fluoxetine and BCM-95.[46] Utilizing the Hamilton Depression Scale, the response rate and mean results were about the same in all three groups, though slightly better in the combination group compared to individual treatment groups.[46] Then 75% of curcumin group and 70% of the fluoxetine group reported "good or excellent" results.[46] The conclusion of the study noted that curcumin was as effective as fluoxetine, with no adverse effects.[46]

Another randomized, double-blind 8-week study with 56 patients diagnosed with major depressive disorder (MDD) was conducted with two arms. Group 1 was placed on BCM-95 curcumin 500 mg twice a day, and group 2 was given placebo twice daily.[47] The Inventory of Depressive Symptomatology was used in a self-rated version.[47] Compared to those on placebo, patients on curcumin experienced improved mood at week 4 and until the end of the study.[47] One interesting finding was that those in the subgroup with atypical depression experienced even greater efficacy.[47]

An open label, 6-week study conducted by Panahi et al. (2014) utilized a curcuminoid-piperine preparation (that would allow for greater absorption of the herb) at a dose of 1000 and 10 mg for a group of 75 patients with MDD and compared results to those of a comparison group of 65 patients with MDD and on antidepressants.[48] Improvements were evident at the end of the 6-week trial in both groups on the Beck Depression Inventory (BDI-II) and the Hospital Anxiety and Depression Scale scores.[48] Significantly, the curcumin group showed greater improvement on both scales except in the affective subscale of the BDI-II.[48] Limitations with these studies include small sample size and relatively short treatment duration. Replications with larger sample sizes and for longer periods of time are needed in future research. Another area requiring further exploration is the optimal dose of curcumin due to concerns of bioavailability of this herb.

DOSAGE AND ADMINISTRATION

The many benefits of curcumin include anti-inflammatory effects, inhibition of enzymes that degrade neurotransmitters, modulation of serotonin, dopamine, and norepinephrine, and promotion of neurogenesis. Curcumin is currently dosed at 500 mg BMD-95 curcumin twice daily. It takes about a month for full benefits to be evident for a sustained improved mood. Ideal treatment duration is unknown at this time, as research is in the early stages. It is important to remember that turmeric, as a cooking herb, has been a part of the cuisine of East India for centuries. Because of its benefits, individuals may wish to add this spice to their daily diets along with a good oil and pepper to maximize absorption.

SAFFRON

The scientific name for saffron is *Crocus sativus* L., a plant that belongs to the Iridaceae family. It is generally referred to as saffron. The commonly used parts of the plant are the dried, orange-colored stigmas and purple petals. Saffron is classified as a bulbous perennial, primarily found in Southern Europe, Turkey, Iran, and Kasmir, India. It grows about 6–8 inches in height and prefers a cool, dry climate. It is harvested in the early morning hours. Of the active constituents present in its petals are flavonoids, tannins, and anthocyanins. Alkaloids and saponins, which are prepared by drying, are present in the stigma. Saffron has a very pleasant sweet aroma, often also utilized in commercial cosmetic and perfume products. It is one of the most expensive spices in the world, partly because of the labor-intensive nature of harvesting the plant. Three parts of the secondary metabolites impact the properties of the spice: crocin, which creates the color of the spice, safranal, which creates the odor, and picrocin, which creates the taste. Saffron possesses antispasmodic and antidepressant properties, increases blood flow, and can facilitate proper digestion. It is available for purchase via standardized capsules that include a ratio of 0.30–0.35 mg of safranal in 15 mg of saffron.

CLINICAL RESEARCH

Research began in 2001 to explore the efficacy of saffron compared to fluoxetine as an antidepressant in animal studies. Results have indicated that the effects of saffron are comparable to the effects of fluoxetine in diminishing depression. The crocin element of saffron alters the 5-HT_{2c} signaling pathway via antagonizing the effects of a piperazine, a serotonin receptor agonist in a rat model. The crocin content is believed to be the active ingredient of saffron as opposed to safranal.[49]

Several human clinical trials have been conducted. In 2005, a 6-week double-blind, randomized trial on 40 adult male and female outpatients ages 18–44 was conducted. Patients were randomly assigned to two different groups for receiving either 30 or 20 mg/day of fluoxetine.[50] The diagnosis was arrived via structured interviews using the HAM-D 17 item.[50] Individuals with mild to moderate depression (score of at least 18) were included.[50] Saffron was shown to be as effective as fluoxetine, and there was no significant difference in side effects between the two groups.[50] A similar 6-week double blinded randomized trial was conducted to compare saffron to imipramine in patients with MDD. Findings showed similar results. Saffron at 30 mg/day was as effective as imipramine at 100 mg/day for treating mild to moderate depression.[51] Saffron was also better toler-ated because it led to fewer side effects.

Saffron compared to standard fluoxetine therapy has been studied more recently (2014) in patients with depression induced by postpercutaneous coronary intervention.[52] No significant difference in the outcomes measured by the HAM-D was found between the group receiving saffron and the group receiving fluoxetine. The dose-dependent nature of saffron's efficacy reported in a 6-week randomized double-blind trial by Moosavi et al. in 2014 looking at efficacy of fluoxetine plus 40 mg of saffron versus fluoxetine plus 80 mg of saffron.[53] Although saffron was found to be effective in both groups, there was a greater decrease in HAM-D scores in the 80-mg saffron group compared to its counterpart receiving only 40 mg. In 2005, a placebo-controlled, double-blind, randomized trial was conducted with 40 patients over 6 weeks.[54] Patients were randomized to receive 30 mg/day of saffron or placebo. HAM-D scores were used to screen people for mild to moderate depression. At 6 weeks, the saffron group had significantly ($P < 0.001$) improved HAM-D scores compared to those patients on placebo.[54] No significant difference was noted in side effects.

Saffron has also been studied for its ability to relieve symptoms of premenstrual syndrome (PMS). In a double-blinded placebo-controlled trial, women received either 30 mg/day of saffron or placebo for two menstrual cycles.[55] Saffron was found to be effective in relieving symptoms of PMS. A significant difference was observed in the efficacy of saffron as measured by the Total Premenstrual Daily Symptoms and HAM-D.[55]

Studies have also been conducted with saffron petals, which are not traditionally used with a medicinal focus. The petals are much less expensive; thus, researchers explored their effective-ness as an antidepressant. In 2006, Moshiri et al. found in a randomized, double-blinded placebo controlled study that the petal was more effective than placebo 2 weeks into the study.[56] In a study comparing the saffron petal to fluoxetine, the petal was found to be as efficacious as fluoxetine, with improvement in both groups at week 1.[57]

Results suggest that saffron is a promising alternative for treating mild to moderate depression. All the trials were done in a relatively rigorous manner. Effect size was significant. In all the trials, nausea and headaches were the most common adverse events reported. As saffron is still in the pre-liminary stages of clinical research, questions remain about the most effective dosing. Each study did, however, limit the dose of saffron monotherapy to 30 mg. Other limitations of the above studies include small sample size, duration of only 6 weeks, site of the study, and third-party verification of composition and potency.[58]

DOSING AND ADMINISTRATION; SIDE EFFECTS AND TOXICITY

Saffron is dosed at 30 mg/day based on the research at this time. Long-term issues with the use of saf-fron beyond 6 weeks are not known for the treatment of mild to moderate depression. Toxicity occurs after ingestion of too high a dose (above 1200 mg/day) and presents with induction of nausea and vom-iting. Overdose has also been connected to stimulating abortions in women; thus, it is contraindicated in pregnancy. At high doses (200–400 mg), saffron has been shown to cause vaginal bleeding.

CONCLUSION

Botanicals contribute in diverse ways to support an individual's return to health. Including herbs in integrative treatment confers considerable benefit. Choosing which herbs to use depends on a number of factors. As research expands our current knowledge, we can expect a growing awareness of how these botanicals influence our physiology. In certain instances, long-term treatment with certain herbs beyond the resolution of depression may be suggested. Long-term use of a combina-tion of adaptogens is often the norm.

Original articles as well as recent meta-analyses make clear that over time the methodology in studying and practicing herbal medicine has improved immensely. The level one evidence for

St. John's wort allows clinicians to consider this botanical as a significant and potent option for the treatment of mild to moderate depression. However, greater replication of studies for the other herbs is needed. Currently only Level 2 evidence supports their use. The safety profile of these herbs suggests that thoughtful prescribing will provide patients with relief of depression with minimal to no adverse effects. Nevertheless, except for St. John's wort, all of the clinical trials testing other herbs have been of relatively short duration and enlisted small numbers of patients. Larger-scale studies of longer duration are needed.

Other factors also need to be addressed. Methods to control the quality and consistency of herbs need to be explored. Better understanding of all the variables that impact the phytochemistry of the plant will help scientists develop treatment profiles and allow for results to be reproduced.[58]

Some issues have not been addressed in randomized, controlled trials. Individualized variations such as age, gender, genetics, general health, and ethnicity are often not analyzed in these studies. Another concern is how to structure blind studies of herbal therapies to avoid biased conclusions. In any treatment protocol, the nutrition and lifestyle of the person also influence the outcome of treatment and may confound the conclusions.

Evidence from traditional medicine and clinical experience add to the valuable information gained from RCTs about botanical remedies. Increasing our knowledge base about these herbs, which have been used around the world since ancient times, will help clinicians better use botanical remedies as part of an integrative approach to treatment for depression and indeed explore their potential for treating other health conditions.

REFERENCES

1. Kessler, R.C., Soukup, J., Davis, R.B. et al. 2001. The use of complementary and alternative therapies to treat anxiety and depression in the United States. *Am J Psychiatry* 158(2): 289–294.
2. Winston, D. 2007. *Adaptogens: Herbs for Strength, Stamina, and Stress Relief.* Rochester, VT: Healing Arts Press.
3. Brekhman, I.I. and Dardymov, I.V. 1968. New substances of plant origin which increase nonspecific resistance. *Ann Rev Pharmacol* 8: 419–430.
4. Sarris, J., Panossian, A., Schweitzer, I. et al. 2011. Herbal medicine for depression, anxiety and insomnia: A review of psychopharmacology and clinical evidence. *Eur Neuropsychopharmacol* 21(12): 841–860.
5. Nierenberg, A.A., Burt, T., Matthews, T. et al. 1999. Mania associated with St. John's wort. *Biol Psychiatry* 46(12): 1707–1708.
6. Guzelcan, Y., Scholte, W.F., Assies, J. et al. 2001. Mania during the use of a combination preparation with St. John's wort (*Hypericum perforatum*). *Nederlands tijdeschrift voor geneeskunde* 145(40): 1943–1945.
7. Houghton, P. 2009. Synergy and polyvalence: Paradigms to explain the activity of herbal products. In *Evaluation of Herbal Medicinal Products.* Eds. P. Mukherjee and P. Houghton. London, UK: Pharmaceutical Press, pp. 85–94.
8. Wong, M.L., O'Kirwan, F., Hannestad, J.P. et al. 2004. St John's wort and imipramine-induced gene expression profiles identify cellular functions relevant to antidepressant action and novel pharmacogenetic candidates for the phenotype of antidepressant treatment response. *Mol Psychiatry* 9: 237–251.
9. Brown, R.P., Gerbarg, P.L., Ramazanov, Z. et al. 2002. *Rhodiola rosea*: A phytomedicinal overview. *Herbal Gram* 56: 40–52.
10. Panossian, A. and Wagner, H. 2005. Stimulating effect of adaptogens: An overview with particular reference to their efficacy following single dose administration. *Phytother Res* 19(10): 819–838.
11. Van Diermen, D., Marston, A., Bravo, J. et al. 2009. Monoamine oxidase inhibition by *Rhodiola rosea* L. roots. *J Ethnopharmacol* 122(2): 397–401.
12. Mattioli, L. and Perfumi, M. 2007. *Rhodiola rosea* L. extract reduces stress- and CRF-induced anorexia in rats. *J Psychopharmacol* 21(7): 742–750.
13. Petkov, V.D., Yonkov, D., Mosharoff, A. et al. 1986. Effects of alcohol aqueous extract from *Rhodiola rosea* L. roots on learning and memory. *Acta Physiol Pharmacol Bulg* 12(1): 3–16.
14. Saratikov, A.S. and Krasnov, E.A. 1987. Chapter III: Stimulative properties of *Rhodiola rosea*. In *Rhodiola rosea is a Valuable Medicinal Plant (Golden Root)*, Ed. A.S. Saratikov and E.A. Krasnov. Tomsk, Russia: Tomsk State University, pp. 69–90.

15. Brichenko, V.S., Kupriyanova, I.E., and Skorokhodova, T.F. 1986. The use of herbal adaptogens together with tricyclic antidepressants in patients with psychogenic depressions. In *Modern Problems of Pharmacology and Search for New Medicines*, Ed. E.D. Goldberg. Tomsk: Tomsk University Press, pp. 58–60.

16. Brichenko, V.S. and Skorokhodova, T.F. 1987. Herbal adaptogens in rehabilitation of patients with depression. In *Clinical and Organizational Aspects of Early Manifestations of Nervous and Mental Diseases*, Ed. E.D. Goldberg. Barnaul, pp. 1897–1815.

17. Darbinyan, V., Aslanyan, G., Amroyan, E. et al. 2007. Clinical trial of *Rhodiola rosea* L. extract SHR-5 in the treatment of mild to moderate depression. *Nord J Psychiatry* 61(6): 503.

18. Fintelmann, V. and Gruenwald, J. 2007. Efficacy and tolerability of a *Rhodiola rosea* extract in adults with physical and cognitive deficiencies. *Adv Ther* 24(4): 929–939.

19. Olsson, E.M., von Scheele, B., and Panossian, A.G. 2009. A randomized, double-blind, placebo-controlled, parallel-group study of the standardized extract shr-5 of the roots of *Rhodiola rosea* in the treatment of subjects with stress-related fatigue. *Planta Med* 75(2): 105–112.

20. Brown, R.P., Gerbarg, P.L., and Graham B. 2004. *The Rhodiola Revolution: Transform Your Health with the Herbal Breakthrough of the 21st Century*. New York, NY: St. Martin's Press, pp. 3–226.

21. Panossian, A. and Wikman, G. 2009. Evidence-based efficacy of adaptogens in fatigue, and molecular mechanisms related to their stress-protective activity. *Curr Clin Pharmacol* 4(3): 198–219.

22. Brown, R.P. and Gerbarg, P.L. 2009. Yoga breathing, meditation, and longevity. *Ann NY Acad Sci* 1172: 54–62.

23. Muller, W.E., Rolli, M., Schafer, C. et al. 1997. Effects of Hypericum extract (LI 160) in biochemical models of antidepressant activity. *Pharmacopsychiatry* 30(2): 102–107.

24. Bouron, A. and Lorrain, E. 2014. Cellular and molecular effects of the antidepressant hyperforin on brain cells: Review of the literature. *Encephale* 40(2): 108–113.

25. Vorbach, E.U., Arnoldt, K.H., and Hübner, W.D. 1997. Efficacy and tolerability of St. John's wort extract LI 160 versus imipramine in patients with severe depressive episodes according to ICD-10. *Pharmacopsychiatry* 30(2): 81–85.

26. Schrader, E. 2000. Equivalence of St John's wort extract (Ze 117) and fluoxetine: A randomized, controlled study in mild-moderate depression. *Int Clin Psychopharmacol* 15(2): 61–68.

27. Kasper, S., Anghelescu, I-G., Szegedi, A. et al. 2006. Superior efficacy of St John's wort extract WS® 5570 compared to placebo in patients with major depression: A randomized, double-blind, placebo-controlled, multi-center trial. *BMC Med* 4: 14.

28. Hypericum Depression Trial Study Group. 2002. Effect of *Hypericum perforatum* (St John's Wort) in major depressive disorder: A randomized controlled trial. *JAMA* 287(14): 1807–1814.

29. Lake, J. 2007. Integrative management of depressed mood. In: *Textbook of Integrative Mental Health Care*. Germany: Thieme. pp. 149–153.

30. Klier, C.M., Schmid-Siegel, B., Schafer, M.R. et al. 2006. St. John's wort (*Hypericum perforatum*) and breastfeeding: Plasma and breast milk concentrations of hyperforin for 5 mothers and 2 infants. *J Clin Psychiatry* 67(2): 305–309.

31. Lee, A., Minhas, R., Matsuda, N. et al. 2003. The safety of St. John's wort (*Hypericum perforatum*) during breastfeeding. *J Clin Psychiatry* 64(8): 966–968.

32. Tierra, M. 1992. Emmenagogues. In: *Planetary Herbology*. Twin Lakes, WI: Lotus Press. p. 274.

33. Lopresti, A.L., Hood, S.D., and Drummond P.D. 2012. Mulitple antidepressant potential modes of action of curcumin: A review of its anti-inflammatory, monoaminergic, antioxidant, immune-modulating and neuroprotective effects. *J Psychopharmacol* 26(12): 1512–1524.

34. Naik, S.R., Thakare, V.N., and Patil, S.R. 2011. Protective effect of curcumin on experimentally induced inflammation hypertoxicity and cardiotoxicity in rats: Evidence of its antioxidant property. *Exp Toxicol Pathol* 63(5): 419–431.

35. Rinwa, P., Kumar, A., and Garg, S. 2013. Suppression of neuroinflammatory and apoptotic signaling cascade by curcumin alone and in combination with piperine in rat model of Olfactory Bulbectomy induced depression. *Plos One* 8(4): 1–12.

36. Lee, K.H., Abas, F., Alitheen, N.B. et al. 2011. A curcumin derivative, 2,6-bis(2,5-dimethoxybenzylidene)-cyclohexanone (BDMC33) attenuates prostaglandin E2 synthesis via selective suppression of cycloxygenase-2 in IFN-γ/LPS-stimulated macrophages. *Molecules* 16(11): 9728–9738.

37. Huang, Z., Zhong, X-M., Li, Z-Y. et al. 2011. Curcumin reverses corticosterone-induced depressive-like behavior and decrease in brain BDNF levels in rats. *Neurosci Lett* 493(3): 145–148.

38. Kulkarni, S.K., Bhutani, M.K., and Bishnoi, M. 2008. Antidepressant activity of curcumin: Involvement of serotonin and dopamine system. *Psychopharmacology* 201(3): 435–442.

39. Xu, Y., Ku, B., Tie, L. et al. 2006. Curcumin reverses the effects of chronic stress on behavior, the HPA axis, BDNF expression and phosphorylation of CREB. *Brain Res* 1122(1): 56–64.

40. Wang, R., Xu, Y., Wu, H-L. et al. 2008. The antidepressant effects of curcumin in the forced swimming test involve 5-HT1 and 5-HT2 receptors. *Eur J Pharmoacol* 578(1): 43–50.

41. Kulkarni, S.K., Dhir, A., and Akula, K.K. 2009. Potentials of Curcumin as an antidepressant. *Sci World J* 9: 1233–1241.

42. Jiang, H., Wang, Z., Wang, Y. et al. 2013. Antidepressant-like effects of curcumin in chronic mild stress of rats: Involvement of its anti-inflammatory action. *Progr Neuro-Psychopharmacol Biol Psychiatry* 47: 33–39.

43. Bhutani, M.K., Bishnoi, M., and Kulkarni, S.K. 2009. Anti-depressant like effect of curcumin and its combination with piperine in unpredictable chronic stress-induced behavioral, biochemical, and neuro-chemical changes. *Pharmacol Biochem Behav* 92(1): 39–43.

44. Hurley, L.L., Akinfiresoye, L., Nwulia E. et al. 2013. Antidepressant-like effects of curcumin in WKY rat model of depression is associated with an increase in hippocampal BDNF. *Behav Brain Res* 239: 27–30.

45. Bergman, J., Miodownik, C., Bersudsky, Y. et al. 2013. Curcumin as an add-on to antidepressive treatment: A randomized, double-blind, placebo-controlled, pilot clinical study. *Clin Neuropharmacol* 36(3): 73–77.

46. Sanmukhani, J., Satodia, V., Trivedi, J. et al. 2014. Efficacy and safety of curcumin in major depressive disorder: A randomized controlled trial. *Phytother Res* 28(4): 579–585.

47. Lopresti, A.L., Maes, M., Maker, G.L. et al. 2014. Curcumin for the treatment of major depression: A randomised, double-blind, placebo controlled study. *J Affect Disord* 167: 368–375.

48. Panahai, Y., Badeli, R., Karami, G-R. et al. 2014. Investigation of the efficacy of adjunctive therapy with bioavailability-boosted curcuminoids in major depressive disorder. *Phytother Res* 29: 17–21.

49. Georgiadou, G., Tarantilis, A., and Pitsikas, N. 2012. Effects of the active constituents of *Crocus sativus* L., crocins, in an animal model of obsessive-compulsive disorder. *Neurosci Lett* 528: 27–30.

50. Noorbalaa, A.A., Akhondzadeha, S., Tahmacebi-Poura, N. et al. 2005. Hydro-alcoholic extract of *Crocus sativus* L. versus fluoxetine in the treatment of mild to moderate depression: A double-blind, randomized pilot trial. *J Ethnopharmacol* 97(2): 281–284.

51. Akhondzadeh, S., Fallah-Pour, H., Afkham, K. et al. 2004. Comparison of *Crocus sativus* L. and imipramine in the treatment of mild to moderate depression: A pilot double-blind randomized trial. *BMC Complement Altern Med* 4(12): 1–5.

52. Shahmansouri, N., Kassaian, S.E., Yekehtaz, H. et al. 2014. A randomized, double-blind, clinical trial comparing the efficacy and safety of *Crocus sativus* L. with fluoxetine for improving mild to moderate depression in post percutaneous coronary intervention patients. *J Affect Disord* 155: 216–222.

53. Moosavi, S.M., Ahmadi, M., Amini, M. et al. 2014. The effects of 40 and 80 mg hydro-alcoholic extract of *Crocus sativus* in the treatment of mild to moderate depression. *J Mazandaran Univ Med Sci* 24(113): 48–53.

54. Akhondzadeha, S., Tahmacebi-Pour, N., Amini, H. et al. 2005. *Crocus sativus* L. in the treatment of mild to moderate depression: A double-blind, randomized and placebo-controlled trial. *Phytother Res* 19(2): 148–151.

55. Agha-Hosseini, M., Kashani, L., Aleyaseen, A. et al. 2008. *Crocus sativus* L. (saffron) in the treatment of premenstrual syndrome: A double-blind, randomized and placebo-controlled trial. *Int J Obstetr Gynecol* 115(4): 515–519.

56. Moshiri, E., Basti, A.A., Noorbala, A.A. et al. 2006. *Crocus sativus* L. (petal) in the treatment of mild-to-moderate depression: A double-blind, randomized and placebo controlled trial. *Phytomedicine* 13(9–10): 607–611.

57. Akhondzadeh Basti, A., Moshiri, E., Noorbala, A.A., Jamshidi, A.H., Abbasi, S.H., and Akhondzadeh, S. 2007. Comparison of petal of *Crocus sativus* L. and fluoxetine in the treatment of depressed outpatients: A pilot double-blind randomized trial. *Prog Neuropsychopharmacol Biol Psychiatry* 31(2): 439–442.

58. Dwyer, A.V., Whitten, D.L., and Hawrelak, J.A. 2011. Herbal medicines, other than St. John's Wort, in the treatment of depression: A systematic review. *Altern Med Rev* 16(1): 40–49.

21 Exercise as an Adjunct to Treating Depression

Ralph E. Carson, LD, RD, PhD

CONTENTS

INTRODUCTION

Eight percent (1 in 12; 20 million) of Americans age 12 and over had moderate to severe depression during 2009–2012.[1] Only one in three of the severely depressed sought the services of a mental health professional. Experts agree that those with severe depression (3%) should be getting psychotherapy (CBT; interpersonal psychotherapy) and/or medication (selective serotonin reuptake inhibitors [SSRIs]). It is not something to be ignored, and a depressive state of mind greatly affects the way a person eats, feels, sleeps, thinks, and interacts with others. Therapy is, however, a long and challenging process. Medications are not always effective and are often fraught with side effects. Often there are problems that do not have solutions, and some forms of severe depression are not amenable to treatment. Exercise, fitness, or physical activity may have one of the widest ranges of effects we see with any treatments for depression.[2] It is worth investigating if exercise could be used together with pharmacotherapy and psychotherapy or as a stand-alone treatment for depression.

CLINICAL BENEFITS OF EXERCISE

A large number of studies over the last 30 years have shown that physical activity may reduce depression in healthy individuals and those diagnosed with major depressive disorder.[3–11] Depression is common in patients with heart disease and heart failure, and exercise resulted in moderate reduction in depressive symptoms.[12,13] Physically active severely obese candidates for gastric bypass surgery were 92% less likely to suffer depression, take antidepressants, or require counseling.[14] Progressive resistance exercise was effective as an anti-depressant in a 10-week randomized controlled trial of 60 and above volunteers with major and minor depression.[15] Many of the studies employ questionnaires such as the Beck Depression Inventory and Hamilton Rate Scale for Depression administered before and after several months of exercise and claim that there is marked improvement. In all reviewed reports, exercise produced meaningful reduction in depressed symptoms compared with psychological therapy (e.g., cognitive behavioral therapy [CBT]).[16–18]

ADOLESCENTS

Depression is the top cause of illness and disability among adolescents, and suicide is the third cause of death.[19] March and his group concluded that the combination of fluoxetine and CBT appears superior to either monotherapy as a treatment for moderate to severe major depressive disorder in adolescents.[20] It is important, however, to investigate alternative interventions in lieu of prescribing medications for depressed youths. Unfortunately there are only a few studies that investigated the effects of exercise in treating depression in 11–19 year olds. A 12-week intervention of supervised and independent aerobic exercise session showed a significant decrease in depressive symptoms of adolescents.[21] In middle-aged girls, fitness may be a strategy that improves self-esteem, weight management, and positive reinforcement.[22] Fitness levels predicted future depression in sixth-grade boys. Physical activity intervention among sedentary adolescent females enhanced global physical self-concept.[23,24] A study by Annesi on 28 girls and 26 boys (93% African American) ages 9–12 years showed that depression tended to decrease with exercise.[25] A study of 81 obese adolescents showed significant changes in physical self-worth, associated measures of self-esteem, and physical activity over time, consistently favoring exercise therapy.[26] An active lifestyle may be important to address in this age group since middle school is the time when fitness levels drop, weight begins to climb, and depression increases. A study by Callister presented at the 2013 Society for Neuroscience reported that physical workouts significantly boosted mood and cut the severity of depression by 63%.[27] It was also reported that 83% of the teens who completed the exercise program were no longer depressed by the end of the study. Together with antidepressant medication and CBT, exercise could contribute significantly to depression. The few existing studies have been criticized because of the small numbers, diversity of participants, and poor methodologies. A review of nine studies drew limited value and concluded that the benefits are unknown as evidence is scarce.[28]

PHARMACEUTICAL THERAPIES

Aerobic exercise has been proposed as a potential treatment for depression and may be comparable with established pharmaceutical therapies. Studies on mice and rats showed better antidepressant effects with exercise than imipramine (TCA; Tofranil®). There were also significant changes in norepinephrine, serotonin, and BDNF similar to those seen with the tricyclic antidepressant.[29,30] In a 1999 Duke study, there was an increase in those no longer having symptoms using either sertraline (Zoloft®) (57%) or exercise (47%) after 4 months of treatment. Both groups had similar improvement in depressive symptoms.[31] In a later study, Blumenthal divided volunteers into four groups. After 4 months researchers recorded those no longer meeting criteria for major depressive disorder (MDD): supervised exercise 45%; home-based exercise 40%, sertraline 47%, and placebo 30%. An earlier study demonstrated exercisers had better long-term outcomes after 10 months than those taking antidepressants.[32] Though a small (17 participant) pilot study showed that exercise is an effective augmentation treatment for antidepressant,[33] most studies do not support the possibility that exercise and medication together have an additive effect.[34] What was notable in the Babyak study was that antidepressant drugs may in fact blunt the benefit of exercise when combined. There was a slight reduction in the remission from depression when sertraline was combined with exercise. Chalder reported in a 2012 study involving 361 adults for 8 months that the addition of physical activity intervention to the usual prescribed care did not improve depression (Beck Depression Inventory) or reduce the use of antidepressants.[35] To date there is no evidence supporting a combination of CBT, antidepressants, and exercise produce greater effectiveness than used individually.

META-ANALYSIS AND REVIEWS

A series of reviews report that exercise produces meaningful reduction in depressed symptoms. Exercise is certainly more effective than no treatment at all and is often reported to be as effective as traditional treatments. The use of exercise in lieu of antidepressants or therapy may appear viable based on the number of studies supporting its value, but researchers warn that we need to exercise caution when interpreting these results.[36] Lawler analyzed 14 studies in 2001 and concluded that exercise's benefit could not be determined due to a lack of quality research.[37] Strothopoulou (11 studies) and Sjosten (13 studies) both concluded that exercise helped in the short term and in older subjects, but more well-controlled studies were needed since the conclusions were unclear and the reliability of the studiers were questionable.[17,38,39] Blake (11 random controlled studies) found that exercise was relevant to the aged, yet there was a need for more long-term studies.[40] Using the Cochrane Database (25 randomly controlled trials) Mead questioned whether exercise was a strong contributor to reducing depressive symptoms and if there was true efficacy.[18] Krough (13 trials) admitted that over the short term, exercise was beneficial, but there was little evidence that the same was true over the long term.[41] Rimer (32 trials) concluded that improvement due to exercise was better than no treatment, but the studies reviewed were too small and not robust.[42] Though several studies reported significant effect of exercise reducing depression, the few high-quality robust studies reviewed were less conclusive. Researchers argued that there was a lack of high-quality robust research and a great need for high-quality rigorously controlled trials.[18] An updated Cochrane Review summarizes these analysis by concluding the overall benefit from exercise is small and when compared to psychological and pharmacological therapies, exercise seems to be no more effective.[18] Mura's review (46 papers reviewed) continues to confirm that there has been little progress in proving that exercise improves depression since Lawler's 2001 meta-analysis.[43] Josefsson (89 reviewed; 13 qualified randomized control trials [RCTs]) showed a large overall effect for exercise in those with mild to moderate depression when participants were willing, motivated, and physically healthy enough to participate.[44] The truth is that exercise is somewhere in the middle, and we are still waiting for quality studies using better methodologies. If exercise is used therapeutically for depression, currently it is better to combine it with other treatments. However, since exercise is better than no treatment at all, it would seem to be a reasonable adjunct to treatment as it costs little, rarely produces harmful side effects, and promotes physical health and well-being.

METHODOLOGY

The problems that arise when reviewing the studies of depression and exercise are the methodological limitations. Many of the studies are either not a blinded design or lack randomization. Often, self-reported questionnaires are used to assess severity of symptoms (mild, moderate, or major depressive disorder) instead of clinical interviews. This prevents the ability to assess adequately the psychiatric disorder. Frequently what was being assessed was mood improvement, quality of life, psychological well-being, anxiety, self-esteem, and/or cognitive capacity. Such measurements may have implications that include depression but are not necessarily clear indicators of depressive symptoms. Depending on the psychometric tool utilized, there can be an overestimation of treatment effects. Furthermore, there are a multitude of complex factors that can contribute to the interpretation of outcomes which include age, gender, genetics, personality, poverty, violence, body image issues, self-esteem, negative thinking patterns, poor coping skills, difficult life events, support or lack thereof from family and friends, psychological co-morbidities, and pre-existing health conditions (i.e., heart condition, obesity, etc.).

A depressed individual's lethargy and lack of interest in anything would be a deterrent to exercising.[45] Having the motivation to engage in exercise may indicate that the depression has begun to subside rather than the exercise improved the depression. It is likely that individuals volunteering for such a study would include those who have a previous interest in activity or are already emerging from their depression. The outcomes may be a product of providing opportunities to master a skill or being associated with a group of like-minded people.

PLACEBO EFFECT

Mild to moderate depression may respond to low levels of activity simply because of placebo effect.[46-48] Mindset is a contributor as indicated by a housekeeping staff that were told that they were satisfying recommendations for an active lifestyle by cleaning hotel rooms. Compared to the control group, they showed a decrease in weight, body fat, waist-to-hip ratio, and body mass index (BMI). Meta-analysis has shown that people get better on both antidepressant medications and placebo, and the difference is small.[49] This mindset could also play a role in the effect of exercise on depression. Hopelessness is at the core of depression, and the potential that exercise frees one from his or her intolerable condition offers hope.

DOSE RESPONSE

In some instances, improvement was directly related to the higher intensity of exercising,[50] or a greater level of fatigue following exercise.[51-53] The higher the dose of exercise (frequency and duration), the lower the relapse rates of patients with MDD.[54,55] One study claimed that a single workout at moderate to high intensity boosted mood (less fatigue, tension, distress, and anger) in depressed patients.[56,57] Ten days was found to be sufficient to achieve substantial improvement in mood.[58] Another study described that exercising three times per week decreased the odds of developing depression by approximately 16%.[59] Every extra weekly activity session the risk drops further by 6% and adds to the overall benefit. The amount of time it takes to see improvement ranged from a single bout,[56] to 10 days,[58] to 6 weeks,[60] to 10 weeks,[61] to 4 months[32] before significant changes in depression occurred.

The improvement in depressive symptoms indicated by most studies was not correlated with either strength training or cardiovascular fitness. Mead suggested that a combination of resistance training and endurance activities reduced depression more than aerobic exercises alone.[18] Supervised (clinically based) had the same effect as unsupervised (home based).[62] The effect of exercise on depression was the same for those in a group setting as in an individual setting.[11] Resistance or aerobic exercises were both equally effective over a 2-month trial.[46,47] In 30 different trials it mattered little how long, how frequently, or the amount of intensity exerted.[45,63] Dunn did show that exercising at a high energy level (17.5 kcal/kg) and high frequency (two to five times per week) reduced depressive symptoms better than less frequent and low energy (<7 kcal/kg).[47] But other studies found that those who engage in leisure time activity at any intensity were less likely to have symptoms of depression.[64] There is no denying that the contribution of exercise results in some improvement of physical and mental health.[65] Poor physical fitness leads to ill health, and ill health can lead to depression. What matters is continued long-term fitness and maintaining a healthy mind and body. For long-lasting results, one will need to make long-term fitness a commitment.[66,67]

Dunn suggests that aerobic exercise at a dose consistent with public health recommendations is an effective treatment for mild to moderately severe depression. A lower dose would be comparable to a placebo.[46,47] The National Institutes of Health support the importance of exercise in managing depression and has established guidelines that call for a structured supervised exercise program. As a step 2 intervention for mild to moderate depression the recommendations are three times a week with each session lasting 45 minutes to an hour.[68,69] Similarly, there are mental health guidelines which recommend either 150 minutes of moderate or 75 minutes of vigorous exercise per week. These sessions should be in bouts of at least 25 minutes over a 3- to 5-day period per week.[70,71]

METHODS OF THERAPEUTIC EFFECT

SEROTONIN

With the advent of microdialysis, researchers have begun to measure neurotransmitter changes in live specimens, including their breakdown (metabolism) and release.[72–74] Serum levels of serotonin (5HT) increase with exercise training.[75–78] Brain serotonergic neurons regulate emotions and produce a calming and centered effect.[79] One possibility is that there is increased synthesis (manufacturing) of serotonin by neurons.[80–82] There may be enhancement of serotonin uptake by the postreceptor neurons as exercise makes them supersensitive to serotonin.[76] At the onset, there is inhibition and reduction of the receptors (5-HT2C) that will take the neurotransmitter back up into the nerve that originally secreted the serotonin.[83] Exercise has been demonstrated to reduce reuptake receptors of the 5-HT2C receptors that play an important role in the pathogenesis of anxiety and depression.[84]

The precursor of serotonin is an amino acid called tryptophan (Jacobs '99[85]; Young '07[86]). Proteins are composed of a string of amino acids much like words are a combination of letters. During exercise there is an increase of the precursor tryptophan that continues to persist after exercise.[87] Motor activity (movement) increases the synthesis and firing rate of serotonin (Reuter '96[88]). There is more of the breakdown product of serotonin (5HIAA) in the cerebral spinal fluid and greater concentrations of serotonin in the hippocampus and frontal cortex.[89–91] At rest, tryptophan competes for entry into the brain with other amino acids (Branch Chain Amino Acids: BCAA [isoleucine, leucine, and valine]). However, the demand for BCAAs when muscles are actively engaged causes the ratio of TRP:BCAA to favor tryptophan.[92]

The decrease in function of serotonin in the hippocampus may be a malfunction of the 5HT-1A receptors in the raphe nucleus.[93] Depression may result from desensitization of these receptors and transmission of serotonin in the hippocampus, prefrontal cortex, and amygdala pathways. Rats were exposed to stress either by forced swimming or elevated plus maze. Depression was ameliorated by administration of exercise. Chronic exercise may improve the disturbances of 5HT-1A regulated signaling in depressed brains and thereby exert antidepressant activity and adaptation to stress.[94]

Exercise increases serotonin levels that last up to one hour after the workout but may not have a long-lasting effect on depression. Recent studies show months after the intervention has ended patients are just as depressed as those who did not participate.[95] This suggests that one must continue to be active to experience the antidepressant effects. In the Duke studies, those who continued to exercise after completion of the initial 16-week study were much less likely to see depression return than other patients.[96,97] Only 8% of the exercise group had their depression return, while 38% of the antidepressant drug only group relapsed. There are numerous studies that suggest that exercise might be considered as a substitute for antidepressants (SSRIs) in mild to moderate depression.[98–103] The advantages of exercise are even more refreshing in light of the risk-benefit profile (antidepressant carry side effects) for some users of the drugs. Yet many experts including the National Institute of Mental Health view the benefit of reducing depression through exercise with skepticism and caution recommending it as a stand-alone treatment for depression.[33,94,104]

NOREPINEPHRINE

Norepinephrine is increased by exercise in several brain areas.[105] The neuromodulator norepinephrine helps the brain deal with stress more efficiently. Scientist think exercise thwarts depression and anxiety by enhancing the body's ability to respond to stress.[106–108] Exercise gives the body the opportunity to deal with a sublethal stress by coordinating the sympathetic nervous system. The more sedentary we are, the less efficient we are at handling stress.

PHENYLETHYLAMINE

Phenyethylamine (PEA) is an endogenous neurotransmitter known to decrease depression and increase energy.[109,110] PEA has been discovered to be decreased in people who are depressed.[111,112] By increasing the release and preventing the reuptake of norepinephrine back into the nerve that releases NOR (presynaptic nerve), there is a cascade effect to the reward pathway that induces feelings of excitement and euphoria through activation of PEA.[113] Moderate exercise raises PEA, and some researchers have linked PEA to the therapeutic effect of exercise on depression and addiction.[111,112]

CORTISOL

Appropriate response to emotional stress is indispensable for humans to avoid threats and survive. Uncontrollable anxiety and chronic stress can induce general anxiety disorders and depression. Corticotrophic-releasing factor (CRF) or corticotrophic-releasing hormone (CRH) may be responsible for the stress response to cope with dangerous situations. CRF is secreted as a result of fear and anxiety rather than the cause.[114] Corticotropin-releasing hormone (CRH) plays a central role in the regulation of the hypothalamic-pituitary-adrenal (HPA) axis (i.e., the final common pathway in the stress response).[115–117] Animal and cell-culture research show very convincingly that cortisol (CRH, glucocorticoids, corticosterone) can increase neurotoxicity.[118–128] Corticotropin-releasing factor (CRF) is considered as the central driving force in the stress response and plays a key role in the pathogenesis of depression.[129] Since the highest cortisol levels and CRF neurons are found in the prefrontal cortex (a brain region that is highly associated with the control of emotion and cognition) and the hippocampus, this may explain the pathogenesis of depression.[130]

Glucocorticoid stress hormones target medial prefrontal cortex (mPfC). Additionally, either chronic stress or chronic administration of glucocorticoids produce rewiring of the circuits (dendritic remodeling).[131,132] The hippocampus of animals (rats and primates) is particularly vulnerable to metabolic insults (prolonged stress, starvation, alcoholism, and drug abuse) and glucocorticoid toxicity.[133,134] This may be a function of cortisol preventing uptake of glucose and glutamate by hippocampal neurons,[135,136] producing damage to nerve branches (dendrites).[137] The hippocampus mediates negative feedback (controls the shutting off of cortisol secretion by the hypothalamus) by turning off further release of cortisol. A reduction of hippocampal neurons would decrease the signal to turn down cortisol production resulting in continuation of neurotoxicity.[138] These findings have significance for disorders such as depression and the presence of elevated glucocorticoids. An inhibitor of CRF (CRFR-1 antagonist) could be useful for treating or preventing the consequences of CRF-mediated stress in depression.[139]

The corticosteroid neurotoxicity hypothesis is not always supported by clinical and experimental observations. Postmortem autopsies in patients treated with corticosteroids (prednisone, cortisone)[138] and patients who had been seriously and chronically depressed showed no indications of massive cell loss or loss of plasticity.[140,141] Particularly absent were massive cell losses in the hippocampus following exposure to stress or steroids.

What may be at play are the same adaptive and reversible changes that were seen in the athlete who is chronically exposed to physical stress. Exercise and cortisol have a complex relationship.[142–144] Both emotional and physical stress can trigger the brain to release more cortisol. Low-intensity exercise decreases circulating cortisol levels, but cortisol may rise after moderate- and high-intensity exercise.[145] Consistent training allows the body (adrenal gland) to adapt to physical stress, so after a bout of intense exercise athletes do not have higher circulating levels of cortisol.[146] Physical activity also helps control cortisol by promoting restful sleep.[147] Exercise combined with stress management (cognitive behavioral therapy, deep breathing, meditation, yoga) are major contributors of reducing stress which are major determinants of cortisol.[148–151] Excess cortisol is responsible for the accumulation of fat around the abdominal organs.[152–154] This distribution of fat is a major contributor to inflammation as a deterrent to brain functioning and repair.[155]

β-Endorphins

β-Endorphins are morphine-like derivatives that are manufactured by human cells. The β-endorphins are manufactured in the pituitary and spinal cord and act peripherally to reduce pain. Within the hypothalamus of the brain there is an area called the arcuate nucleus that produces a substance called POMC (proopiomelanocortin). From this POMC molecule, beta-endorphin is broken off (cleaved) and circulates in the brain capable of attaching to specific receptors (mu-receptors). Once β-endorphin locks onto the mu-receptor it triggers dopamine to be released (actually by inhibiting its inhibitor GABA). The dopamine release is rewarding and often simulates a feeling of euphoria which is referred to by joggers as "runner's high." Exercising continuously for a long time at very high intensity can activate endorphin production.[156,157] Often this level of exercise is at the physical limit when stored muscle energy is depleted (glycogen) and the body is in jeopardy of physical harm. Due to the output of the analgesic endorphins, the runner can continue further without experiencing pain.[158] Treadmill exercise reduced self-administration of morphine (endorphin-like) in male rats.[159] Hippocampal cells which add to neuroplasticity are activated by beta-endorphins during running.[160]

Changes in peripheral beta-endorphins are normally associated with pain perception and mood states. Studies show that exercise above the anaerobic threshold or extended aerobic workout (more than one hour) cause a proportionate increase in lactate, cortisol, and β-endorphins. This combined rise has led some to support a possible link with cortisol and beta-endorphins, though the relationship is not entirely clear.[161]

Changes in mood state occur when a person exercised with an opiate blocker (naloxone or naltrexone) of the mu receptor.[162] Naltrexone is known to block the release of endorphins. Increased endorphins are seen as a response to exercise and in turn produce positive mood changes. However, when preloaded with naltrexone, positive changes in mood were not observed.[163] This supports the theory that mood change was mediated through endogenous endorphins.

There are many that question if endorphins accurately explain how exercise creates the so-called "runner's high." The high may come from completing a challenge or achieving a goal such as finishing a marathon.[164] Usually the effort level (intensity and duration) recommended in treatment programs is not intense enough to trigger endorphin output. These considerations beg one to wonder if it is other neurotransmitters that are more involved: dopamine, serotonin, galanin, or norepinephrine.

DOPAMINE

Physical activity produces beneficial changes in the dopamine system which includes increased dopamine signaling.[165] Invigorating and joy-filled bouts of exercise are beneficial because they stimulate the brain reward pathways, thereby balancing off an unpleasant experience with a pleasant experience. Running is rewarding and has antidepressant effects in rodents.[166] Running causes neurochemical and morphological adaptations in the brain reward pathways of the hippocampus and addictive drugs. In this way exercise has the potential to substitute for inappropriate behaviors (sexual compulsivity, binge eating, alcohol and drug addiction) as a natural substitute because it stimulates many of the same motivational circuits.[167–169] Microdialysis (measuring brain chemicals) studies have found that exercise increases both dopamine levels and the number of dopamine receptors in the rat brain nucleus accumbens (reward center).[170–172] The dopamine system creates an independent positive reinforcement to continue exercise. The increased dopamine availability may pertain to a performance enhancing effect mediated by improvements in heat tolerance. This added heat is due to the increased metabolic rate induced by exercise.[173] The hyperthermic effect also produces a more relaxed peripheral musculature and thus a sense of physical calm that may continue for hours after exercise.[174] There are varying reports of how dopamine response to exercise may play out to curb addictive behaviors. Compulsive exercise is effective in curbing the reward efficacy of Ecstasy, perhaps by reversing the stimulation of dopamine release in the nucleus accumbens.[175] However, in a well-designed study, although subjects exercised vigorously for 30 minutes, no significant changes were observed in the nucleus accumbens that were large enough to detect with positron emission tomography (PET) scan.[176] The dopamine system does not act in isolation and is affected by interaction with other neurotransmitters.

ALTERING BRAIN ARCHITECTURE: NERVE REGENERATION AND NEUROPLASTICITY

Neuroimaging has verified that depression causes the loss (atrophy) of nerve cells and rewiring of circuits throughout the brain. The hippocampus and frontal cortex are critical to mood stabilization, learning, and memory.[177,178] The hippocampus and frontal cortex seem to be particularly susceptible to breakdown during times of stress.[133] Cortisol is a glucocorticoid that mediates and contributes to neural remodeling and ultimately cell death (neurotoxicity).[179–181] Chronic stress keeps our brains continuously exposed to the stress hormones, inhibits neurogenesis,[182] and prunes dendrites.[183] The overall signaling capacity of the neural circuits (synaptic plasticity) is compromised leading to the inability to cope appropriately with stress.

BRAIN-DERIVED NEUROTROPHIC FACTOR AND VGF NERVE GROWTH FACTOR

Alteration of synaptic receptors dictates the strength of communication between two neurons. This synaptic plasticity can be improved at multiple sites throughout the brain, including the hippocampus and frontal cortex.[184–187] Exercise can mend the circuitry and stimulate growth of neurons and its branches (dendrites).[188–193] There is significant increase of growth factors (brain-derived neurotrophic factor [BDNF] and VGF nerve growth factor) that affect nerve signaling and synaptic strength.[194–199] BDNF is a biomarker for depression treatment. Serum BDNF normalizes in depressed humans who have been successfully treated and are no longer depressed. Several studies including the Treatment with Exercise Augmentation for Depression (TREAD) have demonstrated exercise limits the synaptic alteration during stress exposure.

Depressive disorders may be linked to a decrease in hippocampal neurogenesis.[200] Exercise upregulates neurotrophic factor signaling cascades which are implicated in their role as antidepressants.[201,202] The gene that encodes for VGF nerve growth factor influences homeostasis, metabolism, and synaptic plasticity.[197] Peptide precursors of VGF injected into the mouse brain produced antidepressant effects in the animal.[192] Brain-derived neurotrophic factor (BDNF) is a peptide that stimulates cells (stem cells; amplified progenitor cells [AMPC]) in the hippocampus to proliferate and migrate to the left prefrontal cortex (associated with positive mood state).[203–205] An individual can have a more active left prefrontal cortex which makes him or her less apt to be depressed.[206] Through promoting hippocampal neurogenesis, BDNF triggers dendritic remodeling and reduces depression.[207–210] Both exercise and antidepressants produced significant changes when antidepressants alone failed.[201] Together with reboxetine (norepinephrine reuptake inhibitor class of antidepressants), exercise led to rapid (detectable in 2 days and sustained 20 days) increase in hippocampal BDNF mRNA expression in young and aged rats.[211]

ENDOCANNABINOIDS

The endocannabinoid system is best known for its euphoric response resulting from exposure to Δ9-tetra-hydro-cannabinoids or marijuana. Exercise activates the endocannabinoid system. The brain's endocannabinoid system is believed to be a site where exercise induces positive alterations such as an improved sense of well-being, reduction of anxiety, and lowering of pain perception (analgesia).[212] This area of the hypothalamus may also participate in the regulation and motivation of physical activity and hippocampal neurogenesis.[213] When mice were genetically altered so they had no functioning endocannabinoid receptors, they ran half as much as usual. Rats love to run, but apparently, when there is no internal message to the reward pathway, there is less of a thrill and the rats do not indulge as much.[214]

BDNF is a major candidate for exercise-induced neuroplasticity. Endocannabinoid signaling is important for mood improvement. The endocannabinoid system has a positive effect on depression as a result of BDNF.[215] The endocannabinoid (anandamide) and BDNF were highly correlated during and 15 minutes after exercise. Anandamide produced during exercise may be itself initially triggered by cortisol. Since corticosteroids are known to stimulate endocannabinoid synthesis, then exercise may be a stressor that enables the body to increase its peripheral level of anandamide.[216] Thus, exercise and endogenous cannabinoids independently regulate hippocampal plasticity.[217] An increase in endocannabinoid signaling in the hippocampus is required for exercise-induced cell proliferation.[218]

GROWTH HORMONE

Exercise has been effective in increasing synaptic plasticity by directly affecting synaptic structures and potentiating synaptic strength. By strengthening the underlying systems that support plasticity, neurogenesis, metabolism, and vascular function, there is an added resistance to depression. A blunted growth hormone and prolactin response to pharmacological stress test have previously been found in depressed patients. Exercise's influence on growth hormone instructs downstream structural and functional changes. Inflammation impairs growth factor signaling. Patients with mild to moderate depression had a different growth hormone and cortisol response to acute exercise stress compared to healthy controls.[219] Strength training was able to reduce the growth hormone response to acute exercise stress in this patient population.[220]

GALANIN

Beyond the scope of this chapter, there is a known interaction of galanin and norepinephrine that is related to behavioral responses commonly seen with stress and drug abuse.[221] Galanin is known to increase during exercise[222] and may reduce drug cravings by preventing overactivation of norepineph-rine.[223] Any mechanism that lowers cravings would substantially contribute to preventing relapse.

GENETICS

The effect of exercise on depression may not be the same for everyone as genetics may deter-mine who benefits and by how much.[224,225] Looking at pairs of identical twins in which one twin exercises significantly more than the other, there was no significant difference in their level of happiness[226] nor difference in their anxious and/or depressive symptoms.[227] The real possibility exists that depression and anxiety prevent people from exercising. These are not the people who are typically going to volunteer to participate in exercise studies. Those who engage in exercise might provide evidence that the depression has mitigated rather than exercise is the cause of the improve-ment. There were fewer mood symptoms in exercising identical twins than were found in fraternal twins.[228] Depressed patients may need to be screened and prescribed individualized exercise rou-tines that fit their psyche and personality with regard to intensity, competitiveness, and choices. It is clearly important that whatever activity you pursue brings you joy and satisfaction. If you don't enjoy what you are doing, you won't feel better when you are through.[229] Such insight might enhance adherence to fitness recommendations.

INFLAMMATION

Depression has a significant inflammatory component. In any given 5-year span there are ample peer-reviewed scientific journal articles extolling how exercise ameliorates every ailment from the 10 leading causes of death to gum disease and even decreased libido. The mechanism by which exercise acts as a universal healing pathway for almost every chronic ailment is rather simple. It is frequently reported that stress is responsible for 90% of all primary care visits, obesity is the second leading cause of preventable death, and diabetes represents the nation's highest health-care cost. The common link of stress (cortisol), obesity (visceral adipose tissue or VAT), and diabetes (insulin resistance or IR) is that they all trigger "chronic inflammation." Cortisol (stress), excess fat (VAT), and sugar (IR) stimulate receptors on most cells to free up NF-kB (nuclear factor light chain–enhancing kappa B) allowing it to enter the cell nucleus (cytosol) and turn on (gene transcription) the production of inflammatory cytokines (CRP, IL-6, TNF-α, etc.). It follows that as exercise alleviates stress, reduces abdominal fat, and controls blood sugar, there is a clear pathway to its reduction of all chronic debilitating disease. There is evidence that activity reduces production of the inflamma-tory products (eicosanoids and cytokines) as well as reduces the biomarkers for inflammation (such as highly sensitive C-reactive protein).[229] Inflammation can impair growth factor signaling both systemically and in the brain which will eventually have an effect on depression.[186]

KYNURINE

In a study on mice, after 5 weeks of normal stress, the mice developed depression. However, the well-conditioned mice had no depressive symptoms despite being exposed to stress. The finding help explain the protective effect of exercise with regard to depression.[230] The protein kynurine is formed during stress and found in patients with mental illness. The exact function of kynurine is unknown but may have implications for triggering inflammation. KAT is an enzyme that converts kynurine into kynuric acid which cannot cross the blood-brain barrier to produce negative brain changes. By blocking the transport of kynurin, the resulting metabolite cannot cause inflammation with the brain which would lead to depression. High levels of PGC-1α1 in skeletal muscle also show high levels of KAT enzyme. PGC-1α1 increases in skeletal muscles during exercise. In this way, exercise induces changes in skeletal muscle that cause them to perform like the liver or kidney in detoxifying the blood. Ultimately, exercise protects the brain from stress-induced disease.

Tryptophan is the monoamine that is converted to serotonin in the brain. Serotonin allows the body to become calm and centered (antidepressant action). In times of stress, the liver converts more tryptophan to kynurine which can cross the blood-brain barrier to create inflammation. Inflammation can decrease synaptic plasticity and reduce neurotrophic factors (BDNF) that offer resilience to depression. Exercise (resistance training or endurance activation) increases the gene expression of PGC-1α1 gene. The resulting increase in the KAT enzyme converts the kynurine into a product (kynuric acid) that is inhibited from entering the brain.

BEHAVIORAL CHANGES

SLEEP

Slow-wave sleep (delta wave or stages III and IV) is the most reparative type of sleep and can be increased through regular aerobic exercise.[231] When the brain is in slow-wave sleep there is lower energy expenditure, lower oxygen consumption, and lower body heat content.[232] Exercise lowers REM (dream) sleep or keeps it the same while simultaneously increasing deep sleep.[233] Many studies support one major benefit of exercise is enhancing and increasing restorative sleep.[234-237] During restorative sleep the body releases growth hormone which helps the body (and brain) to heal and muscles to grow. Similar improvements in sleep allow the body to truly rest and to feel more awake and energized the following day.

The body generates energy (ATP adenosine triphosphate) by combustion of fuels such as carbohydrates, fat, and protein. As the molecules of adenosine accumulate, they eventually will command the sleep center of the brain to slow down and rest.[238] The more one is active the greater amount of ATP produced. The accumulation over the course of a day contributes to sleep quantity and quality.[239] Another contribution of exercise to sleep concerns its ability to elevate core body temperature. We burn a lot of energy while engaged in exercise, and that energy also generates heat. The elevation of heat by itself may have a calming effect. It takes the body hours to cool down by tiny degrees in order to return to baseline. Yet it is the falling curve of cooling body temperature that invites sleep onset. In a study conducted by Giselle Passo, after moderate aerobic exercise there were reductions in sleep onset latency (40%–54%) and fewer wake time (36%) as well as increase in total sleep time (21%–37%), and improved sleep efficiency (18%).[240]

DISTRACTION HYPOTHESIS, SELF-EFFICACY THEORY, AND MASTERY HYPOTHESIS

Focusing your mind on something other than your problems is going to make you feel better.[18] Exercise is a distraction that can get you away from the cycle of negative thoughts that feed anxiety and depression (Distraction Hypothesis). Participation in various physical outlets is a viable and healthy replacement that generates positive self-worth, self-image, and self-control. Meeting exercise goals or challenges, even small ones, can boost your self-confidence. As one acquires confidence to perform certain physical skills, his or her self-esteem is raised and depression lessons (Self-efficacy Theory).[241] Physical activity activates willpower (desire, motivation) and self-awareness, and commands one's mental resources and strengths. Such accomplishments produce a feeling of mastery (Mastery Hypothesis).[242]

Sometimes this course of events is described as the "positive confidence cycle." Participating in a novel and meaningful activity can produce a sense of accomplishment.[18] Say I begin lifting weights and within a week I can lift 10 pounds more than when I started. The outcome of improved strength is guaranteed. While working out there is the likelihood that I will interact with others at the gym, and mutual sharing of a common interest generates social acceptance. Now that I am lifting weights and feeling better, I also consider quitting smoking, eating better, and reducing stress. This progressive domino effect of lifestyle change is often referred to as the *halo effect*. The cycle is complete when one has acquired self-confidence through self-efficacy.

There are investigations that explain exercise increases sensitivity of the right brain hemisphere which is associated with feelings of tranquility and nonlinear thinking.[243]

Exercise has been demonstrated to stimulate the release of the calming neurotransmitter serotonin and extends the time of attachment to receptors in the emotional (limbic system) area of the brain's meso-cortex. When one participates in boring, monotonous, and repetitive activity, there is a tendency to ventilate negative thoughts. This "letting go" during a conscious state allows us to create solutions to our problems and connect with pleasurable experiences. Failure to release stress by internalizing problems will eventually allow them to surface during the unconscious stages of sleep and disallow proper sleep architecture. This shows up as diminished restorative sleep (stages III and IV) when the body truly rests and repairs.

SOCIALIZATION

Exercise reduces the likelihood of psychological stress, but this may be a result of incidental socialization.[244] Due to the interactive nature of exercising in a group or with friends, one must consider exercise in a social context as contributing to a reduction in depression. Social benefits and the context of exercise participation are important in explaining the relationship of exercise, moods, and depression.[245] One 12-week randomized controlled trial produced improvement in postpartum depression of women in a walking group.[246] Social support might be an important factor to motivate participation in female free clinic patients in order to reduce depression and body esteem.[247]

CONSTANT REPETITIVE MOTION

HYPERKINESIS AND ATTENTION-DEFICIT HYPERACTIVITY DISORDER

Exercise is about movement, and movement is shown to have a calming effect. This has been established in hyperkinesia and children with attention-deficit hyperactivity disorder (ADHD). Children with ADHD are in constant motion (wiggling their bodies, squirming in their seats, jiggling their feet, tapping their pencils, rocking their chairs). ADHD boys were observed moving around the room eight times more and were noted to move their arms twice as much as other students in a classroom.[248–250] Stimulants have a paradoxical effect and are calming in children with ADHD. Hyperkinetic mice lack the gene encoding for the dopamine transporter (DAT) and respond to a novel environment.[251,252] Stimulation of dopamine D4 receptors depresses motor activity. Enhancing dopamine D4 transmission in the basal ganglia and the thalamus is likely part of the mechanism of the therapeutic effects of psychostimulants on ADHD.[253]

Physical movement improves mental focus (ignore distractions), memory, and cognitive flexibility.[254,255] One becomes better able to focus on one thing and is not distracted. This happens because the executive control center of brain is the loci for inhibition (resisting distractions), working memory, and cognitive flexibility (switching between tasks). After 26 minutes of daily physical activity for 8 weeks, ADHD symptoms lessened in grade school children.[256]

Serotonin genes have also been hypothesized to play a role in the etiology of ADHD. It primarily plays a role in emotional dysregulation, impulse control, and aggression. Two variants of the 5HTTLPR (short and long allelic variants) have been linked to the conduct disorder and mood problems in ADHD as a result of either high or low serotonin transporter activity.[257]

OBSESSIVE-COMPULSIVE DISORDER

Many of the antidepressant medications known as *selective serotonin reuptake inhibitors (SSRIs)* have been proven to be effective in treating the symptoms associated with obsessive-compulsive disorder (OCD). Repetitive motion such as walking was found to stimulate the release of serotonin in cats.[85] Patients with OCD are soothed by ritualistic acts and may simply self-medicate to overcome serotonin deficits.

RESILIENCE

Bouncing back in the face of adversity is increased by physical wellness. It protects against the negative effects of stress by enhancing uplifting (dopamine) and calming neurotransmitters (dopamine, serotonin), triggering growth factors (BDNF), mobilizing feel-good neuropeptides (phenylethylamine), while at the same time reducing chronic stress hormones (cortisol and adrenalin).[258,259,260] These neurochemical alterations brought about by physical activity and the consequences of exercise make one less vulnerable to stress and depression.

Exercise toughens the brain so that stress has less of an impact. The mental enrichment brought about by exercise proved a buffer as to how the brain will respond to future stressors. Disrupting metabolically over active subgenual cingulate (Brodmann area 25) white matter using electrical stimulation could reverse symptoms in otherwise treatment-resistant depression.[261] Lehman proposed that exercise may ease depression by acting on Brodmann area 25.[262]

According to research carried out by Michalak, one's attitude while walking has an effect on his or her vulnerability to depression.[263] Depressed individuals move differently than those who are upbeat and positive. It is not unreasonable to speculate that our mood affects how we walk. How we walk in turn affects the way we feel. The difference between recalled positive and recalled negative words was much lower in participants who adapted a depressed walking style as opposed to those who walked as if they were happy. Commuters who stopped driving to work and walked or rode their bikes instead had less stress and were able to concentrate better. The longer we spend commuting in cars, the greater is the toll on psychological well-being.[264]

HEALTH IMPROVEMENT

With regular exercise, one gets stronger, flexible, mobile, and energized. Exercise has long been associated with protecting blood vessels, strengthening the heart, and improving blood flow to the brain. The increased capacity for the cardiovascular system to pump blood improves oxygen transfer and supports healthy brain functioning. Stabilizing blood sugar and controlling insulin delivery are positive attributes of fitness. Keeping inflammation in check and maintaining a healthy immune system contributes to the survival of nervous tissue. There is little debate that a fit body and alert mind contribute to improving our mood on a long-term basis.[265-267] Most importantly, these positive attributes not only make you feel better about yourself but also create a healthier you: regulates blood pressure, keeps inflammation in check, prevents heart disease, lowers cholesterol, improves circulation, bolsters the immune system, manages diabetes, and reduces the risk of cancer.[268-271]

COGNITIVE SKILLS

Cognitive deficits (speed of brain processing and efficiency of the working memory) are core symptoms in patients with MDD.[272] Exercise has been shown to help reduce mental decline and improve cognitive skills. Aerobic fitness is associated with the network underlying cognitive control in adolescent fitness.[273,274] Higher aerobic fitness was related to greater white matter and myelination in children. The creation of more compact fibers provides greater cellular communication resulting in improved learning and memory.[275] Lower fitness levels have been related to decreased cognitive function in tasks requiring cognitive control.

Remaining active throughout our life staves off declining memory and maintains mental sharpness. Cognitive impairment (thinking, learning, memory) is notorious for declining with age. Picture a shoelace with tips at both ends. If that plastic tip cracks and falls off, the shoelace becomes unraveled and frayed. We have these same protective tips on the end of our chromosomes that determine the life span of the cell. These telomeres are tiny pieces of DNA that bind together to keep genes and chromosomes stable. Over time and with added stress, these structures at the ends of chromosomes begin to unravel and get shorter and shorter until they cannot shorten any more. The deterioration and shortening can be mitigated by high intensity or daily short bouts of exercise.[276,277] Merely spending more time on your feet and less time sitting lengthens your telomeres and could possibly increase your life span. Promoting participation in physical activity slows down frontal lobe atrophy and boosted the size of the hippocampus, the opposite of which is observed in dementia, mental decline, and brain aging.[278–283] Exercise might alter people's brain structure by triggering the growth of new nerve cells and blood vessels and increasing production of brain chemicals that promote the growth and repair of brain cells.[284–286]

EXERCISE FOR DEPRESSION

Each of the categories in the description of depression laid out by the NIMH (National Institute of Mental Health) should be included when considering the contribution of exercise as an adjunct to treatment: insomnia, hopelessness, helplessness, loss of pleasure, lack of energy, difficulty remembering and concentrating, issues with appetite, and irritability. Addressing each symptom, it is reasonable to conclude that exercise potentially can reduce the severity of each one of them. Just because there is an association and many people subjectively admit that exercise mitigates their depression does not mean we can assume a causal relationship. Furthermore, proving exercise is therapeutic for depression is not an easy task as demonstrated by the numerous studies that have been attempted for the last three decades. Meta-analysis and review articles continue to caution that there are methodological problems in the designs of many studies which have led to a universal conclusion that the benefits are small and more research is needed.

There is the additional problem when intervening with patients who are so severely depressed they do not want to exercise and hence have poor compliance.[287,288] Depressed individuals are three times more likely not to exercise. To recommend a severely depressed individual undertake an exercise regimen is like prescribing communication to a wife whom is terribly distraught over her husband's illicit affair. If the wife is not able to turn off her emotional pain, discussing the issue may only serve to trigger more guilt, shame, hurt, and self-reproach. Each situation carries with it the need for careful assessment on the part of the health-care professional and willingness of the patient to consider only exercises the patient feels will be of help. Exercises should be chosen so that they produce a positive mood, create a sense of tranquility, incorporate joyful movement, and revitalize the individual. It is a bit paradoxical to expend energy in order to achieve more energy.

Excessive physical activity may lead to overtraining and generate psychological symptoms that mimic depression rather than alleviate them.[289–292] It is equally important that we caution against getting too much exercise which can actually lead to an addiction/compulsion itself. Research has yet to reach a consensus on the definition of exercise dependence. However there is a subset of the exercising population who may develop compulsion to excessive exercise.[292] Exercise activates many neurotransmitter systems involved in the addictive process (dopamine, serotonin, endorphins, glucocorticoids, and endocannabinoids). Rats were shown to decrease morphine administration by exercising. There are several tools to assess exercise addiction: Exercise Dependency Scale[293,294] and the Exercise Addiction Inventory.[295] The typical warning signs of exercise dependence are

1. Using exercise as a form of purging (expending calories to compensate for food consumption)
2. Exercising despite illness (fever) or injury (ankle sprain)
3. Experiencing panic or guilt (unable to relax) when unable to exercise
4. Calculating food consumption based on amount of calories burned
5. Exercising that interferes with social, family, occupational, and recreational activities
6. Having a rigid, uncompromising attitude that makes exercise the priority

7. Keeping a highly detailed performance record
8. Defining one's self-worth by his or her athleticism and exercise achievements
9. Focusing on exercise as work rather than fun and enjoyment

The activity stress paradigm (A-S paradigm) of restrictive feeding and wheel running activity in rats has been studied extensively over the past 40 years.[296,297] Rats are switched from a feeding regimen of 24-hour access to food to one where food is available one hour per day. The animal starts to lose weight before it has adapted to the new schedule. After a while the rat begins to consume more food during the allotted time. If these same rats are given the opportunity to exercise on a running wheel, the rats will never adjust. Instead the rat gets deranged and runs more and more as it eats less and less. Eventually the rodent becomes too scrawny and won't move. Without some external intervention, the animal will starve to death in a few weeks.[298,299] This model permits research on anorexia in animals, but is neither practical nor ethical for studies on humans. The activity stress phenomenon has been referred to as self-starvation, semi-starvation–induced hyperactivity, or anxiety-based anorexia.

CONCLUSION

A thorough investigation on the contribution of exercise on depression includes reviewing articles that do not solely address depression, but expand to include the activity's ability to improve mood, health, well-being, self-esteem, and quality of life.[300–302] Moods refer to a state of prolonged emotions of which depression is included. A mood is generally less specific, less intense, and less likely to be triggered by a particular negative experience. Thirty minutes of moderate intensity on a treadmill was sufficient to improve mood and well-being in patients with MDD. It is noted that there was also improvement in distress, fatigue, tension, confusion, and anger. Psychological well-being is feeling good about yourself and the world around you. It can be thought of as a diversion from negative thinking, possessing a sense of purpose, and a perceived absence of anxiety or depression. Well-being includes having a general satisfaction with life, a sense of coherence (socialization), resilience from adverse situations, and appropriate coping mechanisms. Two to six months of at least 30 minutes a day of exercise significantly improved well-being in participants in a study by Edwards.[303] Exercise produced less tension, less stress, less mental fatigue, improved sleep, less anger, and more joy. Quality of life (QOL) is a state of well-being that encompasses the ability to perform everyday activities that reflect physical, psychological, and social well-being.[304,305] Evidence that QOL is improved by exercise is inconclusive, as very few exercise trials have included QOL outcomes.[306–308] Benefits are subjective and measurements can be difficult due to inconsistencies and poor methodology.[309,310] Historically, promoting exercise for health may be better served from a motivational perspective if directed toward QOL because of the "immediate advantage."[311] Finally, health is defined as the optimal state of physical, mental, and social well-being and not merely the absence of pain and disease. It takes in the ability to do the things you want to do in life in a safe and efficient manner with enthusiasm and energy.

Exercise has so many benefits, that even if it does not produce the ultimate outcome of eliminating depression, there is enough evidence to support its inclusion when appropriate. Physical activity has been shown to improve depressive symptoms to a comparable extent as pharmacotherapy.[312,313] On a molecular level, exercise increases the calming neurotransmitter (serotonin), reward chemicals (dopamine, endocannabinoids, endorphins), mood stabilizers (phenylethylamine), and neuroplasticity (BDNF). At the same time it reduces chemicals associated with stress (cortisol and adrenalin). Exercise has been demonstrated to improve sleep, provide a sense of accomplishment, reduce anxiety, and provide a distraction. The socialization that can be paired with activity is also therapeutic. There are many health benefits that begin with reducing inflammation, which is a process that seems to be involved in all the ills that plague mankind. Advocating exercise helps the young as well as the old. There are no hard and set rules regarding how much, how intense, what type, what supervision, or what frequency is necessary to achieve benefit. Yet despite all of these positive indicators, surveys show that an average of only 40% of patients are counseled by their physician about exercise.[314] According to Pollock, few psychotherapists employ exercise promotion and maintenance as part of their treatment.[315] Research findings over the past two decades strongly indicate that moderate exercise can have a beneficial effect upon depression.[316] These findings strongly support that health-care professionals should recommend exercise for their patients.

REFERENCES

1. NCHS-CDC [Pratt L] National Center for Health Statistics U.S. Center for Disease Control and Prevention (December 2014).
2. Jain, R. Exercise to treat depression. Backed by Biology presentation at the 27th Annual U.S. Psychiatric and Mental Health Congress, Orlando, FL (July 15, 2014).
3. Martinsen, E.W. et al. 1985. Effects of exercise on depression: A controlled study. *Br Med J* 291: 109.
4. Martinsen, E.W. et al. 1989a. Physical fitness levels in patients with anxiety and depressive disorders. *Int J Sports Med* 10: 58–61.
5. Martinsen, E.W. et al. 1989b. Comparing aerobic and nonaerobic forms of exercise in the treatment of clinical depression: A randomized trial. *Compr Psychiatry* 30: 324–331.
6. Martinsen, E.W. et al. 1989c. Exercise adherence and patients' evaluation of exercise in a comprehensive treatment programme for depression. *Nordic J Psychiatry* 43: 521–529.
7. Martinsen, E.W. 1990. Benefits of exercise for the treatment of depression. *Sports Med* 9: 380.
8. Freemont, J. and Craighead, L.W. 1987. Aerobic exercise and cognitive therapy in the treatment of dysphoric moods *Cogn Ther Res* 11: 241–251.
9. Donta, S.T. et al. 2003. Cognitive behavioral therapy and aerobic exercise for Gulf War Veterans' Illnesses: A randomized controlled trial. *JAMA* 289: 1396–1404.
10. Barbour, K.A. et al. 2007. Exercise as a treatment for depression and other psychiatric disorders: A review. *J Cardiopulm Rehab Prev* 27: 359–367.
11. Legrand, F. et al. 2007. Antidepressant effects associated with different exercise conditions in participants with depression: A pilot study. *J Sport Exerc Psychol* 29: 348–364.
12. Blumenthal, A.L. et al. 2012. Effects of exercise training on depressive symptoms in patients with chronic heart failure. The HF-ACTION Randomized Trial. *JAMA* 308: 465–474.
13. Milani, R.V. et al. 2007. Impact of cardiac rehabilitation on depression and its associated mortality. *Am J Med* 120: 799–806.
14. King, W.C. et al. 2013. Associations between physical activity and mental health among bariatric surgical candidates. *J Psychosom Res* 74: 161–169.
15. Singh, N.A. et al. 1997. A randomized controlled trial of progressive resistance training in depressed elders. *J Gerontol* 52: M27–M35.
16. Daley, A.J. et al. 2006. Exercise therapy as a treatment for psychopathologic conditions in obese and morbidly obese adolescents: A randomized, controlled trial *Pediatrics* 118: 2126–2134.
17. Sjosten, N. and Kivela, S.L. 2006. The effects of physical exercise on depressive symptoms among the aged: A systematic review. *Int J Geriatr Psychiatry* 21: 410–418.
18. Mead, G.E. et al. 2009. Exercise for depression. *Cochrane Database Syst Rev* 3:CD004366.
19. WHO. 2014. Health for the World's Adolescents A second chance in the second decade. WHO/FWC/MCA/14.05.
20. March, J. 2006. The Treatment for adolescents with depression study (TADS). *Child Adolesc Psychiatry* 45: 1393–1403.
21. Dopp, R.R. et al. 2012. Exercise for adolescents with depressive disorders: A feasibility study depression. *Res Treat* 2012: ID257472.
22. Ruggero, C. 2014. Does cardiorespiratory fitness protect against depression during middle school? A study presented at the *American Psychological Association's 122nd Annual Conference*, August 7, 2014.
23. Schneider, M. et al. 2008. Physical activity and physical self-concept among sedentary adolescent females: An intervention study. *Psychol Sport Exerc* 9: 1–14.
24. Spence, F.C. et al. 1997. The effect of physical activity participation on self-concept: A meta-analysis. *J Sp Ex Psych* 19: S109.
25. Annesi, J.J. 2004. Relationship between self-efficacy and changes in rated tension and depression for 9 to 12 year old children enrolled in a 12 week afterschool physical activity program. *Percept Motor Skills* 99: 191–194.

26. Daley, A. 2008. Exercise and depression: A review of reviews. *J Clin Psychol Med Settings* 15: 140–147.
27. Callister, R., Giles, A., Nasstasia, Y. et al. 2013. Healthy body healthy mind: Trialing an exercise intervention for reducing depression in youth with major depressive disorder. *Int J Exerc Sci Conf Proc*, 10(1), Article 6.
28. Brown, H.E. et al. 2013. Physical activity interventions and depression in children and adolescents: A systematic review and meta-analysis. *Sports Med* 43: 195–206.
29. Huang, Z.G. et al. 2013. Study on antidepressant effect of kuanxinjieyutang combined aerobic exercise. *Zhong Yao Cai* 36: 1651–1656.
30. van Hoomissen, J.D. et al. 2003. Research report effects of chronic exercise and imipramine on mRNA for BDNF after olfactory bulbectomy in rat. *Brain Res* 974: 228–235.
31. Blumenthal, J.A. et al. 1999. Effects of exercise training on older patients with major depression. *Arch Intern Med* 159: 2349–2356.
32. Babyak, M., Blumenthal, J.A. et al. 2000. Exercise treatment for major depression: Maintenance therapeutic benefit at 10 months. *Psychosom Med* 62: 633–638.
33. Trivedi, M.H. et al. 2006b. Exercise as an augmentation strategy for treatment of major depression. *J Psychiatr Pract* 12: 205–213.
34. Blumenthal, J.A. et al. 2007. Exercise and pharmacotherapy in the treatment of major depressive disorder. *Psychosom Med* 69: 587–596.
35. Chalder, M. et al. 2012. Facilitated physical activity as a treatment for depressed adults: Randomised controlled trial. *BMJ* 344: E2758.
36. Greer, T.L. and Trivedi, M.H. 2009. Exercise in the treatment of depression. *Curr Psychiatry Rep* 11: 466–472.
37. Lawlor, D.A. and Hopker, S.W. 2001. The effectiveness of exercise as an intervention in the management of depression: Systematic review and meta-regression analysis of randomised controlled trials. *BMJ* 322(7289): 763.
38. Stathopoulou, G., Powers, M.B., Berry, A.C., Smits, J.A., and Otto, M.W. 2006. Exercise interventions for mental health: A quantitative and qualitative review. *Clin Psychol Sci Pract* 13(2): 179–193.
39. Georgia, S., Mark, B.P., Angela, C.B. et al. 2006. Exercise interventions for mental health: A quantitative and qualitative review. *Clin Psychol Sci Pract* 13(2): 179–193.
40. Blake, H. et al. 2009. How effective are physical activity interventions for alleviating depressive symptoms in older people? A systematic review. *Clin Rehabil* 23: 873–887.
41. Krogh, J., Nordentoft, M., Sterne, J.A., and Lawlor, D.A. 2011. The effect of exercise in clinically depressed adults: Systematic review and meta-analysis of randomized controlled trials. *J Clin Psychiatry* 72(4): 529–38. doi:10.4088/JCP.08r04913blu.
42. Rimer, J. et al. 2012. Exercise for depression. *Cochrane Database Syst Rev* 7: CD004366.
43. Mura, G. et al. 2014. Efficacy of exercise on depression: A systematic review. *Int J Pscyosocial Rehabil* 18: 23–36.
44. Josefsson, T. et al. 2014. Physical exercise intervention in depressive disorders: Meta-analysis and systematic review. *Scan J Med Sci Sports* 24: 259–272.
45. Anonymous. 2005. Working off depression. *Harvard Mental Health Letter* 22(6): 6–7.
46. Dunn, A.L., Trivedi, M.H. et al. 2002. The DOSE study: A clinical trial to examine efficacy and dose response of exercise as treatment for depression. *Control Clin Trials* 23: 584–603.
47. Dunn, A.L., Trivedi, M.H. et al. 2005. Exercise treatment for depression: Efficacy and dose response *Am J Prev Med* 28: 1–8.
48. Crum, A. and Langer, E.J. 2007. Mind-set matters: Exercise and the placebo effect. *Psychol Sci* 18: 165–171.
49. Kirsch, I. 2008. Challenging received wisdom: Antidepressants and the placebo effect. *McGill J Med* 11: 219–222.
50. Hassmen, P. et al. 2000. Physical exercise and psychological well-being: A population study in Finland. *Prev Med* 30: 17–25.
51. Pardridge, W.M. 1986. Blood brain barrier transport of nutrients. *Nutr Rev* 44 (Suppl), 15–25.
52. Davis, J.M. et al. 2000. Serotonin and central nervous system fatigue: Nutritional considerations. *Am J Clin Nutr* 72(Suppl): 573S–578S.
53. Blomstrand, E. 2001. Amino acids and central fatigue. *Amino Acids* 20: 25–34.
54. Ekkekakis, P. and Petruzzello, S.J. 1999. Acute aerobic exercise and affect: Current status, problems and prospects regarding dose-response. *Sports Med* 28: 337–374.
55. Trivedi, M.H. et al. 2006a. TREAD: Treatment with exercise augmentation for depression: Study rationale and design *ClinTrials* 3: 291–305.

56. Bartholomew, J.B. et al. 2005. Effects of acute exercise on mood and well-being in patients with major depressive disorder. *Med Sci Sports Exercise* 37: 2032–2037.

57. Hamer, M. et al. 2008. Dose response relationship between physical activity and mental health: The Scottish health survey. *Br J Sports Med* 43: 1111–1114.

58. Knubben, K. et al. 2007. A randomized, controlled study on the effects of a short-term endurance training programme in patients with major depression. *Br J Sports Med* 41: 29–33.

59. Pinto Pereira, S.M., Geoffroy, M., and Power, C. 2014. Depressive symptoms and physical activity during 3 decades in adult life: Bidirectional associations in a prospective cohort study. *JAMA Psychiatry* 71(12): 1373–1380.

60. Puetz, T.W. et al. 2008. A randomized controlled trial of the effect of aerobic exercise training on feelings of energy and fatigue in sedentary young adults with persistent fatigue. *Psychother Psychosom* 77: 167–174.

61. Petruzello, S.J. et al. 1991. A meta-analysis on the anxiety-reducing effects of acute and chronic exercise outcomes and mechanisms. *Sports Med* 11: 143–182.

62. Craft, L.L. et al. 2007. Intervention study of exercise for depressive symptoms in women. *J Womens Health* 16: 1499–1509.

63. Lampinen, P. et al. 2000. Changes in intensity of physical exercise as predictors of depressive symptoms among older adults: An eight year follow-up. *Prev Med* 30: 371–380.

64. Harvey, S.B. et al. 2010. Physical activity and common mental disorders. *Br J Psychiatry* 197: 357–364.

65. Hansen, J. et al. 2001. Exercise duration and mood state: How much is enough to feel better. *Health Psychol* 4: 267.

66. De Moor, M.H. et al. 2008. Testing causality in the association between regular exercise and symptoms of anxiety and depression. *Arch Gen Psychiatry* 65: 897–905.

67. Cooney, G.M., Dwan, K., Greig, C.A. et al. 2013. Exercise for depression. *Cochrane Database Syst Rev* (9): 1–142.

68. National Institute for Health and Care Excellence. 2007. Depression: Management of depression in primary and secondary care—NICE guidance. Available at: www.nice.org.uk

69. National Collaborating Centre for Mental Health (UK). 2010. Depression: The Treatment and Management of Depression in Adults (Updated Edition). Leicester (UK): British Psychological Society; 2010 National Institute for Health and Clinical Excellence: Guidance The British Psychological Society & The Royal College of Psychiatrists, 2010 NICE Clinical Guidelines 90 ISBN-13: 978-1-904671-85-5.

70. Otto, M.W., Trivedi, M.H. et al. 2007. Exercise for mood and anxiety disorders. *Prim Care Companion J Clin Psychiatry* 9: 287–294.

71. Otto, M.W. and Smits, J.A. 2009. *Exercise for Mood and Anxiety Disorders*. New York, NY: Oxford University Press.

72. Meeusen, R. et al. 1995. Exercise and brain neurotransmission. *Sports Med* 20: 160–188.

73. Meeusen, R. et al. 1997. Endurance training effects on neurotransmitter release in rat striatum: An *in vivo* microdialysis. *Acta Physiol Scand* 159: 335–341.

74. Meeusen, R. et al. 2001. Brain neurotransmitter levels during exercise. *Dtsch Z Sportmed* 52: 361–368.

75. Dey, S. et al. 1992. Exercise training: Significance of regional alterations in serotonin metabolism of rat brain in relation to antidepressant effect of exercise. *Physiol Behav* 52: 1095–1099.

76. Dey, S. 1994. Physical exercise as a novel antidepressant agent: Possible role of serotonin receptor subtypes. *Physiol Behav* 55: 323–329.

77. Dietrich, A. and McDaniel, W.F. 2004. Endocannabinoid and exercise. *Br J Sports Med* 38: 536–541.

78. Soares, J. et al. 1994. Increased serotonin levels in physically trained men. *Braz J Med Biol Res* 27: 1635–1638.

79. Lowry, C.A. et al. 2009. That warm fuzzy feeling: Brain serotonergic neurons and the regulation of emotion. *J Psychopharmacol* 23: 392.

80. Chaouloff, F. et al. 1986. Motor activity increases tryptophan, 5-hydroxyindoleacetic acid and homovanillic acid in ventricular cerebrospinal fluid of the conscious rat. *J Neurochem* 46: 1313–1316.

81. Chaouloff, F. et al. 1994. Serotonin1C,2 receptors and endurance performance. An illustration of the limits of pharmacological tools in exercise science. *Int J Sports Med* 15: 339–411.

82. Chaouloff, F. 1997. Effects of acute physical exercise on central serotonergic systems. *Med Sci Sp Exerc* 29: 58–62.

83. Millan, M.J. 2005. Serotonin 5-HT2C receptors as a target for the treatment of depressive and anxious states: Focus on novel therapeutic strategies. *Therapie* 60: 441–460.

84. Broocks, A. et al. 2007. Physical training in the treatment of depressive disorders. *Psychiatr Prax* 34:(Suppl 3) S300–S304.

85. Jacobs, B.L. and Fornal, C.A. 1999. Activity of serotonergic neurons in behaving animals. *Neuropsychopharmacology* 21: 9S–15S.

86. Young, S.N. 2007. How to increase serotonin in the human brain without drugs. *J Psychiatry Neurosci* 32: 394–399.

87. Chaouloff, F. et al. 1985. Effects of conditioned running on plasma, liver and brain tryptophan and on brain 5-hydroxytryptamine metabolism of the rat. *Br J Pharmacol* 86: 33–41.

88. Reuter, L.E. and Jacobs, B.L. 1996. A micodialysis examination of serotonin release in the rat forebrain induced by behavioral/experimental manipulation. *Brain Res* 739: 57–69.

89. Wilson, W.M. et al. 1995. Extracellular dopamine in the nucleus accumbens of the rat during treadmill running. *Acra Physiol Scand* 155: 465–466.

90. Wilson, W.M. and Marsden, C.A. 1996. *In vivo* measurement of extracellular serotonin in the ventral hippocampus during treadmill running. *Behav Pharmacol* 7: 101–104.

91. Gomez-Merino, D. et al. 2001. Site dependent effects of an acute intensive exercise on extracellular 5-HT and 5-TIAA levels in rat brain. *Neurosci Lett* 301: 143–146.

92. Davis, C. and Woodside, B.D. 2002. Sensitivity to the rewarding effects of food and exercise in the eating disorders. *Compr Psychiatry* 43: 189–194.

93. Jabeen Haleem, D. 2011. Raphe-hippocampal serotonin neurotransmission in the sex related differences of adaptation to stress: Focus on serotonin-1A receptor. *Curr Neuropharmacol* 9: 512–521.

94. Krogh, J. et al. 2011. The effect of exercise in clinically depressed adults: Systematic review and meta-analysis of randomized controlled trials. *J Clin Psychiatry* 72: 529–538.

95. Blumenthal, J.A. et al. 1999. Effects of exercise training on older patients with major depression. *Arch Intern Med* 159: 2349–2356.

96. Blumenthal, J.A. et al. 2007. Exercise and pharmacotherapy in the treatment of major depressive disorder. *Psychosom Med* 69: 587–596.

97. Dunn, A.L. 1991. Exercise and the neurobiology of depression. *Exerc Sport Sci Rev* 19: 41–98.

98. Nicoloff, G. and Schwenk, T.S. 1995. Using exercise to ward off depression. *Physician Sports Med* 23: 44–58.

99. Sime, W.E. 2007. Exercise therapy for stress management. In *Principles and Practice of Stress Management*, Ed. P.M. Lehrer et al. 3rd ed. Spring Street, NY: Guilford Press, pp. 333.

100. Smith, C. et al. 2007b. A randomized comparative trial of yoga and relaxation to reduce stress and anxiety. *Complement Ther Med* 15: 77.

101. Barbour, K.A. et al. 2007. Exercise as a treatment for depression and other psychiatric disorders: A review. *J Cardiopulm Rehabil Prev* 27: 359–367.

102. Strohle, A. 2009. Physical activity exercise, depression and anxiety disorders. *J Neural Trans* 116: 777.

103. De Matos, M.G. et al. 2009. Effect of physical activity on anxiety and depression. *Presse Med* 38: 734–739.

104. Cooper-Patrick, L. 1997. Exercise and depression in midlife: A prospective study. *Am J Public Health* 87: 670–673.

105. He, S.B. et al. 2012. Exercise intervention may prevent depression. *Int J Sp Med* 33: 525–530.

106. McWilliams, L.A. and Asmundson, G.J. 2001. Is there a negative association between anxiety sensitivity and arousal-increasing substances and activities? *J Anxiety Disord* 15: 161–170.

107. Broman-Fulks, J.J. and Storey, K.M. 2008. Evaluation of a brief aerobic exercise intervention for high anxiety sensitivity *Anxiety Stress Coping* 21: 117–128.

108. Smits, J.A. et al. 2008. Reducing anxiety sensitivity with exercise. *Depress Anxiety* 15: 689–699.

109. Sabelli, H.C. and Javaid, J.I. 1995. Phenylethylamine modulation of affect: Therapeutic and diagnostic implications. *J Neuropsychiatry Clin Neurosci* 7: 6–14.

110. Sabelli, H. et al. 1996. Sustained antidepressant effect of PEA replacement. *J Neuropsychiatry Clin Neurosci* 8: 168–171.

111. Szabo, A. 2000. Physical activity as a source of psychological dysfunction. In *Physical Activity and Psychological Well-Being*, Ed. S.J. Biddle, K.R. Fox, and S.H. Boutcher. London, UK: Routledge, pp. 130–153.

112. Szabo, A. et al. 2001. Phenylethylamine, a possible link to other antidepressant effects of exercise? *Br J Sports Med* 35: 342–343.

113. Ekkekakis, P. and Petruzzello, S.J. 1999. Acute aerobic exercise and affect: Current status, problems and prospects regarding dose-response. *Sports Med* 28: 337–374.

114. Ohmura, Y. et al. 2009. The roles of corticotrophin releasing factor (CRF) in responses to emotional stress: Is CRF release a cause or result of fear/anxiety. *CNS Neurol Disord Drugs Targets* 8: 459–469.

115. Peake, P.M. et al. 1995. Hypercortisolism and obesity. *Ann NY Acad Sci* 29: 665–676.
116. Peake, P.M. *Fighting Fat after Forty.* New York, NY: Viking Press, 2000.
117. Talbot, S., 2002. The cortisol connection. *Why Stress Makes You Fat and Ruins Your Health—and What You Can Do About It,* Alameda, CA: Hunter House.
118. Jensen, C.R. and Schultz, G.W. 1977. *Applied Kinesiology.* New York, NY: McGraw-Hill.
119. Jensen, T.S. 1982. Cerebral atrophy in young torture victims. *NEJM* 307: 1341.
120. Sapolsky, R.M. et al. 1985. A mechanism for glucocorticoid toxicity in the hippocampus: Increased neuronal vulnerability to metabolic insults. *J Neurosci* 5: 1228–1232.
121. Sapolsky, R.M. et al. 1990. Hippocampal damage associated with prolonged glucocorticoid exposure in primates. *J Neurosci* 10: 2897–2902.
122. Sapolsky, R.M. et al. 1996. Why stress is bad for your brain. *Science* 273: 749–750.
123. Sapolsky, R.M. 1999. Glucocorticoids, stress and their adverse neurological effects: Relevance to aging. *Exp Gerontol* 34: 721–732.
124. Sapolsky, R.M. 2001. Depression, antidepressants, and the shrinking hippocampus. *PNAS* 98: 12320–12322.
125. Uno, H. et al. 1994. Neurotoxicity of glucocorticoids in the primate brain. *Horm Behav* 28: 336–348.
126. Piekut, D.T. et al. 1999. Corticotropin-releasing factor—immunolabeled fibers in brain regions with localized kainite neurotoxicity. *Acta Neuropathol* 98: 622–628.
127. Lowery, E.G. et al. 2010. Pre-clinical evidence that corticotropin releasing factor (CRF) receptor antagonists are promising targets for pharmacological treatment of alcoholism. *CNS Neurol Disord Drug Targets* 9: 77–86.
128. Rose, A.K. et al. 2010. The importance of glucocorticoids in alcohol dependence and neurotoxicity. *Alcoholism Clin Exp Res* 34: 2100–2018.
120. QY, M. et al. 2011. Stress and glucocorticoids regulated corticotropin releasing factor in rat prefrotal cortex. *Molecular Cell Endocrinology* 342: 54–63.
130. Linthorst, A.C. et al. 1997. Long term intra-cerebro-ventricular infusion of corticotropin releasing hormone alters neuroendocrine, neurochemical, autonomic, behavioral, and cytokine responses to a systemic inflammatory challenge. *J Neurosci* 17: 4449–4460.
131. Martin, K.P. and Wellman, C.L. 2011. NMDA receptor blockage alters stress-induced dendritic remodeling in medial prefrontal cortex. *Cereb Cortex* 10: 2366–2373.
132. Sterner, E.Y. et al. 2010. Behavioral and neurobiological consequences of prolonged glucocorticoid exposure in rats: Relevance to depression. *Progr Neuro-Psychopharmacol Biol Psychiatry* 34: 777–790.
133. Uno, H. et al. 1989. Hippocampal damage associated with prolonged and fatal stress in primates. *J Neurosci* 9: 1705–1711.
134. Bodnoff, S.R. et al. 1995. Enduring effects of chronic corticosterone treatment on spatial learning, synaptic plasticity, and hippocampal neuropathology in young and mid-aged rats. *J Neurosci* 15: 61–69.
135. Virgin, C.E. et al. 1991. Glucocorticoids inhibit glucose transport and glutamate uptake in hippocampal astrocytes: Implications for glucocorticoid neurotoxicity. *J Neurochem* 57: 1422–1428.
136. Xiao, L. et al. 2010. Glucocorticoid rapidly enhances NMDA-evoked neurotoxicity by attenuating the NR2A-containing NMDA receptor medicated ERK1/2 activation. *Mol Endocrinol* 24: 497–510.
137. Conrad, C.D. et al. 2007. Chronic glucocorticoids increase hippocampal vulnerability to neurotoxicity under conditions that produce CA3 dendritic retraction but fail to impair spatial recognition of memory. *J Neurosci* 27: 8275–8828.
138. Wolkowitz, O.M. 2007. The steroid dementia syndrome: A possible model of human glucocorticoid neurotoxicity. *Neurocase* 13: 189–200.
139. Stahl, S.M. et al. 2008. The potential role of a corticotropin releasing factor receptor-1 antagonist in psychiatric disorders. *CNS Spectr* 13: 467–483.
140. Swaab, D.F. et al. 1994. Increased cortisol levels in aging and Alzheimer's disease in postmortem cerebrospinal fluid. *J Neuroendocrinol* 6: 681–187.
141. Swaab, D.F. et al. 2005. The stress system in the human brain in depression and neurodegeneration. *Ageing Res Rev* 4: 141–194.
142. Hackney, A.C. 2008a. Effects of endurance exercise on the reproductive system of men: The "exercise-hypogonadal male condition." *J Endocrinol Invest* 31: 932–938.
143. Hackney, A.C. et al. 2008b. Research methodology: Endocrinologic measurements in exercise science and sports medicine. *J Athletic Training* 43: 631–639.
144. Hackney, A.C. and Dobridge, J.D. 2009. Thyroid hormones and the interrelationship of cortisol and prolactin: Influence of prolonged, exhaustive exercise. *Pol J Endocrinol* 60: 252–257.

145. Hill, E.E. et al. 2008. Exercise and circulating cortisol levels: The intensity threshold effect. *J Endocrinol Invest* 311: 587–591.

146. Wittert, G.A. et al. 1996. Adaptation of the hypothalamopituitary adrenal axis to chronic exercise stress in humans. *Med Sci Sports Exer* 28: 1015–1019.

147. Reid, K.J. et al. 2010. Aerobic exercise improves self-reported sleep and quality of life in older adults with insomnia. *Sleep Med* 11: 934–940.

148. Jones, D. et al. 2014. The effect of relaxation interventions on cortisol levels in HIV-seropositive women. *J Int Assoc Provid AIDS Care* 13: 328–323.

149. Seekers, J. Stress University of Maryland Medical Centers (June 16, 2013) http://umm.edu/health/medical/reports/articles/stress

150. Cohen, G. and Shamus, E. 2009. Depression, low self-esteem: What can exercise do for you? *Int J Allied Health Sci Pract* 7: 1–5.

151. Rudolf, D. et al. 1998. Cortisol and affective responses to exercise. *J Sport Sci* 16: 121.

152. Epel, E.S. et al. 2000. Stress and body shape: Stress induced cortisol secretion is consistently greater among women with central fat. *Psychosom Med* 62: 623–632.

153. Epel, E. et al. 2001. Stress may add bite to appetite in women: A laboratory study of stress induced cortisol and eating behavior. *Psychoneuroendocrinology* 26: 37–49.

154. Raikkonen, K. et al. 1991. Anger, hostility, and visceral adipose tissue in health postmenopausal women. *Metab Clin Exp* 48: 1146.

155. Rosmond, R. et al. 1998. Stress related cortisol secretion in men: Relationships with abdominal obesity and endocrine, metabolic, and hemodynamic abnormalities. *J Clin Endocrinol Metab* 83: 1853–1859.

156. Goldfarb, A.H. and Jamurtas, A.Z. 1997. Beta-endorphin response to exercise. An update. *Sports Med* 24: 8–16.

157. Pierce, E.F. et al. 1993. Beta-endorphin response to endurance exercise: Relationship to exercise dependence. *Percept Mot Skills* 77: 767–770.

158. Boecker, H. et al. 1991. The runner's high: Opioidergic mechanisms in the human brain. *Cerebral Cortex* 18: 2523.

159. Hosseini, M. et al. 2009. Treadmill exercise reduces self-administration of morphine in male rats. *Pathophysiology* 16: 3–7.

160. Koehl, M. et al. 2008. Exercise induced promotion of hippocampal cell proliferation requires beta-endorphin. *FASEB J* 7: 2253–2262.

161. Helmich, I. et al. 2010. Neurobiological alterations induced by exercise and their impact on depressive disorders. *Clin Pract Epidemiol Ment Health* 6: 115–125.

162. Sparling, P.B. et al. 2003. Exercise activates the endocannabinoid system. *Neuroreport* 14: 2209–2011.

163. Daniel, M. et al. 1992. Opiate receptor blockade by naltrexone and mood state after acute physical activity. *Br J Sports Med* 26: 111–115.

164. Hinton, E. 1986. Taylor does placebo response mediate runner's high? *Percept Mot Skills* 62: 789–790.

165. Knab, A.M. and Lightfoot, J.T. 2010. Does the difference between physically active and couch potato lie in the dopamine system? *Int J Biol Sci* 6: 133–150.

166. Brene, S., Bjornebekk, A. et al. 2007. Running is rewarding and antidepressive. *Physiol Behav* 92: 136–140.

167. Brager, A.J., Glass, J.D. et al. 2010. Chronic ethanol disrupts circadian photic entrainment and daily locomotor activity in the mouse. *Alcohol Clin Exp Res* 34: 1266–1273.

168. Brown, R.A. et al. 2014. A preliminary, randomized trial of aerobic exercise for alcohol dependence. *J Subst Abuse Treat* 47: 1–9.

169. Foley, T.E. and Fleshner, M. 2008. Neuroplasticity of dopamine circuits after exercise: Implications for central fatigue. *Neuromol Med* 10: 67–80.

170. Hattori, S. et al. 1994. Striatal dopamine turnover during treadmill running in the rat: Relation to the speed of running. *Brain Res Bull* 35: 41–49.

171. Wilson, W.M. et al. 1995. Extracellular dopamine in the nucleus accumbens of the rat during treadmill running. *Acra Physiol Scand* 155: 465–466.

172. Meeusen, R. et al. 1997. Endurance training effects on neurotransmitter release in rat striatum: An *in vivo* microdialysis. *Acta Physiol Scand* 159: 335–341.

173. Balthazar, C.H. et al. 2009. Performance enhancing and thermoregulatory effects of intracerebroventricular dopamine in running rats. *Pharmacol Biochem Behave* 93: 465–469.

174. Craft, L.L. and Perna, F.M. 2004. The benefits of exercise for the clinically depressed. *Prim Care Companion J Clin Psychiatry* 6: 104–111.

175. Hi, C. and Kuo, Y.M. 2008. Long term compulsive exercise reduces the rewarding efficacy of 3,4-methylenedioxymethamphetamine. *Behav Brain Res* 187: 185–189.

176. Wang, G.-J., Volkow, N. et al. 2000. PET studies of the effects of aerobic exercise on human striatal dopamine release *Nucl Med* 41: 1352–1356.

177. Czeh, B. 2001. Stress-induced changes in cerebral metabolites, hippocampal volume, and cell proliferation are prevented by antidepressant treatment with tianeptine. *PNAS* 98: 12796–12801.

178. Rajkowska, G. et al. 1999. Morphometric evidence for neuronal and glial prefrontal cell pathology in major depression. *Biol Psychiatry* 45: 1085–1098.

179. Starkman, M.N. 1992. Hippocampal formation volume, memory dysfunction, and cortisol levels in patients with Cushing's syndrome. *Biol Psychiatry* 32: 756–765.

180. Sheline, Y.I. et al. 1996. Hippocampal atrophy in recurrent major depression. *PNAS* 93: 3908–3913.

181. Sheline, Y.I. et al. 1999. Depression duration but not age predicts hippocampal volume loss in medically healthy women with recurrent major depression. *J Neurosci* 19: 5034–5043.

182. Gould, E. et al. 1997. Neurogenesis in the dentate gyrus of the adult tree shrew is regulated by psychosocial stress and NMDA receptor activation. *J Neurosci* 17: 2492–2498.

183. Reagan, L.P. et al. 1997. Controversies surrounding glucocorticoid-mediated cell death in the hippocampus. *J Chem Neuroanat* 13: 149–167.

184. Cotman, C.W. et al. 2002a. Exercise: A behavioral intervention to enhance brain health and plasticity. *Trends Neurosci* 25: 295–301.

185. Cotman, C.W. et al. 2002b. Exercise enhances and protects brain function. *Exerc Sport Sci Rev* 30: 75–79.

186. Cotman, C.W. et al. 2007. Exercise builds brain health: Key roles of growth factor cascades and inflammation. *Trends Neurosci* 30: 464–472.

187. Greenwood, B.N. and Fleshner, M. 2011a. Exercise, stress resistance and central serotonergic systems. *Exerc Sport Sci Rev* 39: 140–149.

188. Rhodes, J.S., Gage, F.H. et al. 2003. Exercise increases hippocampal neurogenesis to high levels but does not improve spatial learning in mice bred for increased voluntary wheel running. *Behav Neurosci* 117: 1006–1016.

189. Adlard, P.A., Cotman, C.W. et al. 2005. The exercise induced expression of BDNF within the hippocampus varies across life span. *Neurobiol Aging* 26: 511–520.

190. Duman, R.S. et al. 2005. Neurotrophic factors and regulation of mood: Role of exercise, diet and metabolism. *Neurobiol Aging* 26 (Suppl 1): 88–93.

191. Broocks, A. et al. 2007. Physical training in the treatment of depressive disorders. *Psychiatr Prax* 34: (Suppl 3) S300–S304.

192. Hunsberger, J.G. et al. 2007. Antidepressant actions of the exercise-regulated gene VGF. *Nature Med* 13: 1476–1482.

193. Tang, S.W. et al. 2008. Influence of exercise on serum brain derived neurotrophic factor concentrations in healthy human subjects. *Neruosci Lett* 431: 62–65.

194. Gerrow, K. et al. 2010. Synaptic stability and plasticity in a floating world. *Curr Opin Neurobiol* 20: 631–639.

195. Bear, M.F., Connors, B.W., and Paradisio, M.A. 2007. *Neuroscience: Exploring the Brain*, 3rd ed. Philadelphia, PA: Lippincott, Williams & Wilkins.

196. Hahm, S. et al. 1999. Targeted deletion of the Vgf gene indicates that the encoded secretory peptide precursor plays a novel role in the regulation of energy balance. *Neuron* 23: 537–548.

197. Alder, J. et al. 2003. Brain-derived neurotrophic factor-induced gene expression reveals novel actions of VGF in hippocampal synaptic plasticity. *J Neuroscience* 23: 10800–10808.

198. Toups, M.S., Trivedi, M.H. et al. 2011. Effects of serum brain derived neurotrophic factor on exercise augmentation of depression. *J Psychiatr Res* 45: 1301–1306.

199. van Praag, H. 1999. Running increases cell proliferation and neurogenesis in the adult mouse dentate gyrus. *Nat Neurosci* 2: 266–279.

200. Bjornebekk, A. et al. 2005. The antidepressant effect of running is associated with increased hippocampal cell proliferation. *Int J Neuropsychopharmacol* 8: 357–368.

201. Russo-Neurstadt, A.A. et al. 2004. Hippocampal brain-derived neurotrophic factor expression following treatment with reboxetine, citalopram, and physical exercise. *Neuropsychopharmacology* 29: 2189–2199.

202. Pereira, A.C. et al. 2007. An *in vivo* correlate of exercise-induced neurogenesis in the adult dentate gyrus. *Proc Natl Acad Sci* 104: 5638–5643.

203. Braun, S. 2000. *The Science of Happiness: Unlocking the Mysteries of Mood*. New York, NY: Wiley.

204. Vogel, G. et al. 2003. Depression drugs powers may rest on new neurons. *Science* 301: 757.

205. Enkiolopov, G. 2006. Research reveals how Prozac triggers new brain cell growth. *Proc Natl Acad Sci* 103: 8233–8238.
206. Kimbrel, T.A. et al. 1999. Frequency dependence of antidepressant response to left prefrontal repetitive transcranial magnetic stimulation (rTMS) as a function of baseline cerebral glucose metabolism. *Biol Psychiatry* 46: 1603–1613.
207. Elder, G.A. et al. 2006. Research update: Neurogenesis in adult brain and neuropsychiatric disorders. *Mt Sinai J Med* 73: 931–940.
208. Marlatt, M.W. et al. 2010. Comparison of neurogenic effects of fluoxetine, duloxetine and running in mice. *Brain Res* 1341: 9399.
209. Yau, Sy et al. 2011. Hippocampal neurogenesis and dendritic plasticity support running-improved spatial learning and depression-like behaviour in stressed rats. *PLoS One* 6: e24263.
210. Lieberwirth, C. and Wang, Z. 2012. The social environment and neurogenesis in the adult Mammalian brain. *Front Hum Neurosci* 6: 118.
211. Garza, A.A. et al. 2004. Exercise, antidepressant treatment, and BDNF mRNA expression in the aging brain. *Pharmacol Biochem Behav* 77: 209–220.
212. Dietrich, A. and McDaniel, W.F. 2004. Endocanabinoid and exercise. *Br J Sports Med* 38: 536–541.
213. Fuss, J. and Gass, P. 2010. Endocannabinoid and voluntary activity in mice: Runner's high and long term consequences in emotional behavior. *Exp Neurol* 224: 103–105.
214. Dubreucq, S. et al. 2010. CB1 receptor deficiency decreases wheel-running activity: Consequences on emotional behaviors and hippocampal neurogenesis. *Exp Neurol* 224: 106–113.
215. Heyman, E. et al. 2012. Intense exercise increases circulating endocannabinoid and BDNF levels in humans—possible implications for reward and depression. *Psychoneuroendocrinology* 37: 844–851.
216. Harte, J.L. et al. 1995. The effects of running and meditation on beta-endorphin, corticotropin-releasing hormone and cortisol in plasma, and on mood. *Biol Psychol* 40: 251–265.
217. Hill, M.N. et al. 2010. Endogenous cannabinoid signaling is required for voluntary exercise-induced enhancement of progenitor cell proliferation in the hippocampus. *Hippocampus* 20: 513–523.
218. Wolf, S.A. et al. 2010. Cannabinoid receptor CB1 mediates baseline and activity-induced survival of new neurons in adult hippocampal neurogenesis. *Cell Comm Signal* 8: 12.
219. Kiive, E. et al. 2004. Growth hormone, cortisol and prolactin responses to physical exercise: Higher prolactin response in depressed patients. *Prog Neuropsychopharmacol Biol Psychiatry* 28: 1007–1013.
220. Krogh, J. et al. 2010. Growth hormone, prolactin and cortisol response to exercise in patients with depression. *J Affect Disord* 125: 189–197.
221. Morilak, D. et al. 2003. Interactions of norepinephrine and galanin in the central amygdala and lateral bed nucleus of the stria terminalis modulate the behavior response to acute stress. *Life Sci* 73: 715–726.
222. Legakis, I.N. et al. 2000. Human galanin secretion is increased upon normal exercise test in middle age individuals *Endocr Res* 26: 357–364.
223. Ogbonmwan, Y.E., Schroeder, J.P., Holmes, P.V., and Weinshenker, D. 2015. The effects of post-extinction exercise on cocaine-primed and stress-induced reinstatement of cocaine seeking in rats. *Psychopharmacology* 232(8): 1395–1403.
224. Blake, H. et al. 2009. How effective are physical activity interventions for alleviating depressive symptoms in older people? A systematic review. *Clin Rehabil* 23: 873–887.
225. Schutte, N.M., Bartels, M., and de Geus, E.C. 2014. Genetic modification of the effects of exercise behavior on mental health. *Front Psychiatry* 3(5): 64.
226. Stubbe, J.H. et al. 2007. The association between exercise participation and well-being: A co-twin study. *Prevent Med* 44: 148–152.
227. Marleen, H.M. et al. 2008. Testing causality in the association between regular exercise and symptoms of anxiety and depression. *Arch Gen Psychiatry* 65: 897–905.
228. De Moor, M.H. et al. 2008. Testing causality in the association between regular exercise and symptoms of anxiety and depression. *Arch Gen Psychiatry* 65: 897–905.
229. Meggs, W.J. 2003. *The Inflammation Cure*. Lincoln, IL: NTC Publishing Group.
230. Agudelo, L.Z. et al. 2014. Skeletal muscle PGC-1α1 modulates kynurenine metabolism and mediates resilience to stress-induced depression. *Cell* 159: 33–45.
231. Jouvet, M. 1994. Paradoxical sleep mechanisms *Sleep* 17: S77–S83.
232. Haskell, E.H. et al. 1981. Metabolism and thermoregulation during stages of sleep in humans exposed to heat and cold. *J Appl Physiol Respirat Environ* 51: 948–954.
233. Brand, S. et al. 2009. High exercise levels are related to favorable sleep patterns and psychological functioning in adolescents: A comparison of athletes and controls. *J Adolesc Health* 46: 133–141.

234. Shapiro, C.M., Bortz, R. et al. 1981. Slow wave sleep: A recovery period after exercise. *Science* 214: 1253–1254.
235. Silva, A., Queiroz, S.S., Winckler, C. et al. 2010. Sleep quality evaluation, chronotype, sleepiness and anxiety of Paralympics Brazilian athletes: Beijing 2008 Paralympics Games. *Br J Sports Med* 46(2): 150–154.
236. Loprinzi, P.D. et al. 2011. Association between objectively measure physical activity and sleep NHANES 2005–2006. *Ment Health Phys Act* 4: 65.
237. King, A.C. et al. 1997. Moderate-intensity exercise and self-rated quality of sleep in older adults: A randomized controlled trial. *JAMA* 227: 32–37.
238. Dworak, M. et al. 2010. Sleep and brain energy levels: ATP changes during sleep. *J Neurosci* 30: 9007–9016.
239. Buman, M.P. and King, A.C. 2010. Exercise as a treatment to enhance sleep. *Am J Lifestyle Med* 4: 500–514.
240. Passos, G.S. et al. 2010. Effect of acute physical exercise on patients with chronic primary insomnia. *J Clin Sleep Med* 15: 270–275.
241. Spence, F.C. et al. 1997. The effect of physical activity participation on self-concept: A meta-analysis. *J Sp Ex Psych* 19: S109.
242. Boggiano, A.K. et al. 1982. The mastery hypothesis and the overjustification effect. *Social Cogn* 1: 38–49.
243. Deslandes, A.C. et al. 2010. Effect of aerobic training on EEG alpha asymmetry and depressive symptoms in the elderly: A 1-year follow-up study. *Braz J Med Biol Res* 43: 585–592.
244. McHugh, J.E. and Lawlor, B.A. 2012. Exercise and social support are associated with psychological distress outcomes in a population of community-dwelling older adults. *J Health Psychol* 17: 833–844.
245. Harvey, S.B. et al. 2010. Physical activity and common mental disorders. *Br J Psychiatry* 197: 357–364.
246. Armstrong, K. and Edwards, H. 2003. The effects of exercise and social support on mothers reporting depressive symptoms: A pilot randomized controlled trial. *Int J Ment Health Nurs* 12: 130–138.
247. Kamimura, A. et al. 2014. The relationship between body esteem, exercise motivations, depression, and social support among female free clinic patients. *Women's Health Issues* 24: 656–662.
248. Barkley, R.A. 1976. Predicting the response of hyperkinetic children to stimulant drugs: A review. *J Abnorm Child Psychol* 4: 327–346.
249. Barkley, R.A. 2000. *Taking Charge of ADHD, Revised Edition: The Complete, Authoritative Guide.* New York, NY: Guilford Press.
250. Hastings, J.E. and Barkley, R.A. 1978. A review of psychophysiological research with hyperkinetic children. *J Abnorm Child Psychol* 6: 13–47.
251. Mitchell, K.J. 2011. The genetics of neurodevelopmental diseases. *Curr Opin Neurobiol* 21: 197–203.
252. Swanson, J. et al. 1998. Cognitive neuroscience of attention deficit hyperactivity disorder and hyperkinetic disorder. *Curr Opin Neurobiol* 8: 263–271.
253. Erlij, D. et al. 2012. Dopamine D4 receptor stimulation in GABAergic projections of the globus pallidus to the reticular thalamic nucleus and the substantia nigra reticulata of the rat decreases locomotor activity. *Neuropharmacology* 62: 1111–1118.
254. Hillman, C.H. et al. 2014. Effects of the FITKids randomized controlled trial on executive control and brain function. *Pediatrics* 134: 1063–1074.
255. Pontifex, M.B. et al. 2013. Exercise improves behavioral, neurocognitive, and scholastic performance in children with attention-deficit/hyperactivity disorder. *J Pediatr* 162: 543–551.
256. Smith, A.L. et al. 2013. Pilot physical activity intervention reduces severity of ADHD symptoms in young children. *J Attention Disord* 17: 70–82.
257. Nikolas, M. et al. 2010. Gene × environment interactions for ADHD: Synergistic effect of 5HTTLPR genotype and youth appraisals of inter-parental conflict. *Behav Brain Funct* 6: 23.
258. Greenwood, B.N. et al. 2011b. Long-term voluntary wheel running is rewarding and produces plasticity in the mesolimbic reward pathway. *Behav Brain Res* 217: 354–362.
259. Terraccuabo, A. et al. 2013. Personality, metabolic rate and aerobic capacity. *PLoS One* 8: e54746.
260. Stine-Morrow, E.A. et al. 2014. Training versus engagement as paths to cognitive enrichment with aging. *Psychol Aging* 29: 891–906.
261. Mayberg, H.S. et al. 2005. Deep brain stimulation for treatment-resistant depression. *Neuron* 45: 651–660.
262. Lehmann, M.L. and Herkenham, M. 2011. Environmental enrichment confers stress resiliency to social defeat through an infralimbic cortex-dependent neuroanatomical pathway. *J Neurosci* 31: 6159–6173.
263. Michalak, J. et al. 2015. How we walk affects what we remember: Gait modifications through biofeedback change negative affective memory bias. *J Behav Ther Exp Psychiatry* 46: 121–125.

264. Martin, A. et al. 2014. Does active commuting improve psychological well-being? Longitudinal evidence from eighteen waves of the British household panel survey. *Prevent Med* 69: 296–303.

265. Otto, M. and Smits, J.A.J. 2011. *Exercise for Mood and Anxiety: Proven Strategies for Overcoming Depression and Enhancing Well-Being.* Oxford University Press.

266. Ransford, H.E. et al. 1996. Aerobic exercise, subjective health and psychological well-being within age and gender subgroups. *Soc Sci Med* 42: 1555–1559.

267. Sears, B. 2002. *The Omega Rx Zone.* New York, NY: Harper Collins.

268. Harvard Men's Health Watch. 2011. Benefits of exercise—reduces stress, anxiety, and helps fight depression. *Harvard Men's Health Watch* (February). Available at: http://www.health.harvard.edu/press_releases/benefits-of-exercisereduces-stress-anxiety-and-helps-fight-depression

269. Harvard Men's Health Watch. 2011. Exercising to relax. Harvard Men's Health Watch (February). Available at: http://www.health.harvard.edu/newsletters/Harvard_Mens_Health_Watch/2011/February/exercising-to-relax?utm_source=mens&utm_medium=pressrelease&utm_campaign=mens0211

270. Plowman, S.A. and Smith, D.L. 2013. *Exercise Physiology for Health Fitness and Performance,* 4th ed. Philadelphia, PA: Lippincott Williams & Wilkins.

271. Maffetone, P. 2012. *Healthy Aging, Illness Prevention, and Sexual Well-Being.* New York, NY: Skyhorse.

272. Oertel-Knochel, V. et al. 2014. Effects of aerobic exercise on cognitive performance and individual psychopathology in depressive and schizophrenia patients. *Eur Arch Psychiatry Clin Neurosci* 264: 589–604.

273. Chaddock, L. et al. 2012. A functional MRI investigation of the association between childhood aerobic fitness and neurocognitive control. *Biol Psychol* 89: 260–268.

274. Voss, M.W. et al. 2011. Aerobic fitness is associated with greater efficiency of the network underlying cognitive control in preadolescent children. *Neuroscience* 199: 166–176.

275. Chaddock-Heyman, L. et al. 2014. Aerobic fitness is associated with greater white matter integrity in children. *Front Hum Neurosci* 8: 584.

276. Puterman, E., Epel, E. et al. 2010. The power of exercise: Buffering the effect of chronic stress on telomere length. *PLoS One* 26: 5.

277. Baker, L.D. et al. 2010. Effects of aerobic exercise on mild cognitive impairment: A controlled trial. *Arch Neurol* 67: 71–79.

278. Andel, R. et al. 2008. Physical exercise at midlife and risk of dementia three decades later. *J Gerontol A Biol Sci Med Sci* 63: 62–66.

279. Yuki, A. et al. 2012. Relationship between physical activity and brain atrophy progression. *Med Sci Sports Exercise* 44: 2362–2368.

280. Erickson, K.I., Gildengers, A.G., and Butters, M.A. 2013. Physical activity and brain plasticity in late adulthood. *Dialogues Clin Neurosci* 15(1): 99–108.

281. Liu, R. et al. 2012. Cardiorespiratory fitness as a predictor of dementia mortality in men and women. *Med Sci Sports Exerc* 44: 253–259.

282. Verdelho, A. et al. 2012. Physical activity prevents progression for cognitive impairment and vascular dementia: Results from the LADIS (Leukoaraiosis and Disability) study. *Stroke* 43: 3331–3335.

283. Gow, A.J. et al. 2012. Neuroprotective lifestyles and the aging brain: Activity, atrophy, and white matter integrity *Neurology* 79: 1802–1808.

284. Voss, M.W. et al. 2013. The influence of aerobic fitness on cerebral white matter integrity and cognitive function in older adults: Results of a one-year exercise intervention. *Hum Brain Mapp* 34: 2972–2985.

285. Leckie, R.L. et al. 2014. BDNF mediates improvements in executive function following a 1-year exercise intervention. *Front Hum Neurosci* 8: 985.

286. Prakash, R.S. et al. 2015. Physical activity and cognitive vitality. *Ann Rev Psychol* 66: 769–797.

287. DiMatteo, M.R. et al. 2000. Depression is a risk factor for noncompliance with medical treatment: Meta-analysis of the effects of anxiety and depression on patient adherence. *Arch Intern Med* 160: 2010–2107.

288. Pinto Pereira, S.M., Geoffroy, M., and Power, C. 2014. Depressive symptoms and physical activity during 3 decades in adult life: Bidirectional associations in a prospective cohort study. *JAMA Psychiatry* 71(12): 1373–1380.

289. Cheney, C.D. 1992. Activity anorexia: Solving the anorexia puzzle: A scientific approach. *Behav Anal* 15: 157–160.

290. Aravich, P.F. et al. 1993. Beta endorphin and dynorphin abnormalities in rats subjected to exercise and restricted feeding: Relationship to anorexia nervosa? *Brain Res* 622: 18.

291. Johnston, O. et al. 2011. Excessive exercise: From quantitative categorization to a qualitative continuum approach. *Eur Eat Disord Rev* 19: 237–248.

292. Demetrovics, Z. and Kurimay, T. 2008. Exercise addiction: A literature review. *Psychiatr Hung* 23: 129–141.

293. Hausenblas, H.A. and Symons Downs, D. 2002a. Exercise dependence: A systematic review. *Psychol Sports Exerc* 3: 89–123.

294. Hausenblas, H.A. Symons Downs, D. 2002b. How much is too much? The development and validation of the exercise dependence scale. *Psychol Health* 3(17): 387–404.

295. Griffiths, M.D. et al. 2005. The exercise addiction inventory: A quick and easy screening tool for health practitioners. *Br J Sports Med* 39: e30.

296. Epling, W.F. and Pierce, W.D. 1984. Activity based anorexia in rats as a function of the opportunity to run on an activity wheel. *Nutr Behav* 1: 37–49.

297. Epling, W.F. and Pierce, W.D. 1996. *Activity Anorexia: Theory, Research and Treatment.* Mahwah, NJ: Lawrence Erlbaum.

298. Beregh, C. and Sodersten, P. 1996. Anorexia nervosa, self-starvation and the reward of stress. *Nat Med* 2: 21–22.

299. Lambert, K.G. 1993. The activity-stress paradigm: Possible mechanisms and applications. *J Gen Psychol* 120: 21.

300. Cooney, G.M., Dwan, K., Greig, C.A. et al. 2013. Exercise for depression. *Cochrane Database Syst Rev* (9): 1–142.

301. Carta, M.G. et al. 2008. Improving physical quality of life with group physical activity in the adjunctive treatment of major depressive disorder. *Clin Pract Epidemiol Ment Health* 26: 4–1.

302. Blake, H. 2012. Physical activity and exercise in the treatment of depression. *Front Psychiatry* 3: 106.

303. Edwards, S. 2006. Physical exercise and psychological well-being. *S Afr J Psychol* 36: 357–373.

304. Gotay, C.C. et al. 1992. Quality-of-life assessment in cancer treatment protocols: Research issues in protocol development. *J Natl Cancer Inst* 84: 575–579.

305. Atlantis, E. et al. 2004. An effective exercise based intervention for improving mental health and quality of life measures: A randomized controlled trial. *Prevent Med* 39: 424–434.

306. Aigner, M. et al. 2006. What does the WHOQOL-Bref measure? Measurement overlap between quality of life and depressive symptomatology in chronic somatoform pain disorder. *Soc Psychiatry Psychiatr Epidemiol* 41: 81–86.

307. Schuch, F.B. et al. 2011. The impact of exercise on quality of life within exercise and depression trials: A systematic review. *Ment Health Phys Act* 4: 43–48.

308. Berlim, M.T. and Fleck, M.P.A. 2003. Quality of life: A brand new concept for research and practice for psychiatry. *Rev Bras Psiquiatr* 25: 249–252.

309. Kerse, N. et al. 2010. Home-based activity program for older people with depressive symptoms: DeLLITE—A randomized controlled trial. *Ann Fam Med* 8: 214–223.

310. McNeil, J.K. et al. 1991. The effect of exercise on depressive symptoms in the moderately depressed elderly. *Psychol Aging* 487–488.

311. Stevens, C.J. and Bryan, A.D. 2012. Rebranding exercise: There's an app for that. *Am J Health Promot* 27: 69–70.

312. Blumenthal, A.L. et al. 2012. Effects of exercise training on depressive symptoms in patients with chronic heart failure the HF-ACTION randomized trial. *JAMA* 308: 465–474.

313. Blumenthal, J.A. et al. 2013. Is exercise a viable treatment for depression? *ACSMs Health Fit J* 16: 17–24.

314. Rethorst, C.D. and Trivedi, M.H. 2013. Evidence-based recommendations for the prescription of exercise for major depressive disorder. *J Psychiatr Pract* 19: 204–212.

315. Pollock, K.M. 2001. Exercise in treating depression: Broadening the psychotherapist's role. *J Clin Psychology/In Session: Psychother Pract* 57: 1289.

316. Pilu, A. 2007. Efficacy of physical activity in the adjunctive treatment of major depressive disorders: Preliminary results. *Clin Pract Epidemiol Ment Health* 3: 8.

22 The Role of Sleep and Light Therapy in Depression

Robin May-Davis, MD

CONTENTS

INTRODUCTION

Humans maintained the solar-based diurnal and seasonal cycles for thousands of years. Since the advent of electric light, we do not follow these environmental cues. Additionally, many of us do not get classic light exposure during the day when it is available, and interior light is of much lower intensity than a sunny day.[1] This shift has likely impacted our health in ways we never considered and are continuing to discover. Changes in light exposure and patterns from travel, computer and cell phone usage, in addition to traditional electric lights may be impacting a number of photosensitive mechanisms in our bodies.[2,3]

One of the most important discoveries of our own internal circadian clocks was the identification of the superchiasmatic nucleus (SCN), a small area of the hypothalamus.[1,4] Neuronal projections come to this area from a specialized region on the retina. The SCN communicates with serotonergic raphe nuclei, located in the brainstem. The raphe provides feedback about level of arousal and threat, and in turn the SCN influences the raphe nuclei's release of serotonin and the sleep–wake cycle. The SCN also regulates the pineal gland and its hormone melatonin, which is essential to our biological clocks and has established diurnal and seasonal variations.[4] As melatonin is released, it signals information about light–dark cycles to a number of sensitive cells in the body.[4] Another critical discovery for sleep is the peptide orexin.[5] Orexin, also known as hypocretin, is produced in the dorsolateral prefrontal hypothalamus and is also thought to have significant impact on the sleep–wake system with projections to both the SNC and portions of the raphe, as well as other regions in the nervous system.[5]

Several theories have been put forward in the literature to account for the impact of light changes and circadian rhythms on mood, and more specifically depression. Research on shift workers clearly identify this group as particularly vulnerable to higher rates of a variety of mental health concerns due in part to circadian "misalignment."[6,7] Studies have identified additional internal "molecular clocks" which are involved in influencing various physiological processes, some of which are considered critical in mood regulation.[5] The impact of these "clocks" can be seen in brain and systemic circuits involving temperature regulation, HPA axis regulation, immunomodular activity, monoamine shifts, mitochondrial activity, and metabolic peptide fluctuations.[8] Many of these areas relate back to explanatory models of mood disorders in current literature.[9] These portions of our internal circadian system, their connections, and their downstream effects provide some potential clues as to how changes in light and sleep might both impact emotional and behavioral conditions.

This background provides a framework relating sleep and light with mood disorders, a complex interaction that continues to be unraveled in greater depth. The clinical identification that light and sleep are important to mood predated much of this more recent molecular work, but these studies continue to reveal the basic science behind what the evidence-based literature has shown. Sleep and light are important factors in mood disorders.

SEASONS, SLEEP, AND DEPRESSION

Seasonal affective disorder (SAD) currently falls within the mood disorders as a modifier to either major depression or bipolar disorder with seasonal pattern.[10] Current epidemiologic studies find a prevalence of 2%–5% of the population as having this variation in mood cycling. There may also be some gender bias; statistically women are even more represented within SAD than in the general unipolar depression. Some studies indicate that this modifier is more common in extreme latitudes,[10,11] but others have found no clear association.[4] Current thinking on SAD has varied on the mechanisms of this pattern, but one common theory is a phase delay between rest and activity cycles.[11]

A relationship between sleep and depression has been long recognized and continues to be complex. Hypersomnia, excessive sleep, can be associated with mood issues and more commonly noted in "atypical" depression states,[10] seen often in SAD and bipolar disorder. Insomnia is difficulty initiating sleep, maintaining sleep, or early awakening if given the opportunity to sleep, and chronic insomnia is that which lasts more than thirty to ninety days, depending on source.[10,12] This condition is most commonly cited with depressive episodes and is reported by one third of the adult population.[13]

Sleep disturbance, included as one of the American Psychiatric Association's DSM criteria for depression,[10] is likely one of the most commonly reported neuro-vegetative symptoms. A quick review of literature is laden with links between insomnia and depression. A 2012 study found that mood and anxiety disorders were associated with 42%–63% of severe insomnia complaints.[14] In an earlier study in 2005, people reporting insomnia had a rate of association with significant depression 9.8 times that of those without sleep concerns.[15] Of note, not all studies have seen this relationship. One found that insomnia more commonly was associated with development of anxiety and not as much with depression.[16] Despite this outlier, the majority of studies see a significant association.

Furthermore, insomnia is associated with the most severe symptom of depression, suicidality. Sleep disturbance appears to be a risk factor for suicidality beyond its association with depression.[17] Decreased sleep was associated with higher suicidal ideation in a survey study of greater than 15,000 Korean residents.[18] In a 2012 review, nightmares as well as insomnia were associated more often with suicidality.[19] Beyond the epidemiologic data, studies using polysomnography have shown that an increase in the rapid eye movement (REM) sleep percentage may engender higher risk for suicidal thoughts.[20] Clearly, understanding factors that might increase suicidal risk is important, and sleep disturbance is among them.

Many of the more recent studies have suggested that rather than sleep disturbance being just another aspect of depression, that sleep disturbance, particularly insomnia, may be a causal factor.[21,22] A 2014 study found that participants with acute insomnia who then transitioned to chronic insomnia, had sleep architecture changes typically seen in depression.[23] They also had higher rates of developing first-onset depression than "normal" sleepers or those for whom acute insomnia resolved.[23] One study found that older adults with insomnia were from four to ten times more likely to be depressed when assessed at future intervals.[19] REM sleep disturbances are even seen in relatives of people with depression, and may precede clinical presentation of this illness.[24]

Despite this trend in data suggesting causality between insomnia and depression, it may not be that simple. Others feel that rather than insomnia causing depression, insomnia and depression are both secondary to some larger physiologic changes creating both sleep and mood disruption. Several researchers are looking at a number of metabolic systems that feed back into brain and hormone regions already identified as critical for mood and sleep.[3,4,8,25] One such study was on the orexinergic system. Animal models implicated that varying levels of light impacted orexinergic signaling in the brain, and reproduced an animal phenotype of depression.[25] This system may be a key mediator of light on mood and is clearly also related to the sleep system. Current investigations into the various links between sleep and depression are expanding our knowledge base rapidly, but we do not have all the answers. Exciting research continues to deepen our understanding of just how these systems interrelate.

BIPOLAR DEPRESSION

For the bipolar patient, circadian-rhythm instability is one of the theories describing what might make an individual more susceptible to mood state switching, mixed symptoms, and more treatment-resistant bipolar depression.[26] Investigations in the "clock gene" mutation and other animal models may shed some light on how sleep relates to bipolar disorder.[8,23] Therefore, interventions that impact circadian rhythms have been a target of therapy for the bipolar depressed patient as well as unipolar patients.

ADDRESSING SLEEP

As in much of medicine, lack of complete understanding of all the biological mechanisms has not impeded applying evidence-based interventions to improve patient care. It is also known that poorly treated sleep issues may result in persistent depression[15] and that optimizing sleep contributes to better outcomes in mood disorders.[27]

Now that we have established the importance of addressing sleep as a means to improve depression, several interventions will be reviewed. This discussion will include a range of conventional and more integrative, complementary options that one might consider when addressing insomnia in the patient with depression. It should be noted that the wealth of information is extensive on the topic of insomnia treatment. Therefore, the overview presented here is not an exhaustive review.

GENERAL MEDICAL ISSUES

One of the first tools in addressing sleep is managing the underlying issues which might make sleep worse. This includes a variety of medical condition such as nocturia, gastro-esophageal reflux, chronic pain, and other conditions that often impact sleep. Management of these issues will not be addressed here, but should be taken into consideration when evaluating the patient with sleep difficulties. Additionally, managing issues such as hormone imbalances, both involving either sex hormones or cortisol, would be critical but will not be explored in this chapter.

There are particular disorders specific to sleep, which seem to have a disproportionate amount of co-morbidity with depression, so these will be explored a bit more in depth.

SLEEP DISORDERS—SLEEP APNEA

Obstructive sleep apnea (OSA) is the most common of sleep breathing disorders and has been long associated with depressive symptoms.[28] OSA is a disorder wherein individuals have abnormalities in ventilation during sleep, resulting in frequent nocturnal awakenings and daytime fatigue.[10] It typically includes snoring, gasping, and pauses in breathing and is often associated with headaches, dry mouth, heartburn, low libido, and at times increased pulmonary hypertension as well as other abnormalities.[10] OSA is typically evaluated and diagnosed by polysomnography.[10,28]

In several studies looking at OSA, higher rates of depressive symptoms are found.[29,30] It is possible that higher depression ratings are associated with more daytime sleepiness, but the relationship is not fully clear.[31] A Centers for Disease Control and Prevention (CDC) epidemiologic study found that even when snorts, gasps, and pauses in breathing are reported by patients, depression was more commonly associated, even in those without a formal sleep study diagnosis.[30] Those who reported issues with these symptoms five nights a week were several times more likely to show signs of depression than those with no snoring or breathing pauses. This study was controlled for weight as well, which is also a common risk factor for sleep apnea.[30] Another cross-sectional study done in Europe found that the odds of having a breathing-related sleep disorder diagnosis was just over five times for those with a major depressive disorder, even after controlling for hypertension and obesity.[29]

The above studies would easily lead to the question whether treating sleep apnea might result in not only better sleep but also better depressive symptom response. A small study rated depression in those with sleep apnea prior to continuous positive airway pressure (CPAP) treatment initiation using both the Hamilton Depression Rating Scale (HDRS) and the Beck scale for depression. After 2 months of CPAP treatment, those who had major depression by structured clinical interview (SCID) had statistically significant responses, with scores nearly cut in half on both ratings scales.[32] In another small study of 37 patients with newly diagnosed sleep apnea, 21 had clinically relevant symptoms by HDRS, and 11 met major depression criteria by SCID. Again, those treated with CPAP had a clinically significant reduction in depressive symptoms.[33]

In contrast, a 2014 study with 300 patients looked at CPAP and depressive symptoms but did not find positive results.[34] Gagnadoux et al. used a self-rated depression scale but no formal diagnosis, and found after one year of CPAP 41% had no clinically significant change. Of note, depressive persistence was highly associated with excessive daytime sleepiness.[34] An older review that looked at a mix of studies evaluating CPAP and its impact on depression noted there were several studies showing improvement or no change.[28] It postulated that some variation in studies might be accounted for by lack of use of "sham-CPAP" as control, adherence issues, variations in duration of treatment, severity of apnea, or even placebo effect. More significantly, the article suggested that more improvement might be seen in those with higher depression scores.[28]

SLEEP DISORDERS—RESTLESS LEG SYNDROME

Restless legs syndrome (RLS), now known as Willis-Ekbom Disease (WED),[35] is a movement-related sleep disorder involving the sensorimotor system that disrupts sleep. Patients report an urge to move their legs associated with an uneasy sensation, which worsens in evening and when lying down, and a relief of sensation by movement.[10] This condition is a fairly prevalent disorder, impacting 2%–7% of the population, and it is common for RLS/WED to be associated with sleep disturbance, low energy, and poor focus.[10] As these symptoms also overlap with depressive complaints, it has been hard to distinguish between major depression and RLS/WED at times. After thorough review of the literature, a 2005 article found that while depressive symptoms are common in WED, there was no consensus of a causal pathway.[36] At that time not enough clear information was known.[36] In 2013, two cohort studies were done which suggested that the relationship might be bidirectional between WED and depression.[37]

In terms of treatment, some studies show that while treating RLS/WED with dopamine agents might lead to depressive symptom improvement,[36,38] treatment of depression in someone with RLS/WED is complicated. Several antidepressants can worsen WED, and it therefore requires careful consideration in management.[35] Serotonin reuptake inhibitors (SSRI) or serotonin-norepinephrine uptake inhibitors (SNRI) may worsen symptoms, while atypical antidepressants might be less likely to do so.[36]

Both of these sleep disorders have a high association with mood, so a quick screening of the patient with fatigue, sleep concerns, and depression should review common symptoms. Once general medical issues and sleep disorders have been ruled out or optimized, further treatment choices need to be taken into account if one desires to manage sleep difficulties.

TREATMENTS FOR INSOMNIA: MEDICATIONS

SEDATIVES

Sedative-hypnotic medications have been used for sleep for several decades. Medications including benzodiazepines as well as the non-benzodiazepine hypnotics are often used both short term and long term for patients with acute and chronic insomnia complaints. Though these at times are used independently, they are often used with antidepressants. These medications are thought to be effective in treating insomnia,[12,39,40] but in choosing medications it is also important to consider other factors. The impact of the medicine on one's mood disorder, as well as safety factors should also play key roles in decision making. These medications can pose a significantly higher risk of harm than placebo.[41] A study reviewed U.S. Food and Drug Administration (FDA) data in 2006 for just over 7000 patients who were randomized to either hypnotic drugs such as zolpidem, eszopiclone, zaleplon, and ramelteon (melatonin agent), or placebo.[42] Among this data set, the incidence of depression was statistically higher in those on sedatives than those randomized to placebo. This study noted that the definition of depression may not have been standardized to major depression per the DSM, but raised an awareness that though effective for sleep, these medications may increase the risk of lowering mood.[42]

Beyond the risks of worsening one's mood, these sedative hypnotic medications have other risks as well. At least one study has shown that a population of patients with depression, but not known sleep apnea, also had statistically more disordered sleep breathing.[43] In a 2014 study, patients who were treated with higher-dose hypnotics had more frequent sleep-related breathing issues as well as worse depression response.[44] Benzodiazepines, and to a lesser extent the "Z-drug" non-benzodiazepine hypnotics, have some habit-forming potential and a risk for both abuse and withdrawal. These are not ideal for patients with comorbid medical and psychiatric conditions, particularly substance use disorders.[45,46]

Even more concerning than worsening mood or addiction, is a potential mortality risk. Kripke et al. in 2012 wrote a paper reviewing patients prescribed hypnotics over two and a half years.[47] Those who had been prescribed a hypnotic had 4.6 times the hazard of dying compared to those who had not received a prescription over the study period.[47] Though correlation is not causation, it raises some suspicion about the safety of these treatments and warrants further exploration.

Sedating antihistamines, or H1 receptor antagonists, such as diphenhydramine and doxylamine, are often used as over-the-counter sleep aids and in combination "PM" medicines. A 2005 review found several studies in support of use of these medications, but suggested data were still preliminary.[48] Subsequent clinical guidelines published in 2008 did not, however, recommend these agents due to lack of evidence for their benefit in insomnia.[12] Not only did they not recommend, but they cautioned against using sedating antihistamines due to their risks, particularly delirium in the elderly.[12]

ANTIDEPRESSANTS

Antidepressants have a variable and complex relationship with sleep physiology. They can have a range of impacts on sleep depending on individual patients' reactions. In general, some of the influence that traditional antidepressants can have on sleep varies from REM suppression to shifting the time it takes to fall asleep, also called sleep onset latency.[49,50] REM sleep suppression is common with tricyclic antidepressants (TCA) and monoamine oxidase inhibitors (MAOIs), but some of these are sedating perhaps due to histaminergic effects. Discontinuation of these medicines can cause a REM rebound which can induce a number of intense dreams. SSRI medications have a variable outcome on sleep but are generally thought to decrease sleep efficiency by both increasing arousals in the night and extending sleep onset latency.[49,50] Antidepressants such as trazodone and mirtazapine are often used for their sedating side effects, but limited long-term data are available on these medications,[12] and they are used off-label. Low-dose doxepin has been FDA approved for insomnia.[50]

PRESCRIPTION MELATONIN AGENTS

It has been suggested that manipulating melatonin might not only be effective for sleep but may also have a role in managing depression.[51] Ramelteon is a prescription medication, which acts at the melatonin receptor and has been FDA-approved for treatment of insomnia in the United States. It is generally thought to be fairly safe and does not have the same concerns of oversedation, tolerance, or withdrawal that can be seen in many other prescription medications for insomnia.[52] Melatonin supplement doses in most studies have been thought to be too low for good comparison to melatonin receptor agonists such as ramelteon.[53] Agomelatine, a melatonin receptor agonist, has been shown to be effective for major depression.[54] It is approved for use in several places outside the United States, but has not gained U.S. approval and has been shown to elevate liver enzymes.[55] It is generally used for depression, rather than for sleep induction. [54]

ATYPICAL ANTIPSYCHOTICS

Some sedating atypical antipsychotics such as quetiapine are used in low doses as an adjunct for sleep, as an alternative to a typical sedative. Per the National Institutes of Health (NIH) statement on insomnia, these are all off-label uses, and due to the considerable health risks of these medications, they are not recommended for insomnia.[12]

ANTICONVULSANTS

The data are fairly limited on the use of anticonvulsants for insomnia, independent of their use for seizures and chronic pain. Gabapentin was shown in a small study of 18 patients with primary insomnia to improve sleep efficiency.[56] It has also been shown to be somewhat effective against perimenopausal hot flashes, which are known to disrupt sleep.[57] Pregabalin has limited data specific to insomnia, but what data were found regarding sleep were positive.[58] Finally, tiagabine had limited data but may play a role in increasing slow-wave or deep sleep, without impact on sleep onset latency or total sleep time.[59]

PSYCHOTHERAPIES AND BEHAVIORAL TREATMENTS

A number of psychological and behavioral methods have been used over the years to tackle insomnia. This heterogeneous group of psychotherapies has resulted in benefits for many patients, but the evidence for them has grown more in recent years as researchers attempt to obtain specific evidence on treatment options. A 2006 review of interventions looked at treatments from 1998 to 2004 which involved behavioral and psychological treatments for individuals with chronic insomnia.[60] This review was supported by the American Academy of Sleep Medicine as a means to update its practice recommendations in this area. The review found that among the 37 studies, five treatments qualified as evidence-based psychotherapy interventions for insomnia, and these in turn were built into their practice updates.[13] These included cognitive behavioral therapy, relaxation, stimulus control therapy (staying out of bed other than for sleep), paradoxical intention (stay awake passively instead of forcing self to sleep to extinguish performance anxiety regarding sleep), and sleep restriction (avoiding spending all day in bed, limiting napping). They found insufficient evidence to recommend imagery or cognitive therapy alone.[13] A meta-analysis also found that several different interventions were helpful for sleep, including behavioral treatment, relaxation, and cognitive-behavioral therapy (CBT).[60]

COGNITIVE-BEHAVIORAL THERAPY AND COGNITIVE BEHAVIORAL THERAPY FOR INSOMNIA (CBT-I)

Cognitive behavioral therapy is a psychotherapeutic modality that has data supporting its use in a number of psychiatric conditions and is one of the current psychotherapies in practice with the largest evidence base for its use.[61] CBT involves being aware of distorted thoughts and behavioral practices that make your condition worse and then changing both thoughts and behaviors to remedy the issue.[62] A review on various approaches of mind-body treatments found cognitive behavioral interventions, including CBT, had robust findings for benefit to sleep, improving both initial and middle insomnia.[63] One study in this review suggested that CBT might reduce sedative use for sleep.

CBT has been tailored specifically to address common thought and behavioral issues in insomnia to improve sleep, commonly called CBT-I.[64] This psychotherapy incorporates various components of behavioral interventions previously reviewed such as stimulus control, sleep restriction, sleep hygiene, and cognitive restructuring, and seems to be more beneficial than any one component of these other behavioral tools. Using CBT-I has been shown in several unbiased studies to be beneficial for sleep and often has a lasting durability of improvement not seen in most other sleep interventions.[12,64] Typically it is delivered in an individual setting, but some data do support its use even as group therapy[65] or online therapy.[66,67] Generally, guidelines and consensus statements currently include CBT-I as a first-line approach for managing insomnia and recommend that those on long-term medications have a trial of therapy to minimize long-term medication exposure.[12,40] There may be some risks with sleep restriction therapy, a component of CBT-I, which has been shown to increase daytime somnolence and impair performance in the short run.[68]

More importantly for the patient with major depression and insomnia, CBT-I was demonstrated as a promising treatment that improved both sleep and depressive symptoms.[27,69] It was studied as an augmentation to the SSRI antidepressant escitalopram, in which 30 subjects found that those using both the medication and CBT-I had double the remission rate of depression over medication alone, and a dramatically higher rate of remission from insomnia, 50.0% versus 7.7%.[27] One article reviewed recommended that CBT-I be broadly disseminated via primary care clinics as a means to help prevent depression.[70]

SLEEP HYGIENE AND SELF-HELP EDUCATION ON SLEEP

One practice that is often recommended by providers for better sleep is called "sleep hygiene." This concept dates back to the mid-1800s.[71] This concept includes a range of self-help behaviors such as creating a comfortable sleep environment, avoiding caffeine and alcohol close to bedtime, sleep scheduling such as setting bedtimes, minimizing naps, increasing exercise, and other behaviors thought to enhance likelihood of sleep improvement.[72,73] The application of "sleep hygiene" is generally done at home independently by the patient. Once educated about recommended changes, he or she applies them on their own without the additional guidance of a professional.

Studies have examined these practices to see if they do indeed improve sleep outcomes. A study by Morin et al. looked at younger patients who complained of sleep issues. Some received educational booklets about insomnia as well as behavioral strategies for sleep, and others were in a control group without education. Those with the sleep hygiene education fared better than a control group by a modest 4% sleep efficiency. These gains were maintained at the 6-month follow-up interval.[73]

Another study involved adults with insomnia but was an open trial. The study had three arms: one with self-help behavioral education, one with therapist-assisted behavioral education, and finally a control wait-list group. Those with the sleep education, either with or without the therapist, improved in sleep-onset latency and insomnia ratings. Though this study had some methodological issues, it suggested that self-help has potential as a low-cost initial intervention.[72] Moving on to larger meta-analyses, two reviews found that self-help therapy for insomnia tended to have small-to-moderate effect size, and did not show an advantage over working with a professional.[74,75] In settings where access might be an issue, however, self-help is a reasonable first approach.

RELAXATION

A review of mind-body approaches in 2010 found that relaxation was one of the approaches in which several studies used decent methodology and found positive results. Typically these included training on progressive relaxation or use of relaxation-guided audio. In this review, relaxation seemed to have a better impact on reducing sleep-onset latency than maintenance of sleep, or staying asleep.[63]

MINDFULNESS MEDITATION AND MINDFULNESS-BASED STRESS REDUCTION

Mindfulness meditation is a style of meditation intended to create awareness of one's existence in the present moment. It is a meditation technique, which has since been expanded into new approaches in behavioral medicine[76] including mindfulness-based stress reduction started by Jon Kabat-Zinn.[77] Use of mindfulness-based meditation has been used in the management of chronic insomnia successfully. One study did an 8-week trial using mindfulness-based stress reduction, mindfulness-based therapy for insomnia, or a self-monitoring group. These two mindfulness-based programs were both shown to have clinically significant improvements in reducing self-reported wake times and insomnia severity, with a slight advantage of the mindfulness-based insomnia treatment group.[78] Another study used mindfulness-based stress reduction and compared with an eszopi-clone 3-mg dose, without placebo arm. This study provided fairly intensive meditation training and had good outcomes for both groups.[79]

INTEGRATIVE SLEEP TREATMENTS

Sarris and Byrne did a review in 2011 to look at the expanding public interest in integrative treatments for chronic insomnia, with a focus mostly on herbs, dietary supplements, and acupuncture.[80] Though some of the studies reviewed were small or flawed, the variety showed a great interest in nonpharmacologic approaches to sleep. Another review on mind-body approaches to sleep also found that while many studies were small and had issues with design, they nonetheless suggested several approaches had promise and further data may help shed light on other options for sleep in the future.[63]

MUSIC

Many people over the years have listened to relaxing music as an aid to facilitate falling asleep. This is an inexpensive and very accessible modality for people to try. There have been studies looking at this approach, and the data may help justify using music in institutional settings such as hospitals or nursing facilities. A review on behavioral interventions for sleep indicated that use of classical music improved sleep quality and depressive symptoms compared to control group.[63] One 2009 meta-analysis was done to evaluate the efficacy of music in sleep quality in individuals with sleep complaints, but of note not necessarily those with defined chronic insomnia. This review found that five studies met their criteria, and music-assisted relaxation was somewhat effective in subjective sleep quality.[81] A more recent meta-analysis looked at 10 adult studies to evaluate the impact of music on sleep quality in those with acute and chronic sleep disorders. This review also found sleep quality improvements but that music seemed to have a cumulative dose and longer follow-up might be needed to fully assess its benefits.[82] These two meta-analyses were geared more toward subjective sleep quality assessments, but there seem to be less data looking at music therapy and more objective measures such as polysomnography and phases of sleep. One study using polysomnography suggested that in patients with long sleep latency, music may increase duration of deep sleep, but did not benefit shortening the sleep latency of any patients.[83] In summary, music appears to benefit subjective sleep quality in several small studies though its mechanism is not fully understood.

ACUPUNCTURE AND ACUPRESSURE

Acupuncture, a key component of traditional Chinese medicine, is a modality used for a variety of acute and chronic medical conditions. Standard acupuncture and electro-acupuncture have been used in several studies to address insomnia.[84,85] In a 2011 study, electro-acupuncture for insomnia associated with depression was done using an active placebo (needling at nonacupuncture sites, as well as noninvasive acupuncture) to enhance the placebo-control design. This study did not find a difference between the active needling at nonspecific sites, and the traditional electro-acupuncture on sleep. Both needling interventions made improvements on subjective sleep over noninvasive placebo.[86] The Cochrane Collaboration, an independent group that systematically reviews the literature and makes evidence-based guidelines, completed a review on acupuncture for insomnia on multiple occasions, in 2007 and again updated in 2012. Their conclusions were that the clinical evidence was just not high-quality enough to support or disprove acupuncture as a method for treating insomnia.[85] Auricular acupuncture has had multiple reviews with various conclusions, including that it appeared to be effective,[87] but another that evidence was too limited.[88] Overall, it appears that the evidence for standard acupuncture, electro-acupuncture, and auricular acupuncture is not yet considered high-quality enough to determine whether it is beneficial.[85] A 36-month trial was started in 2013. This multicenter investigation will see if higher-quality data can shed light on the effectiveness of acupuncture for depression-related insomnia.[89]

Acupressure was included in a 2011 review article and it, on the other hand, was found to have at least two studies of good quality, which showed small-to-moderate effect size of benefit for insomnia.[80]

Limited data currently exist on other interventions such as foot reflexology, massage, and cranial manipulation. There is a suggestion that these might be beneficial, yet more detailed review with improvement in study design is required.[90]

EXERCISE

Many regular exercise practitioners attribute their fitness routines to their good sleep. Studies on exercise and sleep show that aerobic physical activity has sleep benefits that can improve sleep quality and often mood.[91] A meta-analytic study from back in 1996 found that exercise increased slow-wave sleep, improved sleep-onset latency, and improved total sleep time.[92] Even in older adults, who tend to have higher levels of insomnia, aerobic exercise has been self-reported to improve sleep.[94] Additionally, moderate exercise was shown by polysomnography after 4 months to have improved sleep as well as reduced depressive symptoms, and contributed to some improvements in immune and stress hormone markers.[94]

If exercise improves nighttime sleep, does the time of day one exercises matter? For years, exercising too close to bedtime was advised against for fear that it might increase arousal. This assertion likely prompted many not to pursue exercise at a time when it might have been most convenient due to fears that sleep might be worsened. Recent data have come out to refute that assertion. One article was a 2013 Nation Sleep Foundation American Poll, which found that those who performed vigorous evening exercise felt that sleep was often better quality on the days of activity.[92] A further study in 2014 used sleep electroencephalogram (EEG) to assess adults after vigorous evening exercise. In fact, this study found that perceived level of exertion was associated with improved sleep efficiency, shorter time to fall asleep, and deeper sleep in a healthy adult cohort.[95]

Particular types of exercise have been looked at in relation to sleep, particularly in older adults, in whom nonpharmacological options might be more critical to avoid polypharmacy and associated gait and cognitive impairments. Systematic reviews in 2010 and 2011 both agreed yoga and tai chi were among those interventions which had better data for use in chronic insomnia.[63,80] Both reviews included a study of older adults with moderate sleep complaints who used a tai chi intervention compared to a health education intervention for 25 weeks.[96] The tai chi intervention improved sleep duration and yielded less arousal by rating scale. The two systematic reviews also both included a study of yoga in older adults which showed that the active group had shorter sleep onset latency, less arousals, and reported feeling better rested.[97] A more recent 2014 study looked at a yoga intervention, which included yoga postures in a class two times a week and additional daily home yoga meditation compared to a wait-list control group. When used in a group of over 60-year-old adults with insomnia, the intervention group noted improvements in several factors such as subjective sleep quality, decreased fatigue, and even better mood after 12 weeks.[98]

HOMEOPATHY

Homeopathy is the practice of giving remedies which are in extremely diluted amounts, but if given at full strength would create symptoms similar to what it is intending to treat. A 2011 systematic review of various integrative interventions found that there were not an adequate number of randomized trials using homeopathy to evaluate its use.[80] Another specific review of homeopathy for insomnia noted that in 2010, only four randomized, controlled studies compared homeopathic interventions to placebo, and all were of low methodological quality or low number of subjects. Therefore, this review found the evidence was too limited to demonstrate any significant effect.[99] A general review of oral nonprescriptive treatments for insomnia included the homeopathic agent *Natrum muriaticum*, and found lack of adequate information to recommend this remedy.[48] It should be noted that homeopathy is generally individually tailored to the patient, and therefore it does not lend itself as easily to the standard randomized controlled trial utilizing the same intervention for all subjects in a study.

DEVICES (NON-LIGHT)

CRANIAL ELECTROTHERAPY STIMULATION

Cranial electrotherapy stimulation (CES) is a treatment using a FDA-recognized medical device which delivers micro-current electrical stimulation transcutaneously, typically on the head or ears. These devices have been used in studies for pain, anxiety, mood, and sleep.[100] There have been studies reviewing specifically those with insomnia and also some studies looking at sleep as a secondary symptom in another condition such as chronic pain or depression. Many of these studies are favorable, and a meta-analytic review showed a large effect size, with fairly limited reports of side effects.[101] It should be noted that the author of the study appears to have ties to some of the products reviewed.

TRANSCRANIAL MAGNETIC STIMULATION

Repetitive transcranial magnetic stimulation (rTMS) has been used in the treatment of depression.[101] One study looked at its use in the treatment of patients with chronic insomnia. The study compared the treatment to medications and psychotherapy, and after 2 weeks showed improved polysomnographic changes, and better recurrence rates.[102] Of note, 2 weeks is likely too short for a psychotherapy intervention to show benefit, and this intervention for insomnia is likely cost-prohibitive to many.

SUPPLEMENTS

MELATONIN

Melatonin is a hormone found in animals as well as in plants, and in humans plays a role in circadian rhythms as discussed previously in this chapter. Supplemental melatonin hormone has been popular for sleep for many years. A 2002 review looking at the use of integrative treatments found that of over 30,000 individuals, nearly 6% had tried over-the-counter (OTC) melatonin for insomnia.[103] As an OTC supplement, it is not regulated, and there is variability in the quality of the products available. A meta-analysis in 2013 reviewed 19 studies and found that melatonin demonstrated efficacy, which was significant changes in improved total sleep time and reduced sleep latency.[104] Trials with higher doses had greater effects sizes, and impact seemed to persist with continued use.[106] Another prior meta-analysis suggested that melatonin had an impact on lowering sleep latency, but it was just over 10 minutes, so was not clinically helpful.[105] This review found that melatonin's primary role in sleep issues was for those with delayed sleep phase.

As for direct impacts on depression, one older study looked specifically at sleep in major depression, and found that though slow-release melatonin did improve sleep somewhat, it not did impact mood in patients already taking SSRIs.[106] Another review indicated that though a few studies have shown some impact on depression scores, results had been inconsistent, and there was currently no clear evidence for using melatonin specifically for either prophylaxis for depression or depression as a treatment.[107]

Most reviews concluded that though benefit might be more modest than conventional pharmacologic treatments for insomnia, melatonin had a more benign safety profile.[105] Of note, most studies have not looked at long-term use and there also appears to be very limited data as to the risks and impact to one's endogenous melatonin system when exogenous supplement is taken.

HERBAL TREATMENTS (ORAL USE)

As OTC supplements, herbal preparations in the United States are not regulated, and there is variable quality of the products available. A range of herbs have been used in traditional cultures for sleep for centuries, but few of them have been evaluated in the literature.

VALERIAN ROOT

Valerian root is an herbal preparation which has been often used and reviewed, but has very mixed data for sleep. Complementary treatments of over 30,000 individuals were reviewed in interviews in the 2002 National Health interview study, which assessed that 5.9% of these individuals had used valerian previously, but less than half the time this was after consultation with a health provider.[104]

In 2006, Bent et al. did a systematic meta-analysis of 16 randomized studies which concluded that valerian might improve sleep quality with limited side effects.[108] Taibli et al. found, looking at 29 controlled trials and in eight open label trials, that valerian was very safe with limited variation from placebo; the most rigorous studies did not find valerian had significant effects on sleep as a solo agent.[109] A 2010 review looking at 16 studies with both valerian and occasionally with hops noted that though valerian might be associated with improvements in sleep latency or quality of sleep, there was much variation in the study designs.[110] Another study published that year found, after review of 18 randomized, controlled studies, that valerian root had good subjective improvement of insomnia but had not been demonstrated by quantitative or objective measures.[111]

PASSIONFLOWER

Passionflower is another herbal treatment used for anxiety and included in combinations for sleep and relaxation. One study of healthy volunteers found subjective benefit to their sleep quality using passionflower.[112] A more rigorous study combined passionflower with hops and valerian root in a head-to-head comparison with zolpidem for sleep. Both groups had significant improvements, but of note there was no placebo arm. They also found a similar amount of adverse events such as daytime drowsiness.[113]

KAVA KAVA

Prepared from *Piper methysticum*, this herb has been consumed in a variety of cultures to relieve anxiety and facilitate sleep. Much of the data on this herb are related more to anxiety than insomnia, but though limited suggest its possible benefit for sleep.[114] The FDA published an advisory in 2002, which warned of risks to the liver from this supplement. Though many studies looking at its use have not seen this side effect, it is typically recommended with caution, often avoiding in those with preexisting liver disease, and occasionally monitored with liver enzymes. Initial discussion of Kava at that time blamed its preparation or perhaps chemicals used for extraction, but more recent work has suggested agents within the Kava root having hepatotoxic activity.[115]

Many other herbal medicines have been suggested to be useful for sleep and relaxation. These include herbs such as wild lettuce, scullcap, chamomille, Jamaican dogwood, lemon balm, California poppy, hops, St. John's wort, Patrinia root, and traditional Japanese medicine agent Yoku-kan-san-ka-chimpi-hange.[48] A 2005 study done by the American Academy of Sleep Medicine clinical practice review committee found that when reviewing articles between 1980 and 2002, there were very limited well-designed studies for these and several other compounds. Though many individuals may subjectively find these effective, there were limited data to back up these herbal remedies and in the case of Jamaican dogwood, may have some considerable risks.[48]

AROMATHERAPY

Aromatherapy is the use of plant essence and aromatic compounds in a therapeutic setting. The mechanism is the inhalation of volatile molecules via the sense of smell and their impact on the nervous system.[116] Lavender (genus *Lavandula*) is a fragrance used for centuries for its scent and included in many products marketed over the counter for relaxation. Though the volume of more promising data is growing on its use for anxiety in both oral and aromatherapy preparations, limited scientific data are available on lavender for insomnia. One small open study did show benefit for sleep for a small group with mild insomnia.[117] Another small study found that Chinese women with insomnia did better with sleep after 12 weeks of twice-weekly exposure to lavender aromatherapy.[118] Bergamot, ylang ylang, and jasmine are all other scents sometimes recommended for relaxation, but limited data specifically on use in insomnia were available on these scents.

OTHER NUTRACEUTICALS

MAGNESIUM

Magnesium compounds are often suggested as an accessible supplement to consider for sleep. A 2012 double-blind randomized placebo controlled study on primary insomnia in 46 older adults used 500 mg magnesium per night to see if it would benefit their sleep. The results indicated that the magnesium group, though did not differ from control at baseline in magnesium levels, did have changes in subjective insomnia reporting, higher melatonin levels, and lower serum cortisol levels. Total sleep time was not improved, but efficiency was better.[119]

IRON

Although there has been an association found between low ferritin levels and restless legs, studies using supplemental iron have not consistently shown a decrease in symptoms or improvements in sleep overall.[120]

GLYCINE

Glycine is an amino acid that also works as an inhibitory neurotransmitter in the central nervous system of humans. It has been used in supplemental form in a few small studies and shows some promise.[121] One crossover study used 3 g of glycine with 19 females and improved subjective quality of sleeping.[122] A second study was an open trial in which glycine was used in 11 subjects and this small trial found that glycine had beneficial changes both on sleep ratings and polysomnography.[123]

Gamma-Amino Butyric Acid

Gamma-amino butyric acid (GABA) is a primary inhibitory neurotransmitter in humans. Several sedative medications target receptors for this agent. Despite that fact that logically there would be interest in taking exogenous GABA to assist sleep, there are very limited data on supplemental GABA for use in patients with insomnia.[48]

L-Tryptophan

L-Tryptophan is an amino acid, had been a popular choice as an alternative intervention for sleep, and was among several other agents assessed as part of a clinical practice review for the American Academy of Sleep Medicine.[48] They found there was inadequate information for its use in insomnia and additionally some increased risk, presumably related to the eosinophilic myalgia occurrence associated with this supplement.[124] 5-THP, made from L-tryptophan and the precursor to serotonin, is often also recommended for sleep, anxiety, and mood, and though there may be some data relating it to sleep, no controlled studies were found using this intervention with defined insomnia.

Phenibut

Phenibut is sold as a supplement for relaxation. It may have similarities in structure to both baclofen, a muscle relaxer, and pregabalin, an anticonvulsant. It crosses the blood-brain barrier and is reported to work on the GABA receptor.[125] Many accounts of tolerance and withdrawal have been reported, so safety concerns perhaps similar to that of benzodiazepines might be merited.[126]

LIGHT THERAPY

Light Therapy for Sleep

Light therapy has been shown to be effective for a number of sleep-related issues, particularly those related to onset of sleep timing. The American Academy of Sleep Medicine has established practice guidelines for the use of light therapy in sleep. Both delayed and advance sleep phase shift disorders can benefit from bright light therapy, though the timing of the light exposure varies depending on which direction you are trying to shift the sleep cycle.[127] Also, jet lag and shift work have some, though less robust data.[128] There is even a section in the guidelines referring to hypersomnia in SAD, referring to studies suggesting light therapy might be more beneficial for "atypical"-type depressions.[129]

One study looked at amber lenses, which are designed to block blue light, the wavelength thought to make more of an impact on sleep-wake cycles. In this study amber glasses were worn 3 hours prior to sleep and showed significant improvement of sleep quality and improved affect. Of note, the lens groups had poorer quality sleep at outset, and thus had more room for improvement, so this has to be taken into account as a methodological flaw.[130]

There are also "dawn" and "dusk" simulators that work in one's house to fluctuate lighting indoors relating to typical diurnal patterns. There are less data about these, but they may be tools to watch in the future for both sleep and mood.[1]

Light Therapy for Mood

Out of the observation that changes in light exposure might influence seasonal rhythms and mood, came the concept that using light as an intervention might reverse seasonal mood changes. Decades ago this concept was put into use and now bright light therapy has been the treatment of choice for SAD and has expanded to use in a variety of mood and sleep disorders.[4,131]

LIGHT THERAPY FOR SEASONAL AFFECTIVE DISORDER

Bright light therapy has demonstrated its efficacy in treating SAD.[132,133] Some studies using lower-intensity blue wavelength light exposure at lower intensities have also demonstrated a positive effect.[130,131] The 2006 Can-SAD study based out of Canada was a head-to-head comparison with medication. Both 10,000 lux light therapy with placebo and Prozac 20 mg with 100 lux light (placebo) evidence fairly equivalent response and remission rates, but light therapy was reported to have an earlier response and less treatment emergent adverse events.[129]

Light therapy can be used in conjunction with other treatments in a combination approach for both seasonal and nonseasonal depression. A small study of SAD using CBT, light therapy, and their combination noted that CBT may work as good adjuvant treatment to light therapy and seemed to play a role in lower relapse rate the following winter after treatment intervention.[134]

LIGHT THERAPY FOR NONSEASONAL UNIPOLAR DEPRESSION

The literature is fairly clear that light therapy is effective for seasonal depression, but what about for general nonseasonal unipolar depression? A number of studies have been done, but methodological flaws limit the interpretation of several reports.[135,136] Despite these limitations, several meta-analytic reviews investigating primarily bright light interventions have found this treatment to be effective.[137-139] Effect size for light therapy in this group has been considered in the modest range and also comparable to many antidepressant interventions.[137] The Cochrane Review article found that for nonseasonal depression, light therapy does offer modest efficacy, and ideally is administered in the morning, and started at the onset of illness.[139]

Can bright light therapy be added to medications as an augmenting agent? One meta-analysis found that in review of three studies, bright light treatment had modest effect size, but found that bright light as an adjunct to antidepressants was not effective over five studies.[137] Despite this meta-analytic review, several other studies have found that augmenting antidepressant treatment with light therapy did hasten response and increase response rates.[139,140]

LIGHT THERAPY FOR ANTENATAL DEPRESSION

Certainly a group wherein both providers and patients often prefer to avoid medication or even other herbal interventions is the pregnant patient with depression.

Bright light therapy in one small trial was initially done as a randomized, 5-week trial using low-intensity light as their control in a group of pregnant women. The initial 5-week trial showed no difference between the light group and their placebo condition, but did in the 5-week optional extension. Successful treatment was associated with phase advances in melatonin release.[137] The Cochrane database did a meta-analytic review of options for treating antenatal depression. In this review they found that women receiving bright light therapy versus dim light had a significant improvement in depression scores but not necessarily higher remission rates.[133] Therefore, their review stated the evidence was too inconclusive to make a recommendation for use of bright light therapy in pregnancy for depression.[141]

LIGHT THERAPY FOR OLDER ADULTS

Due to concerns of polypharmacy as well as changes in metabolic functioning, nonmedication options are often sought in working with elderly patients suffering from depression. Additionally, the impairment that older adults might have with their SCN-mediated rhythms might also make light therapy a reasonable candidate for intervention. Studies have found that using bright light therapy not only enhanced mood but also improved sleep.[142] One particular study on light therapy also evaluated evening cortisol in their depressed elderly group and found a significant decrease persisted even after discontinuation of the treatment intervention.[142]

PRACTICAL APPLICATIONS—GUIDE FOR USING LIGHT THERAPY

Light therapy involves exposure to a light source, typically a specialized fluorescent lamp. The lamp includes the light source, with a diffusing screen and filter, which protects from UV light. Several units recommend having the light about 1–3 feet away. Eyes should be open, but it is not necessary or even desired to stare into the light source, instead looking at the surface the light is shining on.[1,4] The light source is typically rated in luminous energy, measured in units of lux, rather than radiant energy which is measured in watts. In additional studies investigating varying intensities, the time of daily exposure is also taken into consideration. There are some visors one could wear as the light source, but there are less data on these items.[1] Most studies show a preference for morning exposure to the light.[1,4] While other studies, state time of day was not significant.[138] As for duration of exposure, most studies vary slightly based on luminance, with higher lux ratings having shorter exposures. For example, studies with 10,000 lux emittance may use 15–30 minute exposures, while studies using lower lux ratings used longer exposure time.[1,4] Finally, the time-course of treatment appears to be ongoing, or throughout the winter in the case of seasonal depression, as gains made by exposure in many studies extinguish after termination of regular use.[11]

Alternatively, some studies focus less on luminous emittance and instead on the light wavelength. In the studies which focus on wavelength, primarily they are investigating blue-enriched light, or short wavelength light. Studies using both high lux light as well as low-intensity blue light both have shown antidepressive benefit.[139,140]

Some individuals have speculated that low levels of vitamin D due to lack of sun conversion in areas of extreme latitudes during winter months might be the reason light exposure is important to mood. An older study from 1993 randomized patients with seasonal depression to vitamin D or broad spectrum light of unknown intensity, to allow skin to convert and create vitamin D.[143] Both groups had an increase in vitamin D, and both groups improved their depression scale.[132] Conversely, another study looked at bright light exposure and measured both melatonin and vitamin D, neither of which were associated clearly with the reduction of depressive symptoms which occurred with their intervention.[141]

RISKS OF LIGHT THERAPY

Many studies of light therapy did not report adverse events very systematically.[139] Retinal damage, eyestrain, and perhaps photosensitivity are possible risks, but current thinking is that this is speculative, particularly in the high-quality lamps which filter out UV light. Despite the low likelihood of risks, it is recommended to be avoided in those with retinal disease. As for patients who are known or perhaps unknown to have bipolar disorder, emergent mania is a risk of the treatment.[139] Other than these two primary concerns, various vague complaints have been reported without clear consistency, such as nausea, headache, dizziness, or agitation. Some studies have shown that bright light therapy is not more likely than typical light to induce these vague side effects.[140]

SLEEP RESTRICTION, WAKE THERAPY, AND CHRONOTHERAPY

Sleep deprivation has been a known treatment for rapid intervention in bipolar and unipolar depression.[144,145] This is often done using a combination of three phases: wake therapy, sleep phase advance, and light therapy. Sometimes this combination is referred to as triple chronotherapy.[1] When the wake therapy portion is done, the patient is kept awake all night and into the next day. The sleep phase advance portion comes after the staying awake but requires that the sleep be initiated hours before the typical bedtime. The final portion, light therapy, is timed about an hour prior to typical rising and is a 30-minute light exposure.

This intervention typical acts within 1–2 days, with a positive response in somewhere between 40%–60% of patients.[145,146] For the bipolar patient, this intervention definitely is recommended to be done in the inpatient setting and can induce mania.[1] The difficulty with this intervention has been the lack of sustained response, as though response rates are high, relapses can occur.[145,146] So, what biological changes are seen in responders? Researchers found that of those who responded in one study, there was a distinct pattern change in blood flow detected on fMRI which was also predicted by genotype. Variations in the promoter for the serotonin transporter tended to predict clinical response and reflect the noted fMRI changes.[147]

A study of unipolar inpatients had treatment arms with either three wake therapies in combination with light therapy or an exercise group. The remission rate was just over 58% in the wake treatment group versus 6% in the exercise group, but these responses did not tend to persist.[146]

A 2014 Study by Benedetti et al. used a combination of three cycles of sleep deprivation, morning bright light therapy, and lithium in 141 patients, most of whom had drug-resistant bipolar depression.[147] By one week, 70% responded with a 50% reduction in Hamilton Depression rating (HAM-D), and 55% maintained benefit at one month follow-up. Responses even included those with active suicidal thoughts at time of treatment. Of note, two patients did have emergent mania in the study.[147] Another study used a combination of total sleep deprivation and light therapy in nonresistant versus treatment-resistant bipolar depression patients.[146] Of these groups, 70% nonresistant responded, and 44% treatment-resistant patients responded by a 50% reduction in HAM-D rating. Of these, when followed up 9 months later, 57% of the nonresistant group was still euthymic while 83% of the resistant patients had relapsed into depression.[148] Perhaps one of the keys to maintaining the benefits of this intervention is combining with other treatments. When used in combination with conventional treatments such as lithium versus medication alone, a 2014 study found that these circadian interventions enhanced antidepressant response in bipolar depressed patients, and improvements were seen to persist over a several week period.[146]

Wake therapy or triple chronotherapy seems to be a treatment intervention which has rapid and high response rates, but the tools to maintain these gains merit further study. The more we understand the relationship with sleep, light, and depression, we can better utilize these promising interventions.

CONCLUSION

In summary, poor sleep and depression are highly interrelated. It is likely that chronic insomnia leads to depression, but also possible that larger physiological factors lead to both of these conditions. Treating insomnia benefits depression response, and there are a variety of approaches. Ruling out and treating a variety of medical conditions, such as sleep disorders, are important first steps. Medications can be effective at times, but most have significant safety concerns. Psychotherapies such as CBT-I, relaxation, and mindfulness-based interventions are much safer and have good evidence to support their use. Music and exercise, perhaps particularly yoga and tai chi, may be quite beneficial and are generally safe and good for overall health. Acupuncture is not currently recommended, but future studies are pending to provide more robust data. Medical devices such as CES or TMS are likely effective but may be cost-prohibitive.

Melatonin has some likely benefit, but studies are variable. Oral herbal, aromatherapy, and nutraceutical supplements have some positive studies, and are generally thought to be fairly safe. These have more limited data and are perhaps not clearly as effective as other mind-body choices.

Light therapy is another intervention effective for sleep, especially phase shifted issues. It is also extremely effective for treating major depression with and without seasonal pattern. Finally, chronotherapy is often very effective for treating acute unipolar and bipolar depression, but lasts longer when sleep deprivation is paired with light therapy and possibly medication.

ACKNOWLEDGMENTS

The author of this chapter would like to give a particular thanks to Scott Davis, LCSW, and Jennifer Kramer, LCSW, for their editing and support during this writing. Thanks also to the editors of this book for supporting all of us to look beyond the standard treatments and use the literature to review the best and safest variety of options for our patients.

REFERENCES

1. Terman, M. and McMahan, I. 2012. *Reset Your Inner Clock*. New York: Penguin.
2. Bedrosian, T. and Nelson, R. 2013. Influence of the modern light environment on mood. *Mol Psychiatry* 18(7): 751–757.
3. McClung, C. 2011. Circadian rhythms and mood regulation insights from pre-clinical models. *Eur Neuropsychopharmacol* 21(4): S683–S693.
4. Pail, G., Huf, W., Pjrek, E. et al. 2011. Bright-light therapy in the treatment of mood disorders. *Neuropsychobiology* 64: 152–162.
5. Ebrahim, I., Howard, R., Kopelman, M., Sharief, M., and Williams, A. 2002. The hypocretin/orexin system. *J Roy Soc Med* 95(5): 227–230.
6. Rajarantnam, S., Howard, M., and Grunstein, R. 2013. Sleep loss and circadian disruptions in shift work: Health burden and management. *Med J Aust* 21: S11–S15.
7. Simon, R.D. 2012. Shift work disorder: Clinical assessment and treatment strategies. *J Clin Psychiatry* 73(6): e20. doi:10.4088/JCP.11073br3
8. McClung, C. 2013. How might circadian rhythms control mood? Let me count the ways... *Biol Psychiatry* 74(4): 242–249.
9. Lanfumey, L., Mongeau, R., and Hamon, M. 2014. Biological rhythms and melatonin in mood disorders and their treatments. *Pharmacol Ther* 138(2): 176–184.
10. American Psychiatric Association. 2013. *Diagnostic and Statistical Manual of Mental Disorders*, 5th ed. Arlington VA: American Psychiatric Association.
11. Magnusson, A. and Boivin, D. 2003. Seasonal affective disorder: An overview. *Chronobiol Int* 20(2): 189–207.
12. National Institutes of Health. 2005. State of the science conference statement manifestations and management of chronic insomnia in adults. *Sleep* 28(9): 1049–1057.
13. Morgenthaler, T., Kramer, M., Alessi, C. et al. 2006. Practice parameters for the psychological and behavioral treatment of insomnia: An update. An American Academy of Sleep Medicine Report. *Sleep* 29(11): 1415–1419.
14. Soehner, A. and Harvey, A. 2012. Prevalence and functional consequences of severe insomnia symptoms in mood and anxiety disorders: Results from a national representative sample. *Sleep* 35(10): 1367–1375.
15. Taylor, D., Lichstein, K., Durrence, H., Reidel, B., and Bush, A. 2005. Epidemiology of insomnia, depression, and anxiety. *Sleep* 28(11): 1457–1464.
16. Neckelman, D., Mykeltun, A., and Dahl, A. 2007. Insomnia, anxiety disorders and depression. *Sleep* 30(7): 873–880.
17. Bernert, R. and Joiner, T. 2007. Sleep disturbance and suicide risk: A review of the literature. *Neuropsychiatr Dis Treat* 3(6): 735–743.
18. Kim, H., Park, E., Cho, W., Park, C., Choi, W., and Chang, H. 2013. Association between total sleep duration and suicidal ideation among the Korean general adult population. *Sleep* 36(10): 1563–1572.
19. Pigeon, W., Pinquart, M., and Conner, K. 2012. Meta-analysis of sleep disturbance and suicidal thoughts and behaviors. *J Clin Psychiatry* 73(9): e1160–e1167. doi:10.4088/JCP.11r07586
20. Agargun, M. and Cartwright, R. 2003. REM sleep, dream variables and suicidality in depressed patients. *Psychiatry Res* 119(1–2): 33–39.
21. Staner, L. 2010. Comorbidity of insomnia and depression. *Sleep Med Rev.* 14(1): 35–46.
22. Gillin, J. 1998. Are sleep disturbances risk factors for anxiety, depressive and addictive disorders? *Acta Psychiatr Scand Suppl* 393: 39–43.
23. Ellis, J., Perlis, M., Bastien, C., Gardani, M., and Espie, C. 2014. The natural history of insomnia: Acute insomnia and first onset depression *Sleep* 37(1): 97–106.
24. Pagalini, L., Baglioni, C., Ciapparelli, A., Gemignani, A., and Riemann, D. 2013. REM sleep dysregulation in depression: State of the art. *Sleep Med Rev* 17(5): 377–390.

25. Deats, S., Adidharma, W., Lonstein, J.S., and Yan, L. 2014. Attenuated orexinergic signaling underlies depression-like responses induced by daytime light deficiency. *Neuroscience* 272: 252–260.
26. Lee, H., Son, G., and Geum, D. 2013. Circadian rhythm hypotheses of mixed features, antidepressant treatment resistance, and manic switching in bipolar disorder. *Psychiatry Investig.* 10(3): 225–232.
.27. Manber R., Edinger, J., Gress, J., San Pedro-Salcedo, M., Kuo, T., and Kalista, T. 2008. Cognitive behavioral therapy for insomnia enhances depression outcome in patients with co-morbid major depressive disorder and insomnia. *Sleep* 31(4): 489–495.
28. Schröder, C. and O'Hara, R. 2005. Depression and obstructive sleep apnea (OSA). *Ann Gen Psychiatry* 4: 13.
29. Ohayon, M. 2003. The effects of breathing related sleep disorders on mood disturbances in the general population. *J Clin. Psychiatry* 64(10): 1195–1200.
30. Wheaton, A., Perry, G., Chapman, D., and J Croft. 2012. Sleep disordered breathing and depression among U.S. adults: National Health and Nutrition Examination Survey 2005–2008. *Sleep* 35(4): 461–467.
31. Saunamäki, T. and Jehkonen, M. 2007. Depression and anxiety in obstructive sleep apnea syndrome: A review. *Acta Neurol Scand* 116: 277–288.
32. Elodahdouh, S., El-Habashy, M., and Elbahy, M. 2013. Effect of CPAP on depressive symptoms in OSA *Egypt J Chest Dis Tuberculosis* 63: 389–393.
33. El-Sherbini, A., Bediwy, A., and El-Mitwalli, A. 2011. Association between obstructive sleep apnea (OSA) and depression and the effect of continuous positive airway pressure (CPAP) treatment. *Neuropsychiatr Dis Treat* 7: 715–721.
34. Gagnadoux, F., Le Vaillant, M., Goupil, F. et al. 2014. Depressive symptoms before and after long-term CPAP therapy in patients with sleep apnea. *Chest* 145(5): 1024–1031.
35. Allen, R. 2013. Restless legs syndrome/Willis Ekbom disease: Evaluation and treatment. *Int Rev Psychiatry* 26(2): 248–262.
36. Picchietti, D. and Winkelman, J. 2005. Restless legs syndrome, periodic limb movement in sleep, and depression. *Sleep* 28(7): 891–898.
37. Szentkiralyi, A., Volzke, H., Hoffman, W., Baune, B., and Berger, K. 2013. The relationship between depressive symptoms and restless legs syndrome in two prospective cohort studies. *Psychosom Med* 75(4): 359–365.
38. Hornyak, M. 2010. Depressive disorders in restless legs syndrome: Epidemiology, pathophysiology, and management. *CNS Drugs* 24(2): 89–98.
39. Huedo-Medina, T., Kirsh, I., Middlemass, J., Klonizakis, M., and A.Siriwardena. 2012. Effectiveness of non-benzodiazepine hypnotics in treatment of adult insomnia: Meta-analysis of data submitted to the Food and Drug Administration. *BMJ* 17: doi:10.1136/bmj.e8343.
40. Schuttle-Rodin, S., Broch, L., Buysse, D., Dorsey, C., and Sateia, M. 2008. Clinical guidelines for the evaluation and management of chronic insomnia in adults. *J Clin Sleep Med* 4(5): 487–504.
41. Buscemi, N., Vandermeer, B., Friesen, C. et al. 2007. The efficacy and safety of drug treatments for chronic insomnia in adults: A meta-analysis of RCT's. *J Gen Intern Med.* 22(9): 1335–1350.
42. Kripke, D.F. 2007. Greater incidence of depression with hypnotic used than with placebo. *BMC Psychiatry* 31(7): 42.
43. Cheng, P., Casement, M., Chen, C., Hoffman, R., Armitage, R., and Deldin, P. 2013. Sleep disordered breathing in major depressive disorder. *J Sleep Res* 43(22): 459–462.
44. Li, C., Bai, Y., Lee, Y. et al. 2014. High dosage of hypnotics predicts subsequent sleep-related breathing disorders and is associated with worse outcomes for depression. *Sleep* 37(4): 803–809.
45. Lader, M. 2014. Benzodiazepine harm: How can it be reduced? *Br J Clin Pharmacol* 77(2): 295–301.
46. Hajak, G., Müller, W., Wittchen, H., Pittrow, D., and Kirch, W. 2003. Abuse and dependence potential for the non-benzodiazepine hypnotics zolpidem and zopiclone: A review of case reports and epidemiological data. *Addiction* 98(10): 1371–1378.
47. Kripke, D., Langer, R., and Kline, L. 2012. Hypnotics' associated with mortality or cancer: A matched cohort study. *BMJ Open* 12(1). doi:10.1136/bmjopen-2012-000850
48. Meolie, A., Rosen, C., Kristo, D. et al. 2005. Oral nonprescription treatment for insomnia: An evaluation of products with limited evidence. *J Clin Sleep Med* 1(2): 173–187.
49. Demartinis, N. and Winokur, A. 2007. Effects of psychiatric medications on sleep and sleep disorders. *CNS Neurol Disord Drug Target* (1): 17–29.
50. Wichniak, A., Wierzbicka, A., and Jernajczyk, W. 2012. Sleep and antidepressant treatment. *Curr Pharm Des* 18(63): 5802–5817.
51. Boyce, P. and Hopwood, M. 2013. Manipulating melatonin in managing mood. *Acta Psychitra Scand Suppl.* 444: 16–23.

52. Miyamoto, M. 2009. Pharmacology of remelteon, a selective Mt1/MT2 receptor agonist: A novel therapeutic drug for sleep disorders. *CNS Neuroci Ther* 15(1): 32–51.
53. Cardinali, D., Srinivasan, V., Brzezinski, A., and Brown, G. 2012. Melatonin and its analogs in insomnia and depression. *J Pineal Res* 52(4): 365–375.
54. Fornaro, M., Prestia, D., Colicchio, S., and Perugi, G. 2010. A systematic, updated review on the antidepressant agomelatine focusing on its melatonergic modulation. *Curr Neuropharmacol* 8(3): 287–304.
55. Howland, R. 2009. Critical appraisal and update on the clinical utility of agomelatin, a melotonergic agonist, for the treatment of major depressive disease in adults. *Neuropsych Dis Treat* 5: 563–576.
56. Lo, H.S., Yang, C., Lo, H.G., Lee, C., Ting, H., and Tzang, B. 2010. Treatment effects of gabapentin for primary insomnia. *Clin Neuropharmacol* 33(2): 84–90.
57. Saadati, N., Mohammadjafari, R., Natanj, S., and Abedi, P. 2013. The effect of gabapentin on intensity and duration of hot flashes in postmenopausal women: A randomized controlled trial. *Glob J Health Sci.* Sep 5 (6): 126–130.
58. Roth, T., Arnold, L., Garcia-Borreguero, D., Resnick, M., and Clair, A. 2014. A review of the effects of pregabalin on sleep disturbance across multiple clinical conditions. *Sleep Med Rev.* 18(3): 261–271.
59. Walsh, J., Perlis, M., Rosenthal, M., Krystal, A., Jiang, J., and Roth, T. 2006. Tiagabine increases slow-wave sleep in a dose-dependent fashion without affecting traditional efficacy measures in adults with primary insomnia. *J Clin Sleep Med* 15(2): 35–41.
60. Irwin M., Cole, J., and Nicassio, P. 2006. Comparative meta-analysis of behavioral interventions for insomnia and their efficacy in middle-aged adults and in older adults 55+ years of age. *Health Psychol* 25(1): 3–14.
61. Butler, A., Chapman, J., Forman, E., and Beck, A. 2006. The empirical status of cognitive behavioral therapy: A review of meta-analyses. *Clin Psychol Rev* 26(1): 17–31.
62. Beck, J. 2011. *Cognitive Behavioral Therapy, Second Edition: Basics and Beyond.* New York, NY: Guilford Press.
63. Kozasa, E., Hachul, H., Monson, C. et al. 2010 Mind-body interventions for the treatment of insomnia: A review. *Rev Bras Psiquiatr* 32(4): 437–442.
64. Wang, M., Wang, S., and Tsai, P. 2005. Cognitive behavioural therapy for primary insomnia: A systematic review. *J Adv Nursing* 50(5): 553–564.
65. Koffel, E., Koffel, J., and Gehrman, P. 2014. A meta-analysis of group cognitive behavioral therapy for insomnia. *Sleep Med Rev* 14: 6–16. doi:10.1016/j.smrv.2014.05.001.
66. Thorndike, F., Ritterband, L., Gonder-Frederick, L., Lord, H., Ingersoll, K., and Morin, C. 2013. A randomized controlled trial of an internet intervention for adults with insomnia: Effects on comorbid psychological and fatigue symptoms. *J Clin Psychol* 69(10):1078–1093.
67. van Straten, A., Emmelkamp, J., de Wit, J. et al. 2014. Guided Internet-delivered cognitive behavioural treatment for insomnia: A randomized trial. *Psychol Med.* May 44(7): 1521–1532.
68. Kyle, S., Miller, C., Rogers, Z., Siriwardena, N., MacMahon, K., and Espie, C. 2014. Sleep restriction therapy for insomnia is association with reduced objective total sleep time, increased daytime somnolence, and objectively impaired vigilance: Implications for the clinical management of insomnia disorder. *Sleep* 37(2):229–237.
69. Taylor, D. and Pruiksma, K. 2014. Cognitive and behavioral therapy for insomnia (CBT-I) in psychiatric populations: A systematic review. *Int. Rev Psychiatry* 26(2): 205–213.
70. Baglioni, C., Spiegelhalder, K., Nissen, C., and Riemann, D. 2011. Clinical implications of the causal relationship between insomnia and depression: How individually tailored treatment of sleeping difficulties could prevent onset of depression. *EPMA J* 2(3): 287–293.
71. Gigli, G. and Valente, M. 2013. Should the definition of "sleep hygiene" be antedated of a century? A historical note based on an old book by Paolo Mantegazza rediscovered. To place in a new historical context the development of the concept of sleep hygiene. *Neurol Sci.* 34(5): 755–760.
72. Jernelöv, S., Lekander, M., Blom, K. et al. 2012. Efficacy of behavioral self-help treatment with or without therapist guidance for co-morbid and primary insomnia—A randomized controlled trial. *BMC Psychiatry* 22(12). doi:10.1186/1471-244X-12-5.
73. Morin, C., Beaulieu-Bonneau, S., LeBlanc, M., and Savard, J. 2008. Self-help treatment for insomnia: A randomized, controlled trial. *Sleep* 28(10): 1319–1327.
74. van Straten, A. and Cuijpers, P. 2009. Self-help therapy for insomnia: A meta-analysis. *Sleep Med Rev* 13(1): 61–71.
75. Ho, F., Chung, K., Yeung, W. et al. 2014. Self-help cognitive behavioral therapy for insomnia: A meta-analysis of randomized controlled trials. *Sleep Med Rev* 9: 17–28. Available at: http://dx.doi.org/10.1016/j.smrv.2014.06.010

76. Ong, J. and Sholtes, D. 2010. A mindfulness-based approach to the treatment of insomnia. *J Clin Psychol* 66(11): 1175–1184.

77. Kabatt-Zinn, J. 1991. *Full Catastrophe Living*. New York, NY: Bantam Dell.

78. Ong, J., Manber, R., Segal, Z., Xia, Y., Shapiro, S., and Wyatt, J. 2014. A randomized controlled trial of mindfulness meditation for chronic insomnia. *Sleep* 39(9): 1553–1563.

79. Gross, C., Kreitzer, M., Reilly-Spong, M. et al. 2010. Mindfulness-based stress reduction versus pharmacotherapy for chronic primary insomnia: A randomized controlled clinical trial. *Explore* 7(2): 75–87.

80. Sarris, J. and Byrne, G. 2011. A systematic review of insomnia and complementary medicine. *Sleep Med Rev* 15(2): 99–106.

81. de Niet, G., Tiemens, B., Lendemeijer, B., and Hutschemaekers, G.2009. Music—Assisted relaxation to improve sleep quality: Meta-analysis. *J Adv Nursing* 65(7): 1356–1364.

82. Wang, C., Sun, Y., and Zang, H. 2014. Music therapy improves sleep quality in acute and chronic sleep disorders: A meta-analysis of 10 randomized studies. *Int J Nurs Stud*. 5(1): 51–62.

83. Chen, C., Pei, Y., Chen, N. et al. 2014. Sedative music facilitates sleep in young adults. *J Altern Complement Med* 20(4): 312–317.

84. Cheuk, D., Yeung, W., Chung, K., and Wong, V. 2007. Acupuncture for insomnia. *Cochrane Database Syst Rev* 18(3). doi:10.1002/14651858.CD005472.

85. Ernst, E., Lee, M., and Choi, T. 2011. Acupuncture for insomnia? An overview of systematic reviews. *Eur J Gen Pract* 17(2): 116–123.

86. Yeung, W., Chung, K., Tso, K., Zhang, S., Zhang, Z., and Ho, L. 2011. Electroacupuncture for residual insomnia associated with major depressive disorder: A randomized controlled trial. *Sleep* 34(6): 807–815.

87. Chen, H., Shi, Y., Ng, C., Chan, S., Yung, K., and Zhang, Q. 2007. Auricular acupuncture treatment for insomnia: A systematic review. *J Altern Complement Med* 13(6): 669–676.

88. Lee, M., Shin, B., Suen, L., Park, T., and Ernst, E. 2008. Auricular acupuncture for insomnia: A systematic review. *Int J Clin Pract* 62(11): 1744–1752.

89. Chen, Y., Liu, J., Xu, N.Z. et al. 2013. Effects of acupuncture treatment on depression insomnia: A study protocol of a multicenter randomized controlled trial. *Trials* 14:2. doi:10.1186/1745-6215-14-2.

90. Yeung, W., Chung, K., Poon, M. et al. 2012. Acupressure, reflexology, and auricular acupressure for insomnia: A systematic review of randomized controlled trials. *Sleep Med* 13(8): 971–984.

91. Buman, M., Phillips, B., Youngstedt, S., Kline, C., and Hirshkowitz, M. 2014. Does nighttime exercise really disturb sleep? Results from the 2013 National Sleep Foundation Sleep in American Poll. *Sleep Med* 15(7): 755–761.

92. Reid, K., Baron, K., Lu, B., Naylor, E., Wolfe, L., and Zee, P. 2010. Aerobic exercise improves self-reported sleep and quality of life in older adults with insomnia. *Sleep Med* 11(9): 934–940.

93. Kubitz, K., Landers, D., Petruzzello, S., and Han, M. 1996. The effects of acute and chronic exercise on sleep. A meta-analytic review. *Sports Med* 21(4): 277–291.

94. Passos, G., Poyares, D., Santana, M. et al. 2014. Exercise improves immune function, antidepressive response and sleep quality in patients with chronic primary insomnia. *Biomed Res Int* doi:10.1155/2014/498961.

95. Brand, S., Kalak, N., Gerber, M., Kirov, R., Pühse, U., and Holsboer-Trachsler, E. 2014. Higher self-perceived exercise exertion before bedtime is association with greater objectively assessed sleep efficiency. *Sleep Medicine* 15(19): 1031–1036.

96. Irwin, M., Olmstead, R., and Motivala, S. 2008. Improving sleep quality in older adults with moderate sleep complaints: A randomized controlled trial of Tai Chi Chih. *Sleep* 31(7): 1001–1008.

97. Manjunath, N. and Telles, S. 2005. Influence of yoga and Ayurveda on self-rated sleep in a geriatric population. *Indian J Med Res* 121: 683–690.

98. Halpern, J., Cohen, M., Kennedy, G., Reece, J., Cahan, C., and Baharav, A. 2014. Yoga for improving sleep quality and quality of life for older adults. *Altern Ther Health Med* 20(3): 37–46.

99. Cooper, K. and Relton, C. 2010. Homeopathy for insomnia: A systematic review of research evidence. *Sleep Med Rev* 14(5): 329–337.

100. Kirsch, D. and Gilula, M. 2007. CES in the treatment of insomnia: A review and meta-analysis. *Pract Pain Manage* 7(8): 28–39.

101. Gaynes, B., Lloyd, S., Lux, L. et al. 2014. Repetitive transcranial magnetic stimulation for treatment resistant depression: A systematic review and meta-analysis. *J Clin Psychiatry* 75(5): 477–489.

102. Jiang, C., Zhang, T., Yue, F., Yi, M., and Gao, D. 2013. Efficacy of repetitive transcranial magnetic stimulation in the treatment of patients with chonic primary insomnia. *Cell Biochem Biophys* 67(1): 169–173.

103. Bliwise, D. and Ansari, F. 2007. Insomnia association with valerian and melatonin usage in the 2002 National Health Interview Survey. *Sleep* 30(7): 881–884.

104. Ferracioli-Oda, E., Qawasmi, A., and Bloch, M. 2013. Meta-analysis: Melatonin for the treatment of primary sleep disorders. *PLoS One* 8(5). doi:10.1371/journal.pone.0063773.

105. Buscemi, N., Vandermeer, B., Hooton, M. et al. 2005. The efficacy and safety of exogenous melatonin for primary sleep disorders a meta-analysis. *J Gen Intern Med* 20(12): 1151–1158.

106. Dolberg, O., Hirschmann, S., and Grunhaus, L. 1998. Melatonin for the treatment of sleep disturbance in major depressive disorder. *Am J Psychiatry* 155: 1119–1121.

107. Hansen, M., Danielsen, A., Hageman, I., Rosenberg, J., and Gögenur, I. 2014. The therapeutic or prophylactic effect of exogenous melatonin against depression and depressive symptoms: A systematic review and meta-analysis. *Eur Neuropsychopharmacol* 19: 239–299.

108. Bent, S., Padula, A., Moore, D., Patterson, M., and Mehling, W. 2006. Valerian for sleep: A systematic review and meta-analysis. *Am J Med* 199(12): 1005–1012.

109. Taibi, D., Landis, C., Petry, H., and Vitiello, M. 2007. A systematic review of valerian as a sleep aid: Safe but not effective. *Sleep Med Rev* 11(3): 209–230.

110. Salter, S. and Brownie, S. 2010. Treating primary insomnia—The efficacy of valerian and hops. *Aust Fam Physician* 39(6): 433–437.

111. Fernandez-San Martin, M., Masa-Font, R., Palacios-Soler, L., Sancho-Gomez, P., Calbo-Caldentey, C., and Flores-Mateo, G. 2010. Effectiveness of valerian on insomnia: A meta-analysis of randomized placebo-controlled trials. *Sleep Med* 11(6): 505–511.

112. Ngan, A. and Conduit, R. 2011. A double-blind, placebo controlled investigation of the effects of Passiflora Incarnata (passionflower) herbal tea on subjective sleep quality. *Phytother Res* 25(8): 1153–1159.

113. Maroo, N., Hazra, A., and Das, T. 2013. Efficacy and safety of a polyherbal sedative-hyponotic formulation NSF-3 in primary insomnia in comparison to zolpidem: A randomized controlled trial. *Indian J Pharmacol* 45(1): 34–39.

114. Wheatley, D. 2005. Medicinal plants for insomnia: A review of their pharmacology, efficacy and tolerability. *J Psychopharmacol* 19(4): 414–421.

115. Zhou, R., Gross, S., Liu, J. et al. 2010. Flavokawain B, the hepatotoxic constituent from kava root, induces GSH-sensitive oxidative stress through modulation of IKK/NF-kappaB and MAPK signalling pathways. *FASEB J* 24(12): 4722–4732.

116. Stea, S., Beraudi, A., and De Pasquale, D. 2014. Essential oils for complementary treatment of surgical patients: State of the art. *Evid Based Complement Alternat Med* 726341. doi:10.1155/2014/726341.

117. Lewith, F, Godfrey, A., and Prescott, P. 2005. A single-blinded, randomized pilot study evaluating the aroma of *Lavandula augustifolia* as a treatment for mild insomnia. *J Altern Complement Med* 11(4): 631–637.

118. Chien, L., Cheng, S., and Liu, C. 2012. The effect of lavender aromatherapy on autonomic nervous system in midlife women with insomnia. *Evid Based Complement Alternat Med* 1–8. doi:10.1155/2012/740813.

119. Abbasi, B., Kimiagar, M., Sadeghniiat, K., Shirazi, M., Hedayati, M., and Rashidkhani, B. 2012. The effect of magnesium supplementation on primary insomnia in elderly: A double-blind placebo-controlled clinical trial. *J Res Med Sci* 17(12): 1161–1169.

120. Trotti, L., Bhadriraju, S., and Becker, L. 2012. Iron for restless legs syndrome. *Cochrane Database Syst Rev* 16(5): CD007834. doi:10.1002/14651858.CD007834.pub2

121. Bannai, M. and Kawai, N. 2012. New therapeutic strategy for amino acid medicine: Glycine improves the quality of sleep. *J Pharmacol Sci* 118(2): 145–148.

122. Ingawa, K., Hiraoka, T.R., Tohru, K., Yamadera, W., and Takahashi, M. 2006. Subjective effects of glycine ingestion before bedtime on sleep quality. *Sleep Biol Rhythms* 4(1): 75–77.

123. Yamadera, W., Inagawa, K., Chiba, S., Bannai, M., Takahashi, M., and Nakayama, K. 2007. Glycine ingestion improves subjective sleep quality in human volunteers, correlating with polysomnographic changes. *Sleep Biol Rhythms* 5(2): 126–131.

124. Gordon, M., Lebwohl, M., Phelps, R., Cohen, S., and Fleischmajer, R. 1991. Eosinophilic fascitis associated with tryptophan ingestion. A manifestation of eosinophilia-myalgia syndrome. *Arch Dematol* 127(2): 217–220.

125. Lapin, I. 2001. Phenibut (beta-phenyl- GABA): A tranquilizer and nootropic drug. *CNS Drug Rev* 7(4): 471–481.

126. Samokhvalov, A., Paton-Gay, C., Balchand, K., and Rehm, J. 2013. Phenibut dependence. *BMJ Case Rep* 6. doi:10.1136/bcr-2012-008381.

127. Chesson, A., Littner, M., Davila, D. et al. 1999. Practice parameters for the use of light therapy in the treatment of sleep disorders. *Sleep* 22(5): 641–660.

128. Sack, R., Auckley, D., Auger, R. et al. 2007. Circadian rhythm sleep disorders: Part I, basic principles, shift work and jet lag disorders: An American Academy of Sleep Medicine Review. *Sleep* 30(11): 1460–1483.
129. Lam, R., Levitt, A., and Levitan R. et al. 2006. The Can-SAD study: A randomized controlled trial of the effectiveness of light therapy and fluoxetine in patients with winter seasonal affective disorder. *Am J Psychiatry* 163(5): 805–812.
130. Burkhart, K. and Phelps, J. 2009. Amber lenses to block blue light and improve sleep: A randomized trial. *Chronobiol Int* 26(8): 1602–1612.
131. Terman, M. 2007. Evolving applications of light therapy. *Sleep Med Rev* 11(6): 497–507.
132. Golden, R., Gaynes, B., Ekstrom, R. et al. 2005. The efficacy of light therapy in the treatment of mood disorders: A review and meta-analysis of the evidence. *Am J Psychiatry* 162(4): 656–662.
133. Dennis, C. and Dowswell, T. 2013. Interventions (other than pharmacological, psychosocial or psychological) for treating antenatal depression. *Cochrane Database Syst Rev* 31(7): doi: 10.1002/14651858. CD006795.pub3
134. Rohan, K., Lindsey, K., Roecklein, K., and Lacy, T. 2004. Cognitive-behavioral therapy, light therapy and their combination in treating season affective disorder *J Affect Disord* 80(2–3): 273–283.
135. Even, C., Schröder, C., Friedman, S., and Rouillon, F. 2008. Efficacy of light therapy in nonseasonal depression: A systematic review. *J Affect Disord* 108(1–2): 11–23.
136. Tuunainen A, Kripke, D., and Endo, T. 2004. Light therapy for non-seasonal depression. *Cochrane Database Syst Rev* 2: CD004050.
137. Epperson, C., Terman, M., Terman, J. et al. 2004. Randomized clinical trial of bright light therapy for antepartum depression: Preliminary findings. *J Clin Psychiatry* 65(3): 421–425.
138. Wirz-Justice, A., Graw, P., Kräuchi, K. et al. 1993. Light therapy in seasonal affective disorder is independent of time of day or circadian phase. *Arch Gen Psychiatry* 50(12): 929–937.
139. Anderson, J., Glod, C., Dai, J., Cao, Y., and Lockley, S. 2009. Lux vs wavelength in light treatment of seasonal affective disorder. *Acta Psychiatrica Scand* 120(3): 203–212.
140. Meesters Y., Dekker, V., and Schlangen, L. et al. 2011. Low-intensity blue-enriched white light (750 lux) and standard bright light (10,000 lux) are equally effective in treating SAD. A randomized controlled study. *BMC Psychiatry* 28: 11–17.
141. Partonen, T., Vakkuri, O., Lamberg-Allardt, C., and Lonngvist, J. 1996. Effects of bright light on sleepiness, melatonin, and 25-hydroxyvitamin D (3) in winter seasonal affective disorder. *Biol Psychiatry* 39(10): 865–872.
142. Lieverse, R., Van Someren, E., Nielen, M., Uitdehaag, B., Smit, J., and Hoogendijk, W. 2011. Bright light treatment in elderly patients with nonseasonal major depressive disorder: A randomized placebo-controlled trial. *Arch Gen Psychiatry* 68(1): 61–70.
143. Gloth, F., Alan, W., and Hollis, B. 1999. Vitamin D vs broad spectrum phototherapy in the treatment of seasonal affective disorder. *J Nutr Health Aging* 3(1): 5–7.
144. Wu, J., Kelsoe, J., Schachat, C. et al. 2009. Rapid and sustained antidepressant response with sleep deprivation and chronotherapy in bipolar disorder. *Bio Psychiatry* 66(3): 298–301.
145. Martiny, K., Refsgaard, E., Lund, V. et al. 2013. The day-to-day acute effect of wake therapy in patients with major depression using the HAM-D6 as primary outcome measure: Results from a randomized controlled trial. *PLoS One* 8(6): e67264. doi:10.1371/journal.pone.0067264.
146. Benedetti, F., Riccaboni, R., Locatelli, C., Poletti, S., Dallaspezia, S., and Colombo, C. 2014. Rapid treatment response of suicidal symptoms to lithium, sleep deprivation, and light therapy (chronotherapeutics) in drug-resistant bipolar depression. *J Clin Psychiatry* 75(2): 133–140.
147. Benedetti, F., Bernasconi, A., Blasi, V. et al. 2007. Neural and genetic correlates of antidepressant response to sleep deprivation: A functional magnetic resonance imaging study of moral valence decision in bipolar disorder. *Arch Gen Psychiatry* 64(2):179–187.
148. Benedetti, F., Barbini, B., Fulgosi, M. et al. 2005. Combined total sleep deprivation and light therapy in the treatment of drug-resistant bipolar depression: Acute response and long-term remission rates. *J Clin Psychiatry* 66(12): 1535–1540.

23 The Role of Spirituality and Religion in Depression and Treatment

Natalie L. Hill, M.Div., LICSW

CONTENTS

INTRODUCTION

For as long as people have experienced depression, they have turned to spirituality and religion (S/R) as a source of meaning, solace, and support. Although S/R has lost some of its cultural prominence, it is still the first place many people turn when they become depressed, and it remains a resource for many alongside mental health care. In recent polling, 78% of Americans identified religion as important in their lives, and 87% believe in God.[1] Even more turn to S/R when distressed. Between 80%[2,3] and 90%[4] of people with psychiatric conditions draw on S/R to cope, 65% report that it helps with symptoms, and 30% say it is their most important coping resource, especially when symptoms worsen.[3] Indeed, psychiatric inpatients may devote up to half of the time they spend coping to S/R.[2] When patients were asked to rank their most helpful sources of support, independent S/R activities (such as prayer and meditation) were ranked first, health-care providers were ranked second, and group spiritual activities (such as worship and fellowship) were ranked third; family, friends, and other supports all ranked lower on the list.[5]

These rates contrast sharply with the rates of engagement in formalized treatment. Although depression is widely recognized and the availability of effective treatment has been well publicized, the proportion of people who seek treatment is surprisingly low. In a representative sample of the U.S. population, 50.6% of participants with moderately severe to severe depression had received no treatment, in spite of meeting criteria for antidepressant medication. An additional 17.6% received psychotherapy, but not medication; 17.0% received medication, but not psychotherapy; and only 14.8% received the optimal treatment of both psychotherapy and medication. Furthermore, among those treated with an antidepressant medication, 45.2% continued to experience ongoing symptoms: 26.4% were mildly depressed, 11.9% had moderate depression, 4.9% experienced moderately severe symptoms, and 2.0% continued to experience severe depression.[6]

These data suggest that many people with depression do not receive adequate treatment, but most engage in some form of S/R, and find it helpful in managing their symptoms. Incorporating S/R into treatment for depression may therefore make treatment more acceptable to patients, boost engagement, and enhance treatment response. This chapter explores the potential benefit of including S/R as part of integrative psychiatric treatment for depression, reviewing research on the relationship between S/R and depression, the underlying neurobiology, and the efficacy of S/R interventions in relation to standard treatments.

DEFINITIONS

Spirituality is the experience of connection to the sacred. What is considered sacred is unique to each person, but may include the transcendent (e.g., God, a higher power, the universe, or a sense of common humanity),[7] as well as one's ultimate commitments (e.g., beliefs, social causes, and creative undertakings),[8] and sources of meaning and purpose. *Religion* is a formalized expression of spirituality through specific beliefs and practices as part of a faith tradition or community.[2,8,9] Although both spirituality and religion are complexes of cognition, behavior, and emotion, spirituality places greater emphasis on emotional experience, while religion places greater emphasis on cognitive belief. Behavior is integral to both, though religion is more likely to include group and interpersonal behaviors such as corporate worship and altruistic service.

Both spirituality and religion equally emphasize private behaviors, including prayer, meditation, and reading sacred texts. The central difference between prayer and meditation is that prayer focuses on connecting with a transcendent or divine being, while meditation focuses more broadly on awareness or self-transcendence. Although prayer may involve speech, it need not: contemplative prayer methods focus on listening for or simply sitting in harmony with the divine. Meditation may take one of two forms: open awareness of the present moment, as in mindfulness meditation, or focused awareness of an object of attention such as a mantra or mental image.[10] There is considerable overlap in the techniques and subjective experience of focused meditation and contemplative prayer.

Of course, experiences related to the sacred or transcendent are difficult to operationalize and measure. Therefore, research on these phenomena has had to rely on dimensions of S/R that can be assessed: specific beliefs, and their subjective importance; specific behaviors, their frequency, and the motivation behind them; the subjective sense of meaning and purpose; and subjective perceptions of the divine or transcendent.

THE IMPACT OF SPIRITUALITY AND RELIGION ON DEPRESSION

An extensive body of literature demonstrates that S/R is generally associated with lower rates of depression,[2] lower risk of developing depression,[11-14] reduced severity and duration of depressive episodes,[14] reduced suicidality,[2,9] and faster remission of symptoms.[2] In a systematic review of 850 studies of religion and mental health, religion was associated with greater overall well-being in 79% of relevant studies, lower suicidality in 84%, lower depression in 66%, and lower anxiety in 51%.[15] General measures of religiosity have consistently been found to correlate negatively with depression, ranging from −0.07 to −0.40.[16] In a meta-analysis of 147 studies, a small but reliable negative association was found between S/R and depression, with an omnibus effect size of −0.096.[14] Although this effect size is small, it is comparable to the relationship between depression and gender.[17] It also likely underestimates the effect of certain aspects of S/R, because it combines studies that measured different dimensions of S/R.[15,18] When aspects of S/R are examined separately, it becomes clear that some are associated with decreased depression, while others are neutral, or associated with increased depression. The remainder of this section will examine the most well-researched dimensions of S/R in relation to depression.

INTRINSIC AND EXTRINSIC ORIENTATION

A person's motivation for engaging in S/R, sometimes referred to as their S/R orientation, has been shown to differentially affect mental health. An intrinsic orientation toward S/R describes those for whom S/R is internally valued and personally meaningful; someone with this orientation engages in S/R for its own sake.[19,20] An extrinsic orientation toward S/R describes those who see S/R as a means to an end; they may engage in S/R for belonging, acceptance, social status, support, or comfort.[19] Research consistently demonstrates that an intrinsic orientation is associated with lower levels of depression, while an extrinsic orientation is associated with higher levels of depression.[21,22] The meta-analysis described above found a negative correlation between intrinsic orientation and depression of $r = -0.175$, but a positive correlation between extrinsic orientation and depression of $r = -0.155$, both significantly different than the omnibus effect size.[14] Comparably, a systematic review found a small but reliable positive correlation between extrinsic orientation and depression ($r = 0.03–0.25$), and a slightly larger negative correlation between intrinsic orientation and depression ($r = -0.05$ to -0.36).[16]

Research also suggests that S/R orientation influences the course of major depressive disorder (MDD). Those with an intrinsic orientation are only 55% as likely to experience MDD,[16] and if they do, an intrinsic orientation is associated with less severe symptoms,[23] including less hopelessness[18] and suicidality.[18,24] Intrinsic S/R also contributes to faster remission of symptoms: for example, among depressed, medically ill, older adults, an intrinsic orientation predicted rate of remission from depression, such that a 10-point increase in intrinsic S/R (SD: 8.2) was associated with 70% faster remission.[25] Intrinsic S/R may be beneficial for depression because it provides a source of internal reinforcement, which opens opportunities for pleasure,[21] while cultivating a sense of meaning, purpose, and self-worth. Extrinsic S/R may contribute to depression because people with this orientation engage in S/R behavior in the absence of internal reinforcement.[20] More likely, depression leads to extrinsic S/R when people seek comfort by turning to S/R. In the latter case, the correlation with increased depression should not be a reason to discourage people who are depressed from drawing on S/R as a coping resource.

SPIRITUAL AND RELIGIOUS BELIEFS AND THEIR PERSONAL SALIENCY

Consistent with the link between intrinsic S/R and reduced depression, there is evidence to suggest that stronger beliefs are associated with lower levels of distress than weaker beliefs.[22] Beyond their overall strength, the specific content of beliefs, such as conservative religious beliefs, belief in heaven, hell, and life after death, is largely unrelated to depression.[16] There is one notable exception: believing in God is associated with less severe symptoms in patients with MDD, and believing that one is cared for and supported by God is associated with less depression, due in part to decreased hopelessness.[12]

It is less clear how S/R saliency—the degree of importance one places on S/R—relates to depression. Some studies have found that greater saliency is protective against depression: in a systematic review,[16] those who identified S/R as highly important had 38% odds of developing depression compared to those who did not identify it as important, and among those who were depressed, high importance was associated with only 17% odds of remaining so after 1 year. Another study found that although S/R saliency was unrelated to incidence of depression, it was positively associated with improvement in symptoms over a 1-year period.[26] However, other research has found that higher S/R saliency was associated with increased depression,[27] or curvilinear, with increased depression at the highest and lowest levels of S/R saliency.[28]

One explanation that has been proposed to explain these inconsistent findings is that, rather than directly affecting depression, S/R saliency functions to buffer stress, indirectly reducing depression.[28] For example, research on people with a family history of MDD found that, although S/R saliency reduced the risk of depression, it did so primarily for those experiencing multiple life stressors,[29] or who had a previous history of depression.[30] Thus, there may be an inverse relationship between depression and saliency for those facing increased stress or other risk factors, but no relationship for those without such stressors. Another possibility is that certain beliefs may contribute to depression (e.g., believing oneself to be sinful), creating a positive relationship between S/R saliency and depression for people who hold such beliefs. Finally, depression may cause some people to lose faith, while causing others to place greater importance on S/R,[27] creating the observed curvilinear relationship between the two.

SPIRITUAL AND RELIGIOUS WELL-BEING

Religious well-being (RWB) refers to the quality of one's relationship with God, while spiritual well-being (SWB) refers to a sense of meaning and purpose. SWB decreases a person's odds of experiencing depression by 50%–70%,[31] and is negatively associated with suicidality.[32] Deriving meaning from S/R, an aspect of SWB, has been associated with lower depression in the general population, as well as those with medical illnesses, and caregivers.[18] Furthermore, a greater increase in SWB during depression treatment is associated with greater likelihood of symptom improvement. In contrast, research has generally found that RWB has little to no correlation with depression, although one study found a positive correlation between RWB and depression after controlling for SWB.[31] This finding suggests that a relationship with God may be unhelpful in the absence of a sense of existential meaning as a context for that relationship.

SPIRITUAL AND RELIGIOUS BEHAVIORS

S/R involves not only beliefs, but also practices that people engage in both individually (e.g., meditation, prayer, reading sacred texts) and in groups (e.g., worship services, rituals, classes). These practices involve behaviors and coping responses through which S/R influences mental health.[34] In fact, attending services may be the aspect of S/R most strongly associated with reduced depression, an association that persists after controlling for a range of sociocultural and health factors.[27] In a comprehensive review, 24 of 29 studies linked service attendance to lower rates of depression;[16] attendance is also associated with decreased suicidality.[24,32] Conversely, those who do not attend services have 20%–60% higher odds of experiencing MDD[16]; infrequent attendance is associated with a similar increase in risk of depression.[35]

Service attendance is thought to protect against depression by providing social support from others, connection through shared traditions and values, and meaning through rituals.[28] The negative association between service attendance and depression is partially mediated by increased social support, but depends on the quality of interpersonal interactions at services: positive interactions reduce depression, while negative interactions increase depression.[22] The risk of depression also increases with attendance for those who do not feel accepted, whose spiritual needs are not being met, and who are dissatisfied by decision making or conflict in the community.[35] Actively seeking spiritual support is positively correlated with depression (perhaps because depression motivates help-seeking), but can buffer the impact of stressors on mood, suggesting it may be beneficial when seeking support about a specific problem.[28]

Prayer can be a way for people to seek support from a transcendent power rather than from other people. While frequency of prayer is positively correlated with depression, more sophisticated statistical analysis to identify likely causality suggests that prayer has a null or slightly beneficial effect on depression.[20] This finding is consistent with a systematic review concluding that frequency of private S/R practices is unrelated to depression after controlling for saliency and intrinsic orientation.[16] Thus, when a positive association is found between prayer and depression, it is most likely the result of people turning to prayer when they are depressed.[20]

One explanation for a lack of correlation between private S/R practices and depression is that such practices can be either positive or negative, depending on how they are used. Pargament and colleagues have examined the specific ways people use S/R to cope, and have differentiated between two categories of coping responses, referred to as "positive religious coping" (PRC) and "negative religious coping" (NRC).[36-38] PRC reflects a sense of meaning, spiritual connection, and secure relationship with God. Coping responses that fall into this category include engaging in S/R practices for connection, support, or to take the focus off of problems; giving and receiving support or forgiveness; positively reappraising problems based on S/R beliefs; and trusting God to help resolve problems. NRC, sometimes referred to as "spiritual struggles," includes conflict with God, struggle with belief, interpersonal conflict related to S/R, and internal conflict related to perceived moral imperfections.[39] Coping responses in this category may involve pleading with God to intervene; passively waiting for God to act; expressing feelings of anger or abandonment toward God; and moral scrupulosity.[38]

PRC is associated with decreased depression, distress, helplessness, and stress, along with increased happiness, self-esteem, and quality of life.[19,36] It increases perceived control through reliance on God, and promotes secondary control through adjustment to and acceptance of situations beyond one's control.[40] PRC is also correlated with SWB,[41] which may contribute to its benefit for depression. In contrast, NRC is associated with increased depression,[19] anxiety, and suicidality,[42] and can exacerbate the impact of stress on depression.[43] The most detrimental form of NRC for depression is alienation from God.[42] A meta-analysis of 49 studies found that PRC was consistently associated with positive psychological adjustment (overall effect size = 0.33), while NRC was associated with negative psychological adjustment (overall effect size = 0.22).[44] Other studies suggest that NRC may have a stronger impact on mental health than PRC, but the strength of the relationship depends on how much time one spends on it; specifically, NRC has a stronger impact for those who spend more time in private S/R practice, but a weaker impact for those who spend more time in corporate S/R practice.[42,45] Interestingly, the impact of NRC on mood is independent of religious belief and saliency, meaning that it can contribute to depression even for those who do not identify as religious or spiritual.[46]

In addition to PRC and NRC, there are a few other exceptions to the general finding that private S/R practices are unrelated to depression. Gratitude and forgiveness are both associated with lower levels of depression.[22] In contrast, engaging in behavior incompatible with one's S/R beliefs or faith tradition has a negative impact on mood; for example, unmarried, teenage mothers were more depressed when they were involved in religions opposed to premarital sex.

NEUROBIOLOGICAL EXPLANATIONS

Emerging research has begun to explore possible neurobiological mechanisms behind the link between S/R and depression. Evidence is also building that S/R can actually contribute to structural and functional changes in the brain, suggesting how these practices may be beneficial in the treatment of depression.[47] Findings suggest that neurochemistry, brain activation patterns, and brain structure are all pieces of this puzzle.

NEUROCHEMISTRY

Serotonin, and to a lesser extent, norepinephrine and dopamine, have long been implicated in depression and targeted by antidepressant medication. However, we are learning that S/R practices also modulate the production and release of neurotransmitters. Studies have found that serotonin, dopamine, GABA, and melatonin increase during meditation.[47] In fact, one study found a 65% increase in dopamine release during periods of meditation.[48] The subjective sense of calmness, peace, and well-being associated with such practices is attributable to these neurochemical changes. Furthermore, meditation is associated with increased concentration of gray matter in areas of the brainstem associated with the synthesis and release of serotonin and norepinephrine;[49] this structural change suggests that people may continue to experience neurochemical benefits from meditation even when not in a meditative state. These findings are likely generalizable to any contemplative S/R practice.

ACTIVATION PATTERNS

MDD has been associated with increased activation of the subgenual anterior cingulate cortex (ACC), and decreased activation of the dorsolateral prefrontal cortex (DLPFC),[50] along with disrupted communication between the ACC and the orbitofrontal cortex (OFC).[51] S/R has also been found to affect these brain regions. S/R practices activate the left dorsal and pregenual ACC, while decreasing activation in other areas of the ACC.[52] S/R experiences have been linked to activation of areas of the prefrontal cortex, including the right DLPFC and OFC. Additionally, S/R practices stimulate areas of the hippocampus and amygdala associated with parasympathetic activation;[47] over time, the prefrontal cortex is more readily engaged to modulate amygdala activation, thereby enhancing emotional regulation.[53]

However, the specific brain regions activated during S/R depend on the type of S/R practice involved. The prefrontal cortex demonstrates increased activation in forms of S/R that involve open awareness, but decreased activation during contemplative practices.[47] Similarly, different areas of parietal lobe are activated by specific S/R activities; for example, the somatosensory and visual cortices are activated during practices that involve sensory awareness or imagery, respectively, while deafferentation of the posterior superior parietal lobe is implicated in self-transcendence.

Brain wave frequencies have also been studied in relation to both depression and S/R. In depressed patients, more frequent high-amplitude alpha waves are associated with greater likelihood of remission in response to antidepressant medication.[54] S/R practices such as meditation produce higher-amplitude electroencephalogram (EEG) activity, including alpha waves, as well as increased EEG synchronicity.[55] With ongoing practice, baseline activation patterns during normal daily activities become more similar to the activation patterns elicited by S/R practice, suggesting one mechanism by which S/R practice may contribute to remission of depression.

BRAIN STRUCTURE

Structural differences have been observed in the brains of people with MDD, and those at risk for depression based on a family history of MDD. Both those with active MDD and those with familial risk had less white matter in the subgenual ACC and DLPFC.[56] Furthermore, those with familial risk had significant cortical thinning across a large section of the lateral surface of the right cerebral hemisphere; this cortical thinning was even more significant in people with MDD, who also demonstrated cortical thinning in the same region of the left hemisphere.[57]

In contrast, S/R practices are associated with increased gray matter in the ACC and hippocampus,[58] increased white matter in areas that communicate with the ACC,[59] and decreased gray matter in the amygdala,[53] reflecting emotional resilience. Additionally, S/R salience, but not frequency of participation, was associated with greater cortical thickness bilaterally in the parietal and occipital regions.[57] This relationship was stronger and affected a more expansive region, in those with a familial risk for depression than those without familial risk, particularly in the areas of the left hemisphere where cortical thinning was most associated with MDD. Researchers therefore speculate that there may be a common additive genetic factor of which both depression and S/R salience are expressions.[30] Cortical thickness was also correlated with both degree and duration of sustained

S/R salience, consistent with a model of neuroplasticity where functional changes repeated over time lead to structural changes.[57]

IMPACT OF SPIRITUALITY AND RELIGION ON RESPONSE TO TREATMENT

Since S/R is associated with reduced depression and faster remission, likely due in part to its chemical, functional, and structural effects on the brain, S/R may also impact a patient's response to standard depression treatments through shared neurobiological processes.[53] Preliminary evidence from three studies on treatment response supports such an effect, though the specific mechanisms of action have yet to be identified. Belief in God was associated with lower levels of depression 8 weeks after standard inpatient or outpatient treatment,[60] and greater improvement in depression after an 8-week trial of one of three selective serotonin reuptake inhibitors (SSRIs) (escitalopram, sertraline, or paroxetine).[23] A higher overall level of S/R was also associated with greater improvement in hopelessness and distorted thinking among patients treated with an SSRI, while belief in God was not associated with these outcomes.[23] A positive relationship with God (RWB) predicted response to inpatient or outpatient treatment, with those in the upper tertile for RWB 75% more likely to respond to treatment than those in the lower tertile.[60] However, SWB was not significantly related to treatment response.[61] This finding contrasts with research suggesting SWB is more closely related to depression than RWB. A possible explanation is that SWB (a sense of meaning and purpose) provides greater benefit in preventing depression, while RWB (a positive relationship with God) provides greater benefit after onset of depression. Finally, a curvilinear relationship was found between S/R behavior and symptom improvement following treatment with an SSRI (citalopram): moderate frequencies were associated with 50% greater likelihood of remission than high or low frequencies.[61] This relationship can be explained in terms of PRC and NRC: PRC may increase treatment response, while NRC may decrease treatment response, particularly at high frequencies.

INCORPORATING SPIRITUALITY AND RELIGION INTO TREATMENT

Aspects of S/R are associated with less depression, shorter duration of symptoms, and increased likelihood of remission, to the extent that S/R actually increases the efficacy of standard treatments for depression. It may therefore be beneficial to proactively incorporate S/R into treatment, in order to provide patients with the best chance of full remission. Indeed, evidence suggests that psychotherapeutic interventions based on S/R lead to faster improvements than secular treatments.[2,62] Patients high in S/R saliency, and those experiencing S/R struggles express the desire to address S/R in treatment,[42] and 83% of patients over the age of 55 believe that it is important to discuss S/R in treatment.[63] Therefore, S/R interventions may be particularly relevant for populations who tend to report higher S/R saliency, including women, the elderly, and ethnic groups with strong cultural links to S/R.[64]

EFFICACY OF SPIRITUAL AND RELIGIOUS INTERVENTIONS

Randomized controlled trials comparing S/R and secular interventions have tended to show comparable efficacy between the two approaches. A systematic review concluded that therapies integrating S/R are at least as effective as secular therapies, with better results immediately after treatment, and equivalent results at follow-up, supporting the claim that S/R therapies contribute to faster treatment response.[65] S/R therapies may also make treatment more acceptable to potential patients, and may be more effective than secular therapies for patients with high S/R saliency. When compared to secular therapies in meta-analysis of 5 studies, the mean effect size for S/R therapies was 0.18, which did not reach statistical significance, supporting the conclusion that S/R and secular therapies are equally effective for symptom reduction; however, this analysis also suggested that S/R therapies may yield additional benefits for SWB and treatment satisfaction. A larger meta-analysis including 31 studies of S/R therapies concluded that S/R interventions are effective, with an omnibus effect size (0.56) comparable to that seen in outcome studies of secular therapies (0.48).[66] The most effective interventions in this analysis focused on understanding and applying S/R beliefs to daily behaviors. Finally, preliminary evidence suggests that S/R interventions can be effective even when implemented by clinicians who do not find S/R personally salient.[67]

Although S/R and secular therapies are of comparable efficacy, there are some clear benefits of S/R approaches. Because S/R does not carry the stigma associated with mental health care, incorporating S/R into treatment may increase engagement, acceptability of interventions, and compliance with treatment. It has been shown to increase treatment satisfaction[68] and reduce attrition.[69] S/R interventions are uniquely able to address detrimental aspects of S/R, such as NRC, and may enhance motivation for change. Unique benefits, such as increased SWB, may indirectly contribute to decreasing depression.[33] Finally, because the practice of S/R is ongoing rather than isolated to treatment, it may reduce the risk of relapse.[63]

SPIRITUAL AND RELIGIOUS INTERVENTIONS

S/R interventions can be incorporated into any therapeutic model, alongside traditional interventions. For example, different methods of prayer and meditation can be introduced as coping skills through discussion, psychoeducation, and/or experiential practice. Sacred or spiritual texts consistent with a patient's beliefs may provide resources for discussion, homework, or bibliotherapy.[65] To offset the tendency for depressed patients to selectively attend to negative messages, including S/R messages, clinicians may also draw on positive concepts and beliefs from within a patient's S/R worldview; possible examples include gratitude, forgiveness, unconditional love, help in suffering, and (in cases of bereavement) immortality of the soul.[62]

Other S/R interventions are specific to a given therapeutic approach, with cognitive and behavioral models receiving the most attention in the literature. Cognitive behavioral therapy (CBT) is widely recognized as an effective evidence-based treatment for depression, so S/R adaptations of CBT are promising examples of integrative depression treatment. A core CBT intervention is cognitive restructuring: identifying, challenging, and replacing distorted thoughts that perpetuate depression.[70] S/R contributes to this process in two ways. First, cognitive distortions may involve S/R content:[62] many examples of NRC identified in the literature are also examples of distorted S/R cognitions, such as thinking of oneself as sinful or evil, interpreting experiences as punishment from God or the work of a demonic power.[39] Second, a patient's S/R beliefs can be used to challenge distorted thoughts, whether or not the distortion itself involves S/R content.[63,68] For example, the thought "I am worthless" could be challenged with the thought "God doesn't make junk." When a distortion does contain S/R content, incorporating S/R into the restructuring process is particularly important.[62]

Behavioral activation (BA) has also received extensive attention as an evidence-based treatment for depression; its efficacy was comparable to psychopharmacology, and superior to CBT in at least one study.[71] Based on the theory that depression emerges when the absence of positive reinforcement extinguishes positive behaviors and therefore diminishes opportunities for pleasure,[72] BA seeks to improve mood by increasing valued behaviors that patients find intrinsically reinforcing or that move the patient toward life goals.[21,71] Standard BA targets and gradually increases behaviors in multiple domains, including S/R, based on a patient's values.[73]

A single-session intervention focused exclusively on S/R has also been tested. The BA of religious behaviors (BARB)[73] intervention focused on clarifying participants' S/R beliefs and values, providing psychoeducation about the benefits of S/R for depression, and developing a plan to engage in specific S/R behaviors, with a telephone check-in after 1 week. Participants were assessed at baseline, 2 weeks, and 6 weeks after the session. Compared to supportive treatment, BARB participants showed greater improvement in depression, anxiety, and quality of life, with moderate to large effect sizes. Unsurprisingly, the BARB group also demonstrated greater increases in S/R behaviors, attitudes, and coping. However, the rate and impact of S/R behaviors are surprising: 86.4% adhered to the BA plan developed in session, 84% reported continuing their targeted S/R behaviors 6 weeks after the intervention, and the average pleasurability rating for targeted behaviors was 3.28 on a 1–4 scale, where 4 represented "very pleasurable." It should be noted, however, that S/R behavior in the absence of an intrinsic S/R orientation has been associated with increased depression.[21] Therefore, activation of S/R behaviors should only be used with patients who value S/R. NRC may also influence the impact of S/R behaviors on mood, and should be assessed and addressed as part of any S/R intervention.

CONCLUSIONS, LIMITATIONS, AND FUTURE DIRECTIONS

The vast majority of people who experience depression turn to S/R for help, whether or not they receive psychiatric treatment.[2–4] Patients subjectively report that S/R improves their symptoms,[35] and empirical studies support this claim,[2,11] especially when S/R provides a source of meaning[33] or support.[28] While spiritual struggles, particularly alienation from God, may intensify distress, the positive coping resources available through S/R lessen depression, and foster happiness, self-esteem, and quality of life.[19]

The benefits of S/R are visible in structural, functional, and chemical changes in the brain,[47–57] and preliminary evidence suggests that S/R may enhance the efficacy of standard psychiatric treatment for depression.[60,61] Therapeutic interventions based on S/R are at least as effective as secular interventions, may lead to faster improvements,[65] and have added benefits such as enhanced SWB.[66] S/R interventions may increase the acceptability of treatment, improve satisfaction, reduce attrition,[68] and protect against relapse.[63] Such interventions may be necessary to address spiritual struggles when such struggles are contributing to depression and distress.[69] Therefore, actively integrating S/R into treatment for depression may offer patients the best opportunity for sustainable improvement in mood, functioning, and quality of life.

A limitation of existing research is that the vast majority is correlational and cross-sectional.[20] While some studies do employ a longitudinal model, causation is difficult to assess because important aspects of S/R cannot be experimentally manipulated. The picture is further complicated by the wide range of methods for operationalizing and measuring S/R, which make results difficult to interpret and compare.[18] Where there are inconsistent findings regarding the association between aspects of S/R and depression, a confounding factor may be that some people turn to S/R only during times of hardship or distress; these people may experience less benefit because S/R values may be less intrinsic, and S/R behaviors less well developed.[61] Longitudinal research is needed to examine how S/R may change before, during, and after a depressive episode. Longitudinal research should also be conducted to better understand the neurobiological causes and effects of S/R, depression, and treatment. Larger-scale randomized controlled trials of S/R interventions are needed to better identify what interventions provide added benefit for specific patient populations. Last, there is a need for enhanced training for psychiatric professionals on the impact of S/R on mental health, and how to effectively incorporate it into treatment.

REFERENCES

1. Gallup Poll. Religion. 2013. http://www.gallup.com/poll/1690/%20religion.aspx#1 (accessed December 28, 2014).
2. Koenig, H.G. 2009. Research on religion, spirituality, and mental health: A review. *Can J Psychiatry* 54(5): 283–291.
3. Tepper, L., Rogers, S.A., Coleman, E.M., and Malony, H.N. 2001. The prevalence of religious coping among persons with persistent mental illness. *Psychiatr Serv* 52(5): 660–665.
4. Fitchett, G., Burton, L.A., and Sivan, A.B. 1997. The religious needs and resources of psychiatric inpatients. *J Nervous Mental Dis* 185(5): 320–326.
5. Fallot, R.D. 2007. Spirituality and religion in recovery: Some current issues. *Psychiatric Rehab* 30(4): 261–270.

6. Shim, R.S., Baltrus, P., Ye, J., and Rust, G. 2011. Prevalence, treatment and control of depression symptoms in the United States: Results from the national health and nutrition examination Survey (NHANES), 2005–2008. *J Am Board Fam Med* 24(1): 33–38. doi:10.3122/jabfm.2011.01.100121

7. Walsh, J. 2012. Spiritual interventions with consumers in recovery from mental illness. *J Spirituality Ment Health* 14: 229–241. doi:10.1080/19349637.2012.730462.

8. Worthington, E.L. and Aten, J.D. 2009. Psychotherapy with religious and spiritual clients: An introduction. *J Clin Psychol In Session* 65: 123–130.

9. Chidarikire, S. 2012. Spirituality: The neglected dimension of holistic mental health care. *Adv Ment Health* 10(3): 298–302.

10. Hussain, D. and B. Bhushan. 2010. Psychology of meditation and health: Present status and future directions. *Int J Psychol Psychol Ther* 10(3): 439–451.

11. Murphy, P.E., Ciarrocchi, J.W., Piedmont, R.L., Cheston, S., Peyrot, M., and Fitchett, G. 2000. The relation of religious belief and practices, depression, and hopelessness in persons with clinical depression. *J Consulting Clin Psychol* 68(6): 1102–1106.

12. Pargament, K.I., Koenig, H.G., and Perez, L.M. 2000. The many methods of religious coping: Development and initial validation of the RCOPE. *J Clin Psychol* 56(4): 519–543.

13. Smith, T.B., McCullough, M.E., and Poll, J. 2003. Religiousness and depression: Evidence for a main effect and the moderating influence of stressful life events. *Psychol Bull* 129(4): 614–636.

14. Miller, L. and Kelley, B.S. 2005. Relationships of religiosity and spirituality with mental health and pssychopathology. In *Handbook of the Psychology of Religion and Spirituality*, Ed. R.F. Paloutzian and C.L. Park. New York, NY: Guilford Press, pp. 460–478.

15. Koenig, H.G., McCullough, M.E., and Larson, D.B. *Handbook of Religion and Health: A Century of Research*. New York, NY: Oxford University Press, 2001.

16. McCullough, M.E. and Larson, D.B. 1999. Religion and depression: A review of the literature. *Twin Res* 2: 126–136.

17. Moreira-Almeida, A., Neto, F.L., and Koenig, H.G. 2006. Religiousness and mental health: A review. *Rev Bras Psiquiatr* 28(3): 242–250.

18. Hovey, J.D., Hurtado, G., Morales, L.R.A., and Seligman, L.D. 2014. Religion-based emotional social support mediates the relationship between intrinsic religiosity and mental health. *Arch Suicide Res* 18(4): 376–391. doi:10.1080/13811118.2013.833149.

19. Maltby, J. and Day, L. 2000. Depressive symptoms and religious orientation: Examining the relationship between religiosity and depression within the context of other correlates of depression. *Pers Individ Dif* 28: 383–393.

20. Denny, K.J. 2011. Instrumental variable estimation of the effect of prayer on depression. *Soc Sci Med* 73:1194–1199. doi:10.1016/j.socscimed.2011.08.

21. Agishtein, P., Pirutinsky, S., Kor, A., Baruch, D., Kanter, J., and Rosmarin, D.H. 2013. Integrating spirituality into a behavioral model of depression. *J Cogn Behav Psychother* 13(2): 275–289.

22. Baetz, M. and Toews, J. 2009. Clinical implications of research on religion, spirituality, and mental health. *Can J Psychiatry* 54(5): 292–301.

23. Peselow, E., Pi, S., Lopez, E., Beseda, A., and Ishak, W.W. 2014. The impact of spirituality before and after treatment of major depressive disorder. *Innov Clin Neurosci* 11(3–4): 17–23.

24. Simonson, R.H. 2008. Religiousness and non-hopeless suicide ideation. *Death Studies* 32(10): 951–960. doi:10.1080/07481180802440589

25. Koenig, H.G., George, L.K., and Peterson, B.L. 1998. Religiosity and remission of depression in medically Ill older patients. *Am J Psychiatry* 155(4): 536–542.

26. Braam, A.W., Beekman, A.T.F., Deeg, D.J.H., Smith, J.H., and van Tilburg, W. 1997. Religiosity as a protective or prognostic factor of depression in later life: Results from a community survey in the Netherlands. *Acta Psychiatr Scand* 96(3): 199–205.

27. Baetz, M., Griffin, R., Bowen, R., Koenig, H.G., and Marcoux, E. 2004. The association between spiritual and religious involvement and depressive symptoms in a Canadian population. *J Nervous Mental Dis* 192(12): 818–822.

28. Schnittker, J. 2001. When is faith enough? The effects of religious involvement on depression. *J Sci Study Relig* 40(3): 393–411.

29. Kasen, S., Wickramaratne, P., Gameroff, M.J., and Weissman, M.M. 2012. Religiosity and resilience in persons at high risk for major depression. *Psychol Med* 42: 509–519.

30. Miller, L., Wickramaratne, P., Gameroff, M.J., Sage, M., Tenke, C.E., and Weissman, M.M. 2012. Religiosity and major depression in adults at high risk: A ten-year prospective study. *Am J Psychiatry* 169(1): 89–94.

31. Maselko, J., Gilman, S.E., and Buka, S. Religious service attendance and spiritual well-being are differentially associated with risk of major depression. *Psychol Med* 39: 1009–1017.
32. Taliaferro, L.A., Rienzo, B.A., Pigg Jr., R.M., Miller, M.D., and Dodd, V.J. 2009. Spiritual well-being and suicidal ideation among college students. *J Am Coll Health* 58(1): 83–90.
33. Hawkins, R.S., Tan, S., and Turk, A.A. 1999. Secular versus Christian inpatient cognitive-behavioral therapy programs: Impact on depression and spiritual well-being. *J Psychol Theol* 27(4): 309–318.
34. Fallot, R.D. 2007. Spirituality and religion in recovery: Some current issues. *Psychiatr Rehab J* 30(4): 261–270.
35. Chou, H.G. and Hofer, J.A. 2014. Characteristics of congregations that might increase their participants' risk of depression. *Ment Health Relig Cult* 17(4): 390–399. doi:10.1080/13674676.2013.816940.
36. Abu-Raiya, H. and Pargament, K.I. 2015. Religious coping among diverse religions: Commonalities and divergences. *Psychol Relig Spirituality* 7(1): 24–33, doi:10.1037/a0037652.
37. Pargament, K.I., Smith, B.W., Koenig, H.G., and Perez, L. 1998. Patterns of positive and negative religious coping with major life stressors. *J Sci Study Relig* 37(4): 710–724.
38. Pargament, K.I., Koenig, H.G., and Perez, L.M. 2000. The many methods of religious coping: Development and initial validation of the RCOPE. *J Clin Psychol* 56(4): 519–543.
39. Exline, J.J. 2013. Religious and spiritual struggles. In *APA Handbook of Psychology, Religion and Spirituality (Vol. 1): Context, Theory, and Research*, Ed. K.I. Pargament, J.J. Exline, and J.W. Jones. Washington, DC: American Psychological Association, pp. 459–475.
40. Pargament, K.I., Cole, B., Vandecreek, L., Belavick, T., Brant, C., and Perez, L. 1999. The vigil: Religion and the search for control in the hospital waiting room. *J Health Psychol* 4(3): 327–341.
41. Pieper, J.Z.T. 2004. Religious coping in highly religious psychiatric inpatients. *Ment Health Relig Cult* 7(4): 349–363.
42. Exline, J.J., Yali, A.M., and Sanderson, W.C. 2000. Guilt, discord, and alienation: The role of religious strain in depression and suicidality. *J Clin Psychol* 56(12): 1481–1496.
43. Carpenter, T.P., Laney, T., and Mezulis, A. 2012. Religious coping, stress, and depressive symptoms among adolescents: A prospective study. *Psychol Relig Spirituality* 4(1): 19–30.
44. Ano, G.G. and Vasconcelles, E.B. 2005. Religious coping and psychological adjustment to stress: A meta-analysis. *J Clin Psychol* 61(4): 461–480, doi:10.1002/jclp.20049.
45. Warren, P., Van Eck, K., Townley, G., and Kloos, B. 2015. Relationships among religious coping, optimism, and outcomes for persons with psychiatric disabilities. *Psychol Relig Spiritual* 7(2): 91–99.
46. Rosmarin, D.H., Malloy, M.C., and Forester, B.P. 2014. Spiritual struggle and affective symptoms among geriatric mood disordered patients. *Int J Geriatr Psychiatry* 29: 653–660. doi:10.1002/gps.4052.
47. Newberg, A.B. 2010. Transformation of brain structure and spiritual experience. In *The Oxford Handbook of Psychology and Spirituality*, Ed. L.J. Miller. New York, NY: Oxford University Press, pp. 489–499.
48. Kjaer, T. W., Bertelsen, C., Piccini, P., Brooks, D., Alving, J., and Lou, H.C. 2002. Increased dopamine tone during meditation-induced change of consciousness. *Cogn Brain Res* 13(2): 255–259.
49. Singleton, O., Holzel, B.K., Vangel, M., Brach, N., Carmody, J., and Lazar, S.W. 2014. Change in brainstem gray matter concentration following a mindfulness-based intervention is correlated with improvement in psychological well-being. *Front Human Neurosci* 8: 1–7.
50. Gotlib, I.H. and Hamilton, J.P. 2008. Neuroimaging and depression: Current status and unresolved issues. *Curr Dir Psychol Sci* 17(2): 159–163.
51. Forbes, E.E., May, J.C., Siegle, G.J. et al. 2006. Reward-related decision-making in pediatric major depressive disorder: An fMRI Study. *J Child Psychol Psychiatry* 47(10): 1031–1040.
52. Beauregard, M. 2012. Neuroimaging and spiritual practice. In *The Oxford Handbook of Psychology and Spirituality*, Ed. L.J. Miller, New York, NY: Oxford University Press, pp. 500–513.
53. Chiesa, A., Brambilla, P., and Serretti, A. 2010. Functional neural correlates of mindfulness meditations in comparison with psychotherapy, pharmacotherapy and placebo effect: Is there a link? *Acta Neuropsychiatr* 22(3): 104–117.
54. Tenke, C.E., Kayser, J., Manna, C.G. et al. 2011. Current source density measures of electroencephalographic alpha predict antidepressant treatment response. *Biol Psychiatry* 70(4): 388–394.
55. Mehrmann, C. and Karmacharya, R. 2013. Principles and neurobiological correlates of concentrative, diffuse, and insight meditation. *Harvard Rev Psychiatry* 21(4): 205–218.
56. Amico, F., Meisenzahl, E., Koutsouleris, N., Reiser, M., Moller, H., and Frodl, T. 2011. Structural MRI correlates for vulnerability and resilience to major depressive disorder. *J Psychiatry Neurosci* 36(1): 15–22.

57. Miller, L., Bansal, R., Wickramaratne, P., Hao, X., Tenke, C.E., Weissman, M.M., and Peterson, B.S. 2014. Neuroanatomical correlates of religiosity and spirituality: A study in adults at high and low familial risk for depression. *JAMA Psychiatry* 71(2): 128–135.

58. Luders, E., Thompson, P.M., Kurth, F. et al. 2013. Global and regional alterations of hippocampal anatomy in long-term meditation practitioners. *Human Brain Mapping* 34(12): 3369–3375.

59. Tang, Y., Lu, Q., Fan, M., Yang, Y., and Posner, M.I. 2012. Mechanisms of white matter changes induced by meditation. *Proc Natl Acad Sci* 109(26): 10570–10574.

60. Murphy, P.E. and Fitchett, G. 2009. Belief in a concerned god predicts response to treatment for adults with clinical depression. *J Clin Psychol* 65(9): 1000–1008. doi:10.1002/jclp.20598.

61. Schettino, J.R., Olmos, N.T., Myers, H.F., Joseph, N.T., Poland, R.E., and Lesser, I.M. 2011. Religiosity and treatment response to antidepressant medication: A prospective multi-site clinical trial. *Ment Health Relig Cult* 14(8): 805–818. doi:10.1080/13674676.2010.527931.

62. Vasegh, S. 2011. Cognitive therapy of religious depressed patients: Common concepts between Christianity and Islam. *J Cogn Psychother* 25(3): 177–188. doi:10.1891/0889–8391.25.3.177.

63. Stanley, M.A., Bush, A.L., Camp, M.E. et al. 2011. Older adults' preferences for religion/spirituality in treatment for anxiety and depression. *Aging Ment Health* 15(3): 334–343, doi:10.1080/13607863.2010.5 19326.

64. Hodge, D.R. and Bonifas, R.P. 2010. Using spiritually modified cognitive behavioral therapy to help clients wrestling with depression: A promising intervention for some older adults. *J Relig Spiritual Soc Work Soc Thought* 29(3): 185–206. doi:10.1080/15426432.2010.495598.

65. Paukert, A.L., Phillips, L.L., Cully, J.A., Romero, C., and Stanley, M.A. 2011. Systematic review of the effects of religion-accommodative psychotherapy for depression and anxiety. *J Contemp Psychother* 41(2): 99–108. doi:10.1007/s10879-010-9154-0.

66. Smith, T.B., Bartz, J., and Richards, P.S. 2007. Outcomes of religious and spiritual adaptations to psychotherapy: A meta-analytic review. *Psychother Res* 17(6): 643–655. doi:10.1080/10503300701250347.

67. Propst, L.R., Ostrom, R., Watkins, P., Dean, T., and Mashburn, D. 1992. Comparative efficacy of religious and nonreligious cognitive-behavioral therapy for the treatment of clinical depression in religious individuals. *J Consult Clin Psychol* 60(1): 94–103.

68. Targ, E.F. and Levine, E.G. 2002. The efficacy of a mind-body-spirit group for women with breast cancer: A randomized controlled trial. *Gen Hosp Psychiatry* 24(4): 238–248.

69. Baetz, M. and Bowen, R. Suicidal ideation, affective lability, and religion in depressed adults. *Ment Health Relig Cult* 14(7): 633–641. doi:10.1080/13674676.2010.504202.

70. Beck, J.S. 1995. *Cognitive Therapy: Basics and Beyond.* New York, NY: Guilford Press.

71. Dimidjian, S., Hollon, S.D., Dobson, K.S. et al. 2006. Randomized trial of behavioral activation, cognitive therapy, and antidepressant medication in the acute treatment of adults with major depression. *J Consult Clin Psychol* 74(4): 658–670.

72. Lewinsohn, P.M. 1974. A behavioral approach to depression. In *The Psychology of Depression: Contemporary Theory and Research*, Ed. R.J. Friedman and M.M. Katz. New York, NY: Wiley, pp. 157–185.

73. Armento, M.E.A., McNulty, J.K., and Hopko, D.R. 2012. Behavioral activation of religious behaviors (BARB): Randomized trial with depressed college students. *Psychol Relig Spiritual* 4(3): 206–222.

24 Depression-Specific Yoga and Mindfulness-Based Cognitive Therapy Model

Description, Data on Efficacy, and Differences from Contemporary Models

Basant Pradhan, MD

CONTENTS

INTRODUCTION

As a global burden, depression, one of the most common among all the psychiatric disorders, affects about 121 million people worldwide. Today, depression is the second cause of disability adjusted life-years (DALYs) in the age category 15–44 years.[1] Apart from the huge public health burden, the cost of depression is enormous: workplace costs of over $34 billion per year in direct and indirect costs. People with depression have higher rates of mortality, and over 15% of depressed people take their own lives. This suicide rate is six times higher among men 85 years old and over than it is for the general population. Depression worsens the prognosis for patients with comorbid chronic medical illnesses. In addition, the caregiver burden associated with depression significantly affects workplace performance, and children of mothers who suffer from chronic depression display more behavioral problems at school. Rates of undetected depression among drug and alcohol users are estimated to be as high as 30%.[2] One important clinical issue in treatment of depression is that treatment resistance is relatively common. In cases of depression treated by a primary care physician, 32% of patients partially responded to treatment, and 45% did not respond at all. Rates of total remission following antidepressant treatment are only 50.4%.[3] Nonpharmacological behavioral interventions are attractive because they are potentially more enduring than pharmacological treatments. The lack of side effects and drug–drug interactions, often a concern with pharmacological approaches, may also be more appealing to patients in choosing these interventions.

YOGA, MEDITATION, AND MINDFULNESS: THREE OVERARCHING CIRCLES

It is important to understand that *Yoga, meditation*, and *mindfulness* are conceptually three over-arching circles in the broad scheme of Yoga. Often these three terms are misused colloquially and in the literature. There is considerable confusion around use of the terms *Yoga* and *meditation*: often Yoga is used in physical sense and meditation in mental sense. *Yoga Sutra* (the first text-book of Yoga, based on the *Vedic* philosophy: c. 400 BC)[4] and *Visuddhimagga* (an encyclopedia of meditation and source book of Buddhist doctrine: c. 430 CE),[5] the two classics and primary source textbooks on Yoga and meditation respectively, clearly describe the broad scheme of Yoga that includes meditation. *Yoga Sutra* describes the *Eight-limbed Yoga,* and *Visuddhimagga* describes the *Noble Eightfold Path.* As described in these scriptures, Yoga in its entirety and as it was proposed originally (in ancient India) consists of eight limbs that includes meditation as its two crucial steps (i.e., sixth-step/concentrative-type meditation [Pali: *samatha*, Sanskrit: *dharana*] and seventh-step/ mindfulness-type meditation [Pali: *satipatthana, vipassana,* Sanskrit: *dhyan*]). Thus mindfulness is one among the two types of meditation, the other being *concentration.*[5-7] Meditation is essentially an ongoing *cognitive-emotive-reappraisal process* that takes place within the individual in order to obtain insight and directly experience the personal truths of their life. Technically, meditation involves learning to shift and focus one's attention at will onto an object of choice, such as bodily feelings or an emotional experience, while disengaging from the conditioned or elaborative processing by the mind. Depending on how one's attention is used in the meditative process, the literature broadly classifies meditation into two types: (1) concentrative or focused attention type, and (2) mindfulness or open monitoring (OM) type.[7,8]

In focused attention meditation, attention is focused and sustained on an intended object and involves monitoring the focus of attention, detecting distraction, disengaging attention from the source of distraction, and redirecting attention to the intended object. The open monitoring type, in contrast, involves nonreactive, moment-to-moment monitoring of the content of experience. This monitoring serves to determine the nature of cognitive and emotional patterns. Concentrative medi-tation is often considered as a prerequisite for mindfulness meditation. To practice mindfulness meditation is to become grounded in the present moment; in this process one's role is simply as observer of the arising and passing away of experience. In this, one does not judge the experiences and thoughts, nor does one try to figure things out and draw conclusions, or change anything—the challenge during mindfulness is to simply register the mental events and observe them rather than elaborate them.[9]

YOGA AND (MENTAL) HEALTH

Health is a state of complete physical, mental, and social well-being and not merely the absence of disease or infirmity. The World Health Organization (WHO) defines mental health as a state of well-being in which an individual realizes his or her own abilities, can cope with normal stresses of life, can work productively and fruitfully, and is able to make a contribution to his or her com-munity.[10] In this definition of mental health, emotional well-being, the capacity to live a full and creative life, and the flexibility to deal with life's inevitable challenges are key components. One major objective of Yoga is to acquire deep insights into one's inner self which not only includes one's own abilities and coping but also requires one to use one's spiritual strength for well-being, which are the key elements in the definition of mental health as described above. Yoga and medi-tation can be broadly conceptualized as self-management strategies for gaining insight into the principles of the human mind that explain the nature of its thoughts and experiences. These insights help us realize how to reaccess a natural and positive state of mind, how to experience calmness in a sustained manner regardless of the circumstances we encounter in our daily life, and how to translate these for our well-being.[7] Over the millennia, Yoga and meditation have been advocated as a way of life as well as a kind of psychosomatic preparation for spiritual elevation. In these, one can see that Yoga reflects the basic human goal to transcend the pain, suffering, and uncertainty of human life. In Yoga, maintenance of health is seen as just a preparatory requisite for achieving higher goals of life: thus Yoga sees health not as a goal but rather as an important by-product of the practice of Yoga.[11] In the multiprong approach of Yoga prerequisites for achieving good health are already built-in: in the broad scheme of the *Eight-limbed Yoga* of sage Patanjali or the *Noble Eightfold Path* of Buddha one can see the balanced combination of healthy Yogic lifestyle (includes the balanced way of life, moral behavior, healthy diet, etc.), adequate bodywork through Yogic postures (Sanskrit: *asanas*) and Yogic procedures (Sanskrit: *bandhas, mudras,* and *kriyas*), breath work (Sanskrit: *pranayama*), and techniques of mental development—that is, meditation that leads to elevation of one's consciousness to deeper meditative states (Sanskrit: *samadhis,* Pali: *samapattis*) and eventually self-realization. Being mother to *Ayurveda,* the herbal medicinal system of ancient India, one can clearly see that Yoga does not negate the use of medications and other methods of modern medicine.[12]

Contrary to the beliefs that practice of Yoga and meditation is time consuming or difficult, the authors of one recent study[13] conducted at the Mayo Clinic note that even 15 minutes of daily meditation practice can reduce stress and improve quality of life of the health-care professionals. However, the conventional research methodology employed for the evidence-based study of Yogic interventions is not optimal. As mentioned above, interventions involving Yoga and meditation are complex, consist of a module of many dos and don'ts, and influence almost all aspects of our life that include but are not limited to diet, nutrition, metabolism, physical and social habits, emotional attitudes, and so on. This broad scope makes it rather difficult for researchers to objectively determine the cause and effects of Yoga. So one important fact could be that these interventions are effective, but when we design a trial, we simply do not have adequate methods to measure these experiential parameters. Despite these difficulties in measurements of the effects, Yoga and mindfulness-based interventions have been found to be feasible and effective even in severe illnesses like schizophrenia[14] or attention deficit-hyperactivity disorder (ADHD),[15] both in adults and children alike. Yoga-meditation combines humanistic models with positive psychology and *self-help models* of care. Thus they promote the autonomy of the individual which could decrease the burden of care not only in the caregivers but also in the health-care providers. As mentioned before, these therapeutic methods do not negate the utility of appropriate pharmacological interventions, rather they supplement them. These interventions could provide respite in circumventing some of the difficulties with the health-care access in this managed care era.

USE OF YOGA AND MINDFULNESS IN DEPRESSION

Yoga is probably one of the most ancient mind-body medicines that has shed light on the intricate and complex dynamic interplay between the body and mind, with clear outlines and methods about how one can achieve physical, mental, and spiritual well-being. As elaborated in the meditative philosophies passed down in the past thousand years, when the individual's (Sanskrit: *jiva*) actions are governed by the meditative insights (which results in *wisdom*) rather than just as reactionary responses to the underlying impulses, these *wise actions* do not bring *suffering* (Sanskrit: *dukkha,* which means *sadness* as well).[5] Yoga and meditation, as used in the West, fall under the broad rubric of complementary and alternative medicine (CAM). Utility of Yoga and meditation in depression offers some promise in research studies.[16] In addition to their utility as self-management techniques that empower the person, other benefits are in terms of their low cost and lack of side effects or drug–drug interactions that are concerns typically seen with the pharmacological approaches. Mindfulness/meditation-based interventions represent a group of cognitive and behavioral interventions involving meditation. Historically a Buddhist practice to alleviate suffering,[17] mindfulness approaches have been modified and integrated into present-day therapeutic practices. Mindfulness-based cognitive therapy (MBCT) has been studied and found to be effective in the treatment of depression, both acute phase and relapse preventions.[18] Like cognitive behavioral therapy (CBT), MBCT functions on the theory that when individuals who have historically had depression become distressed, they return to automatic cognitive processes that can trigger a depressive episode. The goal of MBCT is to interrupt these automatic processes and teach the participants to focus less on reacting to incoming stimuli, and instead on accepting and observing them without judgment. This mindfulness practice allows the participant to notice when automatic processes are occurring and to alter their reaction in reflective and nonreactive ways.[19] Although additional controlled clinical trials are needed to document the benefits of programs that combine *pranayama* (breath control), *asanas* (postures), and meditation, there is now emerging evidence to consider yoga and mindfulness-based interventions as potentially beneficial, low-risk adjuncts for the treatment of posttraumatic stress disorder (PTSD), depression, stress-related medical illnesses, and substance abuse.[20]

YOGA AND MINDFULNESS-BASED COGNITIVE THERAPY: USE OF YOGA IN ITS ENTIRETY

The Yoga and Mindfulness-Based Cognitive Therapy (Y-MBCT) models that have been developed by Pradhan (1998 onwards), use Yoga *in its entirety* rather than piecemeal use as just a physical exercise or a breathing technique or only meditation, and so on. Thus the components in the Y-MBCT include all eight steps of Yoga involving body and mind. This broader and integrated application increases not only the scope of these interventions but also their efficacy. These models incorporate *the balanced* lifestyle, posture (asana), yogic procedures (kriya), and of course, meditation in their standardized form. The main meditation methods are the *samyama* [Sanskrit] (the combination of sixth, seventh, and eighth limbs of Yoga) combined with the Buddhist *satipatthana* [Pali] method using the tripartite model of human experience and five-factor model of mind. The theoretical foundation of Y-MBCT derives from the three original scriptural schools of Yoga and mindfulness—that is, the Eight-Limbed Yoga (Sanskrit: *Ashtanga*) of Patanjali (c. fourth century BC), the mindfulness (*satipatthana*) model of Buddha (c. sixth century BC), and the standardizations of the technique-rich style of *Tantra* (second century CE). The cornerstones of the Y-MBCT models are the staged meditation protocols (SMPs), the balanced and meditative lifestyle (Buddha's *Middle Way,* a lifestyle of *moderation* and *compassion*), meditative breathing (calming and energizing types), and symptom-specific Yogic procedures (Sanskrit: *kriyas*).

The main conceptual rationale for therapeutic use of Y-MBCT derives from the mindfulness philosophies that inform us that the locus of all our experiences including the stress or happiness is *inside* (i.e., the mind), but because of the projective (Sanskrit: *vikshepa*) mechanisms, the mind is constantly running away from this inner locus. Because of this projective and centrifugal mechanism of the mind, the experiencer (i.e., ourselves), the things we experience (i.e., the world of our experience with all the objects), and the medium/interface we use to experience these objects (i.e., the mind and the associated sense organs) are not able to work in a harmonious manner. This internal disharmony leads to the distortion of our experience, leading to a state of cognitive-emotive dissonance. Modern science calls it *stress*; Yogic and meditative philosophies call it *dvanda* [Sanskrit] or *klesha* [Pali]. The stress, as we know, leads to poor health. As we see now from cognitive neuroscience research, ancient philosophies of Yoga claim that our experiences are just *representations* in the mind and brain. Representations, as the name suggests, are symbolic (not actual) and dependent on the grade/quality of the mind and brain, and they change with change of the conditions (including the time) that invoked the representations. Our memory (Sanskrit: *smriti, pratyaya*) plays a crucial parameter in shaping these experiences.

Modern cognitive neuroscience agrees that memory is state dependent and changeable,[21] and thus experience is prone to change as well. Meditative wisdom including that of Buddha and Patanjali informs us that amelioration of stress is possible by modification and reappraisal of our internal representations: this is done by achieving the meditative insight about nature of these representations so that premature actions or cognitions (judgments, conclusions, or biases, etc.) are prevented.

Psychotherapeutic use of the Y-MBCT models is based on two major themes in Yoga: (1) Yoga as a profound psychosomatic science, and (2) meditation as a science of attention. Based on translational mindfulness research and recognizing the strengths and limitations of traditional CBT seven manualized Y-MBCT models for *disorder-specific and standardized application* in psychiatric and psychosomatic conditions was developed between 1998 and 2015. These disorder-specific Y-MBCT models are extensions and modifications of the wellness models such as the Standardized Yoga and Meditation Program for Stress Reduction (SYMPro-SR).[7] The seven translational mindfulness models whose efficacy has been tested over 200 multicultural patients from age 7–70 years (in India and the United States) are

1. Model for depression and, non-OCD and non-PTSD types of anxiety disorder (DepS Y-MBCT)
2. Model for refractory OCD (mindfulness-based exposure and response prevention: MB-ERP)
3. Model for refractory PTSD (trauma interventions using mindfulness-based extinction and reconsolidation of trauma memories: TIMBER)
4. Model for ADHD, dyslexia, and cognitive disorders (mindfulness-based remediation of reading and memory: MBR-RAM)
5. Model for chemical addiction and behavioral addiction including impulse control disorder and anger dyscontrol (mindfulness-based inner space technique: M-BIST)
6. Model for somatization/conversion and psychosomatic disorders (mindfulness-based *kriya*: MB-K)
7. Model for psychotic features including hallucinations and delusions (Y-MBCTp)

The Y-MBCT models combine Yogic philosophies, techniques, and practice into pragmatic and user-friendly formats. Recognizing the need and utility of *complementary and alternative medicine* (CAM), more so for youth, Y-MBCT models were initially piloted in children and teens who were thought to be the best meditators. Later, these models were extended to the adult population. The Y-MBCT models have been used in a symptom-specific manner for not only amelioration of symptoms but also for stress reduction, better coping, improvements in quality of life, and functioning and productivity in daily life. All the Y-MBCT models are holistic models of care and can be flexibly combined with other evidence-based treatments including medications and other behavioral interventions and targeted psychotherapies.

The Y-MBCT models are translational, targeted, and standardized. The standardizations involved in the Y-MBCT models include the pragmatism of cognitive behavioral therapy (CBT), neurobiology of human experience and individual disorders, psychosomatics of Yoga, models of mind in the Yogic traditions, five-factor model of human experience as described in the mindfulness philosophies, and the staged meditation protocols and their targeted applications for the symptoms in individual disorders.[7] In addition to the use of disorder-specific rating scales, treatment planning in all the Y-MBCT interventions is guided by use of a quantitative mindfulness scale: ASMI (Assessment Scale for Mindfulness Interventions[7]), which assesses the subject's level of mindfulness in seven dimensions (18 questions, maximum score 90). The higher the ASMI score is, the greater is the level of mindfulness. The outline for the methodology of the depression-specific model of Y-MBCT is described in the following section.

THE Y-MBCT MODEL FOR DEPRESSION AND ITS PSYCHOSOMATIC ADAPTATIONS

The complementary and alternative interventions in depression can be broadly categorized as two types: (1) nontargeted approaches, which as the name suggests employ general or nonspecific use of Yoga and meditation, and (2) targeted approaches that specifically target the individual symptoms of depression. The more well known targeted approaches are *mindfulness-based cognitive therapy*,[18] *dialectic behavioral therapy* (DBT),[22] and *acceptance and commitment therapy* (ACT).[23] As outlined in various recent literature on the therapeutic utility of mindfulness techniques[7,24] the essential elements in mindfulness are focused attention, compassion, empathy, and nonjudgmental attitudes which are therapeutic in patients suffering from depression. Mindfulness interventions typically use these therapeutic elements for treatment of depression. DepS Y-MBCT is a targeted approach and conceptually and methodologically, like the DBT or ACT or MBCT, it falls under the broader category of the *third-wave cognitive therapy*.[25]

Three main tools involved in the DepS Y-MBCT are

1. Calming and energizing breathing meditations to be practiced in sitting/lying down posture
2. Staged meditation protocols (SMPs, levels 1, 2, 3): this involves both the focused attention type of meditation that uses breath and body as the anchors to focus and induce detachment from the symptoms, and the open monitoring (OM) type of meditation empowered by the philosophy of the five-factor model and breathing meditations that maintain the detachment and enhance reappraisal of symptoms (and thus to promote new learning)
3. The *kriyas* ([Sanskrit] the Yogic procedures) and their symptom-specific psychosomatic adaptations for use in the somatic symptoms of depression

Home practice daily (routine and as needed) and flexibly adopting a balanced lifestyle (using the philosophy of Middle Way) provide the matrix for generalization of these interventions to the subject's daily life. Table 24.1 illustrates the components of DepS Y-MBCT.

TABLE 24.1
Symptom-Specific Translational Mindfulness Interventions Targeted for the Various Symptoms of Depression

Cardinal Symptoms of Depression		Targeted Y-MBCT Interventions
Affective	Sadness, anxiety	Detached reappraisal using the five-factor model and four stations of mindfulness
	Anger, impulsivity	Mindfulness Based Inner Space Technique (M-BIST) to decrease expression of anger and impulsivity
Cognitive	Ruminations Negative thinking	Detached reappraisal using the five-factor model and four stations of mindfulness
	Distractions/forgetfulness	Focused attention using breathing and body as anchors
Motivational	Lack of motivation Lethargy	Energizing breathing meditation
Somatic	Headache, pain, constipation	Mindfulness-based *kriya* (MBk)
	Somatic manifestation of panic or anxiety	Mindfulness-based graded exposure therapy (M-BET) and standardized focused attentive-type breathing meditations: For inducing and controlling the arousal process followed by detached reappraisal of the arousal so that new learning and deconditioning are possible

PRELIMINARY DATA ON EFFICACY OF DepS Y-MBCT IN DEPRESSION

As a psychotherapy for depression (with or without comorbid anxiety, the DepS Y-MBCT model has been applied in a multicultural population of 34 patients, age ranging from 14 to 64 years, from both genders and suffering from nonpsychotic depression (both unipolar and bipolar depression). This open trial was done from September 2012 to December 2014 at the Outpatient Psychiatry Clinic of the Cooper University Hospital, Camden, New Jersey. The mean duration of depression in these patients was 11.2 (s.d. 4.3) months, and there was no ongoing substance abuse. In 11 out of 34 patients, at the request of the patient/family, antidepressant medications were continued. Of note, before starting the DepS Y-MBCT interventions, patients were experiencing acute symptoms of depression despite taking these medications in adequate dosage and duration. Throughout the course of DepS Y-MBCT, in these 11 patients the dose of these medications were kept constant and no new antidepressant medications were added. There was high acceptability, feasibility, and patient satisfaction in the patients who continued the DepS Y-MBCT, but two patients dropped out before completing the initial three training sessions and did not return our phone calls asking to let us know about the reasons for the drop out. Out of the rest of the 32 patients, 27 patients completed the whole duration of treatment and have remitted from acute symptoms of depression, and 11 patients have been discharged from care. Remission was defined as reduction of HAM-D scores to ≤7 and the mean number of sessions (45 minutes each) needed for remission was 9.6 (s.d. 3.5) sessions (Table 24.2).

SOME DIFFERENCES OF Y-MBCT MODELS FROM CONTEMPORARY MODELS

As described before, the Y-MBCT models are translational, targeted, and therapeutic and are rooted in the ancient wisdom of the meditative traditions but use the methodology of evidence-based medicine. These models are based on the fundamental philosophies about human experiences and inform us that the pathological experiences in the subjects are deranged, dysfunctional, and exaggerations of the normal human experiences. Thus the disorder-specific models in Y-MBCT are extensions and modifications of the normal experiences—that is, the wellness models (SYMpro-SR). These concepts are derived from the Four Noble Truths in Buddhism (specifically, these are the first and second Noble Truths[26]), and this writer believes that these concepts are less stigmatizing and serve an important purpose of establishing an empathic relationship with the patient and do not alienate the patient from the therapist. Y-MBCT is the use of Yoga in its entirety (all eight limbs) rather than piecemeal. The Y-MBCT model is more experiential, and the therapist needs to be a practitioner, that is he/she practices the wellness model first to acquire the skills of mindfulness and also in the session, the therapist practices with patient. The Y-MBCT interventions are all encompassing and geared toward the whole cluster of symptoms. As described above, the DepS Y-MBCT targets all the cardinal symptoms of depression (psychological as well as somatic), for example, thoughts/ruminations, sad/anger feelings, and the somatic manifestations of depression. This is true for the other Y-MBCT models such as TIMBER (the PTSD version). In daily practice, these interventions are not only done in a standardized way but also have a dosing schedule, for example, routine (longer) practice in morning and night (BID) and symptom-specific p.r.n. (short) practice as needed. These interventions are client centered, and their self-help style includes home practice and daily

TABLE 24.2
Results of the Open Trial of DepS Y-MBCT (*n* = 32)

Study Parameters (Primary Outcome Measures in Italics)	Baseline Scores (mean +/– s.d.)	Scores After Six Sessions (mean +/– s.d.)
Hamilton-Depression Rating Scale (HAM-D, 17 items) scores	24.3 +/– 6.7	16.2 +/– 4.1
Assessment Scale for Mindfulness Intervention (ASMI, 18 items) scores	46.3 +/– 5.3	69.4 +/– 8.5

life applications targeted toward symptoms/dysfunctions. These interventions are feasible and have very low dropout rates. These interventions are feasible in various age groups (when presented in developmentally appropriate language), less stigmatizing, and have been well-accepted by multicultural populations. These interventions offer self-help, promote autonomy of the patient, and foster less dependence. Also as a therapeutic modality, these can be used alone or in combination with psychotropic medications. Preliminary data on their efficacy include both adolescent and adult populations and about 10–12 sessions (individual or group) are needed for induction of remission of symptoms of depression.

CONCLUSIONS, LIMITATIONS, AND FUTURE DIRECTIONS

Although preliminary, these data show that DepS Y-MBCT is feasible, acceptable to patients, and effective in inducing remission of symptoms of depression. Significant limitations of this study include but are not limited to its preliminary nature, open trial design, and small sample size. It is obvious that these findings need replication in larger trials, and DepS Y-MBCT has a long way to go.

ACKNOWLEDGMENTS

This writer acknowledges and deeply appreciates the support of the clinicians, residents, and staff of the Psychiatry Outpatient Department at the Cooper University Hospital, Camden, New Jersey.

REFERENCES

1. Reddy, M.S. 2010. Depression: Disorder and the burden. *Indian J Psychol Med* 32(1): 1–2.
2. NAMI. 2014. The Impact and Cost of Mental Illness: The Case of Depression. Policymakers Toolkit. http://www2.nami.org/Template.cfm?Section=Policymakers_Toolkit&Template=/ContentManagement/ContentDisplay.cfm&ContentID=19043 (accessed February 25, 2014).
3. Papakostas, G.I. and Fava, M. 2010. *Pharmacotherapy for Depression and Treatment-Resistant Depression*. Hackensack, NJ: World Scientific.
4. Satchidananda, S. 1978. *The Yoga Sutras of Patanjali: Translations and Commentary*. Yogaville, VA: Integral Yoga.
5. Buddhaghosa, B. and (translator) Nyanamoli, B. 1975. *The Path of Purification: Visuddhimagga*. Kandy, Sri Lanka: Buddhist Publication Society.
6. Nyanaponika, T. 1954. *The Heart of Buddhist Meditation*. Kandy, Sri Lanka: Buddhist Publication Society.
7. Pradhan, B.K. 2014. *Yoga and Mindfulness Based Cognitive Therapy: A Clinical Guide*. Geneva, Switzerland: Springer.
8. Lutz, A., Slagter, H.A., Dunne, J.D. et al. 2008. Attention regulation and monitoring in meditation. *Trends Cogn Sci* 12(4): 163–169.
9. Kristeller, J. 2004. Meditation: An integrated model across six domains of function. In *The Relevance of the Wisdom Traditions in Contemporary Society: The Challenge to Psychology*. Delft, Netherlands: Eburon.
10. World Health Organization (WHO). 2009. Mental health strengthening our response. Fact sheet 220. http://www.who.int/mediacentre/factsheets/fs220/en/ (accessed February 1, 2011).
11. Iyengar, B.K.S. 2001. *Yoga—The Path to Holistic Health*. London, UK: Dorling Kindersley.
12. Frawley, D. 1999. *Yoga and Ayurveda: Self-Healing and Self-Realization*. Twin Lakes, WI: Lotus Press.
13. Prasad, K., Wahner-Roedler, D.L., Cha, S.S. et al. 2011. Effect of a single-session meditation training to reduce stress and improve quality of life among health care professionals: A dose-ranging feasibility study. *Altern Ther Health Med* 17(3): 46–49.
14. Vancampfort, D., Vansteelandt, K., Scheewe, T. et al. 2012. Yoga in schizophrenia: A systematic review of randomised controlled trials. *Acta Psychiatr Scand* 126(1): 1–9.
15. Zylowska, L., Ackerman, D.L., Yang, M.H. et al. 2008. Mindfulness meditation training in adults and adolescents with ADHD: A feasibility study. *J Atten Disord* 11(6): 737–746.

16. Balasubramaniam, M., Telles, S., and Doraiswamy, P.M. 2013. Yoga on our minds: A systematic review of yoga for neuropsychiatric disorders. *Front Psychiatry* 3: 117.
17. Ludwig, D.S. and Kabat-Zinn, J. 2008. Mindfulness in medicine. *J Am Med Assoc* 300: 1350–1352.
18. Segal, Z.V., Williams, J.M.G., and Teasdale, J.D. 2002. *Mindfulness-Based Cognitive Therapy for Depression: A New Approach to Preventing Relapse.* New York, NY: Guilford Press (2nd and revised edition in 2013).
19. Felder, J.N., Dimidjian, S., and Segal, Z. 2012. Collaboration in mindfulness-based cognitive therapy. *J Clin Psychol* 68(2): 179–186.
20. Brown, R.P. and Gerbarg, P.L. 2005. Sudarshan Kriya yogic breathing in the treatment of stress, anxiety, and depression: Clinical applications and guidelines. *J Altern Complement Med* 11(4): 711–717.
21. Pally, R. 2005. Non-conscious prediction and a role for consciousness in correcting prediction errors. *Cortex* 41: 643–662.
22. Linehan, M.M. 1993. *Skills Training Manual for Treating Borderline Personality Disorder.* New York, NY: Guilford Press.
23. Hayes, S.C., Strosahl, K.D., and Wilson, K.G. 1999. *Acceptance and Commitment Therapy: An Experiential Approach to Behavior Change.* New York, NY: Guilford Press.
24. Lang, A.J., Strauss, J.L., Bomyea, J. et al. 2012. The theoretical and empirical basis for meditation as an intervention for PTSD. *Behav Modif* 36(6): 759–786.
25. Kahl, K.G., Winter, L., and Schweiger, U. 2012. The third wave of cognitive behavioural therapies. *Curr Opin Psychiatry* 25(6): 522–528.
26. Santina, P.D. 1997. *The Tree of Enlightenment: An Introduction to the Major Traditions of Buddhism.* Chico, CA: Buddha Dharma Education Association.

25 Meditation and Mindfulness

Healy Smith, MD, ABIHM and Gregory Thorkelson, MD

CONTENTS

INTRODUCTION

As treatments for depression, mindfulness and meditation might seem to reinforce the very tendencies toward rumination, isolation, and passivity that are symptomatic of depression. The nonjudgmental acceptance that characterizes mindfulness might seem perilously close to the nihilistic resignation of a person suffering from depression. Indeed, a common misconception about meditation is that it offers an escape away from the world and into a literal or metaphorical cave, removed from the stresses and realities of life. Meditation, however, is more accurately understood as exactly the opposite: as a practice of being more present.

The meeting of traditional Eastern contemplative practice and philosophy—from which much of mindfulness and meditation practices are drawn—with contemporary Western scientific models, approach, and technology has opened new doors of insight into our understanding of the mind and consciousness. These differing approaches to understanding the human condition, the self, suffering, and well-being, have complemented each other in ways that can advance both endeavors. But, the encounter between these worlds also carries uncertainties and dilemmas.

While the quantity and quality of research supporting the role of meditation and mindfulness in affecting health and depression, specifically, are among the best among integrative treatments, much of the experience and effect of mindfulness and meditation on any one person is ineffable: beyond quantitative measurement. And yet it is in the encounter between scientific inquiry and cultural practice that extraordinary discoveries about the relationship between the brain and mind have been made.

Since the middle of the twentieth century, well over 2000 articles have been published on mindfulness in the English language. Most of this research has been conducted since the mid-2000s with the bulk of the literature in the areas of mindfulness-based stress reduction (MBSR), mindfulness-based cognitive therapy (MBCT), and transcendental meditation (TM). Of these studies, only a few dozen to date were designed as randomized controlled trials (RCTs), the "gold standard" method of clinical trials, and few were specifically developed to investigate the benefit of mindfulness for depression. As such, much of the research reviewed herein supporting the role of mindfulness for depression is extrapolated from studies on anxiety and from research that illustrates the benefits of mindfulness practices on myriad health conditions.

DEFINITION OF MEDITATION

Meditation can be understood both as a technique, and as a state of being attained through that technique. Meditation has been described in many ways: as a way of life practiced by a devout few (monks, nuns, mystics, ascetics); as a set of techniques available to all with a goal of achieving better health, of attaining enlightenment, or with an emphasis on no goal at all; as a practice engrained in a religious or contemplative way of life; and as a practice situated in manually-based therapies. As discussed below, meditation practices have arisen from and been influenced by many cultures and contexts, and do not resolve into any one unified definition. This "seeming intractability of defining meditation"[1] is acknowledged in the scientific literature, with attempts to correct the "lack of a unified definition and taxonomy."[1]

In the West, meditation is often defined as a mental practice—disciplined yet open and nonjudgmental—involving attention regulation. Other elements common to many definitions of meditation include a defined, self-induced technique, a cultivation of/enhancement of awareness, a state of relaxation, and a suspension of logical thought process.[2]

Meditation is commonly broken down into two main categories based on the direction in which awareness is focused. The first is focused attention, or concentrative meditation, in which attention is focused on a particular object such as the coming and going of the breath or a mantra.[3] When attention wanders, this is recognized, and attention is directed back to the original object of meditation.

The second category is open monitoring meditation in which one cultivates an open, nonreactive, nonjudgmental, moment-to-moment awareness of the sensations and mental events that enter the field of awareness, without focusing on an explicit object. This technique is generally employed after focused attention has been cultivated. Focused attention and open monitoring are often combined into the mindfulness meditation practices commonly taught in the West.

DEFINITION OF MINDFULNESS

Mindfulness is a state of awareness—a way of paying attention—which like meditation, can refer both to a set of techniques and to a state of being. Mindfulness has been defined as bringing one's full attention to the present moment in an accepting, compassionate, nonjudgmental, nonreactive, nonstriving way.[4] Jon Kabat-Zinn, the founder of MBSR and leader in bringing mindfulness meditation into clinical use, defines mindfulness as "paying attention in a particular way: on purpose, in the present moment, and non-judgmentally."[5] Mindfulness can be cultivated through formal meditation practice and through application amid one's daily life, for example, noticing moment-to-moment one's experience while walking, eating, or washing one's hands.

HISTORY

Archaeological records suggest that meditation, in some form, was practiced as early as 2700–5000 BCE; historical consensus suggests that meditation has been practiced for most of human history, dating back to shamanic practices among hunter-gatherer cultures around the world.[6]

Our earliest written records of meditation are found in the teachings of the Hindu Vedas of ancient India, dating back to 1500 BCE, from which breath-work and a devotional focus on the divine evolved. This cultural milieu of the Vedas was foundational to what we now know as Yoga, Buddhism, Tantra, and related systems of belief and practice. Integral to these systems, meditation spread through central and East Asia.

The word *buddha* is a Pali-language term connoting a state of being awake, alert, and perceptive/receptive. Traditionally, the Indian prince who, through renunciation and meditation, attained enlightenment around 500 BCE and began his teachings, has come to be known by the title Buddha.[7] The Buddha taught a philosophy centered on understanding the nature of human suffering, and asserting a path to liberation from that suffering, in which meditation is central. Mindfulness meditation, as we understand it today in the West, has roots in these essential aspects of the Buddha's teachings.[8]

Over time, Buddhism in India branched off into Theravada, the more classical and exclusive tradition, and Mahayana, which opened the practices and possibilities of meditation more widely, and absorbed local influences from Tibetan folklore to Japanese manners. Significant writings discussing meditation dating from 400 BCE to 200 CE include the yoga sutras of Patanjali, and the Bhagavad Gita.[8] Theravada Buddhism extended to Sri Lanka, Burma, Thailand, Laos, Cambodia, and Vietnam. Mahayana Buddhism spread elsewhere through Asia, synthesizing with local religious and cultural practices to develop into Ch'an/Zen in Taoist China and Vajrayana Buddhism in Tibet.[8] In China, Ch'an Buddhism focused highly on meditation, the direct transmission of enlightenment from teacher to student, and koans (paradoxical statements or questions, contemplation of which can bring insight and enlightenment), and spread to Japan by the sixth century CE, developing into the austerely philosophical practice known as Zen by the eighth century CE. Buddhism in Tibet combined with local practices including a mystical pantheon of spirits, energy work, and tantra.

Almost all global cultures and religions have their own traditions of meditative practice that cultivate elevated mind states comparable to Vedic, Yogic, and Buddhist traditions—from the plainsong chant of a Trappist Catholic monk, to *hitbodedut*, the spontaneous personal prayers in a field or forest of a Jewish Chassid, to the intentional silence of a Quaker meeting, to the visionary stillness of an indigenous shaman. While current Western mindfulness meditation as utilized in the therapies described in this chapter bears some resemblance to aspects of all these traditions, and although it is generally deliberately detached from any one cultural or spiritual context, it derives most clearly from Buddhist meditation.[8]

In the early to mid-nineteenth century, early Western interest in this subject was stirred by the Transcendentalists: thinkers like Ralph Waldo Emerson, Henry David Thoreau, and Walt Whitman, who—reading those texts in translation, incorporated Eastern philosophy into their writings, seeking balance in a culture and society that placed increasing value on material worth, industrial and political power, and other signifiers of external achievement.[9] Later in the nineteenth century, the Theosophist movement further popularized Eastern writings and brought Vipassana meditation (insight/mindfulness meditation) to the West.

In 1893, the World Parliament of Religions in Chicago, Illinois, was a landmark in bringing Eastern spiritual leaders to the West.[8] Works like Herman Hesse's *Siddhartha*, and translations of the *Tibetan Book of the Dead*, and, by the 1950s, the writings of Aldous Huxley and Jack Kerouac and other Beat writers, aroused further interest in Buddhism, meditation, and Eastern philosophy. The influential Japanese Zen master D.T. Suzuki taught at Columbia University in the 1950s, collaborated with Carl Jung, and taught Kerouac (and other future beat writers), psychoanalysts Erich Fromm and Karen Horney, and the composer John Cage, among others. He taught with Fromm in a landmark 1957 workshop in Mexico on "Zen Buddhism and Psychoanalysis."[9] Additionally, American soldiers and military psychiatrists were exposed to Eastern thought and Japanese psychotherapy models during World War II, and brought ideas from these models back on their return.[9]

Tibetan Buddhism journeyed West after the exile of the Dalai Lama in 1959, with influential teachers such as Chogyam Trungpa arriving in the United States in 1970, where he established

The Naropa Institute and developed a secular version of his tradition called Shambhala.[8,9] Another influential spiritual leader to come to the West was Thich Nhat Hahn, a Vietnemese monk trained in Zen and Mahayana Buddhism, who became a leading teacher of mindfulness, author, and peace activist (nominated by Martin Luther King Jr. for the Nobel Peace Prize in 1967). Thich Nhat Hahn lectured at Columbia in the early 1960s and established monasteries and retreat centers around the world.

Within the seeking and contrarian mindset of the 1960s counterculture, with its interest in expanded states of consciousness, Yoga and transcendental meditation (TM) became more widely practiced. TM, involving among other things repetition of a personal mantra (a word or phrase), was introduced in the late 1960s by Maharishi Mahesh Yogi and popularized by the Beatles, who studied with him briefly but famously, in 1967.[9]

This popularization attracted the attention of Western medicine and science. As early as the 1930s and 1950s, academic research at Yale University, New Haven, Connecticut, in the United States and Tokyo University in Japan began to measure psychophysiological changes in meditation practitioners.[10] This was followed by a much larger wave of meditation research in the 1970s and 1980s with the study of TM. Reported health benefits included a lowering of blood pressure, heart rate, respiratory rate, oxygen consumption, cholesterol, cortisol, and lactate, as well as fewer doctor visits, longer life span, more alpha rhythms, and some bouts of theta waves. These benefits were largely thought to be due to the brain coherence, or synchrony between different parts of the brain measured by electroencephalogram (EEG), that TM was asserted to elicit.

The validity of this research has been called into question due to the potential bias arising from its being largely funded and conducted by the TM organization itself, and study designs often not being randomized or controlled.[10–12] In the 1970s, Herbert Benson, a cardiologist and professor at Harvard Medical School, directed his research toward meditation, focusing on a version of TM that he separated from its religious roots. In his text *The Relaxation Response*, he identified meditation as an antidote to the stress response, balancing a chronically activated sympathetic nervous system. He found that 20 minutes per day of meditation lowered heart rate, blood pressure, respiratory rate, oxygen consumption, and muscle tension. His research showed that the secular version produced the same physiologic effects as TM.

Other confluences between Eastern meditation traditions and Western psychological practices developed in the 1970s and 1980s. Vipassana meditation, derived from Theravada Buddhism, was further developed in the United States by Joseph Goldstein, Jack Kornfield, and Sharon Salzberg, who formed the Insight Meditation Society in Barre, Massachusetts, in 1975. This is a particularly psychologically framed method; many of its leading teachers are psychotherapists.[9]

In 1979, Jon Kabat-Zinn founded the Mindfulness-Based Stress Reduction program (MBSR) at the University of Massachusetts Medical Center to treat patients with chronic illness, which directed interest in the use of mindfulness and meditation to the medical world. His work brought about a shift in meditation research from TM to mindfulness meditation, and this field of research has since grown exponentially. Like Herbert Benson, Kabat-Zinn secularized mindfulness and meditation, and popularized it for the American public.

In 1987, the Dalai Lama along with Chilean neuroscientist Francisco Varela founded the Mind and Life Institute. Since that time, they have held regular dialogues and interdisciplinary meetings between scientists and spiritual practitioners to better understand the mind and the nature of reality, and to reduce suffering.

By 2007, a study published by the National Center for Complementary and Alternative Medicine (a branch of the NIH) found that the year prevalence of meditation among American adults was 9.4%.[13] Meditation and mindfulness constitute a pioneering mind-body intervention that is being adopted into mainstream health care, sometimes even covered by insurance. Meditation groups have spread to schools, hospitals and medical clinics, yoga studios, corporate wellness programs, and retreat centers.

MINDFULNESS MEDITATION

Contemporary meditation methods range from culturally specific ritual practice like Zen, through such organized movements as Transcendental Meditation, to what has come to be called mindfulness meditation—the method that this chapter chiefly considers, and that is most reliably informed by contemporary research. Mindfulness meditation is a practice or state of moment-to-moment awareness. The technique generally involves first focusing attention, for example, on the breath, quieting the mind, and then extending awareness to whatever thoughts, emotions, or sensations appear.

The stance is open, compassionate, nonjudgmental, accepting: an attitude of observing whatever is happening without trying to change it. This facilitates "direct contact with the experience itself."[14] With experience, one develops insight into the nature of one's thoughts and feelings, which are experienced as transient mental activity rather than as expressions of reality or identity. This process of stepping back and neutrally observing one's thoughts, feelings, and sensations is referred to by some mindfulness meditation researchers as metacognitive awareness, decentering, or cognitive defusion.[15]

Thus, mindfulness facilitates a more direct experience of the world, rather than experience filtered through patterns of reactivity and judgment, or histories and future projections. For example, while sitting in meditation, a feeling of agitation with sitting may arise, and one may have the thought: "I want to stop now." A reactive response could include ending the meditation session early, castigating oneself for being impatient and unable to keep one's mind quiet, or getting lost in thought of how frustrating and difficult meditation practice can be. A mindful approach would involve observing the thought and the feeling, without judging it, getting caught up in it, trying to change it, or reacting to it; perhaps, instead, watching it come and go, noticing the sensations or urges it creates in the moment without getting caught up in its story, without taking it literally, without letting it determine how one feels, or what should be done in the moment. And when one finds oneself carried along the path of, say, self-reproach for not meditating well enough, then one brings mindful attention to that very thought: observing it with compassion and openness, as mental activity, rather than as an expression of absolute truth that dictates how one should feel and live.

While there are useful guides and texts, meditation is ultimately a learning-by-doing phenomenon, and its essential experience is discovered through practice. Mindfulness meditation can be described as shifting one's attention away from content and toward process: away from habituated meaning-making and story-telling, toward more directly observing the trajectories of energy, the textures of feelings and sensations associated with moment-by-moment experience, before rationalizing them into any meaning or story. Applied within a depressive mindset, this story-telling can be especially ruminative and catastrophizing. Consider the example of smiling at a coworker and failing to get a smile in return: one could enter a cycle of overinterpreting the incident as indicating a negative attitude by the coworker, or one could observe one's own overinterpreting thinking from "a step back," recognizing the physical effects of this thinking as tensed muscles or changed posture, without treating the cognitive conclusions of such thinking as unquestionable truths.

Mindfulness meditation is often described within a metaphorical context of the sea and its waves, or the sky and its clouds. On the surface of a metaphorical sea, in high winds or stormy weather, one can be thrown about, rising and falling along forces too strong to resist, with resistance just increasing the blow. One may perceive oneself as falling helplessly and powerlessly to the storm, wishing it to stop. In mindfulness meditation, one may instead identify not just with the waves (that is, not just the workings of one's mind, thoughts, emotions, and sensations), but with the ocean itself—awakening into the deep still waters and seeing that the sea is more than its surface.

Consider the situation from this perspective: the waves do not change the essence of the water. The turbulence and drama of a stormy sea is very real, but it is temporary. The waves pass, and the sea is still the sea. It can be empowering to visualize the waves as seen from a few feet below: experiencing them as energetic expressions, but not as a defining, terrifying, overwhelming entirety.

Conversely and complementarily, one could learn to surf: to approach the waves not as something to be controlled or endured, but to ride. One can cultivate awareness and attunement to their energy; accept and respect what each one is; connect to them in a way that is not about judging them, controlling them, or being controlled by them, but about being with them. From this perspective, one can still be thrown around, underwater, unsure which way is up, but one may experience this in a newly open, nonjudgmental, and fearless way.

BRIEF OVERVIEW OF MINDFULNESS FOR DEPRESSION RESEARCH AND PUTATIVE MECHANISMS

Although literally thousands of publications involving mindfulness have been produced since the middle of the 1950s, few research studies have involved mindfulness specifically for depression and even fewer are carefully designed to minimize bias. As such, findings measuring depression or mood changes must be extracted from studies not designed to formally test improvement in depression from the use of mindfulness techniques.

The primary focus of much of the research has involved targets such as anxiety rather than depression. Indeed, while improved general health and decreased anxiety are among the positive effects of mindfulness that can also mitigate depression, MBSR and other mindfulness approaches appear to directly mediate improvement of depression in a number of ways.

Mindfulness practices have been shown to impact cognitive reactivity, the degree to which a dysphoric or unhappy state enhances negative patterns of thought. MBCT has been shown to decrease cognitive reactivity to sad mood states, which is one mechanism by which it likely exerts its effects of depressive relapse prevention.[16] Mindfulness practices have been shown to improve self-compassion; low levels of self-compassion are associated with rumination, avoidance, and depressive symptoms.[17,18] Other studies suggest that the improvements in mindfulness and decreases in rumination are key factors that inform the benefits of mindfulness techniques particularly for depression relapse prevention in MBCT.[19,20] Mindfulness therapies appear to also exert their antidepressant effects through enhancement of meta-awareness, the ability to take careful note of the contents of consciousness.[21]

In individuals at a high risk of suicidal depression, mindfulness has been shown in EEG studies to promote a balanced pattern of brain activation related to emotion.[22] Though small, another EEG study suggests a shift in EEG patterns to those more consistent with nondepressed individuals after an 8-week MBSR course.[23]

Further research on changes in neural activity suggest that the activity of the insula, an area of the brain associated in part with internally generated emotions, is associated with the creation of a sad mood state in both healthy and depressed individuals.[24] Insular activity is partly modulated by meditation, and the degree of activation has been shown to correlate with amount of meditation practice.[25] MBCT has further been shown to modulate rumination and fear driven by frontal lobular activity through recruitment of the somatosensory cortex and increased interoceptive activation.[26] Newer MBCT imaging research in chronically depressed patients also supports increases in dorsal lateral prefrontal cortex activity to predepression levels with concurrent decreases in ventral lateral prefrontal cortex and amygdala activity after completing an eight week program.[27]

More broadly, mindfulness likely further benefits the individual through modulation of inflammatory pathways. The relationship between inflammation and depression is becoming increasingly clear.[28] Although a direct causal relationship has not been elucidated, mindfulness techniques have been shown in some studies to modulate the expression of pro-inflammatory genes[29] and increase parasympathetic tone[30] which, likely mediated by the vagus nerve, can regulate inflammation. Additionally, mindfulness meditation practices have been shown to modulate the immune system itself, including through increasing CD4+ T lymphocyte counts in HIV-infected adults in direct relationship to the amount of time spent practicing.[31]

Although the research is still in its infancy and a detailed overview is outside the scope of this chapter, there are sufficient mechanistic explanations for the antidepressant and depression relapse prevention effects of mindfulness practices to warrant continued research in this area. The following sections summarize aspects of the extant literature in treating depression.

MINDFULNESS-BASED STRESS REDUCTION

Mindfulness-based stress reduction (MBSR) was developed by Jon Kabat-Zinn, who established his stress reduction clinic at the University of Massachusetts Medical Center in 1979.[32,33] Its initial aim was to help people with chronic pain and serious chronic illness. Its application has since expanded, used in the treatment of many illnesses, as well as for the healthy population seeking better ways to manage stress.

Jon Kabat-Zinn distilled meditation and mindfulness principles from their religious and spiritual roots, making them highly accessible, as well as standardized, and thus amenable to high-quality scientific research. MBSR is an 8-week course led by one to two facilitators in a group of approximately 25–35 people, for 2–2.5 hour weekly sessions, and one full-day mindfulness meditation retreat. Sessions involve formal and informal meditation and mindfulness practices, group sharing, discussion, and psycho-education about stress, coping skills, and assertiveness. The facilitators are encouraged to embody a mindful approach. Mindfulness practices include sitting meditation, mindful hatha yoga, body scan (a guided meditation to focus awareness sequentially on individual parts of the body), and mindful eating. Homework includes about an hour of daily mindfulness practice, requiring real commitment from participants. Participants cultivate openness to present-moment experience, a decentered stance, acceptance of things as they are, and insight into the coming and going of thoughts and sensations, all of which enhance the ability to bear pain and balance stress. These techniques have been widely adopted. Over 700 facilitators have been trained at the University of Massachusetts clinic, there are hundreds of MBSR programs around the world, and over 20,000 people have completed the MBSR course. MBSR programs can now be found in hospitals, schools, prisons, and beyond, and are covered by some insurance companies.

MBSR DEPRESSION RESEARCH

A number of studies have shown improvement in depression with MBSR across diverse groups. As noted previously, nearly all of the studies in the MBSR literature focused on depressive symptoms as secondary outcomes or viewed improvement in mood broadly especially in relationship to significant physical illness. Indeed, the study by Ramel et al. in 2004 investigating MBSR for cognitive processing and measuring affect in patients with a history of depression, one of the studies best able to potentially determine the benefit of MBSR for depression, was unable to draw conclusions about the effectiveness of MBSR as a primary depression treatment.[34] Nevertheless, this study did demonstrate an improvement in rumination and showed benefit with depressive symptoms. The following studies outline some of the support for depressive symptom improvement with MBSR in patients who were often not diagnosed with a major depressive disorder but experienced mood symptoms secondary to health issues or stressors in the environment.

A stressed population of medical students who completed an MBSR course reported improvement in depressive symptoms that continued during the stressful period of examinations.[35] On the other hand, minimally stressed, healthy young adult professional musicians who participated in a 2-month program of thrice weekly courses involving yoga and meditation experienced a decrease in depressive symptoms that appeared to have been directly mediated by the yoga and meditation techniques themselves.[36] Thus, MBSR appears to benefit adults across a range of stress levels.

MBSR exerts antidepressant effects not only in healthy individuals but also in those with serious medical conditions. Patients suffering with multiple sclerosis (MS), an autoimmune disease that damages the protective coating of nerves in the brain and spinal cord, are frequently depressed and experience a rate of suicide seven times higher than the general population. Depression is also a side effect of certain medications used to treat the condition. In multiple studies, MBSR training has been shown to significantly improve depression and previously poor health-related quality of life measures in patients with MS.[37] People with fibromyalgia are also at high risk for depression; over half will experience an episode of major depression. A study using MBSR in firbomyalgia patients demonstrated a decrease in depressive symptoms, a benefit that persisted after the intervention concluded.[38]

Caregivers can also benefit from the use of MBSR. Female caregivers of family members with dementia who participated in a six-session manualized yoga and meditation program experienced statistically significant reductions in depression. This improvement was directly related to the amount of practice time. This dose–response relationship is one of a number of studies underscoring the importance of practice to enhance response.[39]

Regarding randomized control trials with MBSR that assess depression symptoms, a few merit review. In an RCT of 100 women with early stage breast cancer, compared with the nutrition education control group, the MBSR group experienced a nearly 50% improvement on one depression rating scale (SCL-90).[40] Although another group of women with irritable bowel syndrome (IBS) randomized to MBSR versus a support group for 8 weeks did not experience statistically significant improvement in depression after treatment, this was not a primary outcome, and the symptom severity of IBS significantly improved 3 months subsequent to treatment.[41] In a three-arm RCT of women with fibromyalgia, the secondary outcome of depression trended toward improvement, and MBSR-treated patients responded best to the intervention overall; however, these measures did not reach statistical significance.[42] Patients enduring the stresses and medication side effects related to solid organ transplant in a controlled trial with two-stage randomization demonstrated nonstatistically significant improvement in depression only for the MBSR group that was maintained after one year.[43]

THIRD-WAVE BEHAVIORAL THERAPIES

The "third wave" of behavioral therapies introduces new themes to traditional "second-wave" cognitive behavioral therapy (CBT), including the cultivation of acceptance and mindfulness, in part through employing the strategies of metacognitive awareness/decentering/cognitive defusion (a distancing from or dis-identification with one's thoughts).[44,45] As in CBT, thoughts are viewed as mental events that may or may not reflect reality, and maladaptive thoughts are understood to underlie distressing feelings and maladaptive behaviors. Whereas the cognitive focus in CBT is to modify the content of dysfunctional thoughts, the focus in the third-wave therapies is to modify the relationship to, or function of, one's thoughts. MBCT, Dialectical Behavior Therapy (DBT), and Acceptance and Commitment Therapy (ACT) are the best-researched of these therapies for the treatment of depression and will be discussed below.

MINDFULNESS-BASED COGNITIVE THERAPY

Major depressive disorder often follows a chronic course. Based on the high rate of relapse of up to 80% or more,[46-48] increasing risk with more prior episodes, and insufficient maintenance interventions, developing methods of relapse prevention was considered key to reducing the burden of depression.[49] Zindel Segal, J. Mark Williams, and John Teasdale accepted this challenge.

Their development of MBCT was informed by cognitive research on depression relapse vulnerability, which showed that in contrast to subjects with no history of depression, recovered subjects with a history of depression revert to a depressive cognitive processing pattern upon a sad mood induction.[50-52] In remitted depressed patients, normal dysphoric mood reactivated depressive thinking patterns, potentially reinforcing, perpetuating, and intensifying the low mood, and spiraling down into depression. In fact, those with the greatest reactivation of dysfunctional thinking styles upon low mood provocation were found to be at the highest risk of relapse over the next 18 months.[53]

Another well-researched contributor to depression vulnerability is a tendency toward rumination. Though trying to "think one's way out of it" may seem rational, responding to depressive thoughts or feelings with rumination actually perpetuates and worsens depression.[54,55]

Segal, Williams, and Teasdale sought a way to decrease relapse vulnerability by interrupting reactivation of the depressive thinking style, and interfering with the ruminative response. The approach they developed, MBCT, integrates secular meditation and mindfulness practices based on Jon Kabat-Zinn's work in MBSR, with principles of cognitive therapy.[56]

The structure of MBCT mirrors that of MBSR, as an 8-week manualized, skills-based, experiential, weekly group course. Groups run for 2 hours. They are typically composed of 8–15 participants and led by one to two therapists. Therapists are required to have their own mindfulness practices, their embodiment of the mindful approach key to MBCT's efficacy. Course contents include psycho-education, and focus on the practice of meditation and mindfulness skills, including meditation with a focus on the breath and bodily sensations, then extending to an open awareness of the flow of thoughts and feelings. Sitting meditation, mindful movement including walking meditation and mindful yoga, and mindfulness in everyday activities are practiced during the sessions, and applied in daily life. Participants are encouraged to spend 45 minutes per day practicing mindfulness between sessions.

MBCT cultivates in its participants an open, curious, accepting, and compassionate attitude and a decentered stance. These enable depressive thoughts and feelings to be experienced as passing mental events rather than as accurate reflections of one's reality and identity. Instead of being swept into a depressive spiral, one is better equipped to recognize and disengage from depressive and ruminative thinking patterns. One becomes less identified with the content of one's thoughts and feelings, and more identified with their internal observer.

MBCT DEPRESSION RESEARCH

MBCT is a newer therapy, with less research to date, but with encouraging findings in the treatment of depression. Nevertheless, as it composes aspects of both CBT and MBSR, much of the research can be applied to understanding the putative benefit from this newer, structured approach to the clinical use of mindfulness. CBT, developed by Aaron T. Beck and extensively studied since the 1960s, has been repeatedly shown to be an effective, evidence-based treatment for depression. It has a medium to medium-large effect size particularly on chronic depressive symptoms, an impact similar to that of antidepressant medication.[50] In a similar way, MBCT can be helpful for the treatment of depression, but is particularly useful for preventing future episodes of recurrent depression.

In a sample of cancer patients with diverse diagnoses and stages of disease, an MBCT program with the component of a MBSR-like day-long retreat was effective at decreasing symptoms of depression and improving mindfulness with a durability of effect measured at 3 months after treatment.[57] A small pilot trial of caregivers of close relatives with dementia randomized the caregivers to an MBCT-derived program or a nonspecific active control group with equal time and attention. The MBCT group showed a trend toward improvement on the Center for Epidemiologic Studies Depression Scale.[58]

For individuals at risk of depression relapse after at least three previous episodes of depression, MBCT conferred additional benefit to current treatment, resulting in decreased rates of relapse, decreased residual symptoms of depression, and improved quality of life. One RCT of patients in full or partial remission of depression randomized to either maintenance antidepressant medication or MBCT with support to taper medication illustrated that not only was there no cost difference between the usual care group and those additionally receiving MBCT but three quarters of patients treated with MBCT discontinued their maintenance antidepressant medication. Furthermore, there was no statistically significant difference in depression scores or relapse after 15 months despite the lack of antidepressant utilization in most MBCT-treated patients.[59] In another RCT exploring prevention of depressive relapse using MBCT alone versus continued use of antidepressant alone versus switch from antidepressant to placebo, both MBCT and continued antidepressant treatment prevented relapse. Relapse prevention was particularly important for patients with ongoing depressive symptoms who, while no longer meeting criteria for major depressive disorder (MDD), were thus described as having "unstable remission."[60] Further bolstering the benefit of MBCT for preventing depression relapse, chronically depressed adults randomized to treatment versus their perpetually depressed counterparts in a control group improved in appreciation for pleasant activities and experienced an increase in momentary positive emotions.[61]

A small Italian study randomized patients with MDD who had not achieved remission after 2 months of antidepressants to MBCT or a nonspecific active control structurally similar to the MBCT program but devoid of the mindfulness component. Importantly, the MBCT participants who also experienced the mindfulness components had an average decrease on the Hamilton depression rating scale of roughly 50%, a significantly greater improvement than in the control group. The MBCT group also reported a greater improvement on measures of overall well-being.[62] Importantly, when evaluated against maintenance antidepressant treatment of major depression, MBCT compares favorably and is likely more cost effective over time.[63]

It appears that MBCT for relapse prevention in depression is more beneficial in those who have experienced three or more depressive episodes. In patients with only one or two episodes of depression, MBCT may possibly slightly increase the risk for depression relapse although the mechanisms are unclear; furthermore, this finding is not consistent across studies.[64] Along these lines, the National Institute for Clinical and Health Excellence (NICE) in the United Kingdom recommends MBCT for individuals with two or more previous depressive episodes. More recently, MBCT has been studied for the treatment of acute and subacute phases of depressive disorders, predominantly major depressive disorder. As of this publication, since 2009 roughly 10 studies investigated the role of MBCT for patients with depression that did not remit with antidepressant therapy; half of these studies were RCTs. The studies ranged between 18 and 130 participants but all were 8 weeks in duration. Three quarters of these studies showed statistically significant ($p < 0.05$) greater reductions in measurements of depression (primarily as measured by the Beck Depression Index or the Hamilton Rating Scale for Depression) compared to controls.[65] The body of literature on using MBCT for both acute and subacute depression is growing with an increasing body of evidence underscoring the utility of MBCT for both prevention of relapse after three or more episodes and active treatment.

DIALETICAL BEHAVIOR THERAPY

Dialetical behavior therapy (DBT) is a psychotherapy developed by Marsha Linehan in the early 1990s to treat actively suicidal and self-harming patients, many of whom have borderline personality disorder (BPD),[66] and since found efficacious for a range of psychiatric disorders, with a small literature base indicating utility in the treatment of major depressive disorder. DBT blends elements of Buddhist (particularly Zen) mindfulness practice (to facilitate mindful awareness, acceptance of self and the present situation, and distress tolerance) with elements of CBT and assertiveness training (to guide change). Central to its philosophy, DBT teaches and embodies dialectical thinking, a holistic approach to tolerating conflict with awareness and flexibility versus with the rigid and dichotomous thinking commonly found in BPD. The primary dialectic within DBT is in the synthesis of acceptance and change, which are balanced within the skills and strategies taught, as well as in the therapist's stance of accepting patients as they are, and also acknowledging their need for change to attain their goals. DBT diverges from traditional CBT in its emphasis on validating or accepting difficult thoughts versus wrestling with them.

DBT consists of four components: a skills training group, weekly individual psychotherapy, phone coaching, and a consultation team to support the therapist. The skills trained in DBT include mindfulness, distress tolerance, interpersonal effectiveness, and emotion regulation. Mindfulness skills are the first skills taught and are reviewed weekly; they are considered foundational to the other skills. They teach the ability to pay attention nonjudgmentally, moment to moment, and to experience one's emotions fully, without getting stuck in them, being overwhelmed by them, or denying them. Distressing thoughts are accepted, self-destructive urges are tolerated, and the patient becomes increasingly able to act more freely.

DBT DEPRESSION RESEARCH

As DBT was initially developed for adults who are chronically suicidal or self-injurious, many of the research studies are limited to this population and involve depression as a secondary outcome. Indeed, it has been helpful in decreasing depressive symptoms and psychiatric hospitalization in adolescents, female veterans, and adults with BPD. Although thus far limited, recent research suggests that DBT can provide benefit to other populations with depression. In a pilot study of largely chronically depressed individuals over 60 years old and currently taking antidepressants, a 28-week program of DBT was added to the treatment of one cohort while the other group continued to only receive medication. At 6-month follow-up, nearly three times as many patients who also received DBT continued to be in remission compared to those who received medication only; further, only 25% of the patients who received a course of DBT relapsed.[67] Other studies demonstrate large effect sizes for treatment-resistant depression in adults who did not respond adequately to medication.[68] Although further research is needed, the current findings are promising, particularly in cases where pharmacology is inadequate.

ACCEPTANCE AND COMMITMENT THERAPY

Acceptance and commitment therapy (ACT) was developed in 1986 by Steven Hayes.[69] It was not explicitly borne from Buddhism, but rather, from behavioral psychology and a complex and comprehensive theory developed in a basic research program in human language and cognition. This theory, called relational frame theory (RFT), examines the influence of human language on cognition, and guided the development of ACT.[70] ACT is not manualized, and can be used short or long term, in individuals, couples, or groups.

ACT shares important concepts with Buddhism. These include the belief that the normal workings of the human mind can create suffering, and the use of mindfulness techniques to increase psychological flexibility. As with other mindfulness-based therapies, a core focus of ACT is in learning a different, non-content-based way of relating and responding to thoughts and feelings. Most of the vast array of mindfulness techniques utilized in ACT does not involve formal meditation. Creativity is encouraged in finding and developing such techniques. Examples of cognitive defusion techniques include repeating a thought out loud until it becomes just sounds, and introducing before a thought the phrase—"I am having the thought that...."

The six core processes used in ACT include acceptance (opening to and allowing unwanted thoughts and feelings, without attempting to change them), cognitive defusion (a way of recognizing and relating to thoughts and feelings as passing events), being present, self as context (the observing self), values (clarification of the patient's values), and committed action (commitment to change guided by those values).[71]

ACT DEPRESSION RESEARCH

A recent meta-analysis found probable effectiveness of ACT for chronic pain and tinnitus, and possible effectiveness for depression, mixed anxiety, obsessive-compulsive disorder (OCD), substance abuse, psychotic symptoms, and work stress.[72]

Although the body of literature studying the use of ACT for depression is small and growing, available data suggest that ACT is at least similarly efficacious as gold-standard evidence-based therapies such as CBT for depression.[73] It has been used effectively in general outpatients with depression, leading to significant improvement in depression at rates comparable to CBT. Interestingly, the mechanism by which ACT exerts its antidepressant effect appears to differ from CBT. Whereas CBT works through description and observation, ACT appears to mediate depression improvement through the domains of acceptance, awareness, and experience avoidance.[74] Further well-controlled studies focusing on depression as a primary outcome would help to illuminate the benefits of ACT for the treatment of depression.

LOVING-KINDNESS AND COMPASSION MEDITATION

Loving-kindness meditation (LKM) (or *metta* in Pali) and compassion meditation (CM) are intimately related to mindfulness meditation. While mindfulness meditation cultivates the focus needed to practice LKM and CM (and is usually taught first), LKM and CM facilitate the nonjudgmental awareness and compassionate tone integral to mindfulness meditation. Without this nonjudgmental, kind, compassionate approach, it is impossible to open to and mindfully observe one's aversive thoughts, feelings, and sensations.

LKM and CM are inextricably connected, and have at their foundation the belief that all beings are interconnected.[75] LKM refers to the practice of cultivating the intention for "unconditional kindness" to one's self and all beings. CM refers to the practice of cultivating the intention to open to the existence of suffering, and to respond to those who suffer with a nonjudgmental, heartfelt caring, and with the wish that all beings be freed from suffering.

LKM and CM are concentrative types of meditation. In one form of practice, attention is directed to the silent repetition of phrases that express wishes of loving-kindness and compassion, such as phrases invoking safety, happiness, health, and ease, first to oneself, and then extending out to an ever-widening circle of people and beings.

LKM/METTA DEPRESSION RESEARCH

Loving kindness, or *metta*, practices have been shown to improve self-compassion which is associated with a decrease in the number of undesirable emotional states including depression.[76] LKM has also been associated with improvement in depressive symptoms with a concurrent increase in positive emotions in a small study of individuals with high self-critical perfectionism.[77] This is an important finding as self-criticism, a component of a number of psychological disorders, is predictive of a poor treatment response in depression. Furthermore, in a larger study involving working adults, by increasing positive emotions, which enhanced personal resources, LKM appeared to exert its effect in reducing depressive symptoms.[78] Interestingly, even without practice, the effects of increased positive emotions have been shown to persist 15 months after the initial LKM intervention.

CONCLUSION

This chapter has described the practices of mindfulness and meditation, their clinically relevant history, and their use in a variety of therapies for the treatment of depression.

While there have been thousands of studies examining the clinical utility of mindfulness and meditation, a limited number of these studies measure depression as a primary outcome, and few of those are gold-standard RCTs. (MBCT offers the exception: it is the only therapy reviewed in this chapter developed specifically to treat depression, with most of its research oriented around depression as the primary outcome.) Nevertheless, our available data does suggest that the mindfulness-based therapies described can be effective in treating depression. Further research looking at effects specifically on depression is needed.

As noted in this chapter, our understanding of the mechanisms by which meditation and mindfulness exert their effects highlights their wide-reaching benefits across many concerns, symptoms, and illnesses. Benefits are many, and risks low. Large systematic reviews of MBSR and

MBCT have not reported any treatment side effects.[64] Furthermore, a 2014 report from the Agency for Healthcare Research and Quality, the U.S. Department of Health and Human Services section tasked with assessing safety and benefit of healthcare interventions, did not note any harmful outcomes for the meditation programs studied.[79] During treatment, however, awareness training can lead to a transient increase in symptoms, but worsening of depressive symptoms has not been noted in the literature where mindfulness techniques are utilized appropriately. Most of these approaches are associated with high rates of satisfaction and low rates of dropout, usually on the order of 20%.[80]

Mindfulness and meditation training programs emphasize the importance of an active meditation practice for their teachers.[81] On continued mindfulness practice for clinicians, Jon Kabat-Zinn states that mindfulness "cannot be taught to others in an authentic way without the instructor practicing it in his or her own life."[82] Indeed, in one study of MBSR, the clinician's personal experience with meditation was the only predictive factor determining positive clinical outcome.[83] Practice is important for the client as well, as the beneficial effects of treatment appear to taper off over time; however, booster sessions within 9 months to a year after the initial course of therapy can prolong the duration of positive response. Some studies show durability of benefits over one year after initial treatment. Additionally, symptom improvement appears to be dose related; a number of studies across various conditions have shown that those who practice more receive additional incremental health benefit.[84]

Any further conclusion must acknowledge a critique offered by the subject of study itself. Despite the demonstrated benefits just noted, many Buddhist and related traditions explicitly disavow the very idea of utility or usefulness, as what Chogyam Trungpa calls "Spiritual Materialism": the conscious application of spiritual practices for personal betterment—even betterment of physical or mental health. "Ego," Trungpa writes, "is able to convert everything to its own use, even spirituality. For example, if you have learned of a particularly beneficial meditation technique of spiritual practice, then ego's attitude is, first to regard it as an object of fascination and, second to examine it."[85] Conversely, just as a nutrient extracted from a plant does not necessarily contain the powers of the whole plant, so too may appropriated and adapted mindfulness and meditation not necessarily have the same effect as they do when situated within the ancient traditions in which they emerged. And yet, as researchers and clinicians, we are required to extract and synthesize, to examine and treat.

REFERENCES

1. Nash, J. and Newberg, A. 2013. Towards a unifying taxonomy and definition for meditation. *Front Psychol* 4: 1–18.
2. Bond, K., Ospina, M., Hooton, N. et al. 2009. Defining a complex intervention: The development of demarcation criteria for "Meditation." *Psychol Relig Spiritual* 1(2): 129–137.
3. Lutz, A., Slagter, H.A., Dunne, J.D., and Davidson, R.J. 2009. Attention regulation and monitoring in meditation. *Trends Cogn Sci* 12(4): 163–169.
4. Teasdale, J.D., Segal, Z., and Williams, M.G. 1995. How does cognitive therapy prevent depressive relapse and why should attentional control (Mindfulness) training help? *Behav Res Ther* 33(1): 25–39.
5. Kabat-Zinn, J. 1994. *Wherever You Go, There You Are: Mindfulness Meditation in Everyday Life.* New York, NY: Hyperion, p. 4.
6. Monaghan, P. and Viereck, E.G. 2011. *Meditation, The Complete Guide.* Novato, CA: New World Library, pp. 17–20.
7. Smith, B. 2005. Meditation, Eastern. In *New Dictionary of the History of Ideas* (Vol. 4). Ed. M.C. Horowitz. Detroit, MI: Charles Scribner, p. 1414.
8. Morton, S. 2012. Meditation. In *Encyclopedia of Global Religion,* Ed. M. Juergensmeyer and W. Roof. Thousand Oaks, CA: SAGE, pp. 769–772.
9. McCown, D., Reibel, D.K., and Micozzi, M.S. 2011. *Teaching Mindfulness: A Practical Guide for Clinicians and Educators.* New York, NY: Springer, pp. 33, 1533–1535, 1460–1467, 1817, 1680, 1842–1854.
10. West, M. 1979. Meditation. *Br J Psychiatry* 135: 457–467.

11. Canter, P.H. and Ernst, E. 2004. Insufficient evidence to conclude whether or not Transcendental Meditation decreases blood pressure: Results of a systematic review of randomized clinical trials. *J Hypertension* 22(11): 2049–2054.

12. Goldstein, C.M., Josephson, R., Xie, S., and Hughes, J.W. 2012. Current perspectives on the use of meditation to reduce blood pressure. *Int J Hypertens* 2012: 11. Article ID 578397.

13. Barnes, P.M., Bloom, B., and Nahin R.L. 2008. Complementary and alternative medicine use among adults and children: United States, 2007. *Natl Health Stat Rep* 10(12): 1–23.

14. Kabat-Zinn, J. 1994. *Wherever You Go, There You Are: Mindfulness Meditation in Everyday Life.* New York, NY: Hyperion, p. 56.

15. Teasdale, J.D., Moore, R.G., Hayhurst, H. et al. 2002. Metacognitive awareness and prevention of relapse in depression: Empirical evidence. *J Consult Clin Psychol* 70(2): 275–287.

16. Raes, F., Dewulf, D., Van Heeringen, C. et al. 2009. Mindfulness and reduced cognitive reactivity to sad mood: Evidence from a correlational study and a nonrandomized waiting list controlled study. *Behav Res Ther* 47: 623–627.

17. Kuyken, W., Watkins, E., Holden, E. et al. 2010. How does mindfulness-based cognitive therapy work? *Behav Res Ther* 48: 1105–1112.

18. Krieger, T., Altenstein, D., Baettig, I. et al. 2013. Self-compassion in depression: Associations with depressive symptoms, rumination, and avoidance in depressed outpatients. *Behav Ther* 44(3): 501–513.

19. Michalak, J., Ho¨lz, A., and Teismann, T. 2010. Rumination as a predictor of relapse in mindfulness-based cognitive therapy for depression. *Psychol Psychother Theory Res Pract* 84: 230–236.

20. Michalak, J., Heidenreich, T., Meibert, P. et al. 2008. Mindfulness predicts relapse/recurrence in major depressive disorder after mindfulness-based cognitive therapy. *J Nerv Ment Dis* 196: 630–633.

21. Hargus, E., Crane, C., Barnhofer, T. et al. 2010. Effects of mindfulness on metaawareness and specificity of describing prodromal symptoms in suicidal depression. *Emotion* 10: 34–42.

22. Barnhofer, T., Duggan, D., Crane, C. et al. 2007. Effects of meditation on frontal α-asymmetry in previously suicidal individuals. *NeuroReport* 18: 709–712.

23. Davidson, R.J., Kabat-Zinn, J., Schumacher, J. et al. 2003. Alterations in brain and immune function produced by mindfulness meditation. *Psychosom Med* 65(4): 564–570.

24. Liotti, M., Mayberg, H.S., McGinnis, S. et al. 2002. Unmasking disease-specific cerebral blood flow abnormalities: Mood challenge in patients with remitted unipolar depression. *Am J Psychiatry* 159(11): 1830–1840.

25. Brefczynski-Lewis, J.A., Lutz, A., Schaefer, H.S. et al. 2007. Neural correlates of attentional expertise in long-term meditation practitioners. *Proc Natl Acad Sci* 104(27): 1483–1488.

26. Farb, N.A., Anderson, A.K., and Segal, Z.V. 2012. The mindful brain and emotion regulation in mood disorders. *Can J Psychiatry* 57(2): 70–77.

27. Eisendrath, S.J. 2015. A randomized clinical trial of mindfulness-based cognitive therapy for treatment-resistant depression and functional magnetic resonance imaging. *American Psychiatric Association 2015 Annual Meeting.* SCI 2. Presented May 19, 2015.

28. Krishnadas, R. and Cavanagh, J. 2012. Depression: An inflammatory illness? *J Neurol Neurosurg Psychiatry* 83(5): 495–502.

29. Kaliman, P., Alvarez-López, M.J., Cosín-Tomás, M. et al. 2014. Rapid changes in histone deacetylases and inflammatory gene expression in expert meditators. *Psychoneuroendocrinology* 40: 96–107.

30. Ditto, B., Eclache, M., and Goldman, N. 2006. Short-term autonomic and cardiovascular effects of mindfulness body scan meditation. *Ann Behav Med* 32(3): 227–234.

31. Creswell, J.D., Myers, H.F., Cole S.W. et al. 2009. Mindfulness meditation training effects on CD4+ T lymphocytes in HIV-1 infected adults: A small randomized controlled trial. *Brain Behav Immun* 23(2): 184–188.

32. Kabat-Zinn, J. 1996. Mindfulness meditation: What it is, what it isn't, and it's role in health care and medicine. In *Comparative and Psychological Study on Meditation*, Ed. Y. Haruki, Y. Ishii and M. Suzuki. Delft, Netherlands: Eburon, pp. 161–169.

33. Kabat-Zinn, J. 1990. *Full Catastrophe Living: Using the Wisdom of Your Body and Mind to Face Stress, Pain and Illness.* New York, NY: Delacorte.

34. Ramel, W., Goldin, P.R., Carmona, P.E. et al. 2004. The effects of mindfulness meditation on cognitive processes and affect in patients with past depression. *Cogn Ther Res* 28(4): 433–455.

35. Shapiro, S.L., Schwartz, G.E., and Bonner, G. 1998. Effects of mindfulness-based stress reduction on medical and premedical students. *J Behav Med* 21: 581–599.

36. Khalsa, S.B., Shorter, S.M., Cope, S. et al. 2009. Yoga ameliorates performance anxiety and mood disturbance in young professional musicians. *Appl Psychophysiol Biofeedback* 34(4): 279–289.

37. Grossman, P., Kappos, L., Gensicke, H. et al. 2010. MS quality of life, depression, and fatigue improve after mindfulness training: A randomized trial. *Neurology* 75: 1141–1149.
38. Sephton, S.E., Salmon, P., Weissbecker, I. et al. 2007. Mindfulness meditation alleviates depressive symptoms in women with fibromyalgia: Results of a randomized clinical trial. *Arthr Rheumatol* 57: 77–85.
39. Waelde, L.C., Thompson, L., and Gallagher-Thompson, D. 2004. A pilot study of a yoga and meditation intervention for dementia caregiver stress. *J Clin Psychol* 60(6): 677–687.
40. Henderson, V.P., Clemow, L., Massion, A.O. et al. 2012. The effects of mindfulness-based stress reduction on psychosocial outcomes and quality of life in early-stage breast cancer patients: A randomized trial. *Breast Cancer Res Treat* 131(1): 99–109.
41. Gaylord, S.A., Palsson, O.S., Garland, E.L. et al. 2011. Mindfulness training reduces the severity of irritable bowel syndrome in women: Results of a randomized controlled trial. *Am J Gastroenterol* 106(9): 1678–1688.
42. Schmidt, S., Grossman, P., and Schwarzer, B. 2011. Treating fibromyalgia with mindfulness-based stress reduction: Results from a 3-armed randomized controlled trial. *Pain* 152(2): 361–369.
43. Gross, C.R., Kreitzer, M.J., Thomas, W. et al. 2010. Mindfulness-based stress reduction for solid organ transplant recipients: A randomized controlled trial. *Altern Ther Health Med* 16(5): 30–38.
44. Hoffman, S.G., Sawyer, A.T., and Fang, A. 2010. The empirical status of the "new wave" of CBT. *Psychiatr Clin N Am* 33(3): 701–710.
45. Kahl, K. 2012. The third wave of cognitive behavioural therapies: What is new and what is effective? *Curr Opin Psychiatry* 25(6): 522–528.
46. Mueller, T.I., Leon, A.C., Keller, M.B. et al. 1999. Recurrence after recovery from major depressive disorder during 15 years of observational follow-up. *Am J Psychiatry* 156(7): 1000–1006.
47. Judd, L.L 1997. The clinical course of unipolar major depressive disorders. *Arch Gen Psychiatry* 54(11): 989–991.
48. Bauer, M., Whybrow, P.C., Angst, J., Versiani, M., and Möller, H.J. 2002. World Federation of Societies of Biological Psychiatry guidelines for biological treatment of unipolar depressive disorders, Part 1: Acute and continuation treatment of major depressive disorder. *World J Biol Psychiatry* 3(1): 5–43.
49. Vos, T., Haby, M.M., Barendregt, J.J. et al. 2004. The burden of major depression avoidable by longer-term treatment strategies. *Arch Gen Psychiatry* 61(11): 1097–1103.
50. Lau, M. 2004. Teasdale's differential activation hypothesis: Implications for mechanisms of depressive relapse and suicidal behaviour. *Behav Res Ther* 42(9): 1001–1017.
51. Segal, Z.V., Williams, J.M., Teasdale, J.D., and Gemar, M. 1996. A cognitive science perspective on kindling and episode sensitization in recurrent affective disorder. *Psychological Medicine* 26: 371–380.
52. Teasdale, J.D., Segal, Z., and Williams, J.M. 1995. How does cognitive therapy prevent depressive relapse and why should attentional control (mindfulness) training help? *Behavior Research and Therapy* 33: 25–39.
53. Segal, Z.V., Kennedy, S., Gemar, M. et al. 2006. Cognitive reactivity to sad mood provocation and the prediction of depressive relapse. *Arch Gen Psychiatry* 63: 749–755.
54. Nolen-Hoeksema, S. 1991. Responses to depression and their effects on the duration of depressive episodes. *J Abnorm Psychol* 100(4): 569–582.
55. Aldao, A., Nolen-Hoeksema, S., and Schweizer, S. 2010. Emotion-regulation strategies across psychopathology: A meta-analytic review. *Clin Psychol Rev* 30(2): 217–237.
56. Segal, Z.V., Williams, J.M.G., and Teasdale, J.D. 2013. *Mindfulness-Based Cognitive Therapy*, 2nd ed. New York, NY: Guilford Press.
57. Foley, E., Baillie, A., Huxter, M. et al. 2010. Mindfulness-based cognitive therapy for individuals whose lives have been affected by cancer: A randomized controlled trial. *J Consult Clin Psychol* 78: 72–79.
58. Oken, B.S., Fonareva, I., Haas, M. et al. 2010. Pilot controlled trial of mindfulness meditation and education for Dementia Caregivers. *J Altern Complement Med* 16(10): 1031–1038.
59. Kuyken, W., Byford, S., Taylor, R.S. et al. 2008. Mindfulness-based cognitive therapy to prevent relapse in recurrent depression. *J Consult Clin Psychol* 76: 966–978.
60. Segal, Z.V., Bieling, P., and Young, T. 2010. Antidepressant monotherapy vs sequential pharmacotherapy and mindfulness-based cognitive therapy, or placebo, for relapse prophylaxis in recurrent depression. *Arch Gen Psychiatry* 67(12): 1256–1264.
61. Geschwind, N., Peeters, F., Drukker, M. et al. 2011. Mindfulness training increases momentary positive emotions and reward experience in adults vulnerable to depression: A randomized controlled trial. *J Consult Clin Psychol* 79(5): 618–628.
62. Chiesa, A., Mandelli, L., and Serretti, A. 2012. Mindfulness-based cognitive therapy versus psychoeducation for patients with major depression who did not achieve remission following antidepressant treatment: A preliminary analysis. *J Altern Complement Med* 18(8): 756–760.

63. Piet, J. and Hougaard, E. 2011. The effect of mindfulness-based cognitive therapy for prevention of relapse in recurrent major depressive disorder: A systematic review and meta-analysis. *Clin Psychol Rev* 31(6): 1032–1040.
64. Fjorback, L.O., Arendt, M., Ørnbøl, E. et al. 2011. Mindfulness-based stress reduction and mindfulness-based cognitive therapy—A systematic review of randomized controlled trials. *Acta Psychiatr Scand* 124: 102–119.
65. Jain, F.A., Walsh, R.N., Eisendrath, S.J. et al. 2015. Critical analysis of the efficacy of meditation therapies for Acute and Subacute Phase treatment of depressive disorders: A systematic review. *Psychosomatics* 56(2): 140–152.
66. Linehan, M. 1993. *Cognitive-Behavioral Treatment of Borderline Personality Disorder.* New York, NY: Guilford Press.
67. Lynch, T.R., Morse, J.Q., Mendelson, T. et al. 2003. Dialectical behavior therapy for depressed older adults: A randomized pilot study. *Am J Geriatr Psychiatry* 11(1): 33–45.
68. Harley, R., Sprich, S., Safren, S. et al. 2008. Adaptation of dialectical behavior therapy skills training group for treatment-resistant depression. *J Nerv Ment Dis* 196(2): 136–143.
69. Hayes, S.C., Strosahl, K., and Wilson, K.G. 1999. *Acceptance and Commitment Therapy: An Experiential Approach to Behavior Change.* New York, NY: Guilford Press.
70. Barnes-Holmes, Y., Hayes, S.C., Barnes-Holmes, D., and Roche, B. 2001. Relational frame theory: A post-Skinnerian account of human language and cognition. *Adv Child Dev Behav* 28: 101–138.
71. Hayes, S.C., Luoma, J.B., Bond, F.W., Masuda, A., and Lillis, J. 2006. Acceptance and commitment therapy: Model, processes, and outcomes. *Behav Res Ther* 44(1): 1–25.
72. Ost, L.G. 2014. The efficacy of acceptance and commitment therapy: An updated systematic review and meta-analysis. *Behav Res Ther* 61: 105–121.
73. Powers, M.B., Zum Vorde Sive Vording, M.B., and Emmelkamp, P.M. 2009. Acceptance and commitment therapy: A meta-analytic review. *Psychother Psychosom* 78(2): 73–80.
74. Forman, E.M., Herbert, J.D., Moitra, E. et al. 2007. A randomized controlled effectiveness trial of acceptance and commitment therapy and cognitive therapy for anxiety and depression. *Behav Modif* 31(6): 772–799.
75. Salzberg, S. 1995. *Lovingkindness: The Revolutionary Art of Happiness.* Boston, MA: Shambhala.
76. Shapiro, S.L., Warren Brown, K., and Biegel, G.M. 2007. Teaching self-care to caregivers: Effects of mindfulness-based stress reduction on the mental health of therapists in training. *Training and Education in Professional Psychology* 1: 105–115.
77. Shahar, B., Szsepsenwol, O., and Zilcha-Mano, S. 2015. A wait-list randomized controlled trial of loving-kindness meditation programme for self-criticism. *Clin Psychol Psychother* 22(4): 346–356.
78. Fredrickson, B.L., Cohn, M.A., Coffey, K.A. et al. 2008. Open hearts build lives: Positive emotions, induced through loving-kindness meditation, build consequential personal resources. *J Personality Soc Psychol* 95(5): 1045–1062.
79. Goyal, M., Singh, S., Sibinga, E.M.S. et al. 2014. *Meditation Programs for Psychological Stress and Well-Being.* Rockville, MD: Agency for Healthcare Research and Quality.
80. Kabat-Zinn, J., Lipworth, L., and Burney, R. 1985. The clinical use of mindfulness meditation for the self-regulation of chronic pain. *J Behav Med* 8: 163–190.
81. Mccown, D., Reibel, D., and Micozzi, M.S. 2010. *Teaching Mindfulness. A Practical Guide for Clinicians and Educators.* New York, NY: Springer.
82. Kabat-Zinn, J. 2003. Mindfulness-based interventions in context: Past, present, and future. *Clin Psychol Sci Pract* 10: 144–156.
83. Pradhan, E.K., Baumgarten, M., Langenberg, P. et al. 2007. Effect of mindfulness-based stress reduction in rheumatoid arthritis patients. *Arthr Rheumatol* 57: 1134–1142.
84. Carmody, J. and Baer, R.A. 2008. Relationships between mindfulness practice and levels of mindfulness, medical and psychological symptoms and well-being in a mindfulness-based stress reduction program. *J Behav Med* 31(1): 23–33.
85. Trungpa, C. 2002. *Cutting through Spiritual Materialism.* Boston: Shambhala Publications, p. 7.

26 Narrative Therapy

Antolin C. Trinidad, MD, PhD

CONTENTS

INTRODUCTION

To trace the logical relationship of biological processes in depression to its other "half," the act of experiencing its symptoms, the narrative or the story of the one who suffers becomes very important. The biological antecedents of the experience of major depression has been mapped as a disorder of the immune system—such a disorder, with its interlocking physiological mechanisms putatively gone awry, happens invisibly within the organism. In fact, a big part of the stigma attached to mental illnesses stems from its invisibility. On the surface, the sufferer looks "normal," physically unchanged, and showing no outward signs of anatomical abnormality. Instead, the experience of the process comes in the form of its subjective effects, that which are called *vegetative signs*: lethargy, sleep disturbances, and a general malaise slowing down that person's day-to-day activities. That person happens to be human—as such, there is a wider context in which these vegetative experiences are ensconced and the human language functions to give shape to such experiences.

There are effects of these vegetative signs in the ability to perform the sufferer's daily routines. He may become irritable because of the lack of restful sleep—over time, the irritability may negatively affect his family relationships and when that happens, wider ripples emerge in the immediate social fabric of that person. There is now a developing, complex story, a story that branches evermore as time goes by; in fact, the narrative often attains twisting plots and conflicts that often read like a tragedy. One day, an ordinary man lives his life and before he knows it, he develops an alien disorder, an unraveling of his own body processes that leads to drastic consequences. Narrative, the story that accompanies this unravelling, thus inevitably becomes the doppelganger of major depression as a disorder whose early roots may be traceable in biology such as an increase in inflammatory measures. If the biological antecedents may be amenable to therapeutic interventions, can the narrative be equally influenced so that relief from the symptoms, if not an actual recovery, may be possible?

NARRATIVE THERAPY

The fact is that narrative has always been a part of medicine in general, and psychiatry in particular. The standard initial visit of any patient always begins with the "history of the present illness," a narrative reconstruction of the story of the clinical problem as articulated by the patient and subsequently transformed to text by the clinician. Narrative is very much entrenched in the daily practice of medicine. Even in such brief encounters as so-called curbside consults between physicians, the form used is a narrative telling that often begins with something like this: "Hey, let me pick your brain on this difficult case. I have this 33-year-old patient who's as nice as can be, referred to me for headaches, but I've had the most difficult time finding the right treatment." Even the medical record is a coauthored text wherein the doctor or the clinician attains privileged status as someone who shapes the narrative into a form that is proscribed by biomedical conventions—as it were, the clinician acts as the first or the dominant author. In depression, the medical process eventually seeks to place the narrative as a category in the latest edition of the *Diagnostic and Statistical Manual of Mental Disorders*. Without going into the ethics and politics of such diagnostic categories, the medical encounter is an encounter characterized by narrative stilting in that not only do diagnostic categories become the inevitable result, but also the stilting of the individual's own self-description ("I'm a schizophrenic" or "I'm a drug addict"). In other words, biomedical narratives powerfully influence subjectivities. These influences can be enduring and may contribute to the perpetuation of symptoms. Conventional psychotherapy are forms of therapeutic interventions that are meant to restore a more meaningful sense of one's experiences by reviewing the past as sources of insight and strength rather than a source of fatalistic conclusions.

The deployment of narrative as a way of healing is of course not new. Arguably, every form of psychotherapy is narrative therapy—they all require at least two individuals who engage in a series of dialogues, often involving the extensive discussion of life events and the interpretation of these events, a process whose ideal outcome is the improvement of the symptoms of the identified patient in that pairing. In many traditional forms of psychotherapy, a set of theories mediates the dialogue. Rules are set as to how the individuals are to comport themselves in the relationship, and specific agenda are set during sessions, such as cognitive-behavioral therapy (CBT). There are specific theories hypothesized as to the operative mechanisms responsible for change, for example, the hypothesis of a corrective emotional experience in certain forms of psychodynamic therapy, and the changing of dysfunctional, depression-inducing cognitions or automatic thoughts in CBT. Such theories or hypotheses distinguish one form of psychotherapy from another, but in the broadest sense, these therapies all depend on storytelling to understand the problem and to intervene.

THE NARRATIVE TURN IN MEDICINE AND MENTAL HEALTH

A distinction must be made between narrative and narrative therapy. The construction of narratives— accounts of what happens in time, accounts that are made either by oral or written means—is one way by which persons make sense of their experiences and attach meanings to these experiences. Common to most narratives is the temporal dimension. Often, there is an identifiable beginning, middle, and end in the narrative itself. The events recounted themselves happen through time. In the storytelling process, the exact sequencing of these events is chosen by the narrator. These choices make all the difference. Notice for example the change in meaning in the following two ways by which events are sequenced differently:

- A: We fetched mother, and then we held the celebration.
  B: We held the celebration, then we fetched mother.
- A: I was fine, going about my own business when my dog died. He was run over by a truck. My front door was open one morning and he bolted out. I have been blaming myself for it. I feel depressed because I never do anything right, including taking care of the creature that loves me.
  B: I do nothing right. Let me give you an example. I left my front door open one day and my dog ran out. He died. Things got worse when he died. That was when it dawned on me that I can't even take care of the one creature that loves me.

Thus subtle variations in meanings happen with even the slightest changes in temporal sequencing. More variation happens in meaning with additional variations in the choice of words, action sequencing, syntax, and such factors (in oral discourse) as pauses, omissions, and accompanying gestures and facial expressions. It is therefore in the analysis of narratives that one can see the full richness and complexity of human communication.

Many narratives also have dynamics of tension and conflict woven in with the storytelling, elements of what is called a plot. This is illustrated in the following example of a first-person narrative:

> At first I was not aware of what was happening to me. I thought I was just tired, working 60-hour weeks for months on end. Of course I was losing weight and I did not have much of an appetite. I was not concentrating. I had a new boss and I was not getting along with her. However, one day she mentioned that I needed to get help and that I was losing clients because of the way I looked—haggard, thin, five o'clock shadow every day, distracted. I saw my doctor who said I had a hard growth in my tummy. I could not believe it! All I could think about, as I was leaving his office to go to the hospital, paper in my hand to get a scan, was how long I have left to live. I just wish I have enough time left to get to my daughter's college graduation.

The inherent tension here lies on the unknown nature of the condition—one day life seems normal and the next day it is not. Because cancer has been a modern, predictable source of heightened tension in medical encounters, its possibility looms in this vignette providing the source of foreboding and conflict; one conflict is the sudden and acute perception that life is short and limited (existential anxiety). The action of subject or person versus tumor is being played out in the body of this embattled narrator, as if the story unfolds dramatically with his anatomy as the stage on which the action happens.

It is also in narratives that the effects of medical discourse on patient's perception of their own selves become palpable and noticeable. This phenomenon can be seen in the often shocking ways by which patients react to the experience of reading their own medical records. In mentally ill patients, clinicians are often asked whether release of medical records to patients may cause them harm. It is easy to imagine how being described by their doctors or therapists as having borderline personality disorder or having narcissistic traits can affect patient's own self-perception because now, everything will be made to pass through the prism of the medical or psychiatric discourse. Because the narrative as composed by doctors and therapists, often held in authoritative positions, radically differs from patients' own narratives, the discrepancy can yield negative results and reactions. Note for example the following medical record narrative written by a doctor that relates to the previous vignette:

> Fifty year-old Caucasian male with known family history of malignancy, comes in urgently because of dull abdominal pain lasting three months, associated with mood changes (depression and irritability). His vital signs are normal; he appears mildly cachectic. On examination, there is a hard mass in the lower quadrants whose boundaries are not distinct. The plan is to obtain a contrast CT scan of the abdomen to rule out a pancreatic or other malignancy.

The medical way of recounting the cascade of events leading to a diagnostic impression, a "label," is in full display with no attention paid to the affect valence or the effects on the lived life. Greenhalgh and Hurwitz,[1] in expounding on the importance of narrative in the experience of illness and healing, write the following:

> The narrative provides meaning, context and perspective for the patient's predicament. It defines, how, why and in what way he or she is ill. The study of narrative offers a possibility of developing an understanding that cannot be arrived at by any other means. Doctors and therapists frequently see their roles in terms of facilitating 'alternative stories that make sense from the patient's point of view.'

Medical events are significant points or milestones in the life of any individual. The philosopher Paul Ricouer[2] placed significant life events as central to the perception of time—these life events are how we experience the idea of "now." How these life events relate to each other is a function of narrative. It is through narrative that one can see the relationship of these events and through this narrative that the individual can be perceived as moving through time. Ricouer also plants the idea of personal identity firmly with narrative. It is through narrative—like characters in a story—that individuals get a firm sense of who they are especially in relation to time and in relation to other people.[3] Medical events, such as serious illnesses, are events that happen, often abruptly, and must be accommodated into the individual narrative. Because many illnesses are chronic, the identity of that subject is incontrovertibly changed; the narrative now includes a narrative of illness and illness identity.

There are two parallel narratives, therefore, when it comes to illnesses: the individual narrative, and the medical narrative. Of late, the subject of the medical narrative has been the focus of much attention. Critics of medical narratives point out that first of all, the medical point of view has become the privileged point of view when it comes to illness and disease. Modern medical narratives do not provide a space for such existential values as hurt, despair, and grief frequently accompanying illnesses.[4] There is also a potentially adverse effect of such divided, often nonintersecting narratives. One example of this was earlier discussed in a patient's shocked response to reading his or her own medical records. Other ones include the difficulties in the establishment of rapport, imperfect adherences to treatment recommendations, and the specter of malpractice lawsuits, all stemming from communication discontinuities. The crucial role of the doctor in navigating and negotiating with the patient on the future of the interventions on the illness depends on narrative engagement of the doctor. One of the tangible ways by which patient subjectivity affects medical outcome as mediated by poor doctor-patient communication is adherence to medical recommendations. Meta-analysis of physician communication factors to patient adherence shows a strongly positive relationship between the quality of communication and the degree to which patients adhere to treatments.[5] The relationship of doctor-patient communication to narrative is mediated by listening, specifically a type of listening not fettered by the (un)intentional interjection of the medical prerogative or the doctor's presuppositions. Narrative requires a dialogue where the other party is able to receive the narrative through an act of active listening. This is illustrated in the following vignette regarding the re-introduction of medications to a patient who has previously refused such medications for depression:

> **Doctor**: I strongly feel that we should start you on an antidepressant. I know that you have misgivings about this, but it sounds like nothing has helped and you remain significantly depressed. You can't work and your job is in jeopardy.
>
> **Patient**: Okay, I understand, but I told you I am very much afraid of side effects.
>
> **D**: And I told you that we have to weigh the risks and benefits. We can't have you losing your job because you have no energy in the mornings because of your depression.
>
> **P**: I see … let me tell you though. I am starting to feel that my job is defining me—even in this matter. I resent that. I make a good living as a lawyer and I enjoy many benefits from it, but I am a complex person—I have many other facets to me that I would like people to acknowledge. I'm a kind, loving father and I'm one heck of a handball player. In fact, the positive thing about this depression is the fact that I've been off my job and I've had time to think about who I am as a person. You know how your job can swallow you? I think that has happened to me.

The presumption of the doctor in this vignette appears in the notion that the problems with the patient's job performance is a downstream effect of a disease process, whereas the patient saw the time off from his job as a serendipitous opportunity at self-reflection. Indeed, depressive episodes and their attendant effects on behavior have been seen by some scholars as an evolutionary prerogative; it allows the organism to recoup energy and avoid overexertion as a self-protective strategy.[6] For this patient, in some ways, the depressive episode has not been entirely bad when gleaned from the foregoing patient's narrative, a narrative that begs to be given space, time, and careful listening, indeed a proper understanding.

Rita Charon, in her argument to establish the discipline of "Narrative Medicine," points out that narrative analysis has always been important as a source of new knowledge in disciplines that speak to medicine such as anthropology and bioethic.[7] If only mired in scientific knowledge, physicians will be shortchanging their patients, according to Charon:

> Sick people need physicians who can understand their diseases, treat their medical problems, and accompany them through their illnesses. Despite medicine's recent dazzling technological progress in diagnosing and treating illnesses, physicians sometimes lack the capacities to recognize the plights of their patients, to extend empathy toward those who suffer, and to join honestly and courageously with patients in their illnesses. A scientifically competent medicine alone cannot help a patient grapple with the loss of health or find meaning in suffering. Along with scientific ability, physicians need the ability to listen to the narratives of the patient, grasp and honor their meanings, and be moved to act on the patient's behalf. This is narrative competence, that is, the competence that human beings use to absorb, interpret, and respond to stories. ... narrative competence ... enables the physician to practice medicine with empathy, reflection, professionalism, and trustworthiness. Such a medicine can be called narrative medicine.

Narrative competence, as Charon defines it in another article, subsumes critical, nonjudgmental close attention, representation (as in speaking and writing of the encounter), and affiliation, when the physician strives for an authentic connection with the patient.[8] The effects of "honoring" the meanings patients attach to their illnesses and their experiences go beyond the acts of doling out empathy and exhibiting professionalism. They also influence the delivery of care and medical economics. For instance, a big percentage of elderly patients still die in hospitals, and the use of intensive care units continue to occur at high rates toward the end of life.[9]

Patients, and their families, in this situation are then faced with the decision to forego life-prolonging measures or to continue them. This kind of decision, as difficult as it is, not only requires time but also a thoughtful inventory of one's values. It also requires the opportunity to review one's life, accomplishments, and relationships. The narrative journey thus requires much sensitivity and engagement from health-care professionals attending the care of the patient. Individual planning for end-of-life care is an area where personal choice often abuts the availability of sophisticated, life-prolonging technology. Individuals learn, in their own ways, the meaning in the intersecting experiences of suffering and persevering, and they will eventually make their own judgment whether to continue, or not, with obtaining all the evermore sophisticated treatments available to prolong their lives. Health-care providers often are at the bedside and must be ready and must be narratively competent to help in this process. It is hoped that the eventual effects of narrative presence and competence would include a decrease in the cost of health care at the end of life.

DEPRESSION AND NARRATIVE THERAPY

It is not an exaggeration to state that mental illness has been very much "medicalized" insofar as its understanding has been tendentiously dominated by discourse around biomedical models. There have been advantages to this tendency, but there have also been disadvantages, one of which is the tendency for the diagnosis to substitute as an identity for the person. Saying "I'm a schizophrenic," or "I'm ADHD" are commonplace identifiers patients often use in social discourse. The mental illness diagnostic label has morphed into a substitute identity signifier, the effects of which go beyond the labeling. Often, the patient would transduce future experiences through the prism of the diagnostic label(s). Normal life is full of peaks and troughs, but to someone who has been diagnosed with bipolar disorder, those variations can be often conflated as "mood swings," a phrase that has come to be very intimately associated with manic-depressive illness. Other terms have stood in for manic-depressive conceptual stereotyping. Every shopping trip runs the risk of being categorized as a shopping spree, every moment of enjoyment can be confused for "being on top of the world" or an excessively expansive mood possibly indicative of a relapse—life has become a series of increasingly frequent occurrences of symptoms. The patient has *embodied* the diagnosis. Such an embodiment of a diagnostic categorical label in turn runs the risk of prolonging the condition itself because of the further lowering of self-esteem and the decrease in the ability of the patient to enjoy life as it comes, not to mention unnecessary hospitalizations if these descriptors are taken at surface value. The solution to this dynamic does not come as easily as saying "snap out of it" or just forgetting the labels. Often, the label has been seamlessly assimilated by the patient. Scholars of disability are now recognizing the complex interplay of societal forces and mental illness. Disability scholars contend that since the body is both a corporeal and a social construct, identity is also a product of the experience of embodiment.[10] Mental illness may have biological antecedents, but individuals make sense of the experience in unique ways including the adoption of behaviors which may be "non-normative." Societal forces tend to sequester, confine, or exclude these phenomena. The unique experiences of people with mental illnesses as they make sense of their own interior lives thus become even more categorized as signifiers of pathology.

In the 1980s, two family therapists, Michael White and David Epston, formulated a new approach to the treatment of psychological problems presenting in psychotherapy. They called their approach "narrative therapy," whose guiding idea is that psychiatric diagnoses are part of totalizing techniques.[11] The latter phrase came from the philosophy of Michel Foucault who studied the construct of madness and society's effort throughout history to contain and put it under surveillance and later on, its medicalization. The relationship of Foucaldian philosophy to narrative therapy is intimate. For Foucault, power relations and the possession of so-called classificatory knowledge are intertwined—those who classify behaviors (i.e., mental health professionals) are in a powerful position versus those who suffer from madness and who have little to no power. Intrinsic to the maintenance of the power relation are the labels put on categories of madness. In a broader sense, White and Epson's narrative therapy is decidedly poststructuralist in its orientation. It rejects notions of inherent structures (such as the unconscious) in human psychology that breed problematic situations with predictable patterns leading to enduring disease categories. In poststructuralist thought, the concept of the universal is viewed with skepticism. Thus, narratives that purport to provide a one-size-fits-all explanation for problematic situations are narratives that need scrutiny and deconstruction.

In terms of self-narratives, White and Epson suggest that they can be subject to the same intrinsic problems. They are often ingrained and much influenced by dominant and dominating narratives dictated by culture and circumstances. Individuals, thus, do not necessarily author the narratives they have of themselves. They imbibe what is expected, what is customary, or what they imagine the expectations are, culled from their day-to-day realities, often giving in or surrendering their agency to the larger narrative. Again, taking from Foucault, White and Epston suggest that individuals eventually become complicit to their own subjugation by their acceptance of these self-narratives that have not been scrutinized. They give in to the "normalizing" forces that are present in society. As an example, it is no longer normal to be shy and introverted—the onus is on the individual to obtain an evaluation for social phobia and to consider whether drugs can be prescribed for that individual to have a more "normal" social interaction habits. It has been pointed out, as an aside, that the distinction is difficult to make empirically, and that the benefits of drugs is not established.[12] The mental health professionals who define the criteria for social phobia hold the power insofar as they judge whether the condition is normal or abnormal—following Foucault's idea, the one who holds the "knowledge" also holds the power. White and Epston write that the narrative therapists are "consultants" in the effort to re-author the narratives of the lives of "clients." Problems must be externalized and must be viewed as separate from these clients. Efforts are exerted to pinpoint a time in the clients' lives when they were not saddled with these problems and to re-tell the story wherein the client is seen as someone more powerful than the problem. White invites a literary way of reconstructing a narrative that is thick and emplotted. The story extends into a future when the problems are not as big or as overwhelming. It is not only a retelling but a rewriting, inviting significant others to participate and to listen to the new, co-authored story. It is different from psychotherapy in that no assumptions are made about pathological innate structures that are in need of correcting. Rather, what needs correcting is an oppressive story that begs for a rewrite.

CRITIQUE AND OUTCOME STUDIES OF NARRATIVE THERAPY

There are critiques of narrative therapy. One criticism focuses on its embrace of postmodernism as itself a point of view that, while privileging social construction, is suspicious of any metanarrative or a narrative that seeks to explain everything. But even that is tautological. The rejection of meta-narrative, the embrace of postmodernism, is itself a position. Bertrando articulates this problem well[13]:

It is clear, then, that one cannot posit a postmodernism that is in some way positional, that is, in a dialectical relationship to a modernism that cannot be surpassed (it is suggested by the construction of the term, which just adds modernism to the prefix 'post-'). The postmodern narrative therapist enters a similar paradox if he must "see" all narratives as equally valid (Therefore all equally true—or untrue, which would be the same). Not accepting any theory is itself theoretical (or meta-theoretical) position; postmodern therapists thus become self-contradictory, linked to a firm and unmistakable theoretical presupposition: being obliged to disregard any theory. But, for example, what would the majority of postmodern narrative therapists say if someone were to claim that gender, or violence, or abuse problems are "just stories as any other stories', and therefore subject to the very relativism to which the systemic view is subjected?

Bertrando also identifies a potential problem wherein therapists will find it difficult to relate to other professions, such as psychiatry, that use more systematic ways of organizing their knowledge base. Whatever new narrative is produced at the end of narrative therapy is yet again another narrative or discourse, while protesting the idea of grand narratives.[14] Fish points out that only certain works of Foucault and Jacques Derrida informed narrative therapy theory, and that these philosophers' other works (that have been excluded from the discussion) also add to the understanding of social context and power—Fish argues that there is a lopsided consideration of the genealogy of the ideas espoused by narrative therapy, and that there may be inherent political overtones to the idea of therapy itself.[15] But such granular philosophical parsing should not detract from the practical utility of reconsidering patient narratives' centrality to the maintenance, if not the etiology, of their depressive states. The improvement in depression underscores the idea that indeed, the construction of narratives can/will affect mood.

Just like any system of talk therapy, narrative therapy presents difficulties when it comes to empirical, parametric testing of its efficacy. There is predominance of narrative and case-report data in the literature. However, there are two notable reports of prospective studies that suggest efficacy of narrative therapy for depression. An uncontrolled study reports improvement (74%) in depressive symptoms in 47 adults who underwent manualized narrative therapy.[16] A head-to-head comparison between narrative therapy and CBT has also been done.[17] Sixty-three patients were assigned to either NT or CBT. Using the Beck Depression Inventory-II (BDI-II) and Outcome Questionnaire 45.2 (OQ 45.2), both groups showed improvement, but group differences favored CBT using BDI-II but not OQ 45.2. Such comparative results with CBT likely underscores similarities between NT and CBT in that both systems of therapy scrutinize existing negativistic concepts of the self and encourage new and less onerous interpretations not only of events but also the patient's idiosyncratic narrative composition of these events.

CONCLUSION

Narrative has recently become more central to medicine in general and has provided a welcome dialectic to the dominance of biomedical models in the understanding and treatment of medical conditions. Patient narrative has been centralized in this process. In depression, there has been a tendentious dominance of biomedical paradigms, including a discourse revolving around diagnostic categories that can seep into patient's understanding of who they are. They can also often embody these diagnostic categories, using them as the preferred way of understanding the meaning of their experiences. Narrative therapy provides an alternative. It seeks to empower the patient to recreate a different, "re-authored" narrative of their lives that are not only richer and fuller but also more meaningful and nuanced. In the end, what is potentially the most useful feature of narrative therapy is its insistence on a panoramic view of problems that are externalized outside of the person rather than letting diagnostic categories dominate stories patient or clients have constructed of themselves and their trajectories in their lives. Clinical depression is a condition that invites negativistic interpretations and outlooks. Viewed in this way, narrative therapy is one variation in therapeutic endeavors to offer alternatives to the purely medical approach including the use of pharmaceuticals.

REFERENCES

1. Greenhalgh, T. and Hurwitz, B. 1999. Why study narrative? *Br Med J* 318: 48–50.
2. Ricouer, P. 1990. *Time and Narrative (Book 1)*. Chicago, IL: University of Chicago Press.
3. Rasmussen, D. 1995. Rethinking subjectivity: Narrative identity and the self. *Phil Soc Crit* 21(5–6): 159–172.
4. Roberts, G.A. 2000. Narrative and severe mental illness: What place do stories have in an evidence-based world? *Br J Psychiatry Adv* 21(1): 432–441.
5. Haskard-Zolnierek, K.B. and DiMatteo, M.R. 2009. Physician communication and patient adherence to treatment: A meta-analysis. *Med Care* 47(8): 826–834.
6. Nesse, R.M. 2000. Is depression an adaptation? *Arch Gen Psychiatry* 57(1): 14–20.
7. Charon, R. 2001. Narrative medicine: A model for empathy, reflection, profession, and trust. *JAMA* 286(15): 1897–1902.
8. Charon, R. 2007. What to do with stories: The sciences of narrative medicine. *Can Fam Physician* 53(8): 1265–1267.
9. Teno, J.M., Gozalo, P.L., Bynum, J.W. et al. 2013. Change in end-of-life care for medicare beneficiaries: Site of death, place of care, and health care transitions in 2000, 2005, and 2009. *JAMA* 309(5): 470–477.
10. Mulvany, J. 2000. Disability, impairment or illness? The relevance of the social model of disability to the study of mental disorder. *Sociol Health Illness* 22(5): 582–601.
11. White, M. and Epston, D. 1990. *Narrative Means to Therapeutic Ends*. New York, NY: W. W. Norton.
12. Double, D. 2002. The limits of psychiatry. *Br Med J* 324: 900.
13. Bertrando, P. 2002. Text and context: Narrative, postmodernism and cybernetics. *J Fam Ther* 22(1): 83–103.
14. Boston, P. 2000. Systemic family therapy and the influence of post-modernism. *Br J Psychiatric Adv* 21(1): 450–457.
15. Fish, V. 1993. Poststructuralism in family therapy: Interrogating the narrative/conversational mode. *J Marital Fam Ther* 19(3): 221–232.
16. Vromans, L. and Schweitzer, R. 2011. Narrative therapy for adults with major depressive disorder: Improved symptom and interpersonal outcomes. *Psychother Res* 21(1): 4–15.
17. Lopes, R., Gonçalves, M., Machado, P. et al. 2012. Narrative therapy vs. cognitive-behavioral therapy for moderate depression: Empirical evidence from a controlled clinical trial. *Psychother Res*, 24(6), 662–674.

27 Integrative Psychotherapy
Healing the MindBodyMatrix

Martha Stark, MD

CONTENTS

INTRODUCTION

The field of psychiatry has struggled with creating a holistic conceptual framework that captures the essence of what is involved in the process of healing, be it of mind or of body. To that end, the term "MindBodyMatrix" speaks to the complex interdependence of mind and body; it also reflects a keen appreciation for the intimate and precise relationship between the health and vitality of the mind and that of the body. Throughout this chapter, the terms *system, living system, living matrix*, and *MindBodyMatrix* will be used interchangeably.

Stressful stuff happens. But it will be how well we are ultimately able to manage its impact—psychologically, physiologically, and energetically—that will make all the difference. In other words, it will be how well we are ultimately able to cope with the impact of stress in our lives that will either disrupt our growth by compromising our functionality or trigger our growth by forcing us to evolve to a higher level of functionality and adaptive capacity.

The focus here will be on formulating a conceptual framework that captures the essence of what *must* happen if a patient is ever to evolve from less than optimal health to more optimal health. Simply put, for the patient to get better there must be *input from the outside* and the patient must have the capacity *to process, integrate, and adapt to that input*.

More specifically, however, it will actually be *stressful input from the outside* and the patient's *capacity to process, integrate, and adapt to the impact of this stressful input* that will provoke the patient's recovery. In other words, it will be not so much gratification but rather frustration against a backdrop of gratification—to which psychotherapists refer as *optimal frustration*[1]—that will provide the therapeutic leverage needed to provoke, after initial destabilization, the patient's eventual restabilization at a higher level of functionality and adaptive capacity.

This conceptual framework conceives of the healing process—*with respect to both mind and body*—as one that requires the holistic practitioner to be exquisitely attuned to the system's capacity to cope with stress, which in turn will be a story about the system's ability to process and integrate the impact of threatened disruption, which in turn will be a reflection of the underlying orderedness of the MindBodyMatrix and the resultant ease with which information and energy can be transmitted throughout its expanse—lack of order and disrupted ease of flow manifesting as *psychiatric/medical dis-order* and *psychiatric/medical dis-ease*.

But whether the primary involvement is of mind or body, dis-order (that is, disrupted orderedness within the MindBodyMatrix) and dis-ease (that is, disrupted ease of flow within the MindBodyMatrix) are implicated in the generation of chronic health problems.

SELF-ORGANIZING SYSTEMS RESIST CHANGE

In the language of complexity theory, the MindBodyMatrix is a complex adaptive, self-organizing chaotic system.[2,3] The living matrix is *complex* (which speaks to the intricate interdependence of the system's constituent components); *adaptive* (which speaks to the system's capacity to benefit from experience); *self-organizing* (which speaks to the spontaneous emergence of system-wide patterns arising from the interplay of the system's components); and *chaotic* (which speaks to the system's underlying orderedness despite its apparent randomness—an orderedness that will only emerge as the system evolves over time).

How do patients advance from an unhealthy state of *dis-order* (be it psychiatric or medical) to a healthy state of orderedness? Krebs reminds us that we must never lose sight of the fact that self-organizing (chaotic) systems resist perturbation.[4] No matter how compromised they might be, self-organizing systems—fueled as they are by their homeostatic tendency to remain constant over time—are inherently resistant to change; they have an inertia that must be overcome if the system is ever to evolve from impaired capacity to more robust capacity.

The holistic practitioner, in order to expedite advancement of a patient from compromised health to a state of well-being, must *challenge the system* (*whenever possible*) and *support the system* (*whenever necessary*), all with an eye to jump-starting the system's innate ability to self-repair in the face of environmental threat.[5,6] More specifically, in reaction/response to—stressful—therapeutic interventions, the patient will either *react defensively* (when challenged) or *respond adaptively* (when supported) to the impingement, the net result of which will be the therapeutic induction, over time, of healing cycles of defensive collapse and adaptive reconstitution at ever higher levels of resilience, vitality, and integration.

Indeed, the patient's journey from illness to wellness will involve progression through these iterative cycles of disruption and repair as the patient evolves from chaos and dysfunction to coherence and functionality.

This fundamental principle speaks to the almost universal *resistance to change* manifested by psychiatric patients.

Consider a patient who is clinging tenaciously to dysfunctional defenses that had once served her but that have long since outlived their usefulness. As a self-organizing system, the patient must be sufficiently perturbed (that is, impacted) by input from the outside (that is, the therapist's interventions) that there will be impetus (that is, force needed to bring about change) for the patient to relinquish her attachment to these deeply entrenched, maladaptive patterns of acting, reacting, and interacting that have come to define her characteristic (defensive) stance in the world.

In essence, the therapist's interventions must have enough stressful impact that they will challenge the homeostatic balance (that is, the status quo) of the patient's dysfunctional defenses. By the same token, the therapist's interventions must also provide enough support that this input, in combination with the patient's inborn striving toward health (that is, her resilience), will prompt the patient to evolve to ever higher levels of adaptive capacity and wholesome balance. As a result, her dysfunctional actions, reactions, and interactions will become transformed into more functional ways of being and doing.

If the therapist offers only gratification and support, then there will be nothing that needs to be mastered and there will not be much impetus for transformation and growth. But therapeutic input that provides an optimal level of stress (in the form of anxiety-provoking but ultimately health-promoting interventions offering just the right balance of frustration and gratification, just the right combination of challenge and support) will ultimately provoke not only reversal of underlying dysfunction but also optimization of functionality by tapping into the patient's intrinsic striving toward health and inborn ability to self-correct in the face of environmental perturbation.

In truth, support and optimal challenge work in concert. Whereas optimal challenge will trigger recovery and revitalization by prompting the system to adapt, support will facilitate that adaptation by reinforcing the system's underlying resilience and restoring its reserves, thereby *honing the system's ability to cope with—and, even, benefit from—stressful environmental input.*

In sum, challenge is necessary for jumpstarting recovery but it also requires support; by the same token, support is necessary for transformation and growth but it also requires challenge.

THE GOLDILOCKS PRINCIPLE AND OPTIMAL STRESS

The psychiatric patient will respond in any one of three ways to psychotherapeutic interventions that alternately challenge and then support, support and then challenge.

Too much challenge, too much anxiety, too much stress will overwhelm and prompt defense because it will be *too much* to be processed and integrated—in other words, it will be *traumatic stress.*[7]

Too little challenge, too little anxiety, too little stress will offer too little impetus for transformation and growth and will serve, instead, to reinforce the (dysfunctional) status quo.

But just the right amount of challenge, just the right amount of anxiety, just the right amount of stress—to which the father of stress, Hans Selye, referred as *eustress*[8] and to which I refer as *optimal stress*[5,6,9]—will provide just the right amount of therapeutic leverage needed to promote, after initial disruption, reconstitution at a higher level of integration, functionality, and self-regulatory capacity.

The psychotherapist's intent must be to generate an optimal level of anxiety within the patient, anxiety that will then provide the impetus needed to propel the patient, as we shall later see, toward ever higher levels of *awareness* (when the focus is on the patient's internal dynamics), *acceptance* (when the focus is on the patient's affective experience), and *accountability* (when the focus is on the patient's relational dynamics).[10] In essence, the induction of an optimal level of anxiety in the psychiatric patient supports the adage that *no pain, no gain.*

DIFFERENCE BETWEEN A POISON AND A MEDICATION

The noted sixteenth century Swiss physician Paracelsus is credited with having written that the difference between a poison and a medication is the dosage thereof.[11] Equally important is the system's capacity—a function of its underlying resilience—to process, integrate, and ultimately adapt to the impact of that stressor.

Stressful input, therefore, is inherently neither bad (poison) nor good (medication), which is to say that the therapist's interventions are inherently neither toxic (poison) nor therapeutic (medication).

Rather, the dosage of the stressor, the underlying resilience and adaptability of the system (which, as we have seen, is a reflection of its underlying orderedness and fluidity), and the *intimate edge*[12] between stressor and system will determine whether the system, in reaction/response to the environmental stimulus, defends and devolves to ever greater disorganization (dis-order and dis-ease) or adapts and evolves, by way of a series of healing cycles, to ever more complex levels of organization and dynamic balance.

In other words, if the interface between stressor and system is such that the stressor is able to provoke recovery within the system, then what would have been poison becomes medication, what would have constituted toxic input becomes therapeutic input, what would have been deemed traumatic stress becomes optimal stress, and what would have overwhelmed becomes transformative.

Reference is here being made to the therapeutic use of stress to provoke recovery by activating the body's innate ability to heal itself.[13-17] In essence, what doesn't kill you makes you stronger.

THE SANDPILE MODEL AND THE PARADOXICAL IMPACT OF STRESS

Long intriguing to chaos theorists has been the sandpile model, which is believed to offer a dramatic depiction of the cumulative impact, over time, of environmental impingement on open systems.[18] Evolution of the sandpile is governed by some complex mathematical formulas and is well known in many scientific circles; but the sandpile model is rarely applied to living systems and has never been used to demonstrate either the adaptability and resilience of the living system or the paradoxical impact of stress on it.

This simulation model provides an elegant visual metaphor for how we are continuously refashioning ourselves at ever higher levels of complexity and integration—not just in spite of stressful input from the outside but by way of that input.

Amazingly enough, the grains of sand being steadily added to a gradually evolving sandpile are the occasion for both its disruption and its repair. Not only do the grains of sand being added precipitate partial collapse of the sandpile, but also they become the means by which the sandpile will be able to build itself back up—each time at a new level of homeostasis (more specifically, each time at a new allostatic set point).[14] The system will therefore have been able not only to manage the impact of the stressful input but also to benefit from that impact.

And, as the sandpile evolves, an underlying pattern will begin to emerge, characterized by recursive cycles of disruption and repair, destabilization and restabilization, defensive collapse, and adaptive reconstitution at ever higher levels of integration, balance, and harmony.

In essence, the grains of sand represent environmental challenges, the mastery of which will fuel the underlying system's evolution from chaos and dis-order to coherence and orderedness.

TRANSFORMATION OF DEFENSE INTO ADAPTATION

Let us shift now to exploring, more specifically, the process by which stressful psychotherapeutic interventions—specifically designed to create an optimal balance of challenge and support—can facilitate not only reversal of underlying dysfunction (be it in the form of an intractable depression, overwhelming anxiety, unremitting insomnia, knee-jerk irritability, or any other manifestation of unmastered past and present life stressors) but also fine-tuning of functionality.

Well known is Freud's adage[19]: "Where id was, there shall ego be"—relevant for both the child growing up and the patient getting better. Using this premise as a springboard, it will be suggested that both the process of development and the process of getting better ultimately involve "Where defense was, there shall adaptation be."

More specifically, the task of the child and the task of the patient are to evolve from id to ego, that is, from disorganized and chaotic id energy to organized and coherent ego structure; alternatively, it could be said that both of these evolutionary processes involve advancement from *defensive reaction* (when the system is less evolved) to *adaptive response* (once the system has become more evolved).

What this effectively means is that both growing up and getting better are characterized by the transformation of dysfunctional defense (when the impact of an environmental stressor is simply too much to be managed) into more functional adaptation (when the impact of the environmental stressor is able ultimately to be processed and integrated).

Although defenses are less healthy and less evolved and adaptations more healthy and more evolved, both are self-protective mechanisms that speak to the lengths to which a system will go in order to preserve its homeostatic balance in the face of environmental challenge—be that challenge externally or internally derived.

In other words, defense and adaptation are actually flip sides of the same coin; defenses always have an adaptive function, just as adaptations do also serve to defend. As such, defenses and adaptations have a yin-yang relationship, representing, as they do, not opposing but complementary forces. In fact, just as in quantum mechanics, where particles and waves are thought to be different manifestations of a single reality (depending upon the observer's perspective), so, too, defense and adaptation are conjugate pairs demonstrating this same duality (both-and, not either-or).

There is a distinction between, on the one hand, defensive reactions that are mobilized in the immediate aftermath of challenge and are automatic, knee-jerk, stereotypic, and rigid and, on the other hand, adaptive responses that unfold in the aftermath of challenge only over time and are therefore more processed, integrated, flexible, and complex. Defenses are needed to survive, but adaptations enable us to thrive.

As examples of transforming defense into adaptation: If all goes well (whether over the course of growing up or the course of psychotherapy), the need for immediate gratification will become gradually transformed into the capacity to tolerate delay; the need for perfection will become gradually transformed into the capacity to tolerate imperfection; the need for external regulation of the self will become gradually transformed into the capacity for internal self-regulation; and the need to hold on will become gradually transformed into the capacity to let go.

Further examples of transforming defensive reaction into adaptive response include the step-by-step progression from externalizing blame to taking ownership; from cursing the darkness to lighting a candle; from dissociating to becoming more present; from feeling victimized to becoming more empowered; and from being jammed up to channeling energy into the actualization of potential and the pursuit of dreams.

In essence, adaptations involve high-level processing and go hand in hand with a higher level of complexity, whereas defenses involve low-level processing and go hand in hand with a lower level of complexity. A system that *can* will adapt, whereas a system that *can't* will defend. We speak of the *capacity to adapt* but the *need to defend*.

In fact, it could be said that being able to adapt is a story about having the capacity to make a virtue out of necessity (a.k.a. to make a silk purse out of a sow's ear) because it involves managing with finesse—and ultimately to one's benefit—the variety of life stressors to which one will inevitably be exposed over the course of one's life.

THERAPEUTIC INDUCTION OF CYCLES OF DISRUPTION AND REPAIR

As earlier suggested, with respect to the therapeutic process, the catalyst for progressive transformation of less healthy defense into more healthy adaptation will be working through the cumulative impact of optimally stressful therapeutic interventions that afford just the right balance of challenge and support—challenge such that the patient's defenses, no matter how seemingly intractable, will become temporarily destabilized, and support such that the patient, after working through the disruption, will have the opportunity adaptively to restabilize at a higher level of integration, balance, and harmony.

Working through these recursive cycles of disruption and repair will enable the patient ultimately to evolve to a level of functionality, adaptive capacity, and resilience that will render unnecessary the unhealthy defenses to which she had desperately clung in a self-sabotaging attempt to avoid confronting the myriad anxiety-provoking realities in her life—both past and present.

The therapist will be able to facilitate this working-through process by constructing psychotherapeutic interventions strategically designed either to challenge the patient by directing her attention to where she is not (but where the therapist would want the patient to be) or to support the patient by resonating with where she is (and where the patient would seem to need to be).

More specifically, with her finger ever on the pulse of the patient's level of anxiety and capacity to tolerate further challenge, the therapist will therefore alternately challenge (by reminding the patient of what she really does—albeit reluctantly—know) and support (in some situations, by resonating empathically with what the patient finds herself thinking, feeling, or doing in order not to have to know and, in other situations, by resonating empathically with the pain of the patient's grief as she begins to let herself know).

There are several *prototypical psychotherapeutic statements* (including a *conflict statement* and a *disillusionment statement*) that capitalize upon the idea that the *therapeutic use of optimal stress* can indeed expedite the psychotherapeutic endeavor by *precipitating rupture in order to trigger repair.*[9,10,20] These strategically constructed interventions will alternately increase the patient's anxiety (by confronting her with her *knowledge* of some uncomfortable reality) and then decrease the patient's anxiety (by resonating empathically with her *experience* of that uncomfortable reality)—again, all with an eye to generating an optimal level of destabilizing stress and incentivizing anxiety.

Interestingly, the first of these anxiety-provoking but ultimately growth-promoting interventions first names the patient's *adaptive capacity to know an uncomfortable reality* and then resonates empathically with the patient's *defensive need to deny such knowledge.* These conflict statements are specifically designed to call to the patient's attention the conflict that exists within her between, on the one hand, what she really does know and, on the other hand, what she finds herself resorting to in order not to have to know.

The format of these optimally stressful conflict statements is as follows: "You know…, *but* you find yourself thinking, feeling, doing…in order not to have to know." In other words, the patient knows; but, because the anxiety elicited by that knowledge is too much to manage, she finds herself needing to mobilize a (dysfunctional) defense in order not to have to know.

The second of these anxiety-provoking but ultimately growth-promoting interventions also first names the patient's *adaptive capacity to know an uncomfortable reality* but then resonates empathically with the patient's *dawning ability to experience it.* These disillusionment statements are specifically designed to facilitate the patient's grieving by highlighting, on the one hand, the disillusioning reality that the patient is beginning to confront and, on the other hand, the patient's newfound ability to let herself begin to feel the actual pain of her grief about it.

The format of these optimally stressful disillusionment (or grieving) statements is as follows: "You know…, *and* it breaks your heart…" In other words, the patient knows; but, because the anxiety elicited by that knowledge is—for whatever complex mix of reasons—more manageable, she has the adaptive capacity to let herself experience the pain of it.

Whether the therapist utilizes these conflict statements and disillusionment statements or constructs other psychotherapeutic interventions that alternately increase the patient's anxiety (by directing her to where she does not want to be) and then decrease the patient's anxiety (by validating where she is), the underlying principle will be the therapeutic use of stress to provoke recovery.

In whatever ways the therapist alternately challenges and then supports the patient's deeply ingrained defensive patterns, all such interventional efforts—rendered with compassion and without judgment—will reflect a deep appreciation for the patient's ambivalent attachment to these defenses for which she admittedly pays a price but that do also serve her.

In sum, the healing process—to be effective in bringing about deep and lasting change—must involve this *therapeutic induction of healing cycles of disruption and repair* in reaction/response to the therapist's optimally stressful interventions, such that the patient, after initial defensive collapse, will be able subsequently to reconstitute adaptively at ever higher levels of accountability, empowerment, and complex understanding.

PRECIPITATING DISRUPTION IN ORDER TO TRIGGER REPAIR

In essence, the therapeutic intent of the holistic practitioner is to *precipitate disruption in order to trigger repair.* Because, as noted earlier, self-organizing systems resist perturbation, the *provocation of rupture in order to galvanize recovery* must be instigated again and again.

And so it is that the patient's dysfunctional defensive structures must be sufficiently impacted by the therapist's stressful input that their foundation will indeed become weakened. By the same token, however, this unsettling of the foundation will force the patient to tap into underlying resilience in order to restore her homeostatic balance in the face of the optimal challenge—the net result of which will be the eventual emergence of orderedness from chaos as low-level defenses that were dysfunctional become transformed into high-level adaptations that are more functional.

In order to bring about this undermining of the patient's dysfunctional defenses and the subsequent creation of impetus and opportunity for their replacement with more functional self-protective mechanisms, we will repeatedly present the patient with optimally stressful interventions that alternately challenge and then support, support and then challenge. If we want first to increase the patient's anxiety and then to decrease it, we will first challenge and then support. But if we want first to decrease the patient's anxiety and then to increase it, we will first support and then challenge. Either way, our aim is to find that delicate balance between too much anxiety and too little anxiety; it will then be the therapeutic generation within the patient of this incentivizing anxiety that will optimize her potential for transformation and growth.

We will challenge the patient when we sense that we have a window of opportunity to confront the patient about something that we know might make her anxious but that we hope will ultimately provide the impetus for her recovery; we will support the patient when we sense that the patient, made too anxious by our intervention, needs us to back off a bit and, instead, to demonstrate our appreciation for why she is as she is. Again, this dynamic balancing of challenge and support is all being strategically done with an eye to creating within her just the right level of destabilizing tension and stress.

In fact, as we sit with our patients, there is ever tension within us as well—between, on the one hand, our vision of who we think the patient could be (were she but able to make healthier choices) and, on the other hand, our respect for the reality of who she is (and for the choices, no matter how unhealthy, that she is continuously making). And, on some level, we are therefore always struggling to find an optimal balance between challenging the patient with our vision of the choices that we believe she could be making and supporting her through our honoring of the choices that she is making.

So, too, there is ever tension within us between, on the one hand, our investment in helping the patient actualize her inherited potential and realize her dreams and, on the other hand, our sober acceptance of the patient's very real limitations. We are therefore always struggling to find an optimal balance between challenging the patient's dysfunction (in order to spur her on to ever greater heights) and, ever respectfully and nonjudgmentally, supporting the patient's dysfunction (in order to demonstrate our acceptance of the choices she finds herself making).

We must never lose sight of the fact that the patient has come to be as she is and to defend herself in the ways that she does because, at the time of the original privations, deprivations, and injuries, she was simply unable—for whatever complex mix of reasons—to process, integrate, and adapt to their traumatically stressful impact. She was forced instead to cobble together, in order to survive, whatever defenses she possibly could—defenses that then became more firmly entrenched and, over time, crystallized out as her characteristic (defensive) posture in the world.

And so it comes to pass that the patient's dysfunctional defensive structures must be perturbed enough by the therapist's anxiety-provoking interventions that there will be both impetus and opportunity for adaptive reconstitution of these structures at a higher, more functional level.

COMPLEMENTARY MODES OF PSYCHOTHERAPEUTIC ACTION

Psychotherapy affords patients the opportunity for belated mastery of early-on psychological traumas that were simply too overwhelming to be managed at the time they were inflicted. Instead of being processed and gradually organized into healthy psychic structure and adaptive capacity, the unassimilated traumatizing experiences were split off and their chaotic memory traces stored internally, where they then wreaked havoc on the MindBodyMatrix in the form of any number of manifest psychological and physiological symptoms (the aforementioned chronic depression, despair, unremitting anxiety, generalized musculoskeletal pain, adrenal fatigue, brain fog, persistent insomnia, reflexive irritability, and uncontrollable impulsivity, to name but a few).

The therapeutic action of psychodynamic psychotherapy can be conceptualized as having been divided, historically, into roughly three different schools of thought regarding the healing process—schools of thought that are complementary, not conflicting.[10]

As we see, each of the three perspectives focuses on some aspect of the patient's defenses—be it the patient's resistance to acknowledging painful truths about the self (Model 1), the patient's refusal to confront—and grieve—painful truths about her objects (Model 2), or, under the sway of her repetition compulsion, the patient's re-enactment of unmastered childhood dramas on the stage of her life and in the therapy (Model 3). By the same token, each of the three perspectives approaches the healing process somewhat differently—Model 1 is more *cognitive*, Model 2 is more *affective*, and Model 3 is more *relational*.

In any event, the patient's resistances (Model 1), her relentless pursuits (Model 2), and her compulsive and unwitting re-enactments (Model 3) are the dysfunctional defenses to which she clings in order not to have to know, not to have to feel, and not to have to take ownership of what she plays out on the stage of her life. As such, they serve to block out the immediate pain of her grief about all the early on privations, deprivations, and injuries that were simply too overwhelming for her to cope with at the time.

The three schools of psychodynamic thought therefore address different aspects of the therapeutic action; but all three perspectives address transformation of chaotic and less evolved defenses into coherent and more evolved adaptations to the *stress of life*.[21]

Model 1, *enhancement of knowledge within*, is the interpretive perspective of classical psychoanalysis, a drive-defense model that focuses on the patient's unmodulated drives and self-protective defenses, a model that offers the neurotically conflicted patient an opportunity to gain greater self-awareness and insight into her inner workings, so that she can make more informed decisions about her life, become more master of her destiny, and channel her now more modulated energies into actualized potential.

Model 2, *provision of corrective experience for*, is a more contemporary perspective, one that focuses on the patient's psychological deficiencies, these psychic scars the result of early on *absence of good in the form of parental deprivation and neglect*. This deficiency-compensation perspective is one that offers the patient an opportunity in the here-and-now relationship with her therapist both to grieve the early on parental failures and to experience symbolic restitution. As the patient makes her peace with the reality that the people in her world were not, and will never be, all that she would have wanted them to be, she will evolve to a place of greater acceptance and inner peace.

And Model 3, *engagement in relationship with*, is another contemporary perspective, one that focuses on the patient's psychological toxicities, these psychic scars the result of early on *presence of bad in the form of parental trauma and abuse*. The essence of the stance such a patient will come to assume in relation to her therapist is best captured by the late Warren Zevon in a rock song entitled "If You Won't Leave Me I'll Find Someone Who Will."[22] This third model of therapeutic action conceives of the therapy as offering the patient a stage upon which to play out, symbolically, her unresolved childhood dramas but ultimately, as a result of negotiating at the intimate edge of authentic engagement with her therapist, to encounter a different response this time. The outcome will indeed be a better one because the therapist will be able to facilitate resolution by bringing to bear her own, more evolved capacity to process and integrate on behalf of a patient who truly does not know how. As the patient is confronted with the sobering reality of what she has been unconsciously re-enacting in her relationships, she will evolve to a place of greater accountability for her actions, reactions, and interactions.

To summarize, over the course of the treatment, the therapist must remain ever attuned to the dysfunctional defenses that the patient has mobilized as a reaction to life stressors that were simply too much to be processed and integrated at the time. So whether, in the moment, the therapist is focused on the patient's internal dynamics (Model 1), the patient's affective experience (Model 2), or the patient's relational dynamics (Model 3), the therapist will alternately challenge the patient's defensive structures (when possible) and support those structures (when necessary).

These optimally stressful psychotherapeutic interventions, which both challenge and support, will therefore be utilized to provide the impetus for temporary disorganization of the dysfunctional status quo and then compensatory reorganization at a higher level of therapeutic understanding and adaptive capacity. Again and again, these strategically formulated interventions (like the grains of sand in the sandpile model of chaos theory) will prompt destabilization in order to trigger restabilization at ever higher levels of orderedness and complexity.

In essence, the psychotherapeutic process will transform *resistance into awareness* (Model 1), *relentless hope and refusal to grieve into acceptance* (Model 2), and *re-enactment of unresolved childhood dramas into accountability* (Model 3). Growing up (the task of the child) and getting better (the task of the patient) are all about this graduated evolution from defensive dysfunction to ever greater awareness, acceptance, and accountability as the individual incrementally makes her peace with life's harsh realities.

As noted repeatedly throughout this chapter, all three modes of therapeutic action involve transformation of the need to react defensively into the capacity to respond adaptively, and all three evolutionary processes therefore involve the therapeutic induction of healing cycles of defensive collapse and adaptive reconstitution in reaction/response to optimally stressful psychotherapeutic interventions.

But, more specifically, the optimal challenge that will precipitate the disruption and thereby trigger the recovery process will be the result of working through, respectively, the stress of (1) *cognitive dissonance* (Model 1); (2) *affective disillusionment* (Model 2); and (3) *relational detoxification* (Model 3). Perhaps not surprisingly, the stressor in Model 1 will be more cognitive than affective or relational; the stressor in Model 2 will be more affective than cognitive or relational; and the stressor in Model 3 will be more relational than cognitive or affective.[6]

Furthermore, as we see, (1) working through the stress of cognitive dissonance will involve working through the experience of *gain-become-pain* (as a defense once experienced as beneficial becomes increasingly experienced as costly); (2) working through the stress of affective disillusionment will involve working through the experience of *good-become-bad* (as an experience that had once been about positive illusion becomes more about disillusionment); and (3) working through the stress of relational detoxification will involve working through the experience of *bad-become-good* (as an experience that had once been about negative distortion becomes more about reality). All such transformative processes will, of necessity, require that something dysfunctional be relinquished in favor of something more functional; but, even so, the letting go will be experienced as a loss—and must, therefore, be grieved.

In what follows, the focus will be on the therapeutic action in Model 1 (which will result in the transformation of resistance into awareness) and in Model 2 (which will result in the transformation of relentlessness into acceptance).

THE OPTIMAL STRESS OF COGNITIVE DISSONANCE

With respect to creating cognitive dissonance in Model 1, as noted throughout this chapter, the exquisitely attuned therapist—using any of the variety of optimally stressful psychotherapeutic interventions in her armamentarium—will be able to titrate the level of the patient's anxiety. Based on the therapist's moment-by-moment assessment of what the patient can handle, the therapist will therefore either challenge (by way of anxiety-provoking interpretive statements that call into question the dysfunctional defenses to which the patient has long clung in order to preserve her psychological equilibrium) or support (by way of anxiety-assuaging empathic statements that honor these self-protective defenses—a therapeutic stance sometimes referred to as *going with the resistance*).[23,24]

More specifically, the therapist—having donned her Model 1 hat in order to focus, for the moment, on the patient's internal dynamics—will alternately challenge (by highlighting the patient's adaptive capacity to recognize the price she pays for refusing to let go of her dysfunctional defenses) and then support (by resonating empathically with the patient's defensive need to cling to them even so)—all with an eye to creating dissonance within the patient between, on the one hand, her dawning awareness of just how costly her defenses have become and, on the other hand, her newfound understanding of just how invested she has been in holding on to them even so.

The patient is beginning to recognize the price she pays, *but* she finds herself holding on even so and unwilling/unable to let go.

The earlier referenced conflict statements—one of the staples in the Model 1 therapist's armamentarium—are specifically designed to tease out the conflict within the patient between her voice of reality (which is anxiety provoking although ultimately insight promoting and therefore empowering) and the defenses she mobilizes in an effort to silence that voice. As noted earlier, the purpose of Model 1 interventions is to foster the patient's observing (or reflecting) ego so that she can develop a greater awareness of, and appreciation for, the conflict that is being waged within her between her objective knowledge of reality and, fueled as it is by her defensive need not to know, her subjective experience of it.

The following conflict statements first highlight what the patient has the adaptive capacity to acknowledge and then what the patient, made anxious, has the defensive need to protest:

> You know that ultimately you will need to confront, and grieve, the reality that Martin is not emotionally available in the ways that you would have wanted him to be and that until you make your peace with that painful reality you will probably continue to feel angry and depressed; but, in the moment, all you can think about is how desperately frightened and alone you would feel were you to lose him.
>
> You know that if your relationship with Victor is to survive, you will need to take at least some responsibility for the part you're playing in the incredibly abusive fights that you and he have; but you tell yourself it isn't really your fault because if he weren't so provocative, then you wouldn't have to be so vindictive!

Importantly, the therapist's focus must always be on highlighting both what the patient herself is coming to recognize as the price she pays for clinging to her dysfunctional defenses (a *price paid* that fuels the patient's aggressive attachment to her defenses) and what the patient herself is coming to recognize as her investment in maintaining her dysfunctional stance even so (an *investment in* that fuels the patient's libidinal investment in her defenses). Of course it is this ambivalent attachment to the dysfunction—fueled as it is by both aggression and libido—that makes the patient so reluctant to surrender it.

But by locating *within* the patient the conflict between her anxiety-provoking knowledge of an uncomfortable reality and her anxiety-assuaging experience of that reality, the therapist is deftly sidestepping the potential for conflict *between* patient and therapist. In other words, the therapist who is able to resist the temptation to *get bossy* by overzealously advocating for the patient to do the *right thing* will be able masterfully to avoid getting deadlocked in a power struggle with the patient—because such a struggle can easily enough ensue when the therapist takes it upon herself to represent the voice of reality, a stance that then leaves the patient no option but to become the voice of opposition.

In fact, when the therapist introduces the conflict statement with "you know," she is insisting that the patient take responsibility for what the patient really does know. But if the therapist, in a misguided attempt to urge the patient forward, resorts simply to telling the patient what the *therapist* knows, not only does the therapist run the risk of forcing the patient to become ever more entrenched in her defensive stance of opposition, but also the therapist will be robbing the patient of any incentive to take responsibility for her *own* desire to get better.

Again, it is an untenable situation—although it happens all the time—for the psychotherapist to represent the *healthy (adaptive) voice of yes* and for the patient, made anxious, to be then stuck in the position of having to protest the *unhealthy (defensive) voice of no.*

The following presents an example.

Suppose the therapist were to offer her patient the following intervention: "You won't feel any better physically or emotionally until you begin to eat more healthily." Admittedly, there is probably truth in this declaration. But here, by confronting the patient rather boldly with something the therapist has decided the patient needs to know, the therapist will be running the risk of making the patient so anxious that the patient will be unable to take in—or benefit from—the therapist's input.

Indeed, the patient may well react defensively to this anxiety-provoking pronouncement by protesting defiantly "...but the thought of eating more healthily makes me feel so deprived that I don't think I could ever do that!" Unfortunately, now the groundwork has been laid for conflict about eating healthily—which rightfully belongs *in* the patient—to be played out in the space *between* patient and therapist.

But now consider the empowering impact of the following conflict statement, which not only highlights what the patient herself, at least on some level, must already know about the importance of eating healthily but also resonates empathically with what the therapist senses would be the patient's resistance to eating that way: "You know that you won't feel any better physically or emotionally until you begin to eat more healthily; but the thought of actually doing that makes you feel so deprived that, for now anyway, you can't imagine ever being willing or able to make that kind of commitment."

In this latter intervention, the therapist first confronts the patient (by speaking to the patient's ability to recognize the consequences of an unhealthy diet) but then validates the patient (by speaking to the feelings of deprivation the therapist senses the patient would have were the patient to make a commitment to eating more healthily). Here the therapist, by respectfully acknowledging both sides of the patient's ambivalence about letting go of her dysfunction, will be giving the patient space either (1) to reiterate her healthy desire to feel better and to acknowledge her recognition of the price she is paying for continuing to eat unhealthily or (2) to elaborate upon why she is so invested in eating the way she does and therefore upon her resistance to making a commitment to change.

In other words, by way of a conflict statement, not only is the locus of control being named as an internal one but also the patient's ambivalent attachment to her dysfunction is being respectfully acknowledged. Now, instead of creating conflict *between* patient and therapist, the focus can be, appropriately, on conflict *within* the patient.

By repeatedly formulating conflict statements that strategically juxtapose the patient's dawning awareness of just how steep a price she pays for holding on to her defenses and her newfound appreciation for how they have served her, the therapist will be able to create galvanizing tension within the patient—growth-promoting tension that will ultimately become the fulcrum for therapeutic change.

And so it is that the therapist goes back and forth between challenging (by highlighting what the patient is coming increasingly to recognize as the high price she pays for refusing to let go of her dysfunction) and supporting (by articulating, on the patient's behalf, what the therapist senses is the patient's investment in holding on to her dysfunction even so)—all with an eye to making the ambivalently held dysfunction ever less ego-syntonic (that is, ever less consonant with the patient's sense of self) and ever more ego-dystonic (that is, ever more dissonant with her sense of self).

As long as the *gain* (that is, the benefit) is greater than the *pain* (that is, the cost), the patient will *maintain* the defense and *remain* entrenched.

But once the *pain* becomes greater than the *gain*, the stress and *strain* of the cognitive dissonance thereby created between the pain and the gain will prompt the patient ultimately to relinquish the dysfunction.

More specifically, once the *pain* (as a result of all that the patient is coming to recognize as the price she pays for silencing her inner voice of truth) becomes greater than the *gain* (which is becoming ever less compelling as the patient is coming increasingly to understand the defensive nature of her maladaptive ways of being and doing), the stress and *strain* of the cognitive dissonance now being generated within the patient—between her ever greater awareness of the cost and her ever greater appreciation for the defensive nature of the benefit—will provide powerful leverage for the patient gradually to relinquish her attachment to the defense.

In letting go of her dysfunction, the structural (neurotic) conflict within the patient between anxiety-provoking but ultimately empowering forces and anxiety-assuaging but growth-obstructing defensive counterforces will be resolved.

FROM REINING IN TO GIVING FREE REIN

How does this resolution of internal conflict foster growth and recovery of mental health, vitality, and a sense of well-being?

In order to answer this question, it is important to return to the statement of Freud's that was earlier referenced, namely, "Where id was, there shall ego be." A corollary to this adage is Freud's claim that as a result of working through drive-defense conflicts between id drives pressing for release and ego defenses mobilized to thwart them, the *id will be tamed* and the *ego strengthened*— such that no longer will primitive defenses be needed to keep a lid on the id.[19]

In writing about the conflictual relationship between id and ego, Freud likens it to the relationship that exists between a horse and its rider.[19] He suggests that the horse represents the id and its rider the ego. An untamed horse wants no more than to run free; its energy, however, will need to be tamed if that energy is to become available to fuel the progression of horse and rider. Furthermore, the inexperienced rider must become adept at harnessing that energy if horse and rider are to be able to work together so that they can move forward in unison.

As we have just seen in the preceding sections, by progressively working through resistances that had *reined in* both growth-promoting awareness and actualization of potential, Freud's rider (a now stronger and more empowered ego by virtue of having evolved to ever greater insight into its internal workings) will be more skilled at channeling the propulsive power of the horse (a now better regulated and more manageable id by virtue of having had its energy tamed, modified, and integrated)—such that horse and rider will be able to move forward in sync, no longer in conflict but collaboratively.

The defensive need to *rein the horse in* will have become gradually transformed into the adaptive capacity to *give the horse free rein*. More specifically, we could say that the defensive need to curse the darkness will have become gradually transformed into the adaptive capacity to light a candle.

In essence, as the id energies become better modulated and the ego more empowered, the patient will become better able to cope with the various stressors of life by adapting to them instead of defending against them—indeed "Where defense was, there shall adaptation be."

FROM RELENTLESS HOPE TO SERENE ACCEPTANCE

With respect to working through the affective disillusionment of Model 2, let us now look more closely at the transformation *relentless hope* (a defense) into *serene acceptance* (an adaptation).[10,23,24]

A cartoon from *The New Yorker* depicts a restaurant by the name of The Disillusionment Café in which a woman is seated, awaiting the arrival of her order. The waiter returns to her table and announces, "Your order is not ready, and nor will it ever be."

When we don our Model 2 hat, we will need to shift our focus from (1) transformation of resistance into awareness (as a result of working through the stress of cognitive dissonance) to (2) transformation of relentless hope into acceptance (as a result of working through the stress of affective disillusionment). Although, as we see, the language will be different, the concepts are the same; and the net result in both instances will be transformation of dysfunctional defense into more functional adaptation as the patient evolves—through iterative cycles of disruption and repair—from a state of thwarted potential, frustrated desire, and undermining depression to actualization of potential, empowerment, and serene acceptance.

More specifically, many a psychiatric patient, as a child, has suffered great heartache at the hands of a misguided, even if well-intentioned, parent—be it in the form of psychological trauma and abuse (too much bad) or emotional deprivation and neglect (not enough good). Such a patient may never have had occasion to confront the pain of her grief about the parent's unwitting, but devastating, betrayal of her. Instead, the patient has defended herself against the pain of her heartache by pushing it out of awareness and clinging instead to the illusion of her parent (or a stand-in for her parent) as good—and as ultimately forthcoming—if she (the patient) could but get it right.

Under the sway of her repetition compulsion, the patient—as she struggles through life—will find herself delivering into each new relationship her desperate hope that perhaps this time, were she to be but good enough, want it badly enough, or suffer deeply enough, she might yet be able to transform this new object of her relentless desire into the perfect parent she should have had as a child—but never did.[10]

Such a patient, who is relentless in her quest to find that which she can never have, will be at risk for developing an underlying, low-level depression because she has never sufficiently confronted—and grieved—her early on losses or dealt with the pain of her sadness about all the subsequent disappointments she will inevitably have encountered along the way as a result of her constant and relentless pursuit of the unattainable.

In essence, such a patient, who *refuses to grieve*, is effectively *choosing* depression (a defense) over sadness (an adaptation). By *refusing to relinquish her relentless desire*, she is effectively consigning herself to a lifetime of chronic frustration and distress (which is a defensive reaction to disappointments never adequately grieved) instead of accepting that sobering realities are an unavoidable aspect of life (which is the adaptive response to frustration and loss).

Admittedly, the choice is unconscious; but it is a choice nonetheless and one for which the patient must ultimately take responsibility if she is ever to extricate herself from the dysfunctional ties that are binding her to her unmourned past. Only by confronting—and grieving—the multitude of privations, deprivations, and injuries sustained at the hands of her parents will the patient be able, over time, to surrender her attachment to defenses that have admittedly enabled her to avoid feeling the depths of her sadness and grief about those early on parental failures but that have nonetheless left her vulnerable to the development, later on in life, of such symptoms as chronic depression, pervasive anxiety, intractable insomnia, frequent headaches, musculoskeletal tension, knee-jerk impulsivity, bouts of rage, panic attacks, and feelings of helplessness and victimization—all of which are manifestations of unmastered grief.

Indeed, if the patient is ever to relinquish the passionate but self-sabotaging pursuits in which she engages, then she must someday dare to let herself first remember the anguish of just how heartbreaking it really was—both the parental *errors of commission* (presence of bad) and the parental *errors of omission* (absence of good)—and then confront, and mourn, the pain of her grief about the parental betrayals, grief against which she has spent a lifetime unconsciously defending herself. Indeed, until the patient can master her devastation and outrage, their dark presence beneath her surface will taint all subsequent relationships and future endeavors.

If the patient is to be released from the past, then the therapeutic process must be able to provoke transformation of the patient's need to hold on to her relentless hope (a defense against acknowledging the pain of her grief about both past and present objects) into the capacity to confront the pain of her grief and move beyond it to a place of serene acceptance. Simultaneously, if all goes well, the patient's illusions of grandiose omnipotence (a defense against acknowledging the separateness and immutability of her objects) will give way to humble acceptance of the limits of her power to possess and control them (an adaptation to the impact of that sobering reality).

As with the process of working through the patient's resistance, so, too, the process of working through the patient's relentlessness can be facilitated by the therapist's use of optimally stressful interventions designed to precipitate disruption in order to trigger repair. As noted earlier, if, on the one hand, there is no challenge that needs to be mastered, then there will be little impetus for transformation and growth; but if, on the other hand, there is no support, then there will be little opportunity for transformation and growth.

But whereas conflict statements—the staple of the Model 1 therapist—first challenge by addressing the patient's adaptive capacity to know an anxiety-provoking reality and then support by resonating empathically with the patient's defensive need to deny it, disillusionment statements—the staple of the Model 2 therapist—first challenge by addressing the patient's adaptive capacity to know, more specifically, a disillusioning reality and then support by resonating empathically with the patient's adaptive capacity to experience the pain of her grief as she begins to let herself really know—and feel—the full impact of that painful truth.

Furthermore, whereas conflict statements are specifically designed to provoke recovery by challenging the patient to acknowledge the price she is coming to recognize that she pays for holding on to her dysfunction (such that clinging to her dysfunction will become increasingly untenable), disillusionment statements are specifically designed to provoke recovery by challenging the patient to confront the pain of her grief about the people in her world, past and present, who have broken her heart (such that clinging to her relentless hope that they might someday change will become increasingly untenable).

Finally, whereas conflict statements advance the therapeutic process by speaking to an uncomfortable reality that the patient is indeed beginning to acknowledge but then speaking to the defense the patient mobilizes in order not to have to acknowledge it (in other words, the patient knows but denies that she does), disillusionment statements facilitate grieving by speaking to a disillusioning reality that the patient is indeed beginning to acknowledge and then speaking to the devastation the patient experiences as she begins to let that knowledge sink in: "You know that I don't have all the answers, and it upsets and angers you that I don't."

Although disillusionment statements often begin with the more direct challenge of "you know," disillusionment statements can also begin with the less direct challenge of "as you begin to let yourself know" and then go on gently to resonate with the patient's newfound ability to let herself begin to feel the pain of her sadness and grief:

> As you begin to let yourself know that I don't have all the answers, you find yourself getting very upset and angry.
> You know that John will probably never love you in the way that you would have wanted him to, and it breaks your heart.
> As you begin to let yourself know that John will probably never love you in the way that you would have wanted him to, it breaks your heart.
> As you begin to let yourself feel the pain of your disappointment that your father, despite all that you've done for him over the years, still appears to favor your brother over you, the pain of his betrayal goes very deep.
> You know that you can never take back the spiteful things you said to your mother before she died; the pain and guilt of that are so overwhelming that sometimes you find yourself feeling profoundly depressed.

Back and forth, back and forth, the Model 2 therapist will first challenge (when the therapist senses that there is a window of opportunity to confront the patient's refusal to grieve) and then support (in order to create space and opportunity for the patient to delve more deeply into the pain of her grief). It is hoped that the patient, within the context of safety provided by the relationship with her therapist, will be able finally to access the reservoir of tears that have accumulated inside of her over time and to experience the sadness, the anguish, the torment, the fury, and the impotent rage that have been pent up for so long.

THE PROCESS OF GRIEVING

Working through disillusionment is a protracted process, one that requires time, effort, and patience. Whether in relation to past or present objects, grieving must be done in installments. In the psychodynamic literature, it is described as the graduated working through of *optimal disillusionments*.[25] Grieving is a difficult journey that requires the processing and integration of *doses of disappointment* with respect to both *the bad that was* and *the good that was not*.[6]

The patient must come to accept the reality that she is ultimately powerless to do anything to make her objects, both past and present, different. She can, and should, do things to change herself, but she cannot change her objects—and she will have to come to terms with that sobering truth.

As Kopp has written, "Genuine grief is the sobbing and wailing which express the acceptance of our helplessness to do anything about [our] losses."[26]

Also relevant here is the Serenity Prayer (authored by the theologian Reinhold Niebuhr and adopted by 12-step programs): "God grant me the serenity to accept the things I cannot change; courage to change the things I can; and wisdom to know the difference."

The therapeutic action in Model 2 will involve working through the optimal stress of disillusionment, an evolutionary process that will involve processing and integrating the stressful impact of psychotherapeutic interventions that confront the patient's refusal to grieve. The net result will be transformation of the patient's need to defend against the pain of her grief by clinging to her relentless hope into the capacity to adapt by confronting the pain of her grief and coming to a place of serene acceptance with respect to what the object cannot do and of appreciation for what it can.

The bad news, of course, will be the sadness the patient experiences as she begins to accept the sobering reality that disappointment is an inevitable and necessary aspect of relationship. The good news, however, will be the wisdom she acquires as she comes to appreciate ever more profoundly the subtleties and nuances of relationship and begins to make her peace with the harsh reality of life's many challenges. Sadder, yes, but also wiser.

Beckmann poignantly captures the essence of grieving with the following: "Grief is nature's way of healing a broken heart."[27]

Such is the work of grieving—and mastering the experience of loss, disillusionment, heartbreak, and defeat; such is the work of coming to terms with reality and moving on.

In fact, psychological maturity could be described as an adaptation to the impact of disillusioning realities about the self and the world.

Perhaps as we get older, we become sadder; but we also become more aware, more accepting, and more accountable—as we transform the defensive need to have reality be a certain way into the adaptive capacity to accept it as it is.

It will be only once the patient has been able to process and integrate the dissociated grief that she will be able to relinquish her relentless pursuit of the unattainable. The patient will have transformed dysfunctional defense into more functional adaptation once she has grieved and, in the process, developed a more refined awareness of the limitations inherent in relationship and a more evolved capacity to accept that which she cannot change.

More specifically, as the defensive need to hold on becomes transformed into the adaptive capacity to let go, realistic (mature) hope will emerge from relentless (infantile) hope. Along these same lines, Searles has suggested that realistic hope arises in the context of surviving disappointment.[28]

CONCLUSION

Whether resistance (a defense) is transformed into awareness of painful truths about the self (an adaptation), relentlessness (a defense) is transformed into acceptance of painful truths about the object (an adaptation), or cursing the darkness (a defense) is transformed into lighting a candle (an adaptation), the evolutionary process by which a dysfunctional defense is gradually replaced by a more functional adaptation requires that an acute injury be superimposed upon a chronic one, thereby tapping into the innate wisdom of the body and its capacity to self-heal in the face of optimal challenge.

Capitalizing upon this fundamental principle of *controlled damage* (whereby a condition may not heal until it is made acute), the therapist will intervene in ways specifically designed to precipitate rupture in order to trigger repair. More specifically, by providing just the right combination of challenge (to provoke rupture) and support (to allow for repair), the therapist's optimally stressful psychotherapeutic interventions will induce healing cycles of defensive collapse and adaptive reconstitution at ever more complex levels of organization, functionality, and dynamic balance.

Indeed, integrative psychotherapy affords the patient an opportunity—albeit a belated one—to master experiences that had once been overwhelming (and therefore defended against) but that can now, with enough support from the therapist and by drawing upon the patient's underlying resilience and capacity to cope with optimal stress, be processed and integrated (and thereby adapted to).

Again, stressful stuff happens; but whether the primary target is mind or body and the clinical manifestation therefore psychiatric or medical, the critical issue will be the ability of the MindBodyMatrix to handle the impact of the stress through adaptation.

In the poignant words of Ernest Hemingway (1929), "The world breaks everyone, and afterward, many are strong at the broken places."[29]

Is there not a certain beauty in brokenness, a beauty never achieved by things unbroken? If a bone is fractured and then heals, the area of the break will be stronger than the surrounding bone and will not again easily fracture. Are we, too, not stronger at our broken places? And is there not a certain beauty in brokenness, a quiet strength we acquire from having survived adversity and hardship and having mastered the experience of disappointment, heartbreak, and devastation? And, then, when we finally rise above it, don't we rise up in quiet triumph, even if only we notice?

REFERENCES

1. Kohut, H. 1966. Forms and transformations of narcissism. *J Am Psychoanal Assoc* 14(2): 243–272.
2. Strogatz, S. 1994. *Nonlinear Dynamics and Chaos: With Applications to Physics, Biology, Chemistry, and Engineering*. Cambridge, MA: Perseus.
3. Kauffman, S. 1995. *At Home in the Universe: The Search for the Laws of Self-Organization and Complexity*. New York, NY: Oxford University.
4. Krebs, C.T. 2013. *Energetic Kinesiology: Principles and Practice*. Scotland, UK: Handspring Publishing.
5. Stark, M. 2008. Hormesis, adaptation, and the sandpile model. *Crit Rev Toxicol* 38(7): 641–644.
6. Stark, M. 2014. Optimal stress, psychological resilience, and the sandpile model. In *Hormesis in Health and Disease*, Ed. S. Rattan and E. Le Bourg. Boca Raton, FL: CRC Press/Taylor & Francis, pp. 201–224.
7. van der Kolk, B. 2006. *Traumatic Stress: The Effects of Overwhelming Experience on Mind, Body, and Society*. New York, NY: Guilford Press.
8. Selye, H. 1974. *Stress without Distress*. New York, NY: Harper & Row.
9. Stark, M. 2012. The sandpile model: Optimal stress and hormesis. *Dose Response* 10(1): 66–74.
10. Stark, M. 1999. *Modes of Therapeutic Action: Enhancement of Knowledge, Provision of Experience, and Engagement in Relationship*. Northvale, NJ: Jason Aronson.
11. Paracelsus, T. 2004. *The Archidoxes of Magic*. Turner. R. (trans). Temecula, CA: Ibis.
12. Ehrenberg, D. 1992. *The Intimate Edge: Extending the Reach of Psychoanalytic Interaction*. New York, NY: W.W. Norton.
13. Cannon, W.B. 1932. *The Wisdom of the Body*. New York, NY: W.W. Norton.
14. Sapolsky, R.M. 1994. *Why Zebras Don't Get Ulcers*. New York, NY: W.H. Freeman.
15. McEwen, B.S. 1998. Stress, adaptation, and disease: Allostasis and allostatic load. *Ann NY Acad Sci* 840: 33–44.
16. Bland, J. 1999. *Genetic Nutritioneering*. New York, NY: McGraw-Hill.
17. McEwen, B.S. 2002. *The End of Stress as We Know It*. Washington, DC: Joseph Henry Press.
18. Bak, P. 1996. *How Nature Works: The Science of Self-organized Criticality*. New York, NY: Springer-Verlag.
19. Freud, S. 1923. *The Ego and the Id*. New York, NY: W.W. Norton.
20. Stark, M. 2008. Hormesis, adaptation, and the sandpile model. *Crit Rev Toxicol* 38(7): 641–644.

21. Seyle, H. 1978. *The Stress of Life*. New York, NY: McGraw-Hill.
22. Zevon, W. 1996. *I'll Sleep When I'm Dead*. Burbank, CA: Elektra Records.
23. Stark, M. 1994. *Working with Resistance*. Northvale, NJ: Jason Aronson.
24. Stark, M. 1994. *A Primer on Working with Resistance*. Northvale, NJ: Jason Aronson.
25. Kohut, H. 1984. *How Does Analysis Cure?* Chicago, IL: University of Chicago Press.
26. Kopp, S. 1969. The refusal to mourn. *Voices* Spring, 30–35.
27. Beckmann, R. 1990. *Children Who Grieve: A Manual for Conducting Support Groups*. Holmes Beach, FL: Learning Publications, Inc.
28. Searles, H. 1986. *Collected Papers on Schizophrenia and Related Subjects*. London, UK: Karnac Books.
29. Hemingway, E. 1929. *A Farewell to Arms*. New York, NY: Charles Scribner.

28 Integrative Approaches to Perinatal Depression

Vesna Pirec, MD, PhD and Kelly Brogan, MD, ABIHM

CONTENTS

INTRODUCTION

Depressive disorders are the leading cause of mental disability in the modern world[1] where women are affected two to three times more frequently than men.[2] The increased incidence of depressive disorders in women compared to men becomes apparent during puberty and continues until menopause.[3,4] Despite some previously established myths, as well as misleading images created by the media producing false expectations for women and their surroundings of overall well-being in pregnancy, it is now evident that women are not protected from psychiatric illnesses during peripartum. On the contrary, pregnant women are equally susceptible to new-onset depressive illness as well as reoccurrence of previously diagnosed depression as their counterparts, nonpregnant women. It has been shown that depressive symptoms during pregnancy can occur in as many as 20% of women.[2,5] Depression during pregnancy poses a significant risk for development of postpartum depression. The question if depression is more common in postpartum versus other phases of women's life is still a topic of debate, and depending on the inclusion criteria it has been reported in 7%–13% of women.[5,6] In support of the theory about uniqueness of peripartum in relation to the occurrence of perinatal depression, some recent studies demonstrated that the period after giving birth may introduce additional factors of vulnerability in a subset of women, making new moms somewhat more prone to developing various forms of psychiatric conditions, including depression and anxiety.[7] Additionally, reproductive psychiatrists contend that postpartum symptomatology is unique in presentation as well as gravity of risks, including suicide and infanticide. Despite numerous attempts to detect perinatal psychiatric conditions in a timely manner and treat them appropriately, perinatal depression is still a leading cause of maternal morbidity and mortality,[8] and suicide in that period remains one of the most common causes of death in women.[9]

Despite the fact that postpartum depression has been a known entity, described as early as during Hippocrates' times,[10] its etiology is still unclear. In the nineteenth century, the interest for perinatal mental health drastically increased, especially during Marce's time when he dedicated his career to studying it.[11] In the last couple of decades perinatal mental health issues have been drawing particular clinical and research interests, advancing our understanding of the disorder and opening new avenues for its treatment.

Overall, perinatal depression, as DSM-V defines it, is a depressive disorder that can have its onset during pregnancy or within 4 weeks of postpartum. However, most research criteria are guided by the onset of depressive symptoms up to 6 and in some cases 12 months after delivery. The American Congress of Obstetricians and Gynecologists (ACOG) Committee of Obstetric practice (2010) reported that 5%–25% of women are most likely to experience postpartum depression at some point.[12] Consequences of undiagnosed and untreated perinatal depression are numerous for both mother and child. Women who suffer from depression during pregnancy usually do not receive adequate prenatal care, and at times tend to self-medicate by using alcohol and/or drugs which could cause various developmental issues and negatively affect delivery and the entire peripartum period.[13] During pregnancy, depression and stress trigger an increase in maternal cortisol levels, which has the potential to negatively impact obstetrical and infant outcomes, in addition to the potential to initiate fetal programming of adult disease.[14] Furthermore, depressive symptoms during postpartum have been associated with numerous negative outcomes in child development such as temperamental difficulties,[15] insecure attachment,[16] as well as developmental delay.[17] Untreated maternal postpartum depression can adversely affect mother-infant interactions[18] and increase the risk of emotional, cognitive, and behavioral problems in her offspring,[19] including development of depressive disorders in adolescent offspring.[20] Both detection and treatment of perinatal depression remain a challenge with some of the accepted treatment modalities offering less then satisfying results (improvement of symptoms 50% or less), and posing potential risks to mother and to baby, leaving room for additional treatment approaches.

Thus understanding perinatal depression starting with its etiology, potential for implementing preventive measures among women at risk, including adequate screening and timely recognition of symptoms, as well as mindful application of various available treatment modalities are essential steps in providing a better future for new moms and their offspring.

PROPOSED RISK FACTORS AND ETIOLOGIES FOR DEVELOPMENT OF PERINATAL AND POSTPARTUM DEPRESSION

A variety of contributing factors for developing perinatal depression have been studied over the years. While it appears that some genetic vulnerabilities and traumatic and psychosocial circumstances tend to be the most frequent triggers for perinatal and postpartum depression (PPD), not all women with predispositions develop illness. In studies conducted over the last couple of decades, the most commonly identified factors are of psychosocial origin: prior history of depressive illness, co-occurring anxiety and neuroticism, chronic stress during pregnancy, along with marital problems and violence at home.[21–23] It is hard to delineate psychosocial events from changes occurring on a cellular level, as it appears that they are all interconnected creating reciprocal causalities.

Some of those proposed etiologies of perinatal depression will be briefly discussed here. However, based on numerous research findings in the field, it appears that we cannot identify one single cause leading to PPD, yet rather multiple factors tend to co-occur in predisposed individuals which trigger the illness. Yet all potentially contributing factors in the development of PPD open doors to various treatment approaches as well as offer possibilities to apply different preventive measures.

SOCIOCULTURAL

Postpartum depression has been studied in many sociocultural settings over the years. Various observational studies indicated that postpartum depression seems to be less prevalent in cultures where social support is part of regular life expectations, where child care and special food are provided, and upon giving birth the new mother returns to her home of origin and various soothing rituals are implemented.[24] Additionally, more recent studies conducted among multicultural backgrounds in an urban setting (New York City) indicated that identification and organization of social support, even if less spontaneous and given, can still serve as a protective factor from developing postpartum depression.[25]

PSYCHOSOCIAL STRESS IN PREGNANCY

Psychosocial stress has been frequently reported as a significant, yet potentially identifiable and preventive risk factor for perinatal depression. Studies and observations in urban settings demonstrated that the presence of violence at home, being part of certain ethnic groups such as African American, Hispanic, or Asian, as well as dealing with medical comorbidities all play a significant role in development of perinatal depression. Some of those risk factors are identifiable, and thus preventive measures could be put in place.

NEUROENDOCRINE AND PSYCHOIMMUNOLOGICAL CHANGES

In recent years various neuroendocrine and psychoneuroimmunological involvements in the onset of postpartum depression have been reported.[26–28] The leading idea behind this is that labor, delivery, and postpartum period induce multiple inflammatory responses in women, which, in a subset of women could be intensified by genetic predisposition, preexisting inflammatory status, and specific vulnerability leading to depressive symptomatology.[28] Additionally, nutritional status is essential for proper functioning of the hypothalamic-pituitary-adrenal (HPA) axis and adequate immune reactions in the body. During pregnancy due to higher demands for certain nutrients, deficiencies are more likely to occur, leading to dysregulation of immune mechanisms, deprivation of regular cellular mechanisms, and consequently, depressive symptomatology.

INFLAMMATION, TOXINS, AND NEUROAMINES

Reduced monoamine levels (serotonin, dopamine, and norepinephrine) in the brain have been proposed as factors contributing to the neurotransmitter insufficiency responsible for the onset of depressive disorders.[29]

Genetic vulnerability predisposes subgroups of women to develop perinatal depression. Yet it is epigenetics that plays a pivotal role in the development of a majority of illnesses, perinatal depression included. Various external factors influence either triggering or preventing an illness in a predisposed person. Environmental toxins are abundant in our lives and frequently cause oxidative stress, which translates into the inability of the organism to effectively neutralize metabolic products of aerobic oxygenation, leading to different cellular and neuronal damages.

There are numerous toxins such as pesticides, industrial chemicals, carcinogens, and neurotoxic metals that humans are exposed to and ingest on a daily basis. Pregnant women may be especially vulnerable to those exposures, leading to severe physical and mental consequences for both her and her offspring. Significant concern, most likely due to such a massive consumption, has been raised about the negative impact of genetically modified foods that are widely spread in the United States and to a lesser degree in Europe, such as soy, corn, and sugar beets. Those crops are exposed to the pesticide glyphosate, a substance that has been linked to depletion of the serotonin precursor tryptophan, and which also negatively affects gut micro flora, impacting nutrient absorption as well as formation of elements that are crucial for maintaining mood stability and regulated emotions.[30-32] The signal of harm around pesticide exposure likely relates to its endocrine-disrupting properties as well.[33] The effect of trans-species gene insertion is unknown and unstudied.

Furthermore, animal studies showed that some of non-DNA-related phenotypes induced by those environmental toxins could be passed on for several generations, pointing to very powerful negative influence of those exposures to offspring.[34] In addition to nutrient deficiencies, some aspects of modern diet lead to formation of free radicals which are a potential source of inflammation in the body. For example, the abundance of fructose (mainly in the form of fructose syrup which is present in most foods) as well as trans fats which are the product of heat manipulation of vegetable oils have shown to be responsible for the production of free radicals which then trigger inflammation. Several studies examined dietary consumption of casein (dairy products) and gluten related to the development of perinatal depression.

The rationale for that causality discussed in those studies is that the by-product of both casein and gluten is a morphine-like substance, found to be elevated in women with perinatal illness, and thus linked to maternal[35] as well as child psychopathology.[36] Furthermore, autoimmune reactions triggered by environmental toxins causing inflammation have been linked to the onset of autoimmune reactions in perinatal women leading to hypoactivity of HPA in PPD. Hypoactive HPA induces relative reduction of cortisol and corticotropin-releasing factor (CRH), which could then further facilitate inflammatory responses.[37]

HORMONAL DYSREGULATION

Various hormones such as reproductive hormones (progesterone, estradiol), prolactin, oxytocin, as well as thyroid hormones have been linked to the development of perinatal depression.

DYSREGULATION OF HPA AXIS

The dysregulation of the HPA axis has been generally linked to depressive disorders, perinatal depression included.[38-42] In pregnancy, particularly after 36 weeks of gestational age, estrogen and progesterone levels are drastically increased compared to the prepregnancy baseline. During pregnancy, and especially in the third trimester, CRH, which is a driving force for HPA regulation, also increases dramatically due to its secretion from the placenta so that its level may increase up to 100 times at 6–8 weeks prior to delivery.

Consequently, cortisol levels increase significantly as well. However, closer to term, the HPA axis response tends to be blunted due to placental command of feedback. After birth, when levels of estrogen and progesterone, as well as CRH drastically decline, the HPA axis is blunted due to decrease of *hypothalamic* CRH. Rather than representing a temporary transition, in some women, CRH continues to be low for up to 6–12 weeks. It is postulated that this prolongation of blunted HPA could potentially contribute to development of PPD symptoms.[41]

Similar pathophysiological changes have been observed in melancholic depression unrelated to puerperium, and interestingly so, characteristics of perinatal depression largely resemble those of atypical depression. Anxiety in pregnancy has been a well-established risk factor for perinatal depression, the mechanisms of which could also be related to higher sensitivity of cortisol withdrawal upon delivery. Along those lines, a more recent study done by Labad et al.[43] indicated that women who experience intrusive thoughts of harming their children had significantly higher adrenocorticotropic hormone (ACTH) coupled with low CRH and cortisol levels in the morning 2 days after the delivery. ACTH and CRH are produced by the placenta, thus a sharp decrease of CRH can be attributed to delivery of the placenta. However, in this patient group the increase of morning ACTH levels was not coupled with an increase in cortisol levels, which may leave these patients more susceptible to postpartum obsessive, intrusive thoughts.

REPRODUCTIVE STEROID HORMONES

The reproductive hormonal theory is based on the fact that hormonal levels in pregnancy rise significantly during pregnancy, such that estrogen levels in some women increase up to 50–100 times[44,45] and progesterone levels up to 10 times[42,46] as compared to its highest level during the menstrual cycle. Approximately 3–7 days after delivery a drastic drop of those hormones occurs, returning to the prepregnancy levels and potentially attributing to mood disturbances in postpartum. Empirical evidence suggests that reflection of these hormonal changes does not depend on the absolute hormone levels, but rather the fact that a subset of women is more susceptible to those drastic hormonal oscillations,[47] which then lead to multiple depressive and anxiety symptoms. To further support this theory, some indirect evidence suggests that hormonal fluctuation can be responsible for mood changes in peripartum in predisposed women. In a research study this theory was demonstrated by adding and then rapidly withdrawing sex hormones which induced a depressive episode among women who had a previous history of postpartum depression, but not to those who never suffered from this illness.[48] Studies demonstrated that some women with a history of PPD have abnormal responses to fluctuation of estrogen and progesterone, despite having hormonal levels within normal range.[48]

In addition to individual sensitivity to hormonal withdrawal, it has been shown that in the initial postpartum days (3–7) the level of monoamine oxidase A (MAOA), an enzyme found predominantly in the brain and responsible for degrading monoamine-type neurotransmitters, is directly related to estrogen levels.[49] It appears that a drastic decrease in the amount of estrogen increases the levels and activity of MAOA leading to increased degradation of mood-altering neurotransmitters, such as dopamine, norepinephrine, and serotonin. Therefore this finely tuned cascade of hormonal changes during puerperium, when coupled with other risk factors, may contribute to perinatal depression.

THYROID HORMONES

Thyroid hormone instability can also contribute to perinatal depressive illness. It is important to emphasize that some changes in thyroid hormone levels are physiologic during pregnancy and postpartum, such as that during the first trimester in pregnancy thyroid-stimulating hormone (TSH) can decrease and total thyroxin (T4), free T4, and total triiodothyronine (T3) can be slightly elevated without any clinical signs of hyperthyroidism. Thus it appears that pregnancy induces some stimulation of the thyroid gland. Contrary to these expected physiological changes, it has been shown that women who have lower antenatal levels of total and free T4 within euthyroid range, seem to be more predisposed for later development of PPD.[50] Furthermore, autoimmune disorders that are generally more frequent in women than in men tend to occur with even higher frequency in the postpartum period. The presence of thyroid autoantibodies in the antepartum can predict the onset of both postpartum depression and psychosis.[51–54]

OXYTOCIN

Oxytocin (OT) has been studied as a potential etiology factor in perinatal illness, especially with postpartum onset. Oxytocin is directly involved in lactation, and as such plays a pivotal role in the postpartum period. Various observational studies indicated a link between PPD and either early weaning[55,56] or a negative breastfeeding experience.[57,58] Unplanned early breastfeeding discontinuation can lead to myriad neuroendocrine changes, and hormonal disturbances presenting as PPD. A longitudinal study done by Stuebe et al. 2013 demonstrated that lower oxytocin levels in postpartum were directly correlated with more pronounced depressive and anxiety symptoms.[59] Also this study, contrary to previous reports, indicated a protective effect of breastfeeding against development of PPD, showing that exclusive breastfeeding more commonly leads to depressive and anxiety symptoms postpartum. This finding could have been related to poor support systems and lack of adequate education in lactation which in some women can aggravate perinatal depressive symptoms.

Consistent with oxytocin's protective effects is the fact that new moms suffering from perinatal anxiety tend to lose milk faster, as corroborated in animal studies in which chronic stress reduces mothering behaviors.[60] Oxytocin plays a pivotal role in activation of dopaminergic systems in the brain and facilitates mother–infant attachment. Maternal experience upregulates oxytocin receptors allowing oxytocin released during parturition and breastfeeding to affect various brain regions in new moms, inducing anxiolytic effects as well as enhancing bonding. Despite the fact that there are some contradictory findings related to oxytocin's contribution, it is clear that it plays a significant role in physiological and psychological changes occurring postpartum. Further research in this domain is essential as it could shed additional light into breastfeeding practices and its involvement in maternal perinatal illness.

NUTRITION AND NEUROTRANSMITTERS

One of the essential factors for well-balanced neurochemistry of the brain is adequate nutrition. Specific foods, elements, and vitamins are necessary for synthesis and transportation of neurotransmitters in the brain, and are thus indirectly responsible for the maintenance of mood stability.

It appears that the majority of pregnant and nonpregnant women tend to consume suboptimal diets.[61] Pregnancy and lactation during the postpartum period are reproductive phases during which demands for some nutrients drastically increase, posing an even greater risk for nutritional deficiencies to occur. Pregnant women require nutrients not only to support growing fetal tissues, but also to maintain their own enhanced metabolic rate as well as the growth of the placenta and mammary glands. A study conducted by Giddens et al. 2000 demonstrated that pregnant women in the United States tend to consume inadequate amounts of some essential elements such as calcium, magnesium, iron, zinc, vitamin D, and folate, which was associated with increased susceptibility to mood disturbances in the peripartum period.[61]

POLYUNSATURATED FATTY ACIDS

Polyunsaturated fatty acids (PUFAs) are two families of essential fatty acids that cannot be synthesized by the human body and thus have to be obtained through nutrition. Those are the n-3α-linolenic acid (ALA) and the n-6 linoleic acid (LA). Major sources for ALA are soybean oil, fatty fish, some algae, flax seeds, and walnuts and appropriate intake via food of it is essential since the synthesis of n-3 fatty acids from ALA in the body is insufficient. This parent n-3 fatty acid functions in the body through eicosapentaenoic acid (EPA) and its derivative docosahexaenoic acid (DHA). The modern Western diet is abundant in linoleic acid (LA). Major sources of LA are sunflower seeds, lean meats, organ meats, eggs, and vegetable seed oils.

There are two proposed mechanisms of PUFAs, primarily n-3s, involvement in mood stabilization: reduction of inflammation through inhibition of pro-inflammatory substances cytokines and eicosanoids[62] and regulation of synthesis, function, and metabolism of various neurotransmitters in the brain.[63] Out of those two long-chain n-3 free derived fatty acids (FA) EPA and DHA, DHA is more abundant in the brain[64] and tends to accumulate in phospholipids of neuronal cell membrane.[65] EPA and DHA control cell membrane fluidity, receptor binding, transfer of various molecules and nutrients through membranes, as well as various enzymatic reactions.[66] During pregnancy, the development of the fetal central nervous system increases demands for DHA,[67] which is often not met by pregnant women. Fish is an important source of n-3 FA; however, due to concerns raised in the last couple of decades related to mercury and industrial contaminant levels in consumed fish, pregnant women have drastically decreased its consumption, leading to even more significant deficits of DHA and EPA.

HOMOCYSTEINE METABOLISM AND S-ADENOSYL L-METHIONINE (SAMe)

Homocysteine is an amino acid containing sulfur, and is a key component in major cellular pathways including remethylation to methionine, with B12 as a cofactor, prior to methionine's further metabolizing into S-adenosyl methionine (SAMe) with folate as a cofactor. SAMe serves as a major methyl donor during neurotransmitter synthesis, creation of membrane phospholipids, and metabolism of nucleic acids. High levels of homocysteine and low levels of folate have been linked to perinatal depression, as well as numerous problems during labor such as increased incidence of spontaneous abortions and low birth weight, preeclampsia, and placental abruption.[68,69]

VITAMINS B (FOLATE AND B12)

Vitamins B are essential for appropriate metabolism of homocysteine. Folate (vitamin B9) is an important cofactor for monoamine synthesis, reduction of homocysteine (along with B12 as a cofactor) and its derivative L-methylfolate slows down the degradation of tryptophan, which is a precursor for serotonin and melatonin synthesis. There are four transformation steps required to render folic acid a biologically available form of folate that can cross the blood-brain barrier to participate in the production of neurochemicals.

One of these metabolites, 5-MTHF or L-methylfolate, is required for the production of biopterin, a cofactor for neurotransmitter production, and of methionine/S-adenosylmethionine from homocysteine (with B12 as a cofactor), influencing the production and function of neurotransmitters, DNA, and enzymes. In pregnancy the requirement for folate increases 70% compared to nonpregnant and nonlactating women.[70] Genetic vulnerability to perinatal depression has been linked to maternal 5,10 methylene tetrahydrofolate (5MTHF) reductase polymorphism,[71,72] the essential enzyme for converting folate into its brain active form L-methylfolate and consequent inability of the body to synthesize L-methylfolate from folate found in foods (leafy greens, broccoli, sunflower seeds).

VITAMIN D

Vitamin D is a fat-soluble vitamin synthesized in skin as a response to UVB light. In order to be transformed into its biologically functional form, calcitriol, it has to go through two hydroxylation processes in the body. Vitamin D is present in a limited number of foods (eggs, fatty fish, fortified dairy, and beef liver), and its intake mostly depends on fortified foods or supplements. Vitamin D has multiple roles in a human body, including bone formation, suppression of inflammation, as well as modulation of cell growth. Additionally, animal studies demonstrated vitamin D's role on glucocorticoids is that it ultimately reduces and even inhibits the effects of increased glucocorticoids found in stress. Its deficiency is not uncommon in an urban population and is most pronounced among populations at risk, such as darker-skinned people and pregnant women. Despite some controversial findings in the literature, a deficiency in vitamin D has been linked to depressive symptoms in the general population, which can be attributed to its role in the hypothalamus and in synthesis of monoamines.[73,74] The recommended daily dose found in many preparations of multivitamins is usually not sufficient, particularly not for people living in the northern hemisphere. Perinatal depression has been linked to vitamin D deficiency as well, although studies are sparse and additional research is needed. One study conducted among pregnant African American women indicated that decreased levels in 25 hydroxy-vitamin D serum level (25-OH D3, routine indicator of vitamin D levels) in the first trimester were linked to depressive symptoms in the second trimester.[75] Furthermore, a birth cohort study completed in the Netherlands demonstrated a similar relationship between vitamin D deficiency and prenatal depression.[76] Postpartum levels of 25-OH D3 less than 32 ng/mL have been linked with depressive symptoms, yet findings are inconsistent.[77] Supplementation to achieve serum 1,25(OH)D levels above 40 ng/mL often requires more than the recommended dose of 400 IU daily, and in some cases up to 4000 IU daily is required.[78]

NEURONAL PLASTICITY AND BRAIN STRUCTURE CHANGES

Changes in several brain regions including the hippocampus, amygdala, and prefrontal cortex, have been linked to development of PPD in animal models. Additionally in depression the reward system operating via the mesolimbic dopaminergic system and connecting the ventral tegmentum area with the nucleus accumbens (NA) is disrupted. Neuroimaging studies done in women suffering from PPD demonstrated decreased response to reward stimuli via decreased activation of NA[79] and decreased responsiveness to their infant cry.[80] Exposure to chronic stress during pregnancy has been linked to development of PPD. These findings are supported by recent studies, done in rats, which demonstrated that gestational stress significantly changes morphology and neuronal connectives of NA,[81] potentially leading to symptoms of PPD.

PERINATAL DEPRESSION: DIAGNOSIS

In Pregnancy

Due to the overlapping of some depressive symptoms (changes in sleep habits, disturbance in appetite and decreased energy level, decreased sexual drive) with physiological changes frequently occurring during pregnancy, adequate recognition of depressive disorder in this reproductive phase may be challenging, yet is necessary. Additionally, women tend to hide negative feelings and thoughts occurring during this period as they blame themselves for experiences that are very different from the socially accepted standards and expectations linked to this period of women's lives. Thus careful approach and evaluation is essential. If a pregnant women reports one of the following problems, depressive disorder should be suspected: anhedonia or lack of pleasure in previously enjoyable situations (it is helpful to inquire about three activities the woman used to enjoy prior to being pregnant and find out how she feels about them at the time of the encounter with a health provider), hopelessness and helplessness, constant feeling of inadequacy and guilt, as well as self-destructive thoughts or suicidal tendencies.

In Postpartum

Postpartum depression frequently co-occurring with anxiety can start during pregnancy, and could last up to 12 months,[82] or alternatively starts within the first year after the delivery. Despite the fact that official DSM-V[83] criteria for perinatal depression require onset of depressive symptoms within 4 weeks from delivery (and ICD10 within 6 weeks of delivery), in many women symptoms tend to present a couple months later, often between 3 and 6 months postpartum.[5] It appears that women may have some symptoms of depressive disorder prior to being recognized or asking for help, yet they usually attribute most of those feelings to a new stage of their lives, and unless severely disabled and incapable of taking care of the newborn, they would not seek help immediately.

Postnatal mood disturbances can present in various forms. The most common one, for which we rarely see women in our offices, is called *postpartum blues* or *baby blues*. It is important to recognize that postpartum blues have been reported to occur in up to 85% of women in postpartum. Even though the strict criteria of postpartum blues has not been established, it is recognized as a transient and rather self-limited stage with emotional lability being a hallmark symptom, accompanied by dysphoric mood coupled with crying spells, disturbance of sleep and appetite, and irritability, all of which occur soon after the delivery. Symptoms are present in the first postpartum week, with the peak intensity between days 2–5 postpartum, and may be related to hormonal readjustments occurring at that time.[42,46] Most commonly postpartum blues symptoms stabilize by the end of 2 weeks after the delivery, only rarely progressing to PPD.

PPD is a severe mental health condition requiring timely recognition and treatment. Its reported prevalence varies greatly depending on definition criteria and the group studied. For example, a meta-analysis done by Gavin[5] showed a prevalence rate of 19.2%, whereas studies conducted in Italy and Spain[84] demonstrated lower prevalence ranging around 9%. The differences reported can be attributed to study designs, inclusion criteria, and control for other comorbidities.

Clinical presentation of depressive disorder in postpartum tends to be somewhat specific and includes

- Sleep disturbance such as an inability to sleep even if the child is sleeping and other circumstances are conducive to her resting
- Appetite disturbance/decrease
- Feelings of guilt and inadequacy especially related to parenting
- Specific worry/ruminations, often related to her newborn
- Flat mood and anhedonia
- Intrusive thoughts of harm to self and the baby

Anxiety symptoms coupled with intrusive thoughts and ruminations with at times aggressive themes are quite common in perinatal depression and since very disturbing are often a leading cause for seeking help.[85,86] Women tend to report experiencing ego dystonic obsessional intrusive thoughts and/or images related to harming the baby.[87–89] Ego dystonic means that thoughts are unwanted, yet the woman often fluctuates between believing and not believing those intrusions, and her capability to resist them. These findings may be attributed to additional obligations, fatigue, and at times issues with body image, all contributing to feeling overwhelmed. Unless a woman is actively psychotic, thus not having insight into wrongfulness of those thoughts, these women, for the most part, do not harm their babies. However postpartum depression, when severe and untreated, can lead to suicide as well as infanticide.[90–92] Those tendencies are usually described as altruistic in nonpsychotic moms, meaning that a woman, while feeling so miserable, inadequate, and not wishing to continue to live, does not want to abandon her baby.[93]

Interestingly, symptom presentation has been reported to be more severe than in depression unrelated to peripartum.[94] While suffering immensely, these women usually try to hide their symptoms from family and surrounding people due to fear of humiliation. If a woman experiences intrusive thoughts of harming the child and she is not educated that those can occur even in the absence of significant psychopathology, she will continue to suffer silently in fear that if she speaks out and seeks help, her baby may be taken away from her. Yet, lack of appropriate education about feelings and thoughts that may even be considered within a normal range, as well as presenting treatment options when needed in a timely manner leave these women alone in their misery and at times this leads to severe consequences. Thus it is essential that all health professionals who are in contact with perinatal women leave room for open conversation about worries and concerns that they may have, provide adequate education, and discuss treatment options when needed. To better identify women that may be at risk, screening methods are implemented and in several states in the United States and in European countries are required by law.

SCREENING

To appropriately identify women who may be at risk for development of PPD, the American College of Obstetrics and Gynecology (ACOG) strongly recommends perinatal depression screening.[12] To facilitate appropriate detection of perinatal depression, several screening tools have been validated and are widely used throughout many countries worldwide.

The Edinburgh Postnatal Depression Scale (EPDS) is translated in over 30 languages and is used around the globe, whereas The Patient Health Questionnaire (PHQ9) which was created by Pfizer, is often used in U.S. busy primary care settings as well as for research purposes. EPDS is a 10-item self-reported questionnaire that was specifically designed for the peripartum population. It is easy to score, and results above 10 (and/or a positive response to question number 10 which addresses presence of suicidal ideation) warrant further, more detailed assessment by a mental health provider. EPDS should be used several times during peripartum. Ideally, the initial assessment should be done at some point during pregnancy, and two other screenings in postpartum with the last one preferably being done at least 3 months postpartum.

PHQ9 is a nine-item self-reported questionnaire used to assess depression in the general population, and is validated in the peripartum population. Scores above 5 should open a discussion about mood changes with the clinician who sees the woman at the time of screening, and scores above 10 warrant further assessment by a mental health provider.

Despite usefulness of those tools, screening per se cannot substitute for diagnosis and does not always lead to adequate referrals, or to necessarily improved treatment outcomes,[95,96] leaving a huge void and need for improvement. Therefore it is imperative to educate all health professionals encountering the perinatal patient population about PPD symptoms and presentation and how to normalize some symptoms, and encourage women to get professional help when needed, as well as inform women and ideally another family member about available treatments.

Upon detecting positive screening, and referring the patient for further evaluation and potential treatment, it is also important to rule out physical causes that may lead to depressive and anxiety symptoms in peripartum. As was previously discussed in detail, disruption of some hormone levels, as well as nutrient deficiencies and inflammation processes could be responsible for symptom presentation and as such need to be corrected. Therefore once depressive and anxiety symptoms are detected, further assessment geared toward identifying potential deficits should be conducted in order to optimize treatment approaches. These are suggested tests that should be incorporated in the evaluation of PPD:

- Thyroid panel (TSH, free T3, free T4, and thyroid antibodies)
- Vitamin D 25OH level
- Folic acid level
- Vitamin B12 level
- Fasting glucose and HbA1C levels
- hsCRP
- Homocysteine
- CBC with iron panel
- Methylenetetrahydrofolate reductase (MTHFR)

APPROACHES TO TREATMENT SCREENING

Perinatal psychopathology, when present, requires adequate treatment. ACOG recommends psychotherapy to be the initial mode of treatment for mild and moderate perinatal depression. However, more severe presentations of PPD have prompted treatment interventions which include psychopharmacology, a point of debate secondary to sparse data on safety and efficacy of medication interventions in this specific population as well as sparse information on lactation transfer of parent drugs and metabolites. Considering the aforementioned etiological theories, reversal of underlying pathology is a sensible approach.

PSYCHOTHERAPY

The two well-studied and recognized treatment approaches for treatment of PPD are cognitive behavioral therapy (CBT) and interpersonal therapy (IPT).[97-99] Each of these deals with specific issues that may arise in that period of a woman's life. The CBT approach mainly deals with addressing thinking patterns and consequent behaviors that then trigger depressive and anxious emotional reactions. On the other hand, IPT is based on the postulation that issues in relationships that are present in the woman's life could trigger depression, and treatment addresses those. Besides those two evidence-based and accepted treatment approaches for the perinatal population, multiple other psychotherapy modalities have been used with great success, such as mindfulness-based approaches such as dialectical behavioral therapy (DBT), acceptance and commitment therapy (ACT), and mindfulness-based cognitive therapy, as well as group and couples therapy, and therapies geared toward the mother-infant dyad.

PSYCHOPHARMACOLOGY

There is a constant debate about the level of safety for use of antidepressant medication during pregnancy and lactation. The U.S. Food and Drug Administration (FDA) nomenclature used until recently categorized medication use in pregnancy and lactation by labeling them A–D. In November 2014, that nomenclature was removed and a new Pregnancy and Lactation Labeling Rule (PLLR) has been published.[100] This comprehensive document should allow clinicians to create treatment decisions approaching each individual separately while being guided by evidence-based data.

Despite the fact that, due to ethical reasons, double-blind controlled studies cannot be conducted in this patient population, there are numerous reported exposures and studies looking at potential teratogenicity of this medication group concluding that there is no replicable teratogenicity associated with any SSRI or SNRI.[101] Some studies suggest an association between use of SSRIs after 20 weeks of gestation, and pulmonary hypertension in newborns, however those data are inconclusive. Last, postnatal adaptation syndrome (PNAS), a transient, self-limiting occurrence commonly accompanied by increased crying, occasional muscle twitches, decreased feeding and sleep, and in rare cases seizure-like activities has been reported in approximately 30% of infants exposed to SSRIs in pregnancy. Despite the relatively reassuring data related to use of antidepressants in peripartum, the caution is present, and the American Academy of Pediatrics recommends using the lowest effective dose in this patient population.[102]

It is also probable that the risks assessed in the literature are reflective of gross outcomes rather than the impact of epigenetic exposures. These would only be appropriately assessed through evaluation of individual biochemical risk factors and longitudinal outcomes of the offspring, including neurodevelopment, controlling for additional exposures.

There are no specific antidepressants "recommended" for women in peripartum. Rather risks and benefits for each patient based on individual history, presenting symptoms, previous medication exposure and response, as well as personal preference should be carefully considered in order for the most appropriate medication and treatment approach to be suggested. All antidepressant medications are lipophilic and as such cross the placental barrier, meaning that after the first 2 gestational weeks (time needed for placenta to be formed) all medications cross into fetal tissue. One cannot, with any certainty, warrant medication "safety" during pregnancy and lactation, but can, however, present existing data from the literature supported by the fact that to date no teratogenicity has been linked to this medication group. As such, several available antidepressants could be mentioned here as probably used more frequently in this patient population, simply because more data have been available. Thus, based on available data, exposure to nortriptyline, sertraline, and citalopram in utero were not found to have any morphological or behavioral sequelae. If antidepressant administration starts in postpartum and the woman is breastfeeding, passage of nortriptyline, sertraline, or paroxetine into breastmilk is negligible, and they are thus convenient treatment options for lactating mothers. However, regardless of the proposed antidepressant for a particular patient, it is important to remember several key factors:

- The FDA classification for pregnancy and lactation that was guiding practitioners to this date often led to wrong conclusions; the new FDA classification is more promising and will allow the practitioner a better approach while prescribing antidepressants in peripartum.
- Before prescribing any antidepressant medication during pregnancy and lactation, it is essential to educate the woman and her partner if possible, about up-to-date findings reported in the literature, explain some of the information reported by the mass media, and make a treatment plan through dialogue while discussing risks versus benefits.
- In a woman with a history of depressive disorder who becomes pregnant, one should never stop medication abruptly; rather engage a mindful effort at identifying the minimal effective dose or slowly taper the medication administration.
- Pregnancy is not a good time to experiment with new medication only because one would like to place a patient on a medication that is considered "safer." All antidepressant medications enter fetal tissues via the placenta, and no antidepressant medication has been linked to teratogenicity so far.
- Polypharmacy always poses greater risks than a single medication prescribed at one time, thus this should be avoided in peripartum whenever possible.

HORMONAL REPLACEMENT

Potential use of a hormonal preparation in peripartum has been studied for many decades,[103–105] indirectly suggesting that reproductive hormone levels may be responsible for perinatal psychopathology. Additionally, in several studies[106,107] administration of estrogen preparations right after delivery and slowly tapering them off supported the "estrogen withdrawal theory," further pointing out that in a subset of women abrupt change in reproductive hormonal levels could lead to psychopathology in peripartum. Hormonal replacement has been studied by using various estrogen preparations. 17-Beta estradiol, a bioidentical estrogen that highly resembles naturally produced hormone and penetrates the blood-brain barrier well, was found to be the most suitable option. Some studies showed that the 17-beta estradiol patch (100–200 mg/day) applied for up to 6 months postpartum can both prevent the onset and improve already existing PPD symptoms. This approach is contraindicated in women with histories of uterine or breast cancer, as well those that have history of thromboembolic disease. Estradiol administration always has to be paired with a progesterone preparation (available in various forms). One important negative side-effect of hormonal replacement in the postpartum population is that progesterone may decrease milk production, thus making breastfeeding more challenging.

Unfortunately, concerns about potential detrimental effects of hormonal replacement on the endometrium and cardiovascular system have impaired research into hormonal applications for PPD. Interdisciplinary clinics of gynecology and psychiatry would be essential in further studying and implementing this avenue of treatment.

OTHER TREATMENT APPROACHES

SUPPLEMENTS PUFA/OMEGA 3 FA

Omega 3 FA has been extensively studied as a potential treatment for depression, and despite some contradictory results related to variable study populations, ratios of EPA to DHA, as well as the dosages used in those studies, in 2006, the American Psychiatric Association (APA) recommended using PUFA for supplementation during the treatment of depression.[108] Furthermore, the benefits of omega 3 FA have established benefit in obstetrical outcomes and infant health.[109,110] To optimize pregnancy and infant health, one to two servings of oily fish weekly or 200 mg of DHA daily has been recommended. Based on currently available randomized control trials in perinatal depression, the recommended dose for supplementation is 1 g of EPA plus DHA daily.[111] Omega 3 FA are available in various forms, and recommended doses are capsules 2000 mg/day, liquids (2 tbsp/day), or smoothie-type liquid (2 tsp/daily).

VITAMINS B FOLATE

Folate (vitamin B9) found in leafy greens, lentils, broccoli, and sunflower seeds is an important cofactor in the synthesis of monoamines, reduction of homocysteine, and slowing of brain breakdown of tryptophan. The relationship between folate and depression has been studied, and low serum levels were linked to elevated homocysteine, increased depression incidence, and poor treatment response.[112] Additionally augmentation with folate led to increased likelihood of remission.[113]

There are four transformation steps required to render folic acid a biologically available form of folate that can cross the blood-brain barrier to participate in the production of neurochemicals. Recent literature has focused on the role of genetic polymorphism for MTHFR in the metabolism of folate and associations with depressive illness.[114] Bioavailability of folate and its metabolites can theoretically impact homocysteine and neurotransmitter levels as well as global DNA methylation, including placental methylation. Maternal MTHFR polymorphisms are associated with antenatal depression and may influence the fetal programming of serotonin transporter methylation and future functioning.[72] A recent study in the postpartum population demonstrated the benefit of folic acid supplementation during pregnancy for women with low conversion abilities.[71] Bypassing this enzymatic conversion with supplementation of bioactive folate appears to be a potentially important treatment option. Thus it is important to assess individual risk factors in terms of dietary/supplement intake in the first trimester and biomarkers for methylation.

VITAMIN B12

The World Health Organization (WHO) recommends that pregnant women increase their B12 vitamin intake three times (from 0.4 mcg/day to 1.4 mcg/day) in order to compensate for metabolic rate changes during that time.[70]

SAME

Administration of SAMe has been recognized as efficient and is at times used in the treatment of depression.[115,116] Dosing usually starts at 400 mg daily and could gradually be increased to 1600 mg and even 2400 mg daily. SAMe has been used to treat cholestasis in pregnancy, and no adverse effects of its use have been reported. Data related to use of SAMe in PPD are limited, although in one study SAMe was used in postpartum at 1600 mg for a month, and significant reduction of PPD symptoms was recorded.[117] Further investigation of usefulness of SAMe supplementation in the perinatal population is needed.

VITAMIN D

The standard recommendation for vitamin D intake for both pregnancy and lactation are 400 IU/day and 600 IU/day, respectively, based on the evidence that needs do not increase in pregnancy or lactation.[118] Without clear evidence of the beneficial role of vitamin D in perinatal depression, it has been recommended, more as a preventive measure, that the daily intake be 1000 mg or higher (depending on levels) of vitamin D in the diet.[119]

BRIGHT LIGHT

There are several theories as to why exposure to bright light can be beneficial in perinatal depression. It has been shown that lack of light, or exposure to dim light to which women can be increasingly exposed in peripartum, led to depletion of tryptophan which is the main precursor for synthesis of serotonin. In addition, bright light exposure has been postulated to alter estrogen levels in peripartum, indirectly affecting serotonin synthesis. Furthermore, sleep disturbance and fatigue commonly occurring in peripartum could be altered by using bright light, consequently improving mood.

In available studies examining the effect of UV light on depression in peripartum, the lamp strength used was of either 7000 or 10,000 lux and exposures lasted anywhere between 30 and 60 minutes during the morning hours.[120–123] Unfortunately, the efficacy of light therapy in treatment of PPD showed mixed results, leaving this method as a potentially effective but not proven therapeutic modality for this patient population. However, due to growing efficacy, some practitioners recommend initial dosing of 30 minutes beginning within 10 minutes of awakening.[124]

ACUPUNCTURE

In Asian cultures maintenance of the body energy has been considered the main component of optimal health. Blockage of some of those energy paths results in illness. Existing data on both electroacupuncture and noninvasive sham acupuncture in perinatal depression are limiting. Couple studies suggest potential benefits of acupuncture treatment for depression during pregnancy[125,126] as well as postpartum,[127] but further systematic research is essential to determine its efficacy.

PREVENTION OF PERINATAL DEPRESSION

It is believed that perinatal depression leaves significant room for application of preventive methods. Before even examining specific preventive approaches, there are several steps that each health practitioner working with a woman in peripartum could take in order to educate, support, and guide her through that life stage. It is essential to educate women about the necessity of sleep. Lack of sleep or insomnia appears to be a primary trigger of all peripartum mental health illness. New moms should sleep when the baby sleeps. Additionally women in postpartum should be encouraged to delegate tasks even if it is with the help of visiting friends.

The importance of nutrition is significant, and poor nutrition has been demonstrated to have effect sizes as significant as maternal depression for offspring's mental health. The Norwegian Mother and Child Cohort Study examined mothers during pregnancy and again when children were 6 months, 18 months, 3 years, and 5 years old. It was determined that higher scores on an unhealthy dietary pattern during pregnancy predicted externalizing problems among children. A similar trend was observed when the diet of the children in the postnatal period was explored; unhealthy diets predicted higher levels of both internalizing and externalizing problems in children.[128]

In many ways, eating a whole-food, unprocessed, unpackaged, organic diet may be the most robust form of prevention available to us. From a psychosocial perspective, postpartum women tend to be guided by some unwritten social rules where terms such as should, never, and always dominate. It is essential to teach women to let go of those parameters, as most things occur in a specific way for each of them. And last, a new mom should be reminded that doing things for herself, and having her own little pleasures is not just acceptable but needed for her well-being. All practitioners working with women in the perinatal period should, at some point, share the above general messages with their patients. Besides necessary psychoeducation, some more specific approaches for prevention of perinatal depressive illness have been studied.

While psychotherapy has been widely used for treatment of perinatal depression, several studies were looking into potential benefits of psychotherapy in prevention of PPD.[129,130] Adequate social support in postpartum is an instrumental factor for a woman's physical and emotional well-being after childbirth, and consequently lack of it can play a significant role in the onset of PPD.[131] Among different relationships in a woman's life, it appears that the relationship with her partner and the closeness that exists between the two is inversely related to incidence of PPD symptoms.[132–134]

Therefore educating the couple and applying some IPT skills in order to improve the relationship may be one of the essential approaches in prevention of PPD.

CONCLUSION

Perinatal depression is a complex and potentially serious mental health condition. Its etiology is highly multifactorial combining genetic predisposition with various psychosocial, neuroendocrine, psychoimmunological, nutritional, and other factors. Some of the environmental as well as social factors could be modified and potentially either prevent, or at least reduce symptom severity. Additionally, treatment approaches for perinatal depression should closely follow all potential etiological paths, carefully addressing and applying different available techniques in order to assist this patient population. Having said that, it is important to add that many of the mentioned treatment approaches, and some additional ones that have been mentioned in the literature need additional research and observation, so that efficacy as well as safety are better determined.

REFERENCES

1. The World Health Organization. Depression: A Global Public Health Concern. 2012. Available at: http://www.who.int/mental_health/management/depression/who_paper_depression_wfmh_2012.pdf
2. Goldman, L.S., Nielsen, N.H., and Champion, H.C. 1999. Awareness, diagnosis, and treatment of depression. *J Gen Intern Med* 14(9): 569–580.
3. Weissman, M.M., Wickramaratne, P., Nomura, Y., Warner, V., Pilowsky, D., and Verdeli, H. 2006. Offspring of depressed parents: 20 years later. *Am J Psychiatry* 163(6): 1001–1008.
4. Eaton, N.R., Keyes, K.M., Krueger, R.F. et al. 2012. An invariant dimensional liability model of gender differences in mental disorder prevalence: Evidence from a national sample. *J Abnorm Psychol* 121(1): 282–288.
5. Gavin, N.I., Gaynes, B.N., Lohr, K.N., Meltzer-Brody, S., Gartlehner, G., and Swinson, T. 2005. Perinatal depression: A systematic review of prevalence and incidence. *Obstetr Gynecol* 106(5 Pt 1): 1071–1083.
6. O'Hara, M.W. and Swain, A.M. 1996. Rates and risk of postpartum depression—A meta-analysis. *Int Rev Psychiatry* 8(1): 37–54.
7. Vesga-Lopez, O., Blanco, C., Keyes, K., Olfson, M., Grant, B.F., and Hasin, D.S. 2008. Psychiatric disorders in pregnant and postpartum women in the United States. *Arch Gen Psychiatry* 65(7): 805–815.
8. Oates, M. 2003. Perinatal psychiatric disorders: A leading cause of maternal morbidity and mortality. *Br Med Bull* 67: 219–229.
9. Chang, J., Berg, C.J., Saltzman, L.E., and Herndon, J. 2005. Homicide: A leading cause of injury deaths among pregnant and postpartum women in the United States, 1991–1999. *Am J Public Health* 95(3): 471–477.
10. Demand, N.H. 1994. *Birth, Death, and Motherhood in Classical Greece.* Baltimore, MD: Johns Hopkins University Press.
11. Marcé, LV. Treatise on madness in pregnant women, in women who have recently given birth, and in wet nurses, and medical/legal considerations on this subject. [Traité de la folie des femmes enceintes des nouvelles accouchées et des nourrices et considérations médico-légales qui se rattachent à ce sujet] (Paris: JB Baillière et fils, 1858), 394.

12. American College of Obstetricians and Gynecologists. Committee on Obstetric Practice. 2010. Committee opinion No. 453: Screening for depression during and after pregnancy. *Obstetr Gynecol* 115(2 Pt 1): 394–395.

13. Bowen, A. and Muhajarine, N. 2006. Antenatal depression. *Can Nurse* 102(9): 26–30.

14. Davis, E.P. and Sandman, C.A. 2010. The timing of prenatal exposure to maternal cortisol and psychosocial stress is associated with human infant cognitive development. *Child Dev* 81(1): 131–148.

15. Britton, J.R. 2011. Infant temperament and maternal anxiety and depressed mood in the early postpartum period. *Women Health* 51(1): 55–71.

16. Forman, D.R., O'Hara, M.W., Stuart, S., Gorman, L.L., Larsen, K.E., and Coy, K.C. 2007. Effective treatment for postpartum depression is not sufficient to improve the developing mother-child relationship. *Dev Psychopathol* 19(2): 585–602.

17. Deave, T., Heron, J., Evans, J., and Emond, A. 2008. The impact of maternal depression in pregnancy on early child development. *BJOG* 115(8): 1043–1051.

18. Beebe, B., Jaffe, J., Buck, K. et al. 2008. Six-week postpartum maternal depressive symptoms and 4-month mother–infant self- and interactive contingency. *Infant Ment Health J* 29(5): 442–471.

19. Murray, L., Cooper, P.J., Wilson, A., and Romaniuk, H. 2003. Controlled trial of the short- and long-term effect of psychological treatment of post-partum depression: 2. Impact on the mother-child relationship and child outcome. *Br J Psychiatry* 182: 420–427.

20. Pawlby, S., Hay, D.F., Sharp, D., Waters, C.S., and O'Keane, V. 2009. Antenatal depression predicts depression in adolescent offspring: Prospective longitudinal community-based study. *J Affect Disord* 113(3): 236–243.

21. Lancaster, C.A., Gold, K.J., Flynn, H.A., Yoo, H., Marcus, S.M., and Davis, M.M. 2010. Risk factors for depressive symptoms during pregnancy: A systematic review. *Am J Obstetr Gynecol* 202(1): 5–14.

22. Robertson, E., Grace, S., Wallington, T., and Stewart, D.E. 2004. Antenatal risk factors for postpartum depression: A synthesis of recent literature. *Gen Hospital Psychiatry* 26(4): 289–295.

23. O'Hara, M.W. and McCabe, J.E. Postpartum depression: Current status and future directions. *Ann Rev Clin Psychol* 9 2013: 379–407.

24. Wile, J. and Arechiga, M. 1999. Sociocultural aspects of postpartum depression. In *Postpartum Mood Disorders*, Ed. L.J. Miller. Washington, DC: American Psychiatric Press, pp. 83–98.

25. Negron, R., Martin, A., Almog, M., Balbierz, A., and Howell, E.A. 2013. Social support during the postpartum period: Mothers' views on needs, expectations, and mobilization of support. *Matern Child Health J* 17(4): 616–623.

26. Corwin, E.J., Johnston, N., and Pugh, L. 2008. Symptoms of postpartum depression associated with elevated levels of interleukin-1 beta during the first month postpartum. *Biol Res Nurs* 10(2): 128–133.

27. Groer, M.W. and Morgan, K. 2007. Immune, health and endocrine characteristics of depressed postpartum mothers. *Psychoneuroendocrinology* 32(2): 133–139.

28. Maes, M., Lin, A.H., Ombelet, W. et al. 2000. Immune activation in the early puerperium is related to postpartum anxiety and depressive symptoms. *Psychoneuroendocrinology* 25(2): 121–137.

29. Ressler, K.J. and Nemeroff, C.B. 2000. Role of serotonergic and noradrenergic systems in the pathophysiology of depression and anxiety disorders. *Depression Anxiety* 12(Suppl 1): 2–19.

30. Antoniou, M., Habib, M.E.M., Howard, C.V. et al. 2012. Teratogenic effects of glyphosate-based herbicides: Divergence of regulatory decisions from scientific evidence. *J Environ Analyt Toxicol* S4: 006. doi:10.4172/2161-0525.

31. Aris, A. and Leblanc, S. 2011. Maternal and fetal exposure to pesticides associated to genetically modified foods in eastern townships of Quebec, Canada. *Reprod Toxicol* 31(4): 528–533.

32. Samsel, A. and Seneff, S. 2013. Glyphosate's suppression of cytochrome P450 enzymes and amino acid biosynthesis by the gut microbiome: Pathways to modern diseases. *Entropy* 15(4): 1416–1463.

33. Lavezzi, A.M., Cappiello, A., Pusiol, T., Corna, M.F., Termopoli, V., and Matturri, L. 2015. Pesticide exposure during pregnancy, like nicotine, affects the brainstem alpha7 nicotinic acetylcholine receptor expression, increasing the risk of sudden unexplained perinatal death. *J Neurol Sci* 348(1–2): 94–100. doi: 10.1016/j.jns.2014.11.014. Epub: November 18, 2014.

34. Anway, M.D., Cupp, A.S., Uzumcu, M., and Skinner, M.K. 2005. Epigenetic transgenerational actions of endocrine disruptors and male fertility. *Science* 308(5727): 1466–1469.

35. Lindstrom, L.H., Nyberg, F., Terenius, L. et al. 1984. CSF and plasma beta-casomorphin-like opioid peptides in postpartum psychosis. *Am J Psychiatry* 141(9): 1059–1066.

36. Karlsson, H., Blomstrom, A., Wicks, S., Yang, S., Yolken, R.H., and Dalman, C. 2012. Maternal antibodies to dietary antigens and risk for nonaffective psychosis in offspring. *Am J Psychiatry* 169(6): 625–632.

37. Thomson, M. 2013. The physiological roles of placental corticotropin releasing hormone in pregnancy and childbirth. *J Physiol Biochem* 69(3): 559–573.
38. Yim, I.S., Glynn, L.M., Dunkel-Schetter, C., Hobel, C.J., Chicz-DeMet, A., and Sandman, C.A. 2009. Risk of postpartum depressive symptoms with elevated corticotropin-releasing hormone in human pregnancy. *Arch Gen Psychiatry* 66(2): 162–169.
39. Greenwood, J. and Parker, G. 1984. The dexamethasone suppression test in the puerperium. *ANZ J Psychiatry* 18(3): 282–284.
40. Wisner, K.L. and Stowe, Z.N. 1997. Psychobiology of postpartum mood disorders. *Semin Reprod Endocrinol* 15(1): 77–89.
41. Magiakou, M.A., Mastorakos, G., Rabin, D., Dubbert, B., Gold, P.W., and Chrousos, G.P. 1996. Hypothalamic corticotropin-releasing hormone suppression during the postpartum period: Implications for the increase in psychiatric manifestations at this time. *J Clin Endocrinol Metab* 81(5): 1912–1917.
42. Bloch, M., Daly, R.C., and Rubinow, D.R. 2003. Endocrine factors in the etiology of postpartum depression. *Compr Psychiatry* 44(3): 234–246.
43. Labad, J., Vilella, E., Reynolds, R.M. et al. 2011. Increased morning adrenocorticotrophin hormone (Acth) levels in women with postpartum thoughts of harming the infant. *Psychoneuroendocrinology* 36(6): 924–928.
44. Zonana, J. and Gorman, J.M. 2005. The neurobiology of postpartum depression. *CNS Spectrums* 10(10): 792–799, 805.
45. Tulchinsky, D., Hobel, C.J., Yeager, E., and Marshall, J.R. 1972. Plasma estrone, estradiol, estriol, progesterone, and 17-hydroxyprogesterone in human pregnancy. I. normal pregnancy. *Am J Obstetr Gynecol* 112(8): 1095–1100.
46. Glover, V. and Kammerer, M. 2004. The biology and pathophysiology of peripartum psychiatric disorders. *Primary Psychiatry* 11(3): 37–41.
47. Workman, J.L., Barha, C.K., and Galea, L.A.M. 2012. Endocrine substrates of cognitive and affective changes during pregnancy and postpartum. *Behav Neurosci* 126(1): 54–72.
48. Bloch, M., Schmidt, P.J., Danaceau, M., Murphy, J., Nieman, L., and Rubinow, D.R. 2000. Effects of gonadal steroids in women with a history of postpartum depression. *Am J Psychiatry* 157(6): 924–930.
49. Sacher, J., Wilson, A.A., Houle, S. et al. 2010. Elevated brain monoamine oxidase a binding in the early postpartum period. *Arch Gen Psychiatry* 67(5): 468–474.
50. Pedersen, C.A., Johnson, J.L., Silva, S. et al. 2007. Antenatal thyroid correlates of postpartum depression. *Psychoneuroendocrinology* 32(3): 235–245.
51. Bergink, V., Kushner, S.A., Pop, V. et al. 2011. Prevalence of autoimmune thyroid dysfunction in postpartum psychosis. *Br J Psychiatry* 198(4): 264–268.
52. Carle, A., Pedersen, I.B., Knudsen, N. et al. 2014. Development of autoimmune overt hypothyroidism is highly associated with live births and induced abortions but only in premenopausal women. *J Clin Endocrinol Metab* 99(6): 2241–2249.
53. Groer, M.W. and Vaughan, J.H. 2013. Positive thyroid peroxidase antibody titer is associated with dysphoric moods during pregnancy and postpartum. *J Obstetr Gynecol Neonatal Nurs* 42(1): E26–E32.
54. Le Donne, M., Settineri, S., and Benvenga, S. 2012. Early pospartum alexithymia and risk for depression: Relationship with serum thyrotropin, free thyroid hormones and thyroid autoantibodies. *Psychoneuroendocrinology* 37(4): 519–533.
55. Taveras, E.M., Capra, A.M., Braveman, P.A., Jensvold, N.G., Escobar, G.J., and Lieu, T.A. 2003. Clinician support and psychosocial risk factors associated with breastfeeding discontinuation. *Pediatrics* 112(1 Pt 1): 108–115.
56. Chaudron, L.H., Klein, M.H., Remington, P., Palta, M., Allen, C., and Essex, M.J. 2001. Predictors, prodromes and incidence of postpartum depression. *J Psychosom Obstetr Gynaecol* 22(2): 103–112.
57. Stuebe, A.M., Grewen, K., Pedersen, C.A., Propper, C., and Meltzer-Brody, S. 2012. Failed lactation and perinatal depression: Common problems with shared neuroendocrine mechanisms? *J Women's Health* 21(3): 264–272.
58. Watkins, S., Meltzer-Brody, S., Zolnoun, D., and Stuebe, A.M. 2011. Early breastfeeding experiences and postpartum depression. *Obstetr Gynecol* 118(2 Pt 1): 214–221.
59. Stuebe, A.M., Grewen, K., and Meltzer-Brody, S. 2013. Association between maternal mood and oxytocin response to breastfeeding. *J Women's Health* 22(4): 352–361.
60. Nephew, B.C. and Bridges, R.S. 2011. Effects of chronic social stress during lactation on maternal behavior and growth in rats. *Stress* 14(6): 677–684.

61. Giddens, J.B., Krug, S.K., Tsang, R.C., Guo, S., Miodovnik, M., and Prada, J.A. 2000. Pregnant adolescent and adult women have similarly low intakes of selected nutrients. *J Am Diet Assoc* 100(11): 1334–1340.

62. Sontrop, J. and Campbell, M.K. 2006. Omega-3 polyunsaturated fatty acids and depression: A review of the evidence and a methodological critique. *Prevent Med* 42(1): 4–13.

63. Su, K.-P. 2009. Biological mechanism of antidepressant effect of omega-3 fatty acids: How does fish oil act as a "Mind-Body Interface?" *Neurosignals* 17(2): 144–152.

64. Hibbeln, J.R. and Salem, N. Jr. 1995. Dietary polyunsaturated fatty acids and depression: When cholesterol does not satisfy. *Am J Clin Nutr* 62(1): 1–9.

65. Bourre, J.M. 2005. Dietary omega-3 fatty acids and psychiatry: Mood, behaviour, stress, depression, dementia and aging. *J Nutr Health Aging* 9(1): 31–38.

66. Klerman, G.L. and Weissman, M.M. 1989. Increasing rates of depression. *JAMA* 261(15): 2229–2235.

67. Hornstra, G., Al, M.D., van Houwelingen, A.C., and Foreman-van Drongelen, M.M. 1995. Essential fatty acids in pregnancy and early human development. *Eur J Obstetr Gynecol Reprod Biol* 61(1): 57–62.

68. Ray, J.G. and Laskin, C.A. 1999. Folic acid and Homocyst(E)Ine metabolic defects and the risk of placental abruption, pre-eclampsia and spontaneous pregnancy loss: A systematic review. *Placenta* 20(7): 519–529.

69. Picciano, M.F. 2003. Pregnancy and lactation: Physiological adjustments, nutritional requirements and the role of dietary supplements. *J Nutr* 133(6): 1997S–2002S.

70. Allen, L.H. 1994. Vitamin B12 metabolism and status during pregnancy, lactation and infancy. *Adv Exp Med Biol* 352: 173–186.

71. Lewis, S.J., Araya, R., Leary, S., Smith, G.D., and Ness, A. 2012. Folic acid supplementation during pregnancy may protect against depression 21 months after pregnancy, an effect modified by Mthfr C677t genotype. *Eur J Clin Nutr* 66(1): 97–103.

72. Devlin, A.M., Brain, U., Austin, J., and Oberlander, T.F. 2010. Prenatal exposure to maternal depressed mood and the MTHFR C677t variant affect SLC6A4 methylation in infants at birth. *PLoS One* 5(8): e12201.

73. Parker, G. and Brotchie, H. 2011. "D" for depression: Any role for vitamin D? "Food for Thought" Ii. *Acta Psychiatr Scand* 124(4): 243–249.

74. Bertone-Johnson, E.R. 2009. Vitamin D and the occurrence of depression: Causal association or circumstantial evidence? *Nutr Rev* 67(8): 481–492.

75. Cassidy-Bushrow, A.E., Peters, R.M., Johnson, D.A., Li, J., and Rao, D.S. 2012. Vitamin D nutritional status and antenatal depressive symptoms in African American women. *J Women's Health* 21(11): 1189–1195.

76. Brandenbarg, J., Vrijkotte, T.G.M., Goedhart, G., and van Eijsden, M. 2012. Maternal early-pregnancy vitamin D status is associated with maternal depressive symptoms in the Amsterdam born children and their development cohort. *Psychosom Med* 74(7): 751–757.

77. Murphy, P.K., Mueller, M., Hulsey, T.C., Ebeling, M.D., and Wagner, C.L. 2010. An exploratory study of postpartum depression and vitamin D. *J Am Psychiatr Nurses Assoc* 16(3): 170–177.

78. Wagner, C.L., Taylor, S.N., Johnson, D.D., and Hollis, B.W. 2012. The role of vitamin D in pregnancy and lactation: Emerging concepts. *Women's Health* 8(3): 323–340.

79. Moses-Kolko, E.L., Fraser, D., Wisner, K.L. et al. 2011. Rapid habituation of ventral striatal response to reward receipt in postpartum depression. *Biol Psychiatry* 70(4): 395–399.

80. Laurent, H.K. and Ablow, J.C. 2012. A cry in the dark: Depressed mothers show reduced neural activation to their own infant's cry. *Soc Cogn Affect Neurosci* 7(2): 125–134.

81. Haim, A., Sherer, M., and Leuner, B. 2014. Gestational stress induces persistent depressive-like behavior and structural modifications within the postpartum nucleus accumbens. *Eur J Neurosci* 40(12): 3766–3773.

82. Agency for Healthcare Research and Quality. Efficacy and Safety of Screening for Postpartum Depression. 2013. Available at: http://effectivehealthcare.ahrq.gov/ehc/products/379/1437/postpartum-screening-report-130409.pdf

83. American Psychiatric Association (APA). 2013. *Diagnostic and Statistical Manual of Mental Disorders: DSM-5*. Washington, DC: APA.

84. Navarro, P., Garcia-Esteve, L., Ascaso, C., Aguado, J., Gelabert, E., and Martin-Santos, R. 2008. Non-psychotic psychiatric disorders after childbirth: Prevalence and comorbidity in a community sample. *J Affect Disord* 109(1–2): 171–176.

85. Abramowitz, J.S., Meltzer-Brody, S., Leserman, J. et al. 2010. Obsessional thoughts and compulsive behaviors in a sample of women with postpartum mood symptoms. *Arch Women's Ment Health* 13(6): 523–530.

86. Chaudron, L.H. and Nirodi, N. 2010. The obsessive-compulsive spectrum in the perinatal period: A prospective pilot study. *Arch Women's Ment Health* 13(5): 403–410.

87. Jennings, K.D., Ross, S., Popper, S., and Elmore, M. 1999. Thoughts of harming infants in depressed and nondepressed mothers. *J Affect Disord* 54(1–2): 21–28.

88. Abramowitz, J.S., Schwartz, S.A., Moore, K.M., and Luenzmann, K.R. 2003. Obsessive-compulsive symptoms in pregnancy and the puerperium: A review of the literature. *J Anxiety Disord* 17(4): 461–478.

89. Zambaldi, C.F., Cantilino, A., Montenegro, A.C., Paes, J.A., Cesar de Albuquerque, T.L., and Sougey, E.B. 2009. Postpartum obsessive-compulsive disorder: Prevalence and clinical characteristics. *Compr Psychiatry* 50(6): 503–509.

90. Murray, L. and Stein, A. 1989 The effects of postnatal depression on the infant. *Bailliere's Clin Obstetr Gynaecol* 3(4): 921–933.

91. Marmorstein, N.R., Malone, S.M., and Iacono, W.G. 2004. Psychiatric disorders among offspring of depressed mothers: Associations with paternal psychopathology. *Am J Psychiatry* 161(9): 1588–1594.

92. Flynn, H.A., Davis, M., Marcus, S.M., Cunningham, R., and Blow, F.C. 2004. Rates of maternal depression in pediatric emergency department and relationship to child service utilization. *Gen Hospital Psychiatry* 26(4): 316–322.

93. Spinelli, M.G. 2003. *Infanticide: Psychosocial and Legal Perspectives on Mothers Who Kill.* Washington, DC: American Psychiatric.

94. Jacobsen, T. 1999. Effects of postpartum disorders on parenting and on off-spring. In *Postpartum Mood Disorders*, Ed. L.J. Miller. Washington, DC: American Psychiatric Press, 119–139.

95. Flynn, H.A., O'Mahen, H.A., Massey, L., and Marcus, S.M. 2006. The impact of a brief obstetrics clinic-based intervention on treatment use for perinatal depression. *J Women's Health (Larchmt)* 15(10): 1195–1204.

96. Yonkers, K.A., Smith, M.V., Lin, H., Howell, H.B., Shao, L., and Rosenheck, R.A. 2009. Depression screening of perinatal women: An evaluation of the healthy start depression initiative. *Psychiatric Serv* 60(3): 322–328.

97. Segre, L., Stuart, S., and O'Hara, M.W. 2004. Interpersonal psychotherapy for antenatal and postpartum depression. *Primary Psychiatry* 11(3): 52–56, 66.

98. Pearlstein, T. 2008. Perinatal depression: Treatment options and dilemmas. *J Psychiatry Neurosci* 33(4): 302–318.

99. Sockol, L.E., Neill Epperson, C., and Barber, J.P. 2011. A meta-analysis of treatments for perinatal depression. *Clin Psychol Rev* 31(5): 839–849.

100. Food and Drug Administration. 2014. Content and format of labeling for human prescription drug and biological products: Requirements for pregnancy and lactation labeling. Final rule. *Federal Register* 79(233): 72063–72103.

101. Lorenzo, L., Byers, B., and Einarson, A. 2011. Antidepressant use in pregnancy. *Exp Opin Drug Saf* 10(6): 883–889.

102. Committee on Drugs. 2000. American Academy of Pediatrics. Use of psychoactive medication during pregnancy and possible effects on the fetus and newborn. *Pediatrics* 105(4 Pt 1): 880–887.

103. Schmidt, H.J. 1943. The use of progesterone in the treatment of postpartum psychosis. *JAMA* 121(3): 190–192.

104. Bower, W.H. and Altschule, M.D. 1956. Use of progesterone in the treatment of post-partum psychosis. *N Engl J Med* 254(4): 157–160.

105. Kane, F.J. Jr. and Keeler, M.H. 1965. The use of enovid in postpartum mental disorders. *Southern Med J* 58: 1089–1092.

106. Gregoire, A.J., Kumar, R., Everitt, B., Henderson, A.F., and Studd, J.W. 1996. Transdermal oestrogen for treatment of severe postnatal depression. *Lancet* 347(9006): 930–933.

107. Ahokas, A., Kaukoranta, J., Wahlbeck, K., and Aito, M. 2001. Estrogen deficiency in severe postpartum depression: Successful treatment with sublingual physiologic 17beta-estradiol: A preliminary study. *J Clin Psychiatry* 62(5): 332–336.

108. Freeman, M.P., Hibbeln, J.R., Wisner, K.L. et al. 2006. Omega-3 fatty acids: Evidence basis for treatment and future research in psychiatry. *J Clin Psychiatry* 67(12): 1954–1967.

109. McGregor, J.A., Allen, K.G., Harris, M.A. et al. 2001. The omega-3 story: Nutritional prevention of preterm birth and other adverse pregnancy outcomes. *Obstet Gynecol Surv* 56(5 Suppl 1): S1–S13.

110. Hibbeln, J.R., Davis, J.M., Steer, C. et al. 2007. Maternal seafood consumption in pregnancy and neuro-developmental outcomes in childhood (Alspac Study): An observational cohort study. *Lancet* 369(9561): 578–585.

111. Su, K.-P., Huang, S.-Y., Chiu, T.-H. et al. 2008. Omega-3 fatty acids for major depressive disorder during pregnancy: Results from a randomized, double-blind, placebo-controlled trial. *J Clin Psychiatry* 69(4): 644–651.

112. Folstein, M., Liu, T., Peter, I. et al. 2007. The homocysteine hypothesis of depression. *Am J Psychiatry* 164(6): 861–867.

113. Coppen, A. and Bailey, J. 2000. Enhancement of the antidepressant action of fluoxetine by folic acid: A randomised, placebo controlled trial. *J Affect Disord* 60(2): 121–130.

114. Gilbody, S., Lewis, S., and Lightfoot, T. 2007. Methylenetetrahydrofolate reductase (MTHFR) genetic polymorphisms and psychiatric disorders: A huge review. *Am J Epidemiol* 165(1): 1–13.

115. Delle Chiaie, R., Pancheri, P., and Scapicchio, P. 2002. Efficacy and tolerability of oral and intramuscular S-Adenosyl-L-Methionine 1,4-Butanedisulfonate (Same) in the treatment of major depression: Comparison with imipramine in 2 multicenter studies. *Am J Clin Nutr* 76(5): 1172S–1176S.

116. Mischoulon, D. and Fava, M. 2002. Role of S-Adenosyl-L-Methionine in the treatment of depression: A review of the evidence. *Am J Clin Nutr* 76(5): 1158S–1161S.

117. Cerutti, R., Sichel, M.P., Perin, M., Grussu, P., and Zulian, O. 1993. Psychological distress during Puerperium: A Novel Therapeutic approach using S-adenosylmethionine. *Curr Ther Res* 53(6): 707–716.

118. Institute of Medicine. 2011. *Dietary Reference Intakes: Calcium, Vitamin D.* Washington, DC: National Academies Press.

119. Kendall-Tackett, K.A. 2010. *Depression in New Mothers: Causes, Consequences, and Treatment Alternatives.* London, UK: Routledge.

120. Crowley, S.K. and Youngstedt, S.D. 2012. Efficacy of light therapy for perinatal depression: A review. *J Physiol Anthropol* 31: 15.

121. Epperson, C.N., Terman, M., Terman, J.S. et al. 2004. Randomized clinical trial of bright light therapy for antepartum depression: Preliminary findings. *J Clin Psychiatry* 65(3): 421–425.

122. Wirz-Justice, A., Bader, A., Frisch, U. et al. 2011. A randomized, double-blind, placebo-controlled study of light therapy for antepartum depression. *J Clin Psychiatry* 72(7): 986–993.

123. Corral, M., Wardrop, A.A., Zhang, H., Grewal, A.K., and Patton, S. 2007. Morning light therapy for postpartum depression. *Arch Women's Ment Health* 10(5) : 221–224.

124. Deligiannidis, K.M. and Freeman, M.P. 2014. Complementary and alternative medicine therapies for perinatal depression. *Best Pract Res Clin Obstetr Gynaecol* 28(1): 85–95.

125. Manber, R., Schnyer, R.N., Allen, J.J.B., John Rush, A., and Blasey, C.M. 2004. Acupuncture: A promising treatment for depression during pregnancy. *J Affect Disord* 83(1): 89–95.

126. Manber, R., Schnyer, R.N., Lyell, D. et al. 2010. Acupuncture for depression during pregnancy: A randomized controlled trial. *Obstet Gynecol* 115(3): 511–520.

127. Chung, K-F., Yeung, W-F., Zhang, Z-J. et al. 2012. Randomized non-invasive Sham-controlled pilot trial of electroacupuncture for postpartum depression. *J Affect Disord* 142(1–3): 115–121.

128. O'Neil, A., Itsiopoulos, C., Skouteris, H. et al. 2014. Preventing mental health problems in offspring by targeting dietary intake of pregnant women. *BMC Med* 12: 208.

129. Zlotnick, C., Capezza, N.M., and Parker, D. 2011. An interpersonally based intervention for low-income pregnant women with intimate partner violence: A pilot study. *Arch Women's Ment Health* 14(1): 55–65.

130. Wisner, K.L., Perel, J.M., Peindl, K.S., Hanusa, B H., Findling, R.L., and Rapport, D. 2001. Prevention of recurrent postpartum depression: A randomized clinical trial. *J Clin Psychiatry* 62(2): 82–86.

131. Beck, C.T. 2001. Predictors of postpartum depression: An update. *Nurs Res* 50(5): 275–285.

132. Logsdon, M.C. and Usui, W. 2001. Psychosocial predictors of postpartum depression in diverse groups of women. *Western J Nurs Res* 23(6): 563–574.

133. Beck, C.T. 1996. A meta-analysis of predictors of postpartum depression. *Nurs Res* 45(5): 297–303.

134. Banker, J.E. and Yvette LaCoursiere, D. 2014. Postpartum depression: Risks, protective factors, and the Couple's relationship. *Issues Ment Health Nurs* 35(7): 503–508.

29 Integrative Approaches to Adolescent Depression

Amelia Villagomez, MD and Noshene Ranjbar, MD

CONTENTS

INTRODUCTION

There is a high rate of depression among adolescents. Conventional treatment includes cognitive behavioral therapy, psychoeducation, interpersonal therapy, and antidepressant medication. Even after treatment with these approaches, the majority of depressed youth still suffer symptoms. One-third of youth with depression try complementary and alternative approaches. The limited research of integrative approaches for treatment of depression in children and teens is often of poor quality. However, promising research areas exist, and the quantity of research is increasing. This chapter highlights important points to consider during the psychiatric interview and discusses evidence for treatment effectiveness through changes in lifestyle, biological supplements (fish oil, St. John's wort, B12, vitamin D, folic acid, and broad-spectrum micronutrients), and mind-body approaches (meditation, yoga, progressive muscle relaxation, music, and exercise).

CONVENTIONAL TREATMENT APPROACHES

The emotional health of children is of utmost importance to the long-term optimal functioning of a society. Using mathematical models, economists have shown that the most important predictor of adult life satisfaction is childhood emotional health. Although childhood intellectual performance is a good predictor of adult educational achievement and income, it is the least important predictor of adult life satisfaction. Furthermore, adult income only accounts for 0.5% of the variance for adult satisfaction.[1]

In this context, the current emotional health of youth should cause concern. The prevalence of major depressive disorder (MDD) in children is 2%, and the rate increases to 4%–8% among adolescents.[2] An estimated 11% of adolescents will have experienced an episode of depression by the age of 18.[3] The ratio of depression in females to males is 1:1 for children and 2:1 for adolescents.

Current recommended conventional treatments for mild depression consist of supportive psychotherapy, case management, and psychoeducation. Cognitive behavioral therapy (CBT) or interpersonal therapy is recommended for the treatment of mild to moderate depression, and youth with severe depression are treated with an antidepressant with or without CBT.

The efficacy of CBT in combination with an selective serotonin reuptake inhibitor (SSRI) has been studied in depressed adolescents with mixed results. According to the hallmark TADS Study (Treatment of Adolescents with Depression Study), after 12 weeks of treatment, response rates (defined as "very much improved" or "much improved") reached 71% in the group receiving cognitive behavioral therapy (CBT) and fluoxetine; 60.6% in the fluoxetine group; 43.2% in the CBT group; and 34.8% in the placebo group.[2] However, the remission rates (Children's Depression Rating Scale-Revise total score of 28 or below) were as follows: 37% in the combined group, 23% of the adolescents in the fluoxetine group, 16% in the CBT group, and 17% in the placebo group.[4]

Many depressed adolescents do not respond to SSRI treatment even when a second SSRI is tried. Fluoxetine is approved by the U.S. Food and Drug Administration (FDA) for the treatment of MDD for youth 8–18 years old; escitalopram is approved for 12–17 year olds. The TORDIA trial (Treatment of Resistant Depression in Adolescents) showed that 50% of adolescents who did not respond to initial SSRI treatment responded to a different SSRI or venlafaxine. Therefore, approximately 20% of adolescents treated with two different antidepressants will still not have experienced remission. Few high-quality trials of psychotropic medications are available to provide guidance on additional treatment options for these individuals. Treatment guidelines suggest starting pharmacotherapy with an SSRI, then switching to another antidepressant if a response is not achieved. If still no response, an alternate antidepressant from another class (such as bupropion, venlafaxine, or duloxetine) is recommended. Preliminary evidence suggests that repetitive transcranial magnetic stimulation (rTMS) is well tolerated and effective for adolescents with treatment-resistant depression.[5] Some clinicians augment SSRIs with bupropion, mirtazapine, lithium, or an antipsychotic; however, these strategies are derived from *adult* data.[6]

Many depressed adolescents and their families have sought help from complementary and alternative therapies. According to data from the 2007 National Health Interview Survey, 34.8% of youth with anxiety or depression had used complementary and alternative treatments during the past year. Mind-body therapies and biological treatments were the complementary and alternative medicine treatment category most commonly tried. Using the definition from the National Center for Complementary and Alternative Medicine, mind-body therapies include biofeedback, deep breathing exercises, hypnosis, guided imagery, meditation, progressive relaxation, qi gong, support groups, stress management classes, tai chi, and yoga. Biologically based treatments were defined as diets or dietary supplements.[7] Based on adult data, hypothesized reasons parents and children may try complementary and alternative treatments include lack of stigma, desire to avoid consulting a health professional, previous unpleasant experiences with conventional medical therapies, desire for treatment congruent with their own values, and belief that these interventions are "natural."[8,9]

INTEGRATIVE TREATMENTS FOR ADOLESCENT DEPRESSION

During adolescence, neuronal networks are rapidly changing, psychological and behavioral patterns are being formed, and individual identity is taking shape. These changes are highly influenced by genetic, social, and environmental influences. An integrative approach to the treatment of the depressed adolescent takes into account the predisposing, precipitating, perpetuating, and protective factors underlying the depression. It then seeks to help the adolescent and his or her family create and implement a unique, individualized treatment plan, drawing from evidence-based treatment modalities. The integrative treatment model respects individual variability along the dimensions of biology, psychology, and culture; it also takes into account the "biology of belief," the notion that one's response to a certain treatment is highly influenced by one's personal perspective.[10]

INTERVIEW AND FORMULATION

The intake interview yields critical information that will inform treatment planning. The interviewer's demeanor substantially influences the openness of the adolescent or parent(s). Losses, traumatic events, disappointments, conflicts, and failures or the perception of failure are almost always present as possible contributing factors to the depressed mood. Due to shame and/or prior experiences of not feeling heard or validated, many adolescents and parents are reluctant to share these incidents or perceptions.[11] The provider's own sense of self-care, empathy, and intuition can play a significant role in his/her ability to connect with the adolescent and family; a highly skilled and self-aware provider can more easily pick up on psychological or relational nuances that may otherwise go unnoticed.

The provider should be alert to signs of trauma. The works of Scaer, Levine, Van der Kolk, and others in the field of trauma provide valuable insights into the "trauma spectrum."[12-15] Influenced by genetic and epigenetic factors, trauma can be perceived differently by different individuals. Empathic attention to the subjective experience of the adolescent within his/her life context can help the provider become aware of a variety of factors that may lie beneath the depressive symptoms. These factors may include unresolved grief, anger, fear, or other trauma-related responses. Many "treatment-resistant" depression cases have a yet undiscovered trauma that contributes, waiting to be revealed and allowed to heal.

As individuals with depression have often endured traumatic incidents, relationships, and losses, they may "build a wall" to hide vulnerable emotions such as anger, fear, and sadness. An empathic listener can help break a cycle of negative self-talk, self-hatred, and a prolonged lack of self-compassion. This will assist the adolescent in opening up to the beginning of a therapeutic relationship.[16]

Throughout the interview process, the provider can begin to create a bio-psycho-social formulation as an attempt to understand the adolescent and family's condition, including strengths, talents, struggles, and treatment needs. The formulation is then shared in a positive, nonjudgmental, nonpaternalistic way with the adolescent and family. Feedback from the adolescent and parents is welcomed, and their perspectives are honored and heard, while the best interests of the adolescent and family are upheld. The task of the provider, in addition to explaining the formulation, is to help the adolescent and parents recognize the depressive illness and struggle as an opportunity for enhanced self-awareness and self-care, future resilience, and improved emotional, physical, and spiritual well-being.

A collaborative, integrative treatment plan is created using the information revealed by the interview process. The cultural and religious needs of the adolescent and family are taken into account, as well as the community's resources and the family's economic circumstances and means.

PHYSICAL ACTIVITY

Exercise is known to have many health benefits and can be an important part of the integrative treatment of adolescents with depression. A Cochrane Review found that exercise has a small to medium effect on adults with depression, and the effects of exercise on adolescent depression as measured by several small studies suggest a positive correlation.[17,18] A systematic review that included nine trials ($n = 581$), mostly school-based RCTs, reported a small treatment effect for physical activity on depression for adolescents and children.[19] An earlier Cochrane Review reported that exercise has a moderate effect size (SMD: 0.66) for depressive symptoms of children and adolescents in the general population; however, many of the studies were of generally low methodological quality and were heterogeneous.[20] The review found that the level of intensity (high versus low) did not play a role in treatment effect. Exercise is known to have many health benefits and may be used as a useful adjunct to the treatment of adolescents with depression. Clinicians may encourage adolescents to increase exercise and inform patients that even low-intensity exercise is useful.

According to the 2008 Physical Activity Guidelines for Americans published by the Department of Health and Human Services, children ages 6–18 are to engage in 60 minutes or more of physical activity daily. Most of the physical activity is recommended to be either moderate- or vigorous-intensity aerobic physical activity, of which at least three times a week, the activity is of vigorous intensity. Examples of moderate physical activity include brisk walking, dancing, swimming, or bicycling on a level terrain. Examples of vigorous activity include jogging, singles tennis, swimming continuous laps, or bicycling uphill. The 60 or more minutes of daily physical activity must include both muscle-strengthening physical activity (strength training, resistance training, and muscular strength and endurance exercises) and bone-strengthening activity (running, jumping rope, and lifting weights) at least 3 days a week.[21]

Based on the data from the 2003–2004 National Health and Nutritional Examination Survey (NHANES) and data from over 6000 participants who provided data from physical activity monitors, 42% of children ages 6–11 years participate in 60 minutes of physical activity each day, and only 8% of adolescents achieve this goal.[22]

PARENTAL MENTAL HEALTH

The mental and emotional health of parents clearly influences the mental health of their adolescent children. According to data from Star*D, children whose mothers experienced a major depressive episode and comorbid panic disorder with agoraphobia were at an eightfold greater risk of developing a depressive disorder.[23] Star*D also demonstrated that children of depressed mothers have improvement in their psychiatric symptoms when the mother's symptoms remit.[24] Other studies support these findings and underline the importance of parental mental health.

Addressing a parent's mental health may be a sensitive subject given that many parents already have feelings of guilt when presenting to a clinician's office. A nonjudgmental attitude is imperative. To de-stigmatize the question, the clinician may ask the parent, "On a scale of 0–10, how would you rate your own emotional health?" Additionally, in the intake questionnaire, questions about the caregiver's stress can be measured through such scales as the Perceived Stress Scale (PSS).[25] While presenting a formulation and plan to the parents, the clinician can discuss the role of the family's emotional health in the child's improvement, without placing blame on the parents. The clinician can suggest that the adolescent might be more willing to engage in therapy if the parent models his or her own willingness to participate in therapy. The clinician can explain that deep suffering can often be reframed when viewed through the lens of meaning.[26] The parents may consider the adolescent's crisis as an opportunity or catalyst for their own spiritual and emotional development.

IDENTIFYING NUTRITIONAL DEFICIENCIES

Unhealthy dietary patterns and poor mental health appear to be related in adolescents. A systematic review found that the majority of cross-sectional studies have demonstrated a relationship between a poor diet and poor mental health and between a higher-quality diet and better mental health. However, the direction of causality has not been determined.[27] Do depressed individuals seek out high-fat, high-sugar foods as a form of self-medication, or are those who consume poor diets at higher risk of becoming depressed?

It can be challenging for parents to introduce dietary changes for adolescents with depression. Caregivers are encouraged to introduce dietary changes for the entire family. Adolescents may be motived by setting a goal to "eat from the rainbow." This entails daily eating a fruit or vegetable from each of the colors: red (e.g., apples, beets, bell peppers), orange (e.g., apricots, cantaloupe, carrots), yellow (e.g., banana, corn, pineapple), green (e.g., avocado, broccoli, celery), purple (e.g., berries, plums, prunes), and brown/tan/white (e.g., cauliflower, sauerkraut).

In addition to eating a poor-quality diet, depressed adolescents are often deficient in micronutrients. Supplementing the adolescent's diet with micronutrients and herbs will be discussed below.

FOLIC ACID

No trials have yet been conducted to assess the use of folic acid, either as monotherapy or as an augmentation agent, for youth with depression. Low folate levels have been linked to weaker response to SSRI treatment for depression in adults. Five randomized double-blind placebo-controlled trials have examined L-methylfolate augmentation of antidepressants for depressed adults with an effect size of 0.35–0.4; none have yet assessed the use of folic acid as monotherapy for MDD.[28]

VITAMIN D

According to NHANES dates from 2001–2004, 9% of children were vitamin D deficient (25-OH vitamin D < 15 ng/mL) and 61% had insufficient levels (25-OH vitamin D of 15–29 ng/mL). Risk factors for vitamin D deficiency included female gender, ethnicity/race (non-Hispanic blacks, Mexican Americans), obesity, milk less than once per week, and more than 4 hours of television/video/computers per day. Vitamin D deficiency was associated with adverse cardiovascular risks including higher blood pressure and lower HDL.[29]

In youth, the only published study of vitamin D supplementation and depression is a case-control trial using vitamin D for 3 months (4000 IU daily for 1 month, then 2000 IU daily for 2 months) as an augmentative treatment for depressed Swedish adolescents with a serum 25-OH vitamin D of less than 24 ng/mL. There was a positive correlation between vitamin D and well-being and improvement in depressive symptoms after supplementation.[30]

The optimal amount of vitamin D intake and supplementation is controversial. According to the Institute of Medicine report of 2010, 600 IU is the Recommended Dietary Allowance of vitamin D for children under age 18, and the tolerable upper level intake is 3000 IU for 4–8 year olds and 4000 IU for children 9 and above.[31] Strong evidence does not currently exist for vitamin D as a treatment for adolescent depression; however, given its safety in appropriate dosages, importance for bone health, evidence supporting its beneficial effects on the immune system, mental health, and overall life expectancy, clinicians may consider assessing vitamin D levels by ordering a 25-OH vitamin D level and serum calcium level. It is estimated that vitamin D levels increase by 1 ng/mL for every 100 IU of supplementation when given for 3–4 months.[32] Experts have recommended that targeting a 25-OH vitamin D level of 40–70 ng/mL would provide optimal health benefits in children.[33]

Vitamin B12

Vitamin B12 is essential for red blood cell function, and the most severe illness associated with B12 deficiency is megaloblastic anemia. In addition, research suggests that lowering of B12 levels can result in neuropsychiatric symptoms including depression, mania, fatigue, catatonia, irritability, apathy, ataxia, and dementia even in the absence of severe B12 deficiency.[34,35] Sources of dietary B12 include meat, dairy, and eggs, and B12 deficiency is common in vegan and even vegetarian populations.

There have not been any studies examining the effect of B12 on adolescent depression. However, several adult case studies as well as clinical experience with adolescent depression resistant to antidepressant treatment suggest a potentially important role for B12 evaluation and supplementation.[36–38] In children with healthy digestive systems and a diet adequately rich in meats, dairy, and eggs, B12 deficiency or insufficiency is unlikely. In children with inadequate dietary B12, with malabsorptive disorders or taking medications that decrease B12 levels (e.g., valproic acid, oral contraceptives, proton pump inhibitors, metformin), we would recommend screening for B12 insufficiency. Levels of 175–900 pg/mL are considered normal range for B12 levels, but neuropsychiatric signs of deficiency can be manifest with levels higher than 175 pg/mL. Hence, some research is recommending increasing the lower limit to 550 pg/mL.[36]

Omega 3s

Omega 3 and omega 6 polyunsaturated fatty acids (PUFAs) are considered essential fatty acids (EFAs) because they must be ingested through food sources and cannot be synthesized by the body. They are important for the structure and functioning of the central nervous system (CNS). Omega 3 PUFA are involved in many biological mechanisms that may explain their effects on psychiatric disorders; these mechanisms include increased serotonergic neurotransmission, alternations in dopaminergic function, and modulation of heart rate variability.[39]

With the high processed-food content and lack of fish intake in the diets of most adolescents, it is no surprise that the majority of adolescents have suboptimal omega 3 PUFA. In a study published by Harel, total intake by adolescents was only 30% of the Canadian recommended daily allowance of omega 3 PUFA.[40] A study evaluating the food intake of a group of Australian adolescents showed that to meet guidelines for chronic disease prevention, dietary intake of omega 3s would need to increase threefold.[41]

Most studies examining the effect of omega 3 PUFA on mood and behavior have been conducted in adults. A meta-analysis that included 15 adult studies of omega 3 PUFA for primary depression demonstrated that supplements containing 200–2000 mg/day of EPA with the amount of EPA greater than or equal to 60% of total EPA+DHA, had a significant effect on primary depression.[42]

Omega 3 supplementation may benefit youth with depression. A case-control trial of 150 depressed adolescents and 161 healthy controls demonstrated an inverse relationship between the omega 3 index (the percentage of EPA and DHA in RBC membranes) and the risk for unipolar depression.[43]

A cross-sectional study of 6517 Japanese adolescents aged 12 to 15 years showed dietary intake of fish, EPA, and DHA was associated with a lower prevalence of depressive symptoms in males.[44] This finding did not hold for females. The exact reason is not clear but may be related to females' lesser need for essential fatty acids, greater efficiency at converting ALA to DHA, and ability to store essential fatty acids more effectively during times of low intake.[45] As this was a cross-sectional study, only an association was suggested; it cannot be inferred that the lower intake of fish, EPA, and DHA causes the depressive symptoms. Another study initially showed an inverse relationship between omega 3 PUFA intake at age 14 and depressive symptoms; however, this association disappeared when caloric intake and other lifestyle confounders were controlled for.[46]

Numerous studies have assessed the use of omega 3 PUFA for the treatment of ADHD; a mild to modest improvement in symptoms appears to result.[47] However, only two small studies have examined the effect of omega 3s for the treatment of depression for children and adolescents. In an 10-week open-label study, 20 adolescents (ages 8–24) who had not achieved remission with an SSRI (CDRS > 28) were randomized to either omega 3 supplementation low dose (2.4 g/day: EPA 1.6g+DHA 0.8 g) or high dose (16.2 g/day: EPA 10.8g+DHA 5.4 g) in addition to their current SSRI. When compared to healthy controls, these individuals had baseline lower erythrocyte DHA levels but not lower erythrocyte EPA levels. After supplementation, there was a significant increase in erythrocyte EPA and DHA composition. Sixty percent of adolescents in the low-dose group and 100% of patients in the high-dosage group achieved remission (CDRS ≤ 28). Both dosages were well tolerated. Limitations of the study include small sample size, short duration, and lack of a placebo arm.[48]

In a double-blind controlled pilot study, 28 children (ages 6–12) with MDD were randomized to placebo or omega 3 fatty acids (400 EPA+200 mg DHA) for 16 weeks. Among those who completed at least 1 month of supplementation, the group receiving omega 3 had a 70% response (50% reduction in CDRS scores), compared with 0% in the placebo group. Forty percent of those in the omega 3 group and 0% in the placebo group experienced remission (CDRS score < 29). Starting at week 8 and continuing to week 16, omega 3 supplementation was statistically superior to placebo.[49]

In a post hoc analysis of a subset of individuals with borderline personality disorder participating in a double-blind randomized control trial for youth at high risk of developing psychosis ($n = 15$), after 12 weeks, the individuals in the omega 3 group (EPA 700 mg and DHA 480 mg) had significantly lower levels of depression.[50]

Side Effects

Common side effects of omega 3 acids include gastrointestinal effects (loose stools, diarrhea, nausea, vomiting, "fishy burps") and reduced appetite. Omega 3 fatty acids have antithrombotic and antiplatelet effects, and at higher doses increase bleeding time.[51] Very rare but reported side effects include gastrointestinal hemorrhage, hemorrhagic stroke, hemolytic anemia, and urticaria. For adults, the FDA considers omega 3 fatty acids from marine sources in doses up to 3 g to be "Generally Regarded as Safe."

More studies of omega 3s for the treatment of depression are needed in adolescents before exact clinical treatment recommendations can be made. Evidence to date suggests that omega 3 EFA play a role in the treatment of depression for adolescents and are generally safe and relatively inexpensive. Based largely on studies in adults and some studies in children, EPA-rich preparations appear to be more likely effective than DHA-rich ones. The average dosage of omega 3 in the few trials conducted in adolescents is between 1 and 2 g, with more than 60% of total EPA+DHA dosage from EPA. Patients must be advised that quality varies by product. Fish oil can oxidize easily and become rancid, and it is best stored in a cool place away from sunlight.

The potential side effect of "fish burps" may be minimized by storing fish oil capsules in the freezer and taking them with meals. The large size of many fish oil capsule preparations may be too difficult to swallow for some adolescents. In these cases, the practitioner may consider suggesting fish oil in a liquid form mixed in orange juice, flavored yogurt, or smoothies to mask the taste.

BROAD-SPECTRUM MICRONUTRIENTS

Very limited evidence supports supplementing depressed children with a single vitamin/mineral. Vitamins and minerals often work together; therefore, supplementing with only one nutrient may produce suboptimal results and may even cause imbalances in other micronutrients. Broad-spectrum micronutrients product contain a wide variety of vitamins and minerals with the goal of improving the multiple possible nutrient imbalances, insufficiencies, and deficiencies. Four randomized double-blind placebo-controlled trials (RDBPCT) have demonstrated that broad-spectrum micronutrients substantially decrease aggression in young adults and children.[28]

The broad-spectrum micronutrient product that has been most thoroughly studied is EMPowerplus™ (EMP+). EMP+ contains 36 ingredients (16 minerals, 14 vitamins, 3 amino acids, 3 antioxidants). A total of 25 published studies (including two RCTs) of EMP+ have investigated its role in a variety of psychiatric disorders, including bipolar disorder, MDD, anxiety disorders, ADHD, OCD, addictions, and autism.

No RCT has evaluated broad-spectrum micronutrients in adolescents with depression. In adults, a post hoc subgroup analysis applied to data from a RCT of individuals with ADHD treated with EMP+, demonstrated that individuals with ADHD and moderate to severe depression experienced significant improvement in depressive symptoms.[52]

An 8-week open-label feasibility study conducted with 10 children (ages 6–12) with bipolar spectrum disorder showed a 37% decrease in depressive scores and a 45% decrease in mania scores when the children were treated with EMP+.[53] Adverse effects were mild and transient (e.g., initial insomnia or gastrointestinal upset) and improved when children took supplements earlier in the evening and with food.[54]

EMP+ is generally considered safe, and in one naturalistic study of 2 years (ages 2–28), individuals taking EMP+ had fewer side effects than individuals taking conventional psychotropic medications.[55] A systematic review evaluated the biological data from 144 medication-free children and adults and reported no safety concerns and the absence of significant laboratory values changes. Three sources of safety data included in the analysis provided data on long-term exposure (>8 years).[56]

Adverse side effects were transient and minor, and most commonly included headache and gastrointestinal symptoms. An important limitation of this review is that it was unable to assess the safety of EMP+ when combined with psychiatric medications. According to the clinical experience of experts, EMP+ can cause up to a 100-fold potentiation of the CNS effects of lithium and three- to fivefold potentiation for psychotropic medication; it therefore requires significant dosage adjustments when co-administered with CNS-active drugs. It has been recommended that clinicians wishing to start patients on broad-spectrum micronutrients receive additional training and consultation with a specialist. Contraindications include Wilson's disease, hemochromatosis and hemosiderosis, trimethylaminuria, and phenylketonuria.[28]

BOTANICALS: ST. JOHN'S WORT

Extracts of *Hypericum perforatum* (St. John's wort) have been used for centuries in herbal medicine and have received the attention of clinical studies over the past three decades. St. John's wort (SJW) contains at least 10 active constituents that may contribute to its pharmacologic effects, including hyperforin and hypericin. Its efficacy is likely due to a synergistic effect of its multiple constituents and not solely to one component. According to a German study published in 2011 of adolescents treated for depression, 8.5% were prescribed SJW.[57] Two decades ago SJW was prescribed more frequently, but its use has been considerable supplanted by SSRIs.

MECHANISM OF ACTION

SJW's exact mechanism of action has not been clearly defined. SJW has been shown to have antioxidant and anti-inflammatory effects, thereby contributing to the normalization of an overly active hypothalamic-pituitary-adrenal (HPA) axis.[58] SJW's antidepressant properties are also thought to be mediated through inhibiting synaptic uptake of noradrenaline, serotonin, and gamma-aminobutyric acid (GABA), and increasing dopaminergic activity in the prefrontal cortex.[59]

Several trials and meta-analyses have demonstrated the effectiveness of SJW for treating depression in adults. Three open-labeled studies have evaluated SJW for the treatment of depression in children and adolescents; however, there have been no randomized controlled trials.[60–62] Patients in the open-label studies, which lasted between 8 to 10 weeks, showed improvement with SJW, starting as early as week 1. The generalizability of these studies is limited due to their small sample size, lack of strict diagnostic criteria, and lack of placebo arm. Two of the three open-label studies reported a high dropout rate (25%–57%). Adverse events were all mild and transient. Dosages of SJW in the studies ranged from 300–900 mg per day, divided into two to three dosages, and were standardized to contain 0.3% hypericin. One study also standardized SJW to contain 3% hyperforin. No data on long-term use in adults, adolescents, or children are yet available.

SIDE EFFECTS

There have been several case reports of SJW-induced mania in older adults with unipolar depression or bipolar disorder.[63] Side effects are usually mild and transient and may include upset stomach, feelings of restlessness, mild sedation, increased appetite, loose stools, dizziness, constipation, rash, photosensitivity, nausea, dry mouth, and nightmares. The studies in adolescents did not report weight gain, laboratory, or EKG changes with SJW. Photosensitivity has been attributed to the plant's content of hypericin; dosages well beyond recommended amounts for treatment of depression are likely needed to cause phototoxicity. There have only been very few published case reports of photosensitivity.[64] A safety analysis of 594 adult patients treated with SJW for 6 weeks reported that it was well tolerated and side effects were no different from those experienced on placebo; it did not cause sedation, anticholinergic reactions, gastrointestinal disturbances, or sexual dysfunction. The effects of SJW on the developing fetus are not known.

Factors such as where the herb is grown, seasonal conditions, and ripeness at harvest can all affect the quantity of active content in the herb. In a study examining SJW products, some products demonstrated consistent batch-to-batch variability of the amount of hyperforin and hypericin, while others had significant interbatch difference. Therefore, physicians should be aware of significant variability between bottles.[65] Additionally, given that the exact mechanism of action of SJW has not been delineated, it is possible that there are other active components contributing to the antidepressant effect; these components may not be standardized and may vary from bottle to bottle.

DRUG–DRUG INTERACTIONS

SJW affects the pharmacokinetics of many drugs through inducing CYP isoenzymes, especially CYP3A4 and P-glycoprotein. P-glycoprotein is a membrane-associate multidrug efflux pump that serves to protect the body against toxic xenobiotics and metabolites. Many drugs are transported by P-glycoprotein including several HIV protease inhibitors, H2-receptor antagonists, proton pump inhibitors, cardiac glycosides, calcium channel blockers, immunosuppressive agents, corticosteroids, antiemetic and antidiarrheal agents, analgesics, antibiotics, anti-helminthics, anti-epileptics, sedatives, and antidepressants. Therefore, concomitant administration of SJW with a drug transported by P-glycoprotein may result in decreased plasma levels of the drug. For transplant patients taking immune-suppressants such as cyclosporine, the addition of SJW may result in subtherapeutic levels and result in organ rejection. SJW also can induce CYP3A4, CYP2C19, and CPY2C9; it is not thought to significantly affect CYP1A and CYP2D6. SJW has been shown to increase the incidence of intracyclic bleeding episodes and decrease serum concentrations of 3-ketodesogestrel. SJW may increase the risk of unintended pregnancies in individuals taking oral contraceptives. SJW has not been shown to affect the anti-androgenic properties of oral contraceptives and may still be useful to treat acne and hirsutism.[66] There have been no reported cases of SJW causing serotonin syndrome at recommended dosages, but there have been reports when combined with an SSRI or serotonin-norepinephrine reuptake inhibitor (SNRI).[67]

CLINICAL APPLICATION

St. John's wort may be a treatment option for adolescents who prefer botanicals to pharmaceuticals and are not taking medications that may interact with SJW. No data are yet available about optimal dosages in young people, but clinicians working with children often start with 150 mg three times a day and increase up to 300 mg or 600 mg three times a day (plant extracts are usually standardized to 0.3% hypericin). Improvement in symptoms may occur after 1 week, but full response may be seen after 2–8 weeks.[68] Variability of hyperforin and hypericin between batches is a clinical concern. Definitive recommendations cannot be made about the washout period necessary after discontinuing SJW and starting another agent for the treatment of depression; a conservative approach may be to wait 1–2 weeks.[69]

MIND-BODY MEDICINE TECHNIQUES

In addition to supplementation with botanicals and promoting healthy lifestyle factors, an integrative approach to treating depression in adolescents includes mind-body medicine components. Mind-body skill development enhances an adolescent's ability to self-reflect, practice self-care, and become more adept at working through stress. These skills form a repertoire for the adolescent to express emotions in healthier ways, thereby processing anger, grief, disappointment, fear, sadness, and anxiety.

Mind-body skills, especially when practiced in a group setting, contribute to enhanced emotional regulation through many mechanisms, including increased heart rate variability and vagal tone. The continued practice of these skills builds prosocial behavior, empathy, and enhanced self-compassion.[70] Depressive states involve low heart rate variability, poor vagal nerve function, and difficulty regulating emotions, especially under stressful circumstances.[71] Learning about the interrelatedness of mind, body, emotions, and spirit can enhance the adolescent's sense of empowerment during a phase of life when many changes are occurring.

MEDITATION AND MINDFULNESS

Several meditation techniques have been systematically studied in adolescents. Meditation and mindfulness techniques are drawn from ancient contemplative practices known for hundreds of years to enhance resilience in practitioners. Practice of these techniques does not require affiliation with the religious traditions from which they are drawn; they lend themselves well to both clinical use and secular lifestyles. The techniques most studied range from passive to active, and include focused attention, open monitoring, automatic self-transcending, music, creative arts, yoga, tai chi, qi gong, and many forms of meditative movement and dance.[72]

Studies show that meditation and mindfulness techniques play a role in changing neuronal pathways and improving biological and physiological correlates of functioning; these practices show enduring benefits for those who continue to use them on a regular and long-term basis. A few randomized clinical trials have shown significant results in adolescents with depression, and more rigorous research is underway. The training and expertise of the clinician or teacher imparting these techniques to adolescents are critical to the effectiveness of the practices. Given the favorable safety profile of these techniques, effectiveness, low cost, and limited side effects, various meditation and mindfulness skills can help augment a clinical treatment plan for adolescents with depression.[73]

Meditation has been shown to result in many neurophysiological changes including increased parasympathetic activity, reduced locus ceruleus firing and decreased noradrenergic activity, increased GABAergic drive, increased serotonin, and reduced levels of serum cortisol. In addition, the production of endorphins can contribute to the anxiolytic and antidepressant effect of meditation.[74]

A randomized controlled trial of an 8-week mindfulness-based stress reduction (MBSR) intervention in 102 adolescents showed significant reduction of depressive symptoms on self-reported Symptom Checklist-90.[75]

RELAXATION

Relaxation can diminish the stress that often accompanies depression. Relaxation therapy, specifically progressive muscle relaxation (PMR), was studied in comparison to cognitive behavioral therapy (CBT), and the two were found equally effective in improving depressive symptoms as measured by the Beck Depression Inventory Rating Scale (BDI) with $P < 0.001$, the Reynolds Adolescent Depression Scale with $P < 0.05$, and the Beck Depression Index with $P < 0.001$.[76]

A variety of phone and computer applications are available with guided relaxation techniques at low or no cost. Examples include Smilingmind, Headspace®, and Stop, Breathe and Relax.

YOGA

The practice of yoga has its roots in Indian culture, where for millennia it has existed as a complex set of physical, moral, social, and spiritual practices intended to enhance self-awareness and wellness. Researchers have investigated the potential of yoga to reduce depressive symptoms. Various types of yoga have been shown to activate the prefrontal cortex and thalamus, as well as the inhibitory thalamic reticular nucleus, with resulting functional differentiation of the parietal lobe, as visible on neuroimaging. These changes reduce the sensory stimuli to the thalamus, allowing the mind to stay focused with less distractibility. All neurotransmitter systems seem to be affected, contributing to the amelioration of depressive symptoms.[77]

Streeter and colleagues, for example, studied a 12-week yoga intervention, which yielded demonstrable improvements in anxiety and mood, when compared to a metabolically matched exercise program.[78] In this study, yoga postures were correlated with increased thalamic GABA levels and reduced anxiety and depression scores.

Noggle and colleagues investigated a yoga program compared to typical physical education (PE) taken by 11th- and 12th-grade students, exploring feasibility and effect on a self-report format. The study found improved mood in yoga students but a worsened mood in controls. Although the study was small with limitations, the results suggest that yoga may be a helpful alternative to a traditional PE class for adolescents.[79]

CREATIVE ARTS

Creative arts can allow adolescents to express their emotions in healthy, productive, and enjoyable ways. The many types of creative arts include painting, drawing, writing, dance, music, pottery, beading, photography, drama, film, and many others. A study combining group art therapy with breath meditation for adolescents with depression has found this treatment effective in improving participants' subjective sense of well-being by promoting self-expression, self-acceptance, self-growth, self-reflection, and insight.[80]

MUSIC THERAPY

Research suggests that music therapy can affect attention, cognition, emotion processing, stress, and anxiety as part of mental health treatment. Listening to music engages multiple areas of the brain, including cortical, subcortical, and limbic regions, therefore enhancing neuroplasticity. Hudziak and colleagues found an association between playing a musical instrument and increased rate of cortical thickness maturation in brain areas responsible for emotion and impulse regulation, motor coordination and planning, and visuospatial skills.[81] For adults, active participation in music engages more areas of the brain than passive listening.[82]

Some research has focused specifically on music and depressed adolescents. In one study involving 28 depressed adolescent females, Field and colleagues showed significantly reduced right frontal lobe activation and increased left frontal lobe activation, and significantly reduced salivary cortisol in the subjects receiving music therapy; this EEG pattern is consistent with positive affect.[83]

Multiple studies have shown that the musical preference of the individual receiving music therapy makes a significant difference in therapeutic effectiveness. In a study exploring the effect of listening to music on adolescents, Wooten found a significant increase in positive affect but only when the individual listened to preferred music.[84] Some investigators have observed that the music choices of adolescents may indicate their state of emotional vulnerability and mental health; therefore, it is prudent to screen the adolescent's music prior to music therapy intervention.[85]

Hilliard investigated the role of music therapy in reducing grief symptoms in children in a randomized controlled study: findings were significant for the children assigned to the music therapy group, showing improvement in grief and behavior symptoms; children in a wait-list control group did not improve in either grief or behavior symptoms; and children assigned to a social work group showed fewer behavior symptoms with no change in grief symptoms.[86] Research also suggests that dopamine may be involved in socially directed music making, which means that group music therapy may be more effective than individual music therapy in alleviating depression.[87]

A qualitative study performed by Gardstrom investigated the effect of clinical music improvisation on adolescents ages 12–17 with various mental health diagnoses at a partial hospital program; results suggested music is effective in facilitating the expression of emotion.[88]

Despite the lack of more extensive evidence in the effectiveness of music therapy, the safety profile and cost-effectiveness of music therapy makes it a valuable tool for enhancing the treatment of adolescent depression.

DANCE AND MEDITATIVE MOVEMENT

Research suggests that the mirror neuron system is activated when an individual is engaged in movement that is mirroring or mirrored by another. The observation or performance of emotionally charged movements can also enhance limbic brain activation, and studies suggest enhancement of empathy as a result.[89] Impaired ability to regulate emotion, as present during depressive states, makes it difficult for individuals to respond empathically to others and to be self-compassionate.[90]

A small qualitative study by Wall investigated the combination of tai chi and MBSR as part of an educational program for middle-school students. The students reported enhanced calmness, relaxation, well-being, improved sleep, reduced reactivity, enhanced self-care, and heightened self-awareness. Further research with quantitative data is needed to investigate the evidence for incorporating such mindfulness-based programming as part of the educational system.[91]

MIND-BODY SKILLS GROUPS

Mind-body skills groups appear to offer a significant advantage to adolescents in individual treatment. There is a significant advantage to a group program that helps adolescents learn and practice various mind-body skills in a small group. The group model furnishes a structure and sense of safety within which adolescents can explore various mind-body techniques. The group can become a "laboratory" for learning and practicing skills that promote health and self-awareness. The facilitator has the role of a teacher, role model, and therapeutic mentor. As adolescents interact in a safe, supportive setting, they learn to actively listen, set healthier boundaries, and learn more about their common struggles.

Gordon and colleagues studied the use of a 12-week mind-body skills group program for high school students with posttraumatic stress disorder (PTSD) in postwar Kosovo, showing significant reduction of PTSD symptom scores.[92] Another study by Staples showed improvement in both PTSD and depression after a similar mind-body group program; results were largely maintained at 7-month follow up.[93]

CONCLUSION

An integrative approach to the treatment of adolescent depression is a rapidly expanding field. The approach requires open-mindedness, dedication, flexibility, and patience on the part of the provider, adolescent, and caregiver(s); at the same time, it allows for more individualized, comprehensive, empowering, and integrated care of the adolescent and his/her family. Conventional treatment with medications and psychotherapy is embraced according to evidence-based parameters. In addition, health-promoting behaviors such as nutrition and exercise are addressed, and supplementation with omega-3s or other nutrients is suggested based on existing research evidence. Mind-body techniques are taught individually or in groups to enhance self-care, self-awareness, and enhanced emotion regulation, as supported by research in neuroplasticity and resilience. Although many of the modalities discussed in this chapter have not yet been extensively studied, their scientific plausibility, acceptable safety profile, relative affordability, and clinical evidence of their efficacy make them important components of a comprehensive integrative treatment program for adolescents with depression.

ACKNOWLEDGMENTS

We extend heartfelt gratitude to Matthew Erb, P.T., Kurt Kreuger, Janine Walter, Janette Zyriek, Julie Kilpatrik, Talia Rose, Beverly McLean, and Halima Sussman for their unceasing support in our work. We also give thanks to Kathy Smith, M.D., Charles Raison, M.D., Sally Dodds, Ph.D., Mark Gilbert, M.D., and Ole Thienhaus, M.D., of the University of Arizona Department of Psychiatry, for their leadership and mentorship. In addition, we are grateful for the faculty at the Center for Mind Body Medicine, the Arizona Center for Integrative Medicine, and to Enrico Mezzacappa, M.D. and Giulia Mezzacappa, M.D., for their dedication to teaching, mentorship, and modeling. Support was received from the University of Arizona Strategic Priorities Faculty Initiative.

REFERENCES

1. Layard, R., Clark, A.E., Cornaglia, F. et al. 2014. What Predicts a Successful Life? A life-course model of well-being. *Econ J* 124(580): F720–F738.
2. Birmaher, B., Brent, D., and AACAP Work Group on Quality Issues et al. 2007. Practice parameter for the assessment and treatment of children and adolescents with depressive disorders. *J Am Acad Child Adolesc Psychiatry* 46(11): 1503–1526.
3. Merikangas, K.R., He, J. Burstein, M. et al. 2010. Lifetime prevalence of mental disorders in U.S. adolescents: Results from the National Comorbidity Survey Replication–Adolescent Supplement (NCS-A). *J Am Acad Child Adolesc Psychiatry* 49(10): 980–989.
4. March, J., Silva, S. Petrycki, S. et al. 2004. Fluoxetine, cognitive-behavioral therapy, and their combination for adolescents with depression: Treatment for adolescents with depression study (TADS) randomized controlled trial. *JAMA* 292(7): 807–820.
5. Donaldson, A.E., Gordon, M.S. Melvin, G.A. et al. 2014. Brain stimulation. *Brain Stimul* 7(1): 7–12.
6. DeFilippis, M. and Wagner, K.D. 2014. Management of treatment-resistant depression in children and adolescents. *Pediatr Drugs* 16(5): 353–361.
7. Kemper, K.J., Gardiner, P., and Birdee, G.S. 2013. Use of complementary and alternative medical therapies among youth with mental health concerns. *Acad Pediatr* 13(6): 540–545.
8. Badger, F. and Nolan, P. 2007. Use of self-chosen therapies by depressed people in primary care. *J Clin Nurs* 16(7): 1343–1352.
9. Wu, P., Fuller, C. Liu, X. et al. 2007. Use of complementary and alternative medicine among women with depression: Results of a national survey. *Psychiatr Serv.* 58(3): 349–356.
10. Lipton, B. 2007. *The Biology of Belief: Unleashing the Power of Consciousness, Matter and Miracles.* Revised Edition. USA: Hay House.
11. Brown, B. 2012. *Daring Greatly: How the Courage to Be Vulnerable Transforms the Way We Live, Love, Parent, and Lead.* 1st ed. New York, NY: Gotham.
12. Scaer, R. 2005. *The Trauma Spectrum: Hidden Wounds and Human Resiliency.* 1st ed. New York, NY: W.W. Norton.

13. Levine, P. 2010. *In an Unspoken Voice: How the Body Releases Trauma and Restores Goodness.* 1st ed. Berkley, CA: North Atlantic Books.
14. Levine, P. 1997. *Waking the Tiger: Healing Trauma—The Innate Capacity to Transform the Overwhelming Experience.* 1st ed. Berkley, CA: North Atlantic Books.
15. Van Der Kolk, B. 2014. *The Body Keeps the Score: Brain, Mind, and Body in the Healing of Trauma.* 1st ed. New York, NY: Viking Adult.
16. Neff, K. 2010. *Self-Compassion: Stop Beating Yourself Up and Leave Insecurity Behind.* 1st ed. New York, NY: William Morrow.
17. Cooney, G.M., Dwan, K. Greig, C.A. et al. 2013. Exercise for depression. *Cochrane Database Syst Rev* 9: CD004366.
18. Dopp, R.R., Mooney, A.J. Armitage, R. et al. 2012. Exercise for adolescents with depressive disorders: A feasibility study. *Depress Res Treat* 2012(2): 1–9.
19. Brown, H.E., Pearson, N., Braithwaite, R.E. et al. 2013. Physical activity interventions and depression in children and adolescents. *Sports Med* 43(3): 195–206.
20. Larun, L., Nordheim, L. Ekeland, E. et al. 2012. Exercise in prevention and treatment of anxiety and depression among children and young people (Review). *The Cochrane Collaboration* 2012: 1–53.
21. Leavitt, M.O. 2008. *2008 Physical Activity Guidelines for Americans. healthgov.* Available at: http://www.health.gov/paguidelines/pdf/paguide.pdf (accessed January 1, 2014).
22. Troiano, R.P., Berrigan, D. Dodd, K.W. et al. 2008. Physical activity in the United States measured by accelerometer. *Med Sci Sports Exerc* 40(1): 181–188.
23. Pilowsky, D.J., Wickramaratne, P.J. Rush, A.J. et al. 2006. Children of currently depressed mothers: A STAR*D ancillary study. *J Clin Psychiatry* 67(1): 126–136.
24. Wickramaratne, P., Gameroff, M.J., Pilowsky, D.J. et al. 2011. Children of depressed mothers 1 year after remission of maternal depression: Findings from the STAR*D-Child study. *Am J Psychiatry* 168(6): 593–602.
25. Cohen, S., Kamarck, T., and Mermelstein, R. 1983. A global measure of perceived stress. *J Health Soc Behav* 24(4): 385–396.
26. Frankl, V. 2006. *Man's Search for Meaning.* 1st ed. Cutchogue, NY: Beacon Press.
27. O'Neil, A., Quirk, S.E. Housden, S. et al. 2014. Relationship between diet and mental health in children and adolescents: A systematic review. *Am J Public Health* 104(10): e31–42.
28. Popper, C.W. 2014. Single-micronutrient and broad-spectrum micronutrient approaches for treating mood disorders in youth and adults. *Child Adolesc Psychiatry Clin North Am* 23(3): 591–672.
29. Kumar, J., Muntner, P. Kaskel, F.J. et al. 2009. Prevalence and associations of 25-Hydroxyvitamin D deficiency in US children: NHANES 2001–2004. *Pediatrics* 124(3): e362–e370.
30. Högberg, G., Gustafsson, S.A., Hällström, T. et al. 2012. Depressed adolescents in a case-series were low in vitamin D and depression was ameliorated by vitamin D supplementation. *Acta Paediatr* 101(7): 779–783.
31. Ross, A.C., Taylor, C.L. Yaktine, A.L. et al. 2011. Institute of Medicine (US) Committee to review dietary reference intakes for vitamin D and calcium. *Dietary Reference Intakes for Calcium and Vitamin D.* Washington, DC: National Academies Press, pp. 1–4.
32. Heaney, R.P., Davies, K.M. Chen, T.C. et al. 2003. Human serum 25-hydroxycholecalciferol response to extended oral dosing with cholecalciferol. *Am J Clin Nutr* 77(1): 204–210.
33. Weydert, J. 2014. Vitamin D in children's health. *Children* 1(2): 208–226.
34. Bottiglieri, T. 2000. Homocysteine, folate, methylation, and monoamine metabolism in depression. *J Neurol Neurosurg Psychiatry* 69(2): 228–232.
35. Berry, N., Sagar, R., and Tripathi, B.M. 2003. Catatonia and other psychiatric symptoms with vitamin B12 deficiency. *Acta Psychiatr Scand* 108(2): 156–159.
36. Rao, N.P., Kumar, N.C., and Raman, B.R.P. et al. 2008. Role of vitamin B12 in depressive disorder—A case report. *Gen Hospital Psychiatry* 30(2): 185–186.
37. Milanlıoğlu, A. 2011. Vitamin B12 deficiency and depression. *J Clin Exp Invest* 2(4): 455–456.
38. Kate, N., Grover, S., and Agarwal, M. 2010. Does B12 deficiency lead to lack of treatment response to conventional antidepressants? *Psychiatry (Edgmont)* 7(11): 42–44.
39. Freeman, M.P., Hibbeln, J.R. Wisner, K.L. et al. 2006. Omega-3 fatty acids: Evidence basis for treatment and future research in psychiatry. *J Clin Psychiatry* 67(12): 1954–1967.
40. Harel, Z., Riggs, S., Vaz, R. et al. 2001. Omega-3 polyunsaturated fatty acids in adolescents: Knowledge and consumption. *J Adolesc Health* 28(1): 10–15.
41. O'Sullivan, T.A., Ambrosini, G., Beilin, L.J. et al. 2011. Dietary intake and food sources of fatty acids in Australian adolescents. *Nutrition* 27(2): 153–159.

42. Sublette, M.E., Ellis, S.P., Geant, A.L. et al. 2011. Meta-analysis of the effects of eicosapentaenoic acid (EPA) in clinical trials in depression. *J Clin Psychiatry* 72(12): 1577–1584.

43. Pottala, J.V., Talley, J.A., Churchill, S.W. et al. 2012. Prostaglandins, leukotrienes and essential fatty acids. *Prostaglandins Leukot Essent Fatty Acids* 86(4–5): 161–165.

44. Murakami, K., Miyake, Y. Sasaki, S. et al. 2010. Fish and n-3 polyunsaturated fatty acid intake and depressive symptoms: Ryukyus child health study. *Pediatrics* 126(3): e623–e630.

45. Pawlosky, R., Hibbeln, J. Lin, Y. et al. 2003. n-3 fatty acid metabolism in women. *Br J Nutr.* 90(5): 993–4, discussion 994–5.

46. Oddy, W.H., Hickling, S. Smith, M.A. et al. 2011. Dietary intake of omega-3 fatty acids and risk of depressive symptoms in adolescents. *Depress Anxiety* 28(7): 582–588.

47. Bloch, M.H. and Qawasmi, A. 2011. Omega-3 fatty acid supplementation for the treatment of children with attention-deficit/hyperactivity disorder symptomatology: Systematic review and meta-analysis. *J Am Acad Child Adolesc Psychiatry* 50(10): 991–1000.

48. McNamara, R.K., Strimpfel, J., Jandacek, R. et al. 2014. Detection and treatment of long-chain omega-3 fatty acid deficiency in adolescents with SSRI-resistant major depressive disorder. *PharmaNutr* 2(2): 38–46.

49. Nemets, H., Nemets, B. Apter, A. et al. 2006. Omega-3 treatment of childhood depression: A controlled, double-blind pilot study. *Am J Psychiatry* 163(6): 1098–1100.

50. Amminger, G.P., Chanen, A.M., Ohmann, S. et al. 2013. Omega-3 fatty acid supplementation in adolescents with borderline personality disorder and ultra-high risk criteria for psychosis: A post hoc subgroup analysis of a double-blind, randomized controlled trial. *Can J Psychiatry* 58(7): 402–408.

51. Watson, P.D., Joy, P.S., Nkonde, C. et al. 2009. Comparison of bleeding complications with omega-3 fatty acids. *AJC* 104(8): 1052–1054.

52. Rucklidge, J.J., Frampton, C.M., Gorman, B. et al. 2014. Vitamin-mineral treatment of attention-deficit hyperactivity disorder in adults: Double-blind randomised placebo-controlled trial. *Br J Psychiatry* 204(4): 306–315.

53. Frazier, E.A., Fristad, M.A., and Arnold, L.E. 2012. Feasibility of a nutritional supplement as treatment for pediatric bipolar spectrum disorders. *J Altern Complement Med* 18(7): 678–685.

54. Frazier, E.A., Gracious, B., Arnold, L.E. et al. 2013. Nutritional and safety outcomes from an open-label micronutrient intervention for pediatric bipolar spectrum disorders. *J Child Adolesc Psychopharmacol* 23(8): 558–567.

55. Mehl-Madrona, L., Leung, B. Kennedy, C. et al. 2010. Micronutrients versus standard medication management in autism: A naturalistic case-control study. *J Child Adolesc Psychopharmacol* 20(2): 95–103.

56. Simpson, J.S.A., Crawford, S.G., Goldstein, E.T. et al. 2011. Systematic review of safety and tolerability of a complex micronutrient formula used in mental health. *BMC Psychiatry* 11(1): 62.

57. Hoffmann, F., Glaeske, G., Petermann, F. et al. 2012. Outpatient treatment in German adolescents with depression: An analysis of nationwide health insurance data. *Pharmacoepidemiol Drug Saf* 21(9): 972–979.

58. Grundmann, O., Lv, Y. Kelber, O. et al. 2010. Neuropharmacology. *Neuropharmacology* 58(4–5): 767–773.

59. Kasper, S., Caraci, F., Forti, B. et al. 2010. Efficacy and tolerability of hypericum extract for the treatment of mild to moderate depression. *Eur Neuropsychopharmacol* 20(11): 747–765.

60. Findling, R.L., McNamara, N.K., O'Riordan, M. et al. 2003. An open-label pilot study of St. John's wort in juvenile depression. *J Am Acad Child Adolesc Psychiatry* 42(8): 908–914.

61. Hubner, W-D. and Kirste, T. 2001. Experience with St John's Wort (*Hypericum perforatum*) in children under 12 years with symptoms of depression and psychovegetative disturbances. *Phytother Res* 15(4): 367–370.

62. Simeon, J., Nixon, M.K., Milin, R. et al. 2005. Open-label pilot study of St. John's Wort in adolescent depression. *J Child Adolesc Psychopharmacol* 15(2): 293–301.

63. Andreescu, C., Mulsant, B.H., and Emanuel, J.E. 2008. Complementary and alternative medicine in the treatment of bipolar disorder—A review of the evidence. *J Affect Disord* 110(1–2): 16–26.

64. Trautmann-Sponsel, R.D., and Dienel, A. 2004. Safety of hypericum extract in mildly to moderately depressed outpatients. *J Affect Disord* 82(2): 303–307.

65. Wurglics, M., Westerhoff, K., Kaunzinger, A. et al. 2001. Comparison of German St. John's Wort products according to hyperforin and total hypericin content. *J Am Pharm Assoc (Wash)* 41(4): 560–566.

66. Rahimi, R. and Abdollahi, M. 2012. An update on the ability of St. John's Wort to affect the metabolism of other drugs. *Expert Opin Drug Metab Toxicol* 8(6): 691–708.

67. Lantz, M.S., Buchalter, E., and Giambanco, V. 1999. St. John's wort and antidepressant drug interactions in the elderly. *J Geriatr Psychiatry Neurol* 12(1): 7–10.

68. Popper, C.W. 2013. Mood disorders in youth. *Child Adolesc Psychiatry Clin North Am* 22(3): 403–441.
69. Martin, A., ed. 2010. *Pediatric Psychopharmacology*. 2nd ed. New York, NY: Oxford University Press, pp. 356–357.
70. Van Dam, N.T., Sheppard, S.C., Forsyth, J.P. et al. 2011. Self-compassion is a better predictor than mindfulness of symptom severity and quality of life in mixed anxiety and depression. *J Anxiety Disord* 25(1): 123–130.
71. Geisler, F.C.M., Kubiak, T., Siewert, K. et al. 2013. Biological psychology. *Biol Psychol* 93(2): 279–286.
72. Brown, K.W. and Ryan, R.M. 2003. The benefits of being present: Mindfulness and its role in psychological well-being. *J Pers Soc Psychol* 84(4): 822–848.
73. Simkin, D. and Black, N. 2014. Meditation and mindfulness in clinical practice. *Child Adolesc Psychiatry Clin North Am* 23(3): 487–534.
74. Newberg, A.B. and Iversen, J. 2003. The neural basis of the complex mental task of meditation: Neurotransmitter and neurochemical considerations. *Med Hypotheses* 61(2): 282–291.
75. Biegel, G.M., Brown, K.W., and Shapiro, S.L. et al. 2009. Mindfulness-based stress reduction for the treatment of adolescent psychiatric outpatients: A randomized clinical trial. *J Consult Clin Psychol* 77(5): 855–866.
76. Reynolds, W.M. and Coats, K.I. 1986. A comparison of cognitive-behavioral therapy and relaxation training for the treatment of depression in adolescents. *J Consult Clin Psychol* 54(5): 653–660.
77. Mohandas, E. 2008. Neurobiology of spirituality. *Mens Sana Monogr* 6(1): 63–80.
78. Streeter, C.C., Whitfield, T.H., and Owen, L. et al. 2010. Effects of yoga versus walking on mood, anxiety, and brain GABA levels: A randomized controlled MRS study. *J Altern Complement Med* 16(11): 1145–1152.
79. Noggle, J.J., Steiner, N.J., Minami, T. et al. 2012. Benefits of yoga for psychosocial well-being in a US high school curriculum: A preliminary randomized controlled trial. *J Dev Behav Pediatr* 33(3): 193–201.
80. Kim, S., Kim, G., and Ki, J. 2014. Effects of group art therapy combined with breath meditation on the subjective well-being of depressed and anxious adolescents. *Arts Psychother* 41(5): 519–526.
81. Hudziak, J.J., Albaugh, M.D., and Ducharme, S. et al. 2014. Cortical thickness maturation and duration of music training: Health-promoting activities shape brain development. *J Am Acad Child Adolesc Psychiatry* 53(11): 1153–1161.
82. Yinger, O.S. and Gooding, L. 2014. Music therapy and music medicine for children and adolescents. *Child Adolesc Psychiatr Clin North Am* 23(3): 535–553.
83. Field, T., Martinez, A., Nawrocki, T. et al. 1998. Music shifts frontal EEG in depressed adolescents. *Adolescence* 33(129): 109–116.
84. Wooten, M.A. 1992. The effects of heavy metal music on affects shifts of adolescents in an inpatient psychiatric setting. *Music Ther Perspect* 10(2): 93–98.
85. Baker, F. and Bor, W. 2008. Can music preference indicate mental health status in young people? *Australas Psychiatry* 16(4): 284–288.
86. Hilliard, R.E. 2007. The effects of orff-based music therapy and social work groups on childhood grief symptoms and behaviors. *J Music Ther* 44(2): 123–138.
87. Koelsch, S., Offermanns, K., and Franzke, P. 2010. Music in the treatment of affective disorders: An exploratory investigation of a new method for music-therapeutic research. *Music Percept* 27(4): 307–316.
88. Gardstrom, S.C. 2003. An investigation of meaning in clinical music improvisation with troubled adolescents. UMI Dissertations. 79–160.
89. McGarry, L. and Russo, F. 2011. The arts in psychotherapy. *Arts Psychother* 38(3): 178–184.
90. Porges, S. 2011. *The Polyvagal Theory: Neurophysiological Foundations of Emotions, Attachment, Communication, and Self-Regulation (Norton Series on Interpersonal Neurobiology.)* 1st ed. New York, NY: W. W. Norton.
91. Wall, R.B. 2005. Tai Chi and mindfulness-based stress reduction in a Boston Public Middle School. *J Pediatr Health Care* 19(4): 230–237.
92. Gordon, J.S., Staples, J.K., Blyta, A. et al. 2008. Treatment of posttraumatic stress disorder in postwar Kosovar adolescents using mind-body skills groups: A randomized controlled trial. *J Clin Psychiatry* 69(9): 1469–1476.
93. Staples, J.K., Abdel Atti, J.A., and Gordon, J.S. 2011. Mind-body skills groups for posttraumatic stress disorder and depression symptoms in Palestinian children and adolescents in Gaza. *Int J Stress Manage* 18(3): 246.

30 Integrative Approaches for Geriatric Depression

Lewis Mehl-Madrona, MD, PhD,
Barbara Mainguy, MA, and Asha Shah, MD

CONTENTS

INTRODUCTION

Quality of life for the aged includes mental, physical, familial, social, and spiritual elements, all of which must be integrated. Assessment should consider nutrition, supplement and herb intake, medications (and their interactions), movement and exercise, social contacts, presence or absence of community, family conflict, financial resources, spirituality, cognitive impairment, functional independence, abilities to carry out activities of daily life, and issues of purpose and meaning. The geriatrics must be truly integrated—treating body, mind, family, and spirit. This is especially important since nearly two-thirds of elderly patients treated for depression fail to achieve symptomatic remission and functional recovery with first-line pharmacotherapy.[1,2]

Aging has changed in modern times. Descriptions by early European explorers of aging in Native America paint a picture of better nourished, more vigorous, more respected elders than those who live today.[3] These early descriptions portray an elder's role full of meaning and purpose, which is essential to longevity and well-being.[4] The whole is more than the sum of its parts rather than a life stage isolated from others and from one's past self.[5] Through this lens, aging is a complex biopsychosocial and spiritual process that is inextricably linked to every other aspect of society and culture. Re-envisioning aging demands change in the assumptions by which conventional psychiatry is now practiced.[6]

One of the few remaining contemporary examples of indigenous cultures' treatment of aging comes from the hunter-gatherer societies of the Inglalik people of Alaska, representing a culture in which the elderly were deeply honored, integral members of the society. The Inglalik strongly promoted and supported cooperation and mutual dependence among men and women, young and old. Their primary foods and sources of materials for artifacts were wild species. Manufacturing involved hand labor and individual skills applied to locally available raw materials. Little differentiation existed in social roles by age or sex.[3] Meaning and purpose were not denied to the elderly through forced retirement. Rather, the elders were venerated for their knowledge of habitats, weather patterns, and their memory of recent and remote events. One might anticipate many fewer diseases of meaning (e.g., cancer, heart disease, diabetes, and depression), as the community system affects the individual's health. Skeletal remains largely confirm this absence.

INTEGRATIVE TREATMENT OF GERIATRIC DEPRESSION

Depression in older adults carries significant risk for decline in health functioning, morbidity, and mortality, including suicide.[8–10] Past research has suggested that old age is etiologically related to depression[11]; however, new studies are casting doubt on this hypothesis.[12] Cui and Vaillant[13] tested 113 male college graduates biennially from age 26 until age 62, when they were asked to retrospectively assess 16 major negative life events on a self-report checklist, which included antecedent variables (family history of depression, social class of parent, psychosocial "soundness" in college) and outcome variables (marital adjustment, physical health at age 65 years, affective spectrum disorder). The researchers found that psychological health is affected more by negative life events than by adverse physical health associated with aging.

Additional studies further question the existence of a predictable relationship between old age and depression. Among 113 patients with major depressive disorder (MDD) at the Duke University Clinical Research Center, a higher percentage of older adults reported complete recovery from their depression than younger adults, and a much higher percentage of younger adults reported additional episodes of depression compared to older adults, even though the older adults were also coping with an increased number of chronic health conditions.[14] The positive correlation between age and unipolar depression disappeared when potentially confounding variables were controlled for, including female gender, lower income, physical disability, cognitive impairment, and social support; the oldest actually had the fewest depressive symptoms.[11] Practitioners may have low expectations for recovery from depression of patients with medical problems. Practicing psychologists were asked to read a vignette about a potential client in which age (either 37 years or 70 years) and health (unremarkable or poor) were manipulated. Participants were then asked to diagnose the client and to predict the therapeutic response.[15] Strong health biases against recovery existed regardless of age of the client. Older adults more often present in poor health and may receive biased treatment given the expectation that they will not fare well. Doctors' expectations may play a role in determining the outcome of treatment.

Late-life depression has a neurodegenerative component that leads to impaired executive function and increases in subcortical white matter hyperintensities.[16] Phosphorus magnetic resonance spectroscopy (MRS) can quantify several important phosphorus metabolites in the brain, particularly the anabolic precursors and catabolic metabolites of the constituents of cell membranes, which could be altered by neurodegenerative activity.[17] Ten patients with late-life major depression who were medication free at the time of the study and 11 aged normal comparison subjects were studied using ^{31}P MRS three-dimensional chemical shift imaging at 4 Tesla.[18] Phosphatidylcholine and phosphatidylethanolamine comprise 90% of cell membranes in brain but cannot be quantified precisely with ^{31}P MRS. Phosphocholine and phosphoethanolamine, which are anabolic precursors, as well as glycerophosphocholine and glycerophosphoethanolamine, which are catabolic metabolites of phosphatidylcholine and phosphatidylethanolamine, were measured. Glycerophosphoethanolamine was elevated in the white matter of depressed subjects, suggesting an enhanced breakdown of cell membranes in these subjects. Glycerophosphocholine did not show any significant difference between comparison and depressed subjects, but both showed an enhancement in white matter compared with gray matter. These findings support the hypothesis that neurodegenerative processes are increased in the white matter of patients with late-life depression compared to the normal elderly population.

INDIGENOUS HEALTH SYSTEMS

Chinese, Native American, Ayurvedic, and other indigenous systems of healing share with emerging integrative geriatrics the idea that a given disease may manifest spiritually as well physically.[19] This worldview believes that the most effective interventions must address the spiritual disturbance as a source for the physical manifestation.[20] Integrative geriatrics proposes that the origins of disease are multifactorial rather than hierarchical, and include genetic, physical, emotional, psychological, and spiritual issues. This does not necessarily imply that spiritual imbalances or deficiencies are the root cause. Integrative geriatrics assumes that the individual has the potential for healing at the spiritual level, even when physical cure does not take place.[21,22]

ACUPUNCTURE

Traditional Chinese geriatrics focuses on the preventive elements of connection with nature and the mind-body relationships.[23] Harmony between man and nature requires coordinating daily activities with the seasons and with circadian rhythm. Integration of the mind and body demands moderation in physical and emotional activities and the practice of moderate exercise. Traditional Chinese treatments seek balance, harmony, and proper energy flow throughout the person. Systemic patterns of dysfunction are diagnosed, leading to person-centered treatment more than disease-specific treatment.[24]

Forty-eight community-dwelling elderly were randomized into true or placebo acupuncture, and intervention consisted of 10 sessions.[25] Sleep quality, depression, and stress scores were evaluated by the Pittsburgh Sleep Quality Index (PSQI), Beck Depression Inventory (BDI II), and Perceived Stress Scale (PSS), respectively, before and after the intervention. Acupuncture was highly effective for improving sleep quality (−53.23%; $p < 0.01$), depression (−48.41%; $p < 0.01$), and stress (−25.46%; $p < 0.01$).

TAI CHI

Exercises like Tai Chi, which encompass both mental and physical elements, facilitate a peaceful and serene mind during the performance of gentle and flexible movements. Its movements are thought to stimulate the flow of chi (vital energy, or life-giving force) through the body's energy meridians. Restoring balance and vitality to the energy body (as manifested in the meridians) can slowly but surely restore balance and vitality to the physical body, and affect mental health.[26] Tai Chi is often called "moving meditation" since a goal is to banish extraneous thoughts and to focus upon relaxation, balance, and harmony.[27] Tai Chi embodies an integrated mind-body approach to healing.

A meta-analysis examined 35 articles published before April 1, 2013, involving 2765 participants.[28] Hedges d effect sizes were calculated, and random effects models were used to estimate population variance of the observed effects and its moderators using meta-regression analysis. Tai Chi training reduced depression by a heterogeneous standardized mean effect size 0.36 (95% CI, 0.19–0.53); reductions were larger in participants having elevated symptoms at baseline. Studies with blinded allocation of participants had smaller effects. The homogeneous mean effect of Qigong on depression was 0.38 (95% CI = 0.25–0.51). The heterogeneous mean effect of Tai Chi on anxiety was 0.34 (95% CI = 0.02–0.66); reductions were larger when participants were Asian and smaller when they were older. The heterogeneous mean effect of Qigong on anxiety was 0.72 (95% CI = 0.4–1.03); reductions were inversely related to age and positively related to session duration and weekly frequency. Tai Chi and Qigong exercises were concluded to have small-to-moderate efficacy for reducing symptoms of depression and anxiety.

The relationship between long-term Tai Chi training and depressive symptoms was investigated among 529 Japanese Tai Chi practitioners.[29] Tai Chi training information, including total training time and a Tai Chi grade, was assessed using a structured questionnaire, and depressive symptoms were evaluated using the 15-item Geriatric Depression Scale (GDS) for subjects aged ≥65 and the 20-item Self-rating Depressive Scale (SDS) for subjects aged <65 with cut-off points: GDS ≥5 and SDS ≥11. The prevalence of depressive symptoms was 15.9%. After adjustments for potential confounding factors, the odds ratios of having depressive symptoms by increasing levels of Tai Chi training time were 1.00, 0.64 (0.37–1.11), 0.65 (0.37–1.13), 0.34 (0.18–0.65) (P for trend <0.01). This study demonstrated that long-term Tai Chi training was independently related to a lower prevalence of depressive symptoms.

Among 112 adults with major depression, age 60 years and older, who had been treated with escitalopram for approximately 4 weeks, 73 partial responders to escitalopram continued to receive escitalopram daily and were randomly assigned to 10 weeks of adjunctive use of either (1) Tai Chi (TC) for 2 hours per week or (2) health education (HE) for 2 hours per week.[30] Subjects in the escitalopram and TC condition were more likely to show greater reduction of depressive symptoms and to achieve a depression remission as compared with those receiving escitalopram and HE. Subjects in the escitalopram and TC also showed significantly greater improvements on the 36-Item Short Form Health Survey of physical functioning and in cognitive tests, and a decline in the inflammatory marker, C-reactive protein, compared with the control group. This study is especially interesting in showing the role that complementary therapies could play as adjunctive treatments in nonresponders or poor responders to conventional treatments.

QIGONG

Practicing Qigong exercises may favorably affect many functions of the body, permit reduction of the dosage of drugs required for health maintenance, and provide greater health benefits than the use of drug therapy alone.[31] In a randomized controlled single blind study, 58 adults over age 50 were admitted to a post-acute intermediate care rehabilitation facility, to receive a 90 minute, biweekly, 4-week structured Qigong intervention plus usual care and rehabilitation ($N = 29$) or usual care and rehabilitation alone ($N = 29$).[28] Outcomes included quality of life (0–100 points visual analogical scale), pain (0–10 points scale), and depressive symptoms (five-item modified Yesavage Geriatric Depression Scale). Of the enrolled 58 participants (mean age ±SD = 74.3 ± 8.2 years, 88% women), four in the control group dropped out. No statistically significant differences in baseline characteristics were shown between groups, including age, gender, marital status, education, comorbidity, functional status, main diagnosis at admission, and number of rehabilitation sessions. In an intention-to-treat analysis (repeated measures ANOVA), the intervention group experienced a significant improvement in quality of life (mean increase of 19 points versus 2.6 points for controls, $p = 0.002$). Pain and depressive symptoms improved in both groups. Adherence was good (79% of participants completed the whole program). No adverse events were reported. The authors concluded that a structured Qigong intervention, together with usual care, could contribute to improve quality of life of patients admitted to a postacute intermediate care rehabilitation unit, compared to usual care.

SPIRITUALITY

There is growing interest in examining the implications of spirituality for mental health.[32] Spiritual experiences have been associated with psychological and physical well-being.[33–39] Spirituality has been gaining recognition as a legitimate and important aspect of human functioning, related reliably to both physical and mental health, even though the mechanisms behind the positive outcomes cannot be readily explained.[40,41] Ample evidence supports an association between psychological functioning with measures of religious commitment.[40] Religious behavior (for example, church attendance) has been shown to be a highly reliable predictor of mental health in over 1000 studies. Spirituality appears to be robustly associated with lower levels of substance abuse, depression, and suicide, with improved treatment outcomes and higher levels of life satisfaction and general well-being.[41] Meaning and purpose in life are central to many extant models and measures of spirituality and have been proposed as one of the main mechanisms through which spirituality affects mental health.[42,43]

Conversely, boredom and boredom proneness are negatively associated with perceived meaning and purpose in life and self-actualization.[44–48] Among retired persons, boredom is associated with ill health.[44] Transforming boredom is therefore a potential means to improve geriatric mental health. One of the means for this transformation is through volunteerism. Activities derived from spiritual development and spiritual practice (e.g., feeding the homeless) provide important avenues for the transformation of boredom. Research has yet to document the relationship between boredom and falls, but we suspect it exists. Boredom arises in the absence of purpose, meaning, and self-actualization. Therefore, geriatrics must cultivate these traits.

Among 157 Korean elder-family caregiver dyads in Seoul, Korea, both caregivers' and elders' self-transcendence was positively related to their own sense of purpose in life.[49] However, only elders' spiritual perspective was related to purpose in life. Also, elders' purpose in life was positively associated with caregivers' purpose in life. There was a strong negative relationship between elders' purpose in life and their depressive symptoms, but there was not a significant negative relationship between caregivers' purpose in life and elders' depressive symptoms. Elders' purpose in life mediated the negative effects of elders' self-transcendence and spiritual perspective and of caregivers' self-transcendence and purpose in life on elders' depression. The findings suggested that purpose in life for both the caregiver and elder played an important role in elders' depression.

NUTRITION AND BRAIN FUNCTION

An inadequate dietary supply of any of a number of essential micronutrients (some 40 vitamins, minerals, and other small molecule essential nutrients) can adversely affect brain function.[50–53]

In 2013, Donini et al. evaluated the change in eating habits occurring in 526 elderly (age 65 and older) subjects in four regions of Italy.[54] The authors concluded that the high prevalence of senile anorexia in the geriatric population and its impact on nutritional status merited research to establish an intervention.[55] Two hundred seventeen lived in their homes; 213 were residents in nursing homes; and 93 lived in rehabilitation or acute wards. All subjects underwent a multidimensional geriatric evaluation of nutritional status, anthropometric parameters, health and cognitive status, depression, taste, chewing and swallowing function, and some hormones related to appetite. In anorexic elderly subjects, the global food intake was reduced, and the eating pattern was characterized by reduced consumption of meat, eggs, fish, fruit, and vegetables. The consumption of milk and cereals remained unchanged from earlier dietary patterns. Nutritional parameters were significantly better in normal eating subjects and correlated with diet variety.[56]

The Quebec Longitudinal Study on Nutrition and Aging (NuAge) collected social, health, and biological data of 1793 community-dwelling men and women aged 68–82 years at recruitment for

4 years.[57] The incidence of depression was defined by scores in the 30-item Geriatric Depression Scale greater than or equal to 11 or antidepressant medication use over the 3 years of follow-up. Those deemed "depressed" at baseline were excluded. Dietary patterns were created through principal component analysis on amount (grams) of food items consumed in each of the 32 predefined food categories. Tertiles of B-vitamin intake were created from the mean of three nonconsecutive 24-hour recalls. Multiple logistic regression models were adjusted for several demographic, health, and social confounders. For the study of the reverse causality hypothesis, the authors conducted a nested case-control study. Participants, free of depression at baseline, who developed depression at some point of follow-up, were matched by age group and sex with nondepressed participants. The intakes of energy, protein, saturated fat, dietary fiber, B6, B12, and folate at the time of depression were compared with intakes the year prior between depressed and nondepressed groups using mixed-model repeated measures ANCOVA. The incidence of depression was 12.5% ($n = 170$, 63% women). Principal component analysis revealed three dietary patterns: varied diet, traditional diet, and convenience diet. Only varied diet was protective of depression incidence before adjustment for confounders. None of the three patterns were associated with the outcome in fully adjusted models. Tertiles of total energy intake were, however, inversely and independently associated with depression incidence. Men in the highest tertile of B12 intake from food had lower risk of depression compared with those in the lowest tertile. Higher B6 intake from food was protective among women, but the effect was dependent on total energy intake. Neither intakes from food and supplements (total) nor folate intake showed detectable benefits. Differences in quantity of food (energy intake) were more strongly associated with the likelihood of developing depression in the following years among generally healthy seniors living in the community than small differences in quality (dietary patterns). Nutrients were thought to predict depression better than food items, particularly non-energy-adjusted B6 in women and energy-adjusted B12 in men, whose lower intakes were associated with increased risk for depression.

MICRONUTRIENTS AND DEPRESSION

Some studies suggest positive effects of multivitamin and mineral supplementation on cognitive function, both mild cognitive impairment (MCI) and Alzheimer's disease (AD).[58,59] Bruce Ames has shown how deficiencies in several micronutrients are associated with chromosome breaks and disease in humans.[60] According to his triage theory, scarce micronutrients present in states of hidden malnutrition are used for short-term survival at the expense of long-term survival, so that when an additional insult comes later during the course of susceptible life, pathology occurs. The "latent early life-associated regulation" (LEARn) model suggests that environmental stress and/or nutritional imbalance marks a gene which later during life and in the presence of a secondary trigger will be expressed aberrantly causing overt pathology.[61,62] The epigenetic oxidative redox shift (EORS) theory of aging proposes that sedentary behavior associated with age triggers an oxidized redox shift and impaired mitochondrial function inducing epigenetic changes.[63] For these reasons, Ames proposes a role for comprehensive, high-dose, high-potency micronutrient supplements for a number of psychiatric conditions in the elderly.[60]

In another study, participants over age 65 completed a validated food frequency questionnaire at baseline between 2001 and 2003.[64] Factor analysis was used to identify three dietary patterns: "vegetables-fruits" pattern, "snacks-drinks-milk products" pattern, and "meat-fish" pattern. Depressive symptoms were measured at baseline and 4 years using the validated Geriatric Depression Scale. Multiple logistic regression was used for cross-sectional analysis ($n = 2902$) to assess the associations between dietary patterns and the presence of depressive symptoms, and for longitudinal analysis on their associations with 4-year depressive symptoms, with adjustment for sociodemographic and lifestyle factors. The highest quartile of "vegetables-fruits" pattern score was associated with reduced likelihood of depressive symptoms compared to the lowest quartile at baseline. A similar inverse trend was observed for the highest quartile of "snacks-drinks-milk products" pattern score compared to the lowest quartile. There was no association of "meat-fish" pattern with the presence of depressive symptoms at baseline. None of the dietary patterns were associated with subsequent depressive symptoms at 4 years. Higher "vegetables-fruits" and lower "snacks-drinks-milk products" pattern scores were associated with reduced likelihood of baseline depressive symptoms in Chinese older people in Hong Kong. The longitudinal analyses failed to show any causal relationship between dietary patterns and depressive symptoms in this population, suggesting that the effects of diet unfold over many years and not acutely.

VITAMIN D

Vitamin D deficiency is one of the postulated links between diabetes and depression and dementia.[65–69] Hypovitaminosis D is commonly observed in the elderly population. A restricted ultraviolet light exposure, low vitamin D intake, and decreased skin synthesis capacity may be related to the development of vitamin D deficiency in aging populations. In NHANES III, Martins and colleagues observed lower 25(OH)D levels in women, persons over 60 years, and obese and diabetic participants.[70] In 1984, a study among middle-aged and elderly English men and women showed that postprandial glucose levels were highest during the winter.[71] The presence of 1-alpha-hydroxylase in cerebrospinal fluid and the existence of vitamin D receptors (VDRs) on various brain structures supports the hypothesis that vitamin D is involved in mental health.[72] While animal experiments point toward a protective effect of vitamin D against several age-related diseases,[73] population-based studies have not yet provided conclusive evidence of an association with diabetes,[65,74] cognitive functioning, and depression.[67–69,75–78] The European SENECA study found an inverse relationship between both 25-hydroxy-vitamin D levels and glucose levels with depression and dementia.[73,79–87]

In a cross-sectional study involving 21 men (mean age of 75.4 ± 6.8 years) and 96 women (mean age of 75.0 ± 6.8 years), body mass index, percent body fat, and waist circumference were measured along with functional physical fitness, including strength, cardiorespiratory endurance, agility, dynamic balance, and flexibility.[88] Serum levels of vitamin D, lipoprotein lipids, fasting glucose, and insulin were measured. The Korean form of the Geriatric Depression Scale (K-GDS) was used to assess depression level and status. Pearson correlation analyses were used to calculate bivariate correlations between measured variables. Multiple linear regression analyses were used to identify any independent predictors for K-GDS-based depression score. Depression scores were significantly and inversely associated with functional physical fitness including strength ($P < 0.001$), cardiorespiratory endurance ($P < 0.001$), agility ($P = 0.002$), and dynamic balance ($P < 0.001$). A similar trend in correlation was observed between depression and serum vitamin D level. Multiple linear regression analyses showed that strength ($P < 0.001$), cardiorespiratory endurance ($P = 0.005$), and percent body fat ($P = 0.045$) were significant independent predictors of depression in this study population. The finding of this study suggested that fitness promotion along with a healthy diet habit should be a key component of intervention against depression in elderly persons.

DIHYDROEPIANDOSTERONE

Dihydroepiandosterone (DHEA) supplementation has been shown to be beneficial in treating major depression, though the exact physiological mechanism is unknown.[89] One study reported positive effects of DHEA administration in healthy women over age 70 on several neuropsychological symptoms. Positive effects on sexual interest and satisfaction and sense of well-being are more consistent in elderly women than in men. The recommended administered dose is 25–50 mg once a day in women and 100 mg in men. Androgenic side effects (greasy skin, acne, increased growth of body hair) are frequent but reversible. The treatment should be taken under close medical supervision in order to detect a possible hormone-dependent cancer such as breast cancer in women and prostate cancer in men. Many authorities recommend active screening for breast and prostate cancers before starting DHEA, as well as ongoing monitoring.

In a population-based cohort longitudinal study in the general community, 789 older participants without depression and cognitive impairment at the baseline were included among 3099 screened subjects.[90] Serum DHEAS levels were determined based on blood samples; incident depression and severe depression were diagnosed by means of the Geriatric Depression Scale (GDS) and confirmed by geriatricians skilled in psychogeriatric medicine. No baseline differences were found in GDS across age- and gender-specific tertiles of serum DHEAS. Over 4.4 years of follow-up, 137 new cases of depression were recorded. Of them, 35 among men and 64 in women were cases of incident severe depression. Cox's regression analysis, adjusted for potential confounders, revealed that higher DHEAS levels were associated with reduced risk of incident depression irrespective of gender and of severe incident depression only in men. Higher serum DHEAS levels were found to be significantly protective for the onset of depression irrespective of gender, whereas only in men was this association found also for incident severe depression.

S-Adenosylmethionine

S-Adenosylmethionine (SAMe), a substance found naturally in the human body, may contribute to an increase in the levels of certain neurotransmitters when given in supplement form. Although definitive data on efficacy are still lacking, SAM-e appears to have enough of an antidepressant effect to warrant further research. In a 2001 review, the authors found considerable variability in trial sample sizes and dose administration.[91] Several reviews and at least two meta-analyses of trials completed prior to 1994 concluded that SAMe was superior to placebo in treating depressive disorders and approximately as effective as standard tricyclic antidepressants. Although these results come from small clinical trials, SAMe appears to be well tolerated, with the majority of adverse effects presenting as mild to moderate gastrointestinal complaints. In a pilot study of SAMe in 13 depressed patients with Parkinson's disease, all of whom had been previously treated with other antidepressant agents without significant benefit or with intolerable side effects, SAMe was administered in doses of 800–3600 mg per day for a period of 10 weeks.[92] Of the 11 patients who completed the study, 10 had at least a 50% improvement on the 17-point Hamilton Depression Scale (HDS). Although uncontrolled and preliminary, this study suggested that SAMe may be a safe and effective alternative to the antidepressant agents currently used in patients with Parkinson's disease.

Another study examined a subsample from one site of a two-site study of adults with diagnosed MDD, recruited from 2005 to 2009.[93] After washout, eligible subjects were randomized to SAMe (1600–3200 mg/daily), escitalopram (10–20 mg/daily), or matching placebo for 12 weeks of double-blind treatment (titration at week 6 in nonresponse). On the primary outcome of the Hamilton Depression Rating Scale (HAMD-17), a significant difference in improvement was observed between groups from baseline to week 12 ($p = 0.039$). The effect size from baseline to endpoint was moderate to large for SAMe versus placebo ($d = 0.74$). SAMe was superior to placebo from week 1, and to escitalopram during weeks 2, 4, and 6. No significant effect was found between escitalopram and placebo or SAMe. Response rates (HAMD-17 $\geq$ 50% reduction) at endpoint were 45%, 31%, and 26% for SAMe, escitalopram, and placebo, respectively; while remission rates (HAM-D $\leq$ 7) were 34% for SAMe ($p = 0.003$), 23% for escitalopram ($p = 0.023$), and 6% for placebo.

Vitamin B12 and Folate

In a randomized, double-blind, placebo-controlled trial of citalopram (20–40 g) together with 0.5 mg of vitamin B12, 2 mg of folic acid and 25 mg of vitamin B6 for 52 weeks among community-dwelling adults aged 50 years or over with DSM-IV-TR major depression, measured with the Montgomery-Åsberg Depression Rating Scale (MADRS) with a primary outcome of remission of the depressive episode after 12, 26 and 52 weeks and with secondary outcome measures of reduction of MADRS scores over time and relapse of major depression after recovery by week 12, 153 people were randomized (76 placebo, 77 vitamins).[94] Remission of symptoms was achieved by 78.1% and 79.4% of participants treated with placebo and vitamins by week 12 ($P = 0.840$), by 76.5% and 85.3% at week 26, and 75.8% and 85.5% at week 52 (effect of intervention over 52 weeks: odds ratio [OR] = 2.49, 95% CI 1.12–5.51). Group differences in MADRS scores over time were not significant ($P = 0.739$). The risk of subsequent relapse among those who had achieved remission of symptoms at week 12 was lower in the vitamins than placebo group (OR = 0.33, 95% CI 0.12–0.94). B vitamins did not increase the 12-week efficacy of antidepressant treatment, but enhanced and sustained antidepressant response over 1 year.[95] Many vitamin studies are short term, which may explain their lack of efficacy.

Besides preventing macrocytic anemia, vitamin B12 is important for transmethylation of neuroactive compounds.[96] Disruption of methylation in the central nervous system (CNS) could increase homocysteine levels resulting in direct neurotoxic effects.[97] Hyperhomocysteinemia has also been reported to have a neurotoxic action independent of its vascular effects by overstimulation of N-methyl-D-aspartate receptors or by increasing hippocampal neuron vulnerability to excitotoxic insults and amyloid-β peptide toxicity.[98] Elevated homocysteine has been associated with increased risk for AD and with faster cognitive decline.[99]

The prevalence of vitamin B12 deficiency has been estimated at 15%–44% in the elderly.[97] It is often overlooked due to its multiple clinical manifestations that can affect the blood, neurological, gastrointestinal, and cardiovascular systems, and skin and mucous membranes.[100] The various presentations of vitamin B12 deficiency are related to the development of geriatric syndromes like frailty, falls, cognitive impairment, and geriatric nutritional syndromes like protein-energy malnutrition and failure to thrive, in addition to enhancing aging anorexia and cachexia. Lower levels of serum vitamin B12 were predictive of cognitive decline ($p < 0.05$).[101]

One-third of depressed patients have low folic acid levels. Studies show that repleting folate levels also improve symptoms of depression.[102–104] In the Women's Health and Aging Study,[105] serum levels of vitamin B12, folate, methylmalonic acid, and total homocysteine were measured in 700 disabled, women aged 65 years and over, living in the community, and without dementia. Depressive symptoms were measured with the Geriatric Depression Scale and categorized as absent, mild, moderate, or severe. Homocysteine levels, folate levels, folate deficiency, and anemia were not associated with depression status. The depressed subjects, especially those with severe depression, had a significantly higher serum methylmalonic acid level and a nonsignificantly lower serum vitamin B12 level than the nondepressed subjects. Metabolically significant vitamin B12 deficiency was present in 14.9 of the 478 nondepressed subjects, 17.0% of the 100 mildly depressed subjects, and 27.0% of the 122 severely depressed women. After adjustment for sociodemographic characteristics and health status, the subjects with vitamin B12 deficiency were 2.05 times as likely to be severely depressed as were nondeficient subjects. Therefore, in community-dwelling older women, metabolically significant vitamin B12 deficiency is associated with a twofold risk of severe depression.

Among inpatients with severe depression, 52% had raised total plasma homocysteine accompanied by significant lowering of serum, red cell, CSF folate, CSF S-adenosylmethionine, and all three CSF monoamine metabolites. Total plasma homocysteine was significantly negatively correlated with red cell folate in depressed patients, but not in controls.[106] In one representative study, fluoxetine at a dose of 20 mg/day for 8 weeks was given to 213 outpatients with MDD. Subjects with low serum folate levels were more likely to have melancholic depression and were significantly less likely to respond to fluoxetine.[107]

The psychiatric symptoms of folate deficiency are found among 25% of hospitalized patients, and include anorexia, insomnia, fatigue, hyperirritability, apathy, withdrawal, confusion, lack of motivation, anxiety, depression, delusions, dementia, slowed cerebration, forgetfulness, and disorientation. Prevention requires 50–1000 mcg/day and oral treatment consists of 2–5 mg/day.

Folate requires enzymatic conversion to L-methylfolate, which is the biologically active form of folic acid and can be prescribed as a prescription medical food.[108] The enzyme MTHFR, which catalyzes the rate-determining step in L-methylfolate synthesis, is subject to a common polymorphism rendering the enzyme less effective. This can lead to lower levels of L-methylfolate being available to activate tetrohydropbiopterin for serotonin production in the raphe nucleus. Recent data strongly suggest that L-methylfolate is an effective augmentation strategy for major depression at both the initial onset of symptoms and in patients with treatment-resistant depression. Patients with a combination of genetic mutations at *MTHFR*, early life adversity, and/or obesity are potentially excellent candidates for L-methylfolate augmentation.

MELATONIN

Melatonin has been reported effective with 84% of depressed patients showing abnormal levels.[109] Daylight is the necessary ingredient, which keeps the melatonin cycle in time with the real world. Without daylight, the body adjusts naturally to a 25-hour rhythm, and it is the light reaching the eyes, which, in humans, is required for this process. Melatonin administration or light therapy or both can correct these difficulties.[110] Circadian and sleep disturbances may be central for understanding the pathophysiology and treatment of depression. The effect of melatonin on depression/depressive symptoms has been investigated previously. A systematic review assessed the current evidence of a therapeutic and prophylactic effect of melatonin in adult patients against depression or depressive symptoms. A search was performed in the Cochrane Library, PubMed, EMBASE, and PsycINFO for published trials on November 14, 2013. Inclusion criteria were English language, RCTs, or crossover trials. Ten studies of 486 patients were included in the final qualitative synthesis, and four studies, 148 patients, were included in two meta-analyses. Melatonin doses varied from 0.5 to 6 mg daily, and the length of follow-up varied from 2 weeks to 3.5 years. Three studies were done on patients without depression at inclusion, two studies in patients with depression, and five studies included a mixture. Six studies showed an improvement in depression scores in both the melatonin and placebo groups, but there was no significant difference. One study showed a significant prophylactic effect and another found a significant treatment effect on depression with melatonin compared to placebo. The two meta-analyses did not show any significant effect of melatonin. No serious adverse events were reported. Although some studies were positive, there was no clear evidence of a therapeutic or prophylactic effect of melatonin against depression or depressive symptoms.

AMINO ACIDS

Amino acid supplementation has been reported helpful in some patients with depression. In one open trial of 351 depressed patients who had failed antidepressant drug treatment, 85% experienced significant improvement in 2 weeks from a combination of amino acids, which included tryptophan and taurine.[111] Seventy percent remained consistently improved, based on scores on the Zung Depression Test. The authors also included vitamin B6 and magnesium. Tryptophan has long been reported effective for depression, often in combination with vitamins B3 and B6.[112] Tryptophan has been compared to amitriptyline in a randomized, controlled trial.[113] In one study, 115 general practice patients were enrolled in a 12-week double-blind study using the Hamilton Depression Scale before and after treatment to assess the level of depression. The four treatment groups were (1) tryptophan 1 gm t.i.d.; (2) tryptophan 1 gm t.i.d. and amitriptyline 25 mg t.i.d. raised later to 50 mg t.i.d.; (3) amitriptyline 25 mg t.i.d., later raised to 50 mg t.i.d.; and (4) placebo t.i.d. All treatments were significantly better than placebo ($p < 0.05$). Far more of the placebo group withdrew during the study than the other three groups ($p < 0.0004$). Amitriptyline significantly relieved depression ($p < 0.001$) as did tryptophan ($p < 0.01$). The combination was better than either alone ($p < 0.05$), demonstrating synergy. Side effects of tryptophan were significantly less than with amitriptyline.

ACETYL-L-CARNITINE

Acetyl-L-carnitine (ALC) is a potential antidepressant with novel mechanism of action because of its diverse functions related with neuroplasticity.[114] Animal and cellular models suggest that ALC's neuroplasticity effect, membrane modulation, and neurotransmitter regulation may play an important role in treatment of depression. Four randomized clinical studies (RCTs) demonstrated the superior efficacy of ALC over placebo in patients with depression. Two RCTs showed its superior efficacy over placebo in dysthymic disorder, and two other RCTs showed that it is equally effective as fluoxetine and amisulpride in treatment of dysthymic disorder. ALC was also effective in improving depressive symptoms in patients with fibromyalgia and minimal hepatic encephalopathy. It was also found to be equally tolerable to placebo and better tolerable than fluoxetine and amisulpride. ALC may be potentially effective and tolerable, in particular, for older populations and patients with comorbid medical conditions who are vulnerable to adverse events from antidepressants.

OMEGA-3 FATTY ACIDS

Omega-3 fatty acids have been considered as treatment for depression. Phospholipids make up 60% of the dry weight of the brain. They are essential for neuronal and especially for synaptic structure and play key roles in the signal transduction responses to dopamine, serotonin, glutamate, and acetylcholine. The unsaturated fatty acid components of phospholipids are abnormal in depression, with deficits of eicosapentaenoic acid and other omega-3 fatty acids and excesses of the omega-6 fatty acid arachidonic acid.[115] Correction of this abnormality by treatment with eicosapentaenoic acid improves depression.[116] The fatty acid abnormalities also provide a rational explanation for the associations of depression with cardiovascular disease, immunological activation, cancer, diabetic complications, and osteoporosis. The abnormalities cannot be explained by diet, although diet may attenuate or exacerbate their consequences. A number of enzyme abnormalities could explain the phenomena with phospholipase A(2), and coenzyme A-independent transacylase being strong candidates. Nevertheless, the field is still unfolding. A review of five omega-3 studies for depression found no effectiveness for omega-3 as a therapeutic agent, though all studies confirmed lowered omega-3 levels in depression.[117] Further research is ongoing.

Specific research findings include the association of depression with a lowered degree of esterification of serum cholesterol, an increased C20:4 omega 6/C20:5 omega 3 ratio alongside the decreases in omega-3. In one study, there was no significant effect of antidepressive treatment on any of the fatty acids. The authors concluded that major depression is associated with a deficiency of omega-3 polyunsaturated fatty acids and a compensatory increase in MUFAs and C22:5 omega 6 in phospholipids. They believe that the fatty acid alterations in depression are related to an inflammatory response in that illness; and that this disorder may persist despite successful antidepressant treatment.[118]

EXERCISE

More than 1000 trials have explored the relationship between depression and exercise.[119] Regularly performed exercise is as effective as pharmacotherapy or psychotherapy. In a representative study from 2002 for geriatric depression, patients were randomized to attend either exercise classes or health education talks for 10 weeks.[120] Assessments were made "blind" at baseline, and at 10 and 34 weeks. The primary outcome was seen with the 17-item Hamilton Rating Scale for Depression (HRSD). Secondary outcomes were seen with the Geriatric Depression Scale, Clinical Global Impression, and Patient Global Impression. At 10 weeks a significantly higher proportion of the exercise group (55% versus 33%) experienced a greater than 30% decline in depression according to HRSD (OR = 2.51, $P = 0.05$, 95% CI 1.00–6.38). The authors concluded that because exercise was associated with a modest improvement in depressive symptoms at 10 weeks, older people with poorly responsive depressive disorder should be encouraged to attend group exercise activities.

In a 2014 systematic review of exercise programs as interventions to decrease depressive symptoms and to improve quality of life and self-esteem in older people, exercise therapy in older people was shown to be effective, as evidenced by a decrease in depressive symptoms [standardized mean difference (SMD) −0.36; 95% confidence interval (CI) −0.64, −0.08], and improvements in quality of life (SMD 0.86; 95% CI 0.11, 1.62) and self-esteem (SMD 0.49; 95% CI 0.09, 0.88). The changes were statistically significant.[121]

However, the "Older People's Exercise intervention in Residential and nursing Accommodation" (OPERA) study found no benefit of a training program for nursing home staff together with twice-weekly, physical therapist–led exercise classes upon depressive symptoms. The OPERA trial included over 1000 residents in 78 nursing homes in the United Kingdom. The overall attendance rate at group exercise sessions was low (50%) as were levels of staff training. Few staff in the nursing home were enthusiastic about the intervention, and the nursing home culture prioritized protecting residents from harm over encouraging activity. The trial team delivered 3191 exercise groups, but only 36% of participants attended at least one group per week, and depressed residents attended significantly fewer groups than those who were not depressed. Residents were frail so that most groups included only seated exercises. The intervention did not change the culture of the homes and activity levels did not change outside the exercise groups. Residents did not engage in the exercise groups at a sufficient level, and this was particularly true for those with depressive symptoms at baseline. The physical and mental frailty of care home residents may make it impossible to deliver a sufficiently intense exercise intervention to impact on depressive symptoms.

A systematic review and meta-analysis of studies that examined the effects of structured exercise on depressive symptoms in stroke patients found 13 acceptable studies ($n = 1022$) for inclusion.[122] Exercise resulted in less depressive symptoms immediately after the exercise program ended, standardized mean difference = −0.13 [95% CI = −0.26, −0.01], $I^2 = 6\%$, $p = 0.03$, but these effects were not retained with longer-term follow-up. Exercise appeared to have a positive effect on depressive symptoms across both the subacute (≤6 months post-stroke) and chronic stage of recovery (>6 months). There was a significant effect of exercise on depressive symptoms when higher-intensity studies were pooled, but not for lower-intensity exercise protocols. Antidepressant medication use was not documented in the majority of studies, and thus its potential confounding interaction with exercise could not be assessed. This review coupled with the OPERA trial, suggests that staff enthusiasm is essential and that there is a minimal required dose of exercise to produce an effect.

BOTANICALS AND DEPRESSION

St. John's Wort

St. John's wort has been shown effective for depression in a number of studies;[123–130] however, since none were specifically directed toward a geriatric population, we will not review it further.

Gingko Biloba and Valerian

Extracts of ginkgo biloba leaves, standardized to contain 24% gingko flavonoglycosides and 6% terpenoids, exert antidepressant effects, especially in people over 50 years of age.[131] Ginkgo biloba has been shown to counteract one of the major changes in brain chemistry associated with aging—reduction in the number of serotonin receptor sites in brain cells. Because of the reduced number of serotonin receptor sites, the elderly are thought to be more susceptible to depression, impaired mental function, insomnia, and sleep disturbances. A study to determine alterations in the number of serotonin receptors in old and young lab rats given the extract showed a statistically significant increase (by 33%) in the number of binding sites in older but not in younger rats. Accordingly, gingko biloba may counteract at least some age-dependent reduction of serotonin binding sites in the aging human brain.[132,133] Although the exact mechanism of action is unclear, the extract may address two issues that cause serotonin receptors to decline with age: impaired receptor synthesis, and changes in cerebral neuronal membranes or receptors as a result of free radical damage. The extract has demonstrated the ability to increase protein synthesis and is known to be a potent antioxidant.

In another representative study, gingko biloba also proved to diminish depression. In a double-blind, placebo-controlled trial of 40 elderly people, randomized to treatment groups given standard drug or a combination of standard drug plus 240 mg ginkgo treatment, the group that received gingko biloba had a decreased score on the Hamilton Depression Scale (HAM-D) of 50% versus 7% in the control group.[134] It has been used as an adjunct in people over age 50 who do not respond to conventional treatment (treatment-resistant depression). The dosage is 40–80 mg PO daily of extract, standardized to 24% gingko flavoglycosides and 6% terpenoids. A response is expected within 2–3 weeks, but it may take 3 months for full effects. Rare cases of mild gastrointestinal upset have been noted, along with headache, allergic skin reactions, and mild antiplatelet effects, which dictate some care in patients on anticoagulants.[135]

Valerian is used as a sedative in the treatment of insomnia.[136] It can also be used in the treatment of stress and anxiety. Two controlled human studies in geriatric subjects with sleep disturbances have provided evidence to suggest that *Valeriana officinalis* may have antidepressant effects.[137,138] In the former study, participants reported significant improvements in mood and well-being after only 2 weeks of treatment, whereas the full sleep-promoting effects were not experienced until the end of 4 weeks. Together, these studies suggest that valerian may also have intrinsic antidepressant effects.

BALNEOTHERAPY

Balneotherapy is the use of hot and cold baths containing different types of minerals for treating illnesses, which dates back to early civilization. These baths include sulfur springs and concentrated salt water pools from drying lakebeds, such as the Dead Sea in Israel. One study with 52 elderly adults from different areas of Spain participated in a balneotherapy program funded by the government's Institute for Elderly and Social Services, known as IMSERSO. The group included 23 men (age, 69.74 ± 5.19 years) and 29 women (age, 70.31 ± 6.76 years), and pain was analyzed using the visual analogue scale.[139] Mood was assessed using the Profile of Mood Status. Sleep was assessed using the Oviedo Sleep Questionnaire. Depression was assessed using the Geriatric Depression Scale. The balneotherapy program was undertaken at Balneario San Andrés (Jaén, Spain). The water at Balneario San Andrés, according to the Handbook of Spanish Mineral Water, is a hypothermic ($\geq 20°C$) hard water of medium mineralization, with bicarbonate, sulfate, sodium, and magnesium as the dominant ions. Balneotherapy produced significant improvements ($P < 0.05$) for all variables (pain, mood state, sleep, and depression) in the total sample. A differential effect was found between the sexes regarding pain improvement, with men, but not women, having significantly improvement ($P < 0.01$) after treatment. With regard to improving mood, sex differences were also shown, with women, but not men, significantly improved ($P < 0.05$) in both depression and fatigue. A 12-day balneotherapy program had a positive effect on pain, mood, sleep quality, and depression in healthy older people.

SOCIAL INTERACTIONS

Socialization improves depression, even when people socialize with animals and robots. In a study from Auckland, New Zealand, 40 nursing home residents were randomized to either a group who interacted with a seal robot, or to a control group that attended normal activities.[140] Sessions took place twice a week for 1 hour over 12 weeks. Based on observation and patient surveys, the investigators found that residents who interacted with the robot experienced significantly less loneliness over the period of the trial. The robot and the facility's resident dog appeared to influence the social environment, but the robot was observed to have a more positive effect than the dog. The robot was a positive addition to the nursing home environment.

Another study examined the relationship between social support, depression, instrumental activities of daily living (IADLs), and utilization of in-home and community-based services.[141] The sample included 39 adults age 65 years and older. Depression levels significantly decreased as levels of social support increased. IADLs functioning significantly decreased as depression levels increased. In addition, the number of in-home services significantly increased as IADLs functioning lessened. More services were needed as levels of social support declined.

Another study assessed the relationships between older patients' social support resources with depressive symptoms and psychosocial functioning at 6 months following a psychiatric hospital discharge.[142] The data used in this study were extracted from a prospective study conducted by the NIMH (National Institute of Mental Health-56208). The sample included 148 older patients who participated in both the initial and the 6-month follow-up assessments. Patients' depressive symptoms were related to availability of a confidant and time spent in the company of others.

PSYCHOTHERAPY

The efficacy of psychotherapy has been studied as an intervention for treating depression in geriatric patients. A 2014 systematic review and meta-analysis of randomized controlled psychotherapy trials for late-life depression identified 27 trials with 37 therapy-control contrasts and 2245 subjects.[141] Trials utilized five types of control groups (waitlist, treatment-as-usual, attention, supportive therapy, placebo). In the combined contrasts, psychotherapy was effective (SMD: 0.73; 95% confidence interval [CI]: 0.51, 0.95; $z = 6.42$, $p < 0.00001$). Supportive psychotherapy appeared to best control for the nonspecific elements of psychotherapy and was associated with considerable change itself, but few trials have utilized it as a control. Despite its efficacy, use of psychotherapy is low.[143] A 2014 study of psychotherapy utilization patterns for community-dwelling older adults with depressive symptoms showed that 27% received psychotherapy; nearly two-thirds of these residents reported four or fewer visits. Mental health counselors were the most frequently reported service providers (50%–62.5%). The benefits of particular types of psychotherapy have been studied. Behavioral activation methods have been shown to be effective for older adults with depression, and manuals have been adapted for geriatric populations.[144]

In 2013, 221 adults aged 60 years and older participated in a randomized clinical trial comparing the efficacy of Problem Solving Therapy (PST) and Supportive Therapy (ST) for geriatric depression.[145] Performance on a measure of executive functioning with a significant information processing speed component (Stroop Color and Word Test) improved after treatment, $F (1, 312) = 8.50$, $p = 0.002$, and improved performance was associated with a reduction in depressive symptoms but not treatment type. Performance on other measures of executive functioning, verbal learning, and memory did not change significantly after 12 weeks of psychotherapy treatment.

Niemeyer et al. assessed whether systematic reviews investigating psychotherapeutic interventions for depression were affected by publication bias.[146] They used 31 data sets reported in 19 meta-analyses and detected significant bias in five (16.13%; rank correlation test) and six (19.35%; Egger's regression analysis) of the data sets. Applying the trim and fill procedure to amend presumably missing studies rarely changed the assessment of the efficacy of therapeutic interventions, with two exceptions. In one data set psychotherapy was no longer found more efficacious than pharmacotherapy in reducing the dropout rate at post-treatment when publication bias was taken into account. In the second data set, after correcting for publication bias, there was no longer evidence that depressed patients without comorbid personality disorder profited more from psychotherapy and pharmacotherapy than patients with comorbid personality disorder. Thus, findings that psychotherapy has efficacy in treating geriatric depression would appear robust. Yoga, either in conjunction with psychotherapy, or by itself, has also been shown to be effective.[147–153]

NEUROFEEDBACK AND COGNITIVE REMEDIATION

Executive dysfunction is common in geriatric depression and predicts poor clinical outcomes, often persisting despite remission of symptoms. A neuroplasticity-based computerized cognitive remediation-geriatric depression treatment (nCCR-GD) was developed to target this executive dysfunction.

The treatment was compared to the drug escitalopram, given 20 mg for 12 weeks.[154] Ninety-one percent of participants completed nCCR-GD, which was equally effective at reducing depressive symptoms as escitalopram in 4 weeks. At 12 weeks, the nCCR-GD treatment showed greater executive function improvement compared to escitalopram.

HOMEOPATHY

Homeopathy is one of the most frequently used but controversial forms of complementary and alternative medicine (CAM).[155] It is based on the ancient "principle of similars." Highly diluted preparations of substances that cause symptoms in healthy individuals are used to stimulate healing reactions in patients who display similar symptoms when ill.[156] In classical homeopathy, a single remedy is selected based on a patient's total spectrum of symptoms.[157]

The number of patients using homeopathy in the United States has quadrupled from 1990 to 1997 and continues to rise.[158] In Germany about 10% of men and 20% of women used homeopathy in the year 2002.[159] The constitutional remedies, in particular, are similar conceptually to what psychology has termed *temperaments*, or Jungian analysts call *archetypes*. There are no randomized, controlled trials of homeopathy for depression. A 2-year prospective study of homeopathic treatment of elderly patients of which depression was one commonly occurring condition was published in 2013.[155] For all 200 patients over age 70 in their cohort, severity of disease decreased significantly from 6.2 (SD ± 1.7) to 3.0 (±2.2), the initial improvement maximized in 3 months and remained stable during the 24-month follow-up. Virtually all of the elders were using homeopathy to treat a chronic medical condition. This was a prospective, multicenter, cohort study involving 38 primary care practices with additional specialization in homeopathy, in Germany and Switzerland. Data were gathered from all patients of 70 years or older consulting the physician for the first time. Patients were included consecutively at their first consultation with a participating physician and were followed up for a total of 24 months. Patients were included in the study regardless of their diagnosis; 68% of all patients agreed to participate in the study. In order to participate in the study, physicians were required to have certified training in classical homeopathy and at least 3 years of practical experience. They all followed the principles of classical homeopathy. All homeopathic physicians worked in their own doctor's offices; hospital services were not included. A total of 187 physicians belonging to four different working groups were contacted either by post or telephone and informed about the study. Of these, 103 physicians chose to participate. To reflect usual care, all homeopathic physicians were completely free to choose a treatment. Outcome questionnaires documented sociodemographic data, prior medical history, patient symptoms and complaints, quality of life, and other treatments. Independently of their physicians, patients rated the severity of their complaints as they experienced them on a numeric rating scale (NRS, 0 = no complaints, 10 = maximum severity of complaints the patient could imagine for this disease).[160] All complaints listed by patients in their baseline questionnaire were transferred to their follow-up questionnaires by the study office personnel, which ensured that each baseline complaint was assessed at each subsequent follow-up. General health-related quality of life was assessed using the MOS SF-36 questionnaire.[161] Major improvements in quality of life were not observed.

CONCLUSION

Synergy between therapeutic interventions and between the different "levels of healing" plays a critical role in integrative geriatric psychiatry. One study showed that a home-based intervention for depression implemented by a psycho-geriatric team provided more benefit than was provided by medication alone.[162] The team provided individualized care optimized for each client, focused upon problem-solving psychotherapy, development of social support, and community intervention. Fifty-eight percent of the intervention group recovered compared with only 25% of the control group, a difference of 33%. Even after the researchers controlled for possible confounders using logistic regression analysis, patients of the geriatric team were nine times more likely to recover than patients receiving medication alone. The support provided by the geriatric team contributed to patient improvement, underscoring the importance of the human aspect of care.

Another study examined the feasibility and acceptability of a 6-month interprofessional (IP) nurse-led mental health promotion intervention among older home care clients (over age 70) using personal support services.[163] Of 142 eligible and consenting participants, 98 (69%) completed the 6-month and 87 (61%) completed the 1-year follow-up. Of the 142 participants, 56% had clinically significant depressive symptoms, with 38% having moderate to severe symptoms. The intervention was feasible and acceptable to older home care clients with depressive symptoms and was effective in reducing these symptoms and improving health-related quality of life at 6-month follow-up, with small additional improvements 6 months after the intervention. The intervention also reduced anxiety at 1-year follow-up. Significant reductions were observed in the use of hospitalization, ambulance services, and emergency room visits over the study period.

Geriatrics presents unique opportunities for integrative psychiatry. Geriatric patients tend to have more than one impaired organ system, complicating their care over that of younger, healthier, or less frail people. Because of the relation of depression to many medical conditions, geriatric medicine and psychiatry must work together more closely than many other specialties of medicine. The art of geriatric psychiatry is to use the least toxic and interventionist means to protect and promote mental health.

Integrative geriatric psychiatry, therefore, is the treatment of systems—humans, families, and communities—with potentially multiple modalities and levels of entry, ranging from nutritional, energetic, physical, psychological, molecular, familial, community, and spiritual. Its goal is to reduce suffering and promote well-being among the elderly by whatever means possible while limiting side effects. If movement therapies, for example, decrease falls, we can better prevent the depression that comes from lack of mobility.

Integrative geriatric psychiatry must focus on restoring health more than treating disease, compatible with the World Health Organization's definition of health as "a state of complete physical, mental, and social well-being and not merely the absence of disease or infirmity".[7] Despite the exciting developments in neuroscience and psychiatry, time, attention, and community have been shown to be key ingredients in recovery from geriatric depression. Teamwork is the essential concept in the care of geriatric patients who are depressed.

ACKNOWLEDGMENTS

The authors acknowledge the patients and their families with whom they have had the opportunity to work, and who have led to the insights and experiences expressed in this chapter.

REFERENCES

1. Charney, D.S., Nemeroff, C.B., and Lewis, L. 2002. National depressive and Manic-Depressive Association consensus statement on the use of placebo in clinical trials of mood disorders. *Arch Gen Psychiatry* 59: 262–270.
2. Thase, M.E. 2003. Achieving remission and managing relapse in depression. *J Clin Psychiatry* 64(Suppl 18): 3–7.
3. Mehl-Madrona, L. 2003. Native American Medicine: Herbal pharmacology, therapies, and elder care. In *Medicine Across Cultures: The History of Non-Western Medicine*, Ed. H. Selin. Lancaster, UK: Kluwer, pp. 253–270.
4. Cunningham, A.J. et al. 1998. A randomized controlled trial of the effects of group psychological therapy on survival in women with metastatic breast cancer. *Psycho-Oncology* 7: 508–517.
5. Bell, I.R. et al. 2002. Integrative medicine and systemic outcomes research: Issues in the emergence of a new model for primary health care. *Arch Intern Med* 162: 133–140.
6. Zollman, C. and Vickers, A. 1999. What is complementary medicine? *BMJ* 319: 693–696.

7. World Health Organization (WHO). 2001. About WHO: Definition of health. [cited 2001, October 9]; Available at: http://www.who.int/aboutwho/en/definition.html.

8. Wang, P.S. et al. 2005. Twelve-month use of mental health services in the United States: Results from the National Comorbidity Survey Replication. *Arch Gen Psychiatry* 62(6): 629–640.

9. White House Conference on Aging. 2005. *Report of the 2005 White House Conference on Aging.* Washington, DC: Superintendent of Documents.

10. Institute of Medicine. 2008. *Retooling for an Aging America: Building the Health Care Workforce.* Washington, DC: National Academies Press.

11. Blazer, D. et al. 1991. The association of age and depression among the elderly: An epidemiologic exploration. *J Gerontol* 46(6): M210–M215.

12. Pochert, A. 1997. Depression. A natural aspect of aging? 2 October 1997 [cited 2010, December 14]; Available at: http://www.hope.edu/academic/psychology/335/webrep/depress.html

13. Cui, M.D., Xing-jai, D., and Vaillant, G.E. 1996. Antecedents and consequences of negative life events in adulthood: A longitudinal study. *Am J Psychiatry* 153(1): 21–26.

14. Hughes, R.N., DeMallie, D.C., and Blazer, D.G. 1993. Does age make a difference in the effects of physical health and social support on the outcome of a major depression: A natural aspect of aging? *Am J Psychiatry* 150(5): 728–733.

15. James, J.W. and Haley, W.E. 1995. Age and health bias in practicing clinical psychologists. *Psychol Aging* 10(4): 610.

16. Harper, D.G. et al. 2014. Tissue-specific differences in brain phosphodiesters in late-life major depression. *Am J Geriatr Psychiatry* 22(5): 499–509.

17. Busse, M. et al. 2014. Decreased quinolinic acid in the hippocampus of depressive patients: Evidence for local anti-inflammatory and neuroprotective responses? *Eur Arch Psychiatry Clin Neurosci* 1–9.

18. Ray, A. et al. 2014. ABCB1 (MDR1) predicts remission on P-gp substrates in chronic depression. *Pharmacogenom J* 15(4): 332–339.

19. Fulder, S. 1996. *The Handbook of Alternative and Complementary Medicine.* 3rd ed. Oxford, England: Oxford University Press.

20. Bell, C.C. 2004 *Sanity of Survival: Reflections on Community Mental Health and Wellness.* Chicago, IL: Third World Press.

21. Maizes, V. and O. Caspi. 1999. The principles and challenges of integrative medicine. *West J Med* 171: 148–149.

22. Gaudet, T.W. 1998. Integrative medicine. *Integr Med* 1: 67–73.

23. Da-hong, Z. 1982. Preventive geriatrics: An overview from traditional Chinese medicine. *Am J Chin Med* 10: 32–39.

24. Ernst, E. and White, A. 1998. *Acupuncture: A Scientific Appraisal.* Oxford, England: Butterworth Heinemann.

25. Zuppa, C. et al. 2015. Acupuncture for sleep quality, BDNF levels and immunosenescence: A randomized controlled study. *Neurosci Lett* 587: 35–40.

26. Wolf, S.L., Barnhart, H.X., and Kutner, N.G. 1996.Reducing frailty and falls in older persons: An investigation of Tai Chi and computerized balance training. *JAGS* 44: 489–497.

27. Koh, T.C. 1982. Tai Chi and ankylosing spondylitis. A personal experience. *Am J Chin Med* 10: 59–61.

28. Yin, J. and Dishman, R.K. 2014.The effect of Tai Chi and Qigong practice on depression and anxiety symptoms: A systematic review and meta-regression analysis of randomized controlled trials. *Ment Health Phys Act* 7(3): 135–146.

29. Li, Y. et al. 2014. Long-term Tai Chi training is related to depressive symptoms among Tai Chi practitioners. *J Affect Disord* 169: 36–39.

30. Lavretsky, H. et al. 2011. Complementary use of tai chi chih augments escitalopram treatment of geriatric depression: A randomized controlled trial. *Am J Geriatr Psychiatry* 19(10): 839–850.

31. Sancier, K.M. 1999. Therapeutic benefits of qigong exercises in combination with drugs. *J Altern Complement Med* 5(4): 383–389.

32. MacDonald, D.A. and Holland, D. 2002. Examination of the psychometric properties of the temperament and character inventory self-transcendence dimension. *Personality Individ Diff* 32: 1013–1027.

33. Hood, R.W. et al. 1979. Personality correlates of the report of mystical experience. *Psychol Rep* 44(3): 804–806.

34. Hood, R.W. 1977. Eliciting mystical states of consciousness with semi-structured nature experiences. *J Scient Study Relig* 16(2): 155–163.

35. Hood, R.W. 1977. Differential triggering of mystical experience as a function of self-actualization. *Rev Relig Res* 18(3), 264–270.

36. Hood, R.W. 1974. Psychological strength and the report of intense religious experience. *J Scient Study Relig* 13(1): 65–71.

37. Maslow, A. 1962. *Toward a Psychology of Being*. New York, NY: Start Publishing Co.

38. Murphy, M. 1992. *The Future of the Body: Explorations into the Further Evolution of Human Nature*. Los Angeles, CA: Tarcher Perigee.

39. Maslow, A. 1970. *Religions, Values, and Peak-Experiences*. New York, NY: Viking.

40. George, L.K. et al. 2000. Spirituality and health: What we know, what we need to know. *J Soc Clin Psychol* 19(1): 102–116.

41. Gartner, J. 1996. Religious commitment, mental health, and prosocial behavior: A review of the empirical literature. In *Religion and the Clinical Practice of Psychology*, Ed. E.P. Shafranske. Washington, DC: American Psychological Association, pp. 187–214.

42. Ellison, C.W. 1983. Spiritual well-being: Conceptualization and measurement. *J Psychol Theol* 11(4): 330–340.

43. Elkins, D.N. et al. 1988. Toward phenomenological spirituality: Definition, description, and measurement. *J Human Psychol* 28(4): 5–18.

44. Weinstein, L., Xie, X., and Cleanthouse, C.C. 1995. Purpose in life, boredom, and volunteerism in a group of retirees. *Psychol Rep* 70: 688–690.

45. Wink, P. and Donahue, K. 1997. The relation between two types of narcissism and boredom. *J Res Personality* 31(1): 136–140.

46. Tolor, A. and Siegel, M.C. 1989. Boredom proneness and political activism. *Psychol Rep* 65(1): 235–240.

47. Barghill, R.W. 2000. The study of life boredom. *J Phenomenologic Psychol* 31(2): 188–219.

48. McLeod, C.R. and Vodanovich, S.J. 1991. The relationship between self-actualization and boredom proneness. *J Soc Behav Personality* 6(5), 137–146.

49. Kim, S.S., Hayward, R.D., and Reed, P.G. 2014. Self-transcendence, spiritual perspective, and sense of purpose in family caregiving relationships: A mediated model of depression symptoms in Korean older adults. *Aging Ment Health* 18(7): 905–913.

50. Bryan, J., Osendarp, S., Hughes, D., Calvaresi, E., Baghurst, K., and van Klinken, J.W. 2004. Nutrients for cognitive development in school-aged children. *Nutr Rev* 62: 295–306.

51. McCann, J.C. and Ames, B.N. 2005. Is docosahexaenoic acid, an n-3 long chain polyunsaturated fatty acid, required for the development of normal brain function? An overview of evidence from cognitive and behavioral tests in humans and animals. *Am J Clin Nutr* 82: 281–295.

52. McCann, J.C., Hudes, M., and Ames, B.N. 2006. An overview of evidence for a causal relationship between dietary availability of choline during development and cognitive function in offspring. *Neurosci Biobehav Rev* 30: 696–712.

53. McCann, J.C. and Ames, B.N. 2007. An overview of evidence for a causal relationship between iron deficiency during development and cognitive or behavioral function in children. *Am J Clin Nutr* 85: 931–945.

54. Lai, J.S., Hiles, S., Bisquera, A., Hure, A.J., McEvoy, M., and Attia, J. 2014. A systematic review and meta-analysis of dietary patterns and depression in community-dwelling adults. *Am J Clin Nutr* 99: 181–197.

55. Biessels, G.J., Staekenborg, S., Brunner, E., Brayne, C., and Scheltens, P. 2006. Risk of dementia in diabetes mellitus: A systematic review. *Lancet Neurol* 5: 64–74.

56. Anderson, R.J., Freedland, K.E., Clouse, R.E., and Lustman, P.J. 2001. The prevalence of comorbid depression in adults with diabetes: A meta-analysis. *Diabetes Care* 24: 1069–1078.

57. Gougeon, L. 2014. Nutritional predictors of depression in a cohort of community-dwelling elderly Canadians: NuAge cohort. *Appl Physiol Nutr Metab* 39(12): 1412.

58. Benton, D. 2001. Micro-nutrient supplementation and the intelligence of children. *Neurosci Biobehav Rev* 25: 297–309.

59. TheNemoGroup. 2007. Effect of a 12-mo micronutrient intervention on learning and memory in well-nourished and marginally nourished school-aged children: Two parallel, randomized, placebo-controlled studies in Australia and Indonesia. *Am J Clin Nutr* 86: 1082–1093.

60. Ames, B. 2006. Low micronutrient intake may accelerate the degenerative diseases of aging through allocation of scarce micronutrients by triage. *Proc Natl Acad Sci USA* 103: 17589–17594.

61. Lahiri, D.K., Zawia, N.H., Greig, N.H., Sambamurti, K., and Maloney, B. 2008. Early-life events may trigger biochemical pathways for Alzheimer's disease: The "LEARn" model. *Biogerontology* 9(6): 375–379.

62. Lahiri D.K. and Maloney, B. 2010. The "LEARn" (latent early-life associated regulation) model integrates environmental risk factors and the developmental basis of Alzheimer's disease, and proposes remedial steps. *Exp Gerontol* 45(4): 291–296.

63. Brewer, G.J. 2010. Epigenetic oxidative redox shift (EORS) theory of aging unifies the free radical and insulin signaling theories. *Exp Gerontol* 45: 173–179.

64. Chan, R., Chan, D., and Woo, J. 2014. A prospective cohort study to examine the association between dietary patterns and depressive symptoms in older Chinese people in Hong Kong. *PloS One* 9(8): e105760.

65. Alvarez, J.A. and Ashraf, A. 2010. Role of vitamin D in insulin secretion and insulin sensitivity for glucose homeostasis. *Int J Endocrinol* 2010: 351–385.

66. Annweiler, C. et al. 2009. Vitamin D and cognitive performance in adults: A systematic review. *Eur J Neurol* 16: 1083–1089.

67. Hoogendijk, W.J. et al. 2008. Depression is associated with decreased 25-hydroxyvitamin D and increased parathyroid hormone levels in older adults. *Arch Gen Psychiatr* 65: 508–512.

68. May, H.T. et al. 2010. Association of vitamin D levels with incident depression among a general cardiovascular population. *Am Heart J* 159: 1037–1043.

69. Milaneschi, Y. et al. 2010. Serum 25-hydroxyvitamin D and depressive symptoms in older women and men. *J Clin Endocrinol Metab* 95: 3225–3233.

70. Martins, D., Pan, W.M., Zadshir, D. et al. 2007. Prevalence of cardiovascular risk factors and the serum levels of 25-hydroxyvitamin D in the United States: Data from the third national health and nutrition examination survey. *Arch Intern Med* 167: 1159–1166.

71. Jarrett, R.J., Murrells, T.J., Shipley, M.J., and Hall, T. 1984. Screening blood glucose values: Effects of season and time of day. *Diabetologia* 27: 574–577.

72. Eyles, D.W. et al. 2005. Distribution of the vitamin D receptor and 1 alpha-hydroxylase in human brain. *J Chem Neuroanat* 29: 21–30.

73. Brouwer-Brolsma, E.M., Feskens, E.J., Steegenga, W.T., and de Groot, L.C. 2013. Associations of 25-hydroxyvitamin D with fasting glucose, fasting insulin, dementia and depression in European elderly: The SENECA study. *Eur J Nutr* 52:917–925.

74. Mitri, J., Muraru, M.D., and Pittas, A.G. 2011. Vitamin D and type 2 diabetes: A systematic review. *Eur J Clin Nutr* 65: 1005–1015.

75. Chan, R. et al. 2011. Association between serum 25-hydroxyvitamin D and psychological health in older Chinese men in a cohort study. *J Affect Disord* 130: 251–259.

76. Nanri, A. et al. 2009. Association between serum 25-hydroxyvitamin D and depressive symptoms in Japanese: Analysis by survey season. *Eur J Clin Nutr* 63: 1444–1447.

77. Pan, A. et al. 2009. Association between depressive symptoms and 25-hydroxyvitamin D in middle-aged and elderly Chinese. *J Affect Disord* 118: 240–243.

78. Wilkins, C.H., Sheline, Y., Roe, C.M., Birge, S.J., and Morris, J.C. 2006. Vitamin D deficiency is associated with low mood and worse cognitive performance in older adults. *Am J Geriatr Psychiatr* 14: 1032–1040.

79. Annweiler, C. et al. 2010. Association of vitamin D deficiency with cognitive impairment in older women: Cross-sectional study. *Neurology* 74: 27–32.

80. Buell, J.S. et al. 2010. 25-Hydroxyvitamin D, dementia, and cerebrovascular pathology in elders receiving home services. *Neurology* 74: 18–26.

81. Buell, J.S. et al. 2009. Vitamin D is associated with cognitive function in elders receiving home health services. *J Gerontol A Biol Sci Med Sci* 64: 888–895.

82. Lee, D.M. et al. 2009. Association between 25-hydroxyvitamin D levels and cognitive performance in middle-aged and older European men. *J Neurol Neurosurg Psychiatr* 80: 722–729.

83. Llewellyn, D.J. et al. 2010. Vitamin D and cognitive impairment in the elderly US population. *J Gerontol A Biol Sci Med Sci* 66: 59–65.

84. Llewellyn, D.J., Langa, K.M., and Lang, I.A. 2009. Serum 25-hydroxyvitamin D concentration and cognitive impairment. *J Geriatr Psychiatr Neurol* 22: 188–195.

85. McGrath, J. et al. 2007. No association between serum 25-hydroxyvitamin D3 level and performance on psychometric tests in NHANES III. *Neuroepidemiology* 29: 49–54.

86. Llewellyn, D.J. et al. 2010. Vitamin D and risk of cognitive decline in elderly persons. *Arch Intern Med* 170: 1135–1141.

87. Slinin, Y. et al. 2010. 25-Hydroxyvitamin D levels and cognitive performance and decline in elderly men. *Neurology* 74: 33–41.

88. Lee, I.H. et al., 2014. Association between depression and physical fitness, body fatness and serum Vitamin D in elderly population. *Korean J Obesity* 23(2): 125–130.

89. Cogan, E. 2001. DHEA: Orthodox or alternative medicine? *Rev Med Brux* 22(4): A381–A386.
90. Veronese, N. et al. 2014. Serum dehydroepiandrosterone sulfate and incident depression in the elderly: The Pro. VA study. *Am J Geriatr Psychiatry* 23(8): 863–871.
91. Fetrow, C.W. and Avila, J.R. 2001. Efficacy of the dietary supplement S-adenosyl-L-methionine. *Ann Pharmacother* 35(11): 414–425.
92. Di Rocco, A. et al. 2000. S-Adenosyl-Methionine improves depression in patients with Parkinson's disease in an open-label clinical trial. *Mov Disord* 15(6): 1225–1229.
93. Sarris, J. et al. 2014. S-adenosyl methionine (SAMe) versus escitalopram and placebo in major depression RCT: Efficacy and effects of histamine and carnitine as moderators of response. *J Affect Disord* 164: 76–81.
94. Leeton, J. 1974. Depression induced by oral contraception and the role of vitamin B6 in its management. *ANZ J Psychiatry* 8(2): 85–88.
95. Almeida, O.P. et al. 2014. B vitamins to enhance treatment response to antidepressants in middle-aged and older adults: Results from the B-VITAGE randomised, double-blind, placebo-controlled trial. *Br J Psychiatry* 205(6): 450–457.
96. Wolters, M., Ströhle, A., and Hahn, A. 2004. Age-associated changes in the metabolism of vitamin B (12) and folic acid: Prevalence, aetiopathogenesis and pathophysiological consequences. *Z Gerontol Geriatr* 37(2): 109–135.
97. Neugroschl, J.A.K.E., Samuels, S.C., and Martin D.B. 2005. Dementia, *Comprehensive Textbook of Psychiatry*, Eds. B.J. Sadock and V. Sadock. Baltimore, MD: Lippincott Williams and Wilkins, pp. 1068–1092.
98. Agarwal, R. et al. 2010. Role of vitamin B12, folate, and thyroid stimulating hormone in dementia: A hospital-based study in north Indian population. *Ann Indian Acad Neurol* 13(4): 257–262.
99. Davis, S.R, Quinlivan, E.P., Shelnutt, K.P et al. 2005. The methylenetetrahydrofolate reductase 677C->T polymorphism and dietary folate restriction affect plasma one-carbon metabolites and red blood cell folate concentrations and distribution in women. *J Nutr* 135: 1040–1044.
100. Ocampo Chaparro, J.M. 2013. Vitamin B12 deficit and development of geriatric syndromes. *Colombia Médica* 44(1): 43–47.
101. Dahal, A. et al. 2014. The status of vitamin B12 in elderly persons suffering from dementia. *IAJPR* 4(4): 2057–2063.
102. Howard, J.S. 1975. Folate deficiency in psychiatric practice. *Psychosomatics* 18(3): 112–115.
103. Mischoulon, D. et al. 2000. Anemia and macrocytosis in the prediction of serum folate and vitamin B12 status, and treatment outcome in major depression. *J Psychosom Res* 49(3): 183–187.
104. Coppen, A. and Bailey, J. 2000. Enhancement of the antidepressant action of fluoxetine by folic acid: A randomised, placebo controlled trial. *J Affect Disord* 60(2): 121–130.
105. Penninx, B.W., Guralnik, J.M., Ferrucci, L., Fried, L.P., Allen, R.H., and Stabler, S.P. 2000. Vitamin B12 deficiency and depression in physically disabled older women: Epidemiologic evidence from the women's health and aging study. *Am J Psychiatry* 157(5): 715–721.
106. Bottiglieri, T. et al. 2000. Homocysteine, folate, methylation, and monoamine metabolism in depression. *J Neurol Neurosurg Psychiatry* 69(2): 228–232.
107. Fava, M. et al. 1997. Folate, vitamin B12, and homocysteine in major depressive disorder. *Am J Psychiatry* 154(3): 426–428.
108. Rabjohn, P. 2014. The role and postulated biochemical mechanism of L-methylfolate augmentation in major depression: A case-report. *Psychiatr Ann* 44(4): 197–204.
109. Shealy, C.N. 1991. *Neurochemical Substrates of Depression and Their Relation to Cardiac Disease*. Springfield, MO: Holistic Press.
110. Hansen, M.V., Danielsen, A.K., Hageman, I., Rosenberg, J., and Gögenur, I. 2014. The therapeutic or prophylactic effect of exogenous melatonin against depression and depressive symptoms: A systematic review and meta-analysis. *Eur Neuropsychopharm* 24(11): 1719–1728.
111. Mauri, M.C. et al. 1998. Plasma and platelet amino acid concentrations in patients affected by major depression and under fluvoxamine treatment. *Neuropsychobiology* 37(3): 124–129.
112. Young, S.N., Chouinard, G., and Annable, L. 1981. Tryptophan in the treatment of depression. *Adv Exper Med Biol* 133: 727–737.
113. Thomson, J. et al. 1982. The treatment of depression in general practice: A comparison of L-tryptophan, amitriptyline and a combination of L-tryptophan and amitriptyline with placebo. *Psychol Med Nov* 12(4): 741–751.
114. Wang, S.M. et al. 2014. A review of current evidence for acetyl-l-carnitine in the treatment of depression. *J Psychiatr Res* 53: 30–37.

115. Peet, M. et al. 1998. Depletion of omega-3 fatty acid levels in red blood cell membranes of depressive patients. *Biol Psychiatry* 43(5): 315–319.
116. Horrobin, D.F. 2001. Phospholipid metabolism and depression: The possible roles of phospholipase A2 and coenzyme A-independent transacylase. *Hum Psychopharmacol* 16(1): 45–52.
117. Maidment, I.D. 2000. Are fish oils an effective therapy in mental illness–an analysis of the data. *Acta Psychiatr Scand* 102(1): 3–11.
118. Maes, M. et al. 1999. Lowered omega3 polyunsaturated fatty acids in serum phospholipids and cholesteryl esters of depressed patients. *Psychiatry Res* 85(3): 275–291.
119. Rakel, D. 2007. *Integrative Medicine*. Philadelphia, PA: Saunders Elsevier.
120. Mather, A.S. et al. 2002. Effects of exercise on depressive symptoms in older adults with poorly responsive depressive disorder. Randomised controlled trial. *Br J Psychiatry* 180(5): 411–415.
121. Park, S.H., Han, K.S., and Kang, C.B. 2014. Effects of exercise programs on depressive symptoms, quality of life and self-esteem in older people: A systematic review of randomized controlled trials. *Appl Nurs Res* 27(4): 219–226.
122. Eng, J.J. and Reime, B. 2014. Exercise for depressive symptoms in stroke patients: A systematic review and meta-analysis. *Clin Rehabil* 28(8): 731–739.
123. Pizzorno, J.E., Michael, N., and Murray, T. 2013. *Textbook of Natural Medicine*. St. Louis, MO: Elsevier.
124. Gaster, B. and Holroyd, J. 2000. St John's wort for depression: A systematic review. *Arch Intern Med* 160(2): 152–156.
125. Harrer, G.S.V. 1994. Clinical investigation of the antidepressant effectiveness of Hypericum. *J Geriatr Psychiatry Neurol* 7(suppl 1): S1–S8.
126. Morazzoni, P.B.E. 1995. *Hypericum perforatum*. *Fitoterapia* 66: 43–68.
127. De Smet, P.A. 1996. St. John's Wort as an antidepressant. *BMJ* 313: 241–242.
128. Kirsch, I. 2014. Antidepressants and the placebo effect. *Zeitschrift für Psychologie* 222(3): 128–134.
129. Kirsch, I. et al. 2008. Initial severity and antidepressant benefits: A meta-analysis of data submitted to the Food and Drug Administration. *PLoS Med* 5(2): e45.
130. Russo, E. et al. 2014. *Hypericum perforatum*: Pharmacokinetic, mechanism of action, tolerability, and clinical drug–drug interactions. *Phytother Res* 28(5): 643–655.
131. de Souza Silva, J.E. et al. 2014. Use of herbal medicines by elderly patients: A systematic review. *Arch Gerontol Geriatr* 59(2): 227–233.
132. Varteresian, T. and Lavretsky, H. 2014. Natural products and supplements for geriatric depression and cognitive disorders: An evaluation of the research. *Curr Psychiatry Rep* 16(8): 1–9.
133. Huquet, F., Drieu, K., and Piriou, A. 1994. Decreased cerebral 5-HT1a receptors during aging: Reversal by Ginkgo biloba. *J Pharm Pharmacol* 46: 316–318.
134. Mullaicharam, A. 2014. A review on evidence based practice of ginkgo biloba in brain health. *Int J Chem Pharm Anal* 1(1): 24–30.
135. Brian-Quinn, C.S.W. 1997. *The Depression Sourcebook*. Los Angeles, CA: Lowell House.
136. Jonathan, R.T. et al. 2000. *Herbs for the Mind*. New York, NY: Guilford Press.
137. Vorbach, E. and Gortelmayer, R.B.J. Therapie von insomnien: Wiksamkeit und vertraglichkeit eines Baldrian-Praparates. *Psychopharmakotherapie* 3: 109–115.
138. Kamm-Kohl, A.V., Jansen, W., and Brockmann, P. 1984. Modern valerian therapy of nervous disorders in elderly patients. *Medwelt* 35: 1450–1454.
139. Latorre-Román, P.Á. et al. 2015. Effect of a 12-day balneotherapy programme on pain, mood, sleep, and depression in healthy elderly people. *Psychogeriatrics* 5(1): 14–19.
140. Robinson, H. et al. 2013. The psychosocial effects of a companion robot: A randomized controlled trial. *J Am Med Directors Assoc* 14(9): 661–667.
141. Lam, B.T., Cervantes, A.R. Lee, W.K. 2014. Late-life depression, social support, instrumental activities of daily living, and utilization of in-home and community-based services in older adults. *J Human Behav Soc Env* 24(4): 499–512.
142. Li, H. et al. 2013. Social support resources and post-acute recovery for older adults with major depression. *Comm Ment Health J* 49(4): 419–426.
143. Gum, A.M. et al. 2014. Six-month utilization of psychotherapy by older adults with depressive symptoms. *Comm Ment Health J* 50(7): 759–764.
144. Pasterfield, M. et al. 2014. Adapting manualized behavioural activation treatment for older adults with depression. *Cogn Behav Ther* 7: e5.
145. Mackin, R.S. et al. 2013. Cognitive outcomes after psychotherapeutic interventions for major depression in older adults with executive dysfunction. *Am J Geriatr Psychiatry* 22(12): 1496–1503.

146. Niemeyer, H., Musch, J., and Pietrowsky, R. 2013. Publication bias in meta-analyses of the efficacy of psychotherapeutic interventions for depression. *J Consult Clin Psychol* 81(1): 58.

147. Yuan, C.S. and Bieber, E.J. 2006. *Textbook of Complementary and Alternative Medicine.* Andover, UK: Informa UK.

148. Jain, F.A. et al. 2014. Critical analysis of the efficacy of meditation therapies for acute and subacute phase treatment of depressive disorders: A systematic review. *Psychosomatics* 56(2): 140–152.

149. Louie, L. 2014. The effectiveness of yoga for depression: A critical literature review. *Issues Ment Health Nurs* 35(4): 265–276.

150. Cramer, H. et al. 2013. Yoga for depression: A systematic review and meta-analysis. *Depress Anxiety* 30(11): 1068–1083.

151. Janakiramaiah, N. et al. 2000. Antidepressant efficacy of Sudarshan Kriya Yoga (SKY) in melancholia: A randomized comparison with electroconvulsive therapy (ECT) and imipramine. *J Affect Disord* 57(1): 255–259.

152. Balasubramaniam, M., Telles, S., and Doraiswamy, P.M. 2012. Yoga on our minds: A systematic review of yoga for neuropsychiatric disorders. *Front Psychiatry* 3: 117. doi: 10.3389/fpsyt.2012.00117.

153. D'Silva, S., Poscablo, C.H. R.2012. Mind-body medicine therapies for a range of depression severity: A systematic review. *Psychosomatics* 53: 407–423.

154. Morimoto, S.S. et al. 2014. Neuroplasticity-based computerized cognitive remediation for treatment-resistant geriatric depression. *Nature Comm* 5: 1239–1247. doi: 10.1038/ncomms5579.

155. Teut, M. et al. 2010. Homeopathic treatment of elderly patients—A prospective observational study with follow-up over a two year period. *BMC Geriatrics* 10: 10. doi: 10.1186/1471-2318-10-10.

156. Jonas, W. and Jacobs, J. 1996, *Healing With Homeopathy.* Los Angeles, CA: Warner Books.

157. Linde, K. et al. 1997. Are the clinical effects of homeopathy placebo effects? A meta-analysis of placebo controlled trials. *Lancet* 350: 834–843.

158. Eisenberg, D.M. et al. 1998. Trends in alternative medicine use in the United States, 1990–1997: Results of a follow-up national survey. *JAMA* 280: 1569–1575.

159. Härtel, U. and Volger, E. 2003. Inanspruchnahme und Akzeptanz von klassischen Naturheilverfahren und alternativen Heilmethoden in Deutschland. Ergebnisse einer repräsentativen Bevölkerungsstudie. *Das Gesundheitswesen* 65.

160. Huskisson, E.C. and Scott, J. 1993. *VAS Visuelle Analog-Skalen; auch VAPS Visual Analogue Pain Scales, NRS Numerische Rating-Skalen; Mod. Kategorialskalen, in Handbuch psychosozialer Meßinstrumente—ein Kompendium für epidemiologische und klinische Forschung zu chronischer Krankheit,* Ed. G. Westhoff. Hogrefe: Göttingen. pp. 881–885.

161. Bullinger, M. and Kirchberger, I. 1998. SF-36 Fragebogen zum Gesundheitszustand. *Handbuch für die deutschsprachige Fragebogenversion.* Göttingen: Hogrefe.

162. Banerjee, S. et al. 1996. Randomised controlled trial of effect of intervention by psychogeriatric team on depression in frail elderly people at home. *BMJ* 313(7064): 1058–1061.

163. Markle-Reid, M. et al. 2014. An interprofessional nurse-led mental health promotion intervention for older home care clients with depressive symptoms. *BMC Geriatr* 14(1): 62.

31 Clinical Case Studies
Putting It All Together

Kat Toups, MD, DFAPA

CONTENTS

Now, the fun part! How do we put all of these ideas together in clinical practice?

One thing is clear—with integrative or functional medicine, each case is different.

Some features of Integrative Psychiatry include the following:

- Search for the root cause
- Find out a person's story
- Search for sources of inflammation
- Investigate factors, and put together a timeline of events that led up to the current state
- Explore diet, nutrients, lifestyle, stress, beliefs, gastrointestinal (GI) health, hormones, genetics, and toxins

As you will see from the case studies that follow, there are a variety of different approaches to healing available when one incorporates Integrative Psychiatry into the paradigm.

The shared feature in all of these case studies is healing. This means doing whatever it takes in the service of the patient to help the patient get well, rather than accepting the traditional status quo belief that an improvement in symptoms is good enough.

The aim here is not just to reduce suffering, but to help people get well.

I hope these cases will catalyze some new ways of approaching healing in Psychiatry for you.

DIETARY INTERVENTION FOR DEPRESSION AND SOMATIC COMPLAINTS

Cynthia Gariépy, ND
Clinique Cynthia Gariépy
Québec City, Canada

A 38-year-old woman presented with:

- Fatigue
- Depression
- Digestive problems
- Intense pruritus
- No libido
- Chronic vaginosis

I saw this patient a few months ago after her doctor told her that "conventional" medicine could no longer help her. In the 10 years prior to her first visit, she had been on antibiotics to treat various mild infections but always seemed to be sick or on the verge of becoming sick.

Different antibiotics and antifungals were used to try to get the vaginosis under control, without success. The woman had two small boys and feared not being able to fully take care of them because of her illness. She was having marital problems due to her low libido, fatigue, and the constant feeling of depression. At the time I first evaluated her, she was on Effexor 75 mg.

INITIAL INTERVENTION

- Due to financial restrictions, I did not run any functional tests initially.
- I started her on a very low sugar diet.
- We added probiotics: Lactobacillus rhamnosus GG (LGG), 10 billion CFU twice a day.

ONE-MONTH FOLLOW-UP

- The vaginosis was much reduced, and she had no more intense pruritus.
- Digestive issues were also much better.
- She still had loose stool, but had no more abdominal distention and flatulence.

NEXT INTERVENTIONS

- We initiated a gluten-free/casein-free diet for the next 3 months.
- Since money was an issue, I decided to make dietary changes and keep the supplements to a minimum.
- I designed a meal plan to introduce omega-3s with the following:
  - Chia seed oil daily
  - Turmeric with pepper daily
  - Two servings of colored fish every week
  - Sprouted seeds from the cabbage family at the beginning of every meal
- I recommended an increased intake of water
- I recommended betaine-HCL with pepsin at every meal as a digestive enzyme aid
- I recommended continuing the LGG probiotics for an additional 3 months

SECOND FOLLOW-UP

- She was completely changed!
- She had more energy, felt less depressed, and had very few digestive issues remaining.

- She had no recurrence of the vaginosis.
- She had not fought the flu in 3 months.
- Her libido was slowly coming back.

I then added dietary sources of folates and suggested a B-complex vitamin along with 500 mg of *Rhodiola rosea*.

FINAL FOLLOW-UP

- I last saw her 6 months after the second follow-up.
- She had been diagnosed with celiac disease 1 month prior (she had to reintroduce gluten temporarily for the test), and was now feeling great.
- She has tried reintroducing dairy, but felt her digestive issues returning, so she decided to remain dairy free.
- Her general practitioner had decided to gradually stop the Effexor.
- Her libido returned to normal, and she had a lot more energy.
- She had stopped taking the probiotic, but continued to take the vitamin B with *Rhodiola*.

DIETARY PEPTIDES AND FOOD HYPERSENSITIVITIES

Cynthia Gariépy, ND
Clinique Cynthia Gariépy
Québec City, Canada

This is a patient I saw a few years ago, before non-celiac gluten sensitivity was described.
   She was a 42-year-old woman who presented with the following symptoms:

- Loose stools, sometimes diarrhea
- Fatigue
- Depression
- Anxiety
- Difficulty falling asleep, and frequent waking due to abdominal pain
- Headaches
- Abdominal distention
- Gas
- Heartburn, reflux
- Feeling of being full after a few bites of food
- Always felt better when she had not eaten in a few hours

The patient saw her general practitioner (GP) when the symptoms started at the age of 24.
   The GP referred her to a gastroenterologist for a colonoscopy—the results were negative.
   Blood studies were done. Iron was a bit low but not enough to raise further suspicions. She was advised to eat liver once a week. No medications were prescribed, and she was asked to follow-up 3 months later.
   At the 3-month follow-up, the GP asked if there were any benefits from eating liver.
   When told no, the GP prescribed diazepam 2 mg at bedtime. Three months later, the patient came back for a follow-up visit. At that time, the anxiety had not changed, sleep was slightly better, and the rest of her symptoms were not altered. The loose stools were now replaced by three to four episodes of diarrhea a day, and the fatigue was worse than ever. The woman also now had terrible back pains and restless leg syndrome. The GP asked the patient if she would consider discussing issues of her life to explore whether the whole picture might possibly be related to stress.

Insulted by that comment and feeling that her symptoms were not between her ears, the patient abandoned the GP and tried to explore alternate avenues. She consulted a chiropractor, who worked on her back problems. After six treatments, the back pain was noticeably improved, so the woman never went back. The rest of her symptoms remained the same.

At the age of 28, the woman got pregnant after 3 years of trying to conceive, but she lost the baby at 13 weeks. After the miscarriage, the feelings of depression became worse, and she finally agreed to consult a psychologist. After 2 years of psychotherapy, the symptoms of depression were slightly better, but the fatigue, anxiety, and the feeling of always having something wrong were present more than ever.

In psychotherapy, an issue arose that the woman had been sexually abused at the age of 17. Although explored at length in psychotherapy, the feeling of being faulty and dirty was still present. Her libido was much affected by this, and she seldom had sexual relations with her husband of many years.

At the age of 32, the woman again consulted with the GP, who now diagnosed irritable bowel syndrome (IBS), and sent her to consult with a nutritionist. Legumes, cruciferous vegetables, and coffee were stopped; however, the woman had rarely eaten cruciferous vegetables in the last few years and never ate legumes. She stopped the coffee, and the diarrhea went from three to four episodes per day to two to three episodes per day. The other symptoms remained unchanged. She was told to persevere on this diet and to give it time. After a year of not drinking coffee, the symptoms remained unchanged.

She then started researching the Internet about special diets, and tried a raw food diet for 6 months. For the first 2 months, her level of energy increased but by month 3 had returned to the baseline low levels. At the 6-month mark, she stopped the diet when she noticed that she now had five to six episodes of diarrhea a day.

She again consulted her GP, and he prescribed loperamide (Imodium®) for the diarrhea for 3 months. After 10 days, the diarrhea decreased from five to six episodes per day to two to three per day. At the 3-month follow-up visit, the loperamide dose was increased. The diarrhea stopped, but then the woman started having bouts of constipation. The loperamide dose was then decreased, but the constipation now alternated with diarrhea. The woman started having more feelings of depression and now began having suicidal thoughts.

She decided to go back to psychotherapy, and after another year in therapy, her feelings of depression and her suicidal thoughts had diminished, but they were not completely gone.

At the age of 36, she was prescribed lubiprostone (Amitiza®) for the constipation and her other IBS symptoms. After 3 weeks, the woman experienced less constipation, less abdominal pain, and less distention. The lubiprostone medication was continued. After a year on lubiprostone, the symptoms of fatigue, depression, suicidal thoughts, insomnia, and a general sense of being always affected with digestive issues, although less intense, were still present.

At the age of 38, the patient and her husband decided to adopt a child. When they returned from Asia with their adoptive baby, the digestive issues became worse than ever, and the fatigue intensified.

Considering the demanding dimensions of taking care of a child, as well as the physical demands and jet lag experienced from the international travel, the cause of the increased fatigue was attributed to the whole adoption story. She was told that with time, everything would get better.

At the age of 40, feeling worse than ever before, the woman was diagnosed with severe burnout and put on sick leave for 3 months. After 3 months, nothing had changed, and a prescription for venlafaxine (Effexor®) 37.5 mg was given. After 3 months the venlafaxine dose was increased to 75 mg. At 75 mg, the feelings of depression and suicidal thoughts improved, but the digestive issues were still very much present.

At age 41, she consulted the GP again, and this time a panel for celiac disease was ordered. The results came back negative. The woman and her husband then decided that she would quit her job and stay at home to regain her strength.

I saw this patient at age 42. When I opened her medical file, the doctor had written: "Somatization, possible IBS, sexual abuse, refusal to undertake long-term antidepressant therapy."

The first step I undertook was to run an IgG antibody food panel that tested reactivity toward 93 foods and *Candida*. I also ordered a comprehensive stool analysis.

The results for the IgG panel came back as follows:

Gluten IgG: Moderate elevation
Dairy: Moderate to severe elevation
Egg white: Moderate elevation
Almonds: Moderate elevation

The results from the comprehensive stool analysis came back as follows:

+ *Cryptococcus albidus* (Yeast)
+ *Rhodotorula glutinis/mucilaginosa* (two other species of yeast)
Pancreatic elastase 172 ʋg/mL (this digestive enzyme should be at least >200, but higher than this is optimal)
Valerate 0.5% (this short-chain fatty acid level should be higher)

The first step I undertook was to ask the patient to eliminate dairy for a period of 2 months.
At the 2-month follow-up visit, the digestive-related symptoms were down by 30% to 40%.
The second step was to eliminate gluten for a 2-month period.
At the following visit, the woman was very much encouraged and reported that her digestive issues were almost completely gone. She was also feeling much less fatigued, less anxious, and less depressed. I then asked her to eliminate eggs for 1 month, followed by the elimination of almonds. After all reactive foods were eliminated, the patient decided to stop treatment because she felt better than ever, and she was scared to do anything else because of a fear that her symptoms might reappear.

I had not seen the patient for 8 months when she came back with symptoms of vaginal candidiasis, a skin rash, and light sleep.
I then tackled the yeast issue.
After several months on natural antifungals and a low-sugar diet, she was better than ever.
She had no symptoms of a digestive nature, and she was sleeping well throughout the night. There were no more skin rashes.
She remains gluten and dairy free.
She eats eggs only rarely and keeps her sugar intake low.
Editor's Note: This was an 18 year saga of depression and medical issues with a significant impact on this young woman's quality of life and functioning in multiple domains. This all resolved in a few months with elimination of a few reactive foods and healing her gut infections.

SAME + *RHODIOLA* FOR DEPRESSION WITH SUICIDAL IDEATION
Richard M. Carlton, MD
Psychiatry
New York, New York

KATERINA: DEPRESSION WITH SUICIDAL IDEATION

Katerina was a 41-year-old divorced woman living with her 10-year-old son. She had acute and highly active suicidal ideation. An ex-pat from Sweden, she had been living in New York City with her son, trying to make it as a freelance writer. Unsuccessful and not making a living, she had become suicidal and stated she would definitely have jumped off the roof of her building were it not for her son. She did not want to inflict psychological damage on him. Years earlier, when she was a young girl, her own mother had made an extremely serious suicide attempt, surviving only because she was accidentally found in the bathtub after having taken an overdose, about to go under.

Katerina's past bouts of depression had responded fairly well to a selective serotonin reuptake inhibitor (SSRI) available in Sweden, but it always took that medication a month or two to work. This time around she could not wait that long for relief, and she could not afford hospitalization. I proposed that we start with SAMe (starting at 400 mg/d and building quickly to 1600 mg/d). I explained that this nutrient boosts the synthesis of several neurotransmitters, and that it has been documented to work as well as prescription antidepressants, but far more quickly, and with far fewer side effects. I told her we would add in the herbal adaptogen *Rhodiola rosea* (100 mg once per day) to enhance the release of dopamine and thus energize her and further brighten her mood. We agreed that if this regimen did not work within a few days, we would add in an SSRI antidepressant to augment the nutrients, and vice versa.

The SSRI was never necessary. She called 3 days later to let me know that she no longer felt suicidal. She said that although nothing had changed in her very difficult economic circumstances, nevertheless, she no longer felt that she had to kill herself over it.

Still euthymic a few months later, she and her son went home to Sweden for the summer. There she enjoyed the embrace of a warm circle of friends and family and received several job offers. When she and her son returned to New York City in September, and she needed help from friends about whether or not to return to Sweden for good, these "friends" were destructive instead of being supportive. She collapsed emotionally in response, and once again had a desire and determination to kill herself.

In the intervening months she had greatly reduced her dose of SAMe and *Rhodiola*, so I told her to go right back up to the previous levels and to see me in 2 days. In those 2 days, the increased dosages of the nutrients had already kicked in, completely alleviating her suicidal ideation, and helping to clear her mind. No longer "paralyzed" by doubt, she had decisively made the (sensible) decision to return to Sweden to take a full-time job in a loving and supportive environment.

This case illustrates that a strategy to *increase* neurotransmitter synthesis:

- Can often work as well as prescription antidepressants (which scavenge whatever amounts of neurotransmitter have already been made and have been released into the synapse).
- This approach can work rapidly, sometimes in just days (in contrast to the month or more that it can often take for prescription antidepressants to work).

L-PHENYLALANINE AND NUTRIENTS IN SUBSTANCE ABUSE AND DEPRESSION

Richard M. Carlton, MD
Psychiatry
New York, New York

PETER: ANHEDONIC DEPRESSION FOLLOWING DECADES OF SUBSTANCE ABUSE

Peter was a 60-year-old man who was divorced three times. He was referred by his psychologist for treatment of severe depression with marked anhedonia that was not responding adequately to the duloxetine (Cymbalta®) 60 mg/d that he had been taking for 10 years.

Peter had started abusing alcohol at age 16, and cocaine at age 22. He used these drugs steadily until becoming sober at age 50. While on these drugs, he was outgoing and charismatic. He had been the informal "mayor" at some popular dance clubs in New York City, introducing people to each other and wheeling and dealing. He made millions of dollars in the jewelry industry, enough to retire comfortably at about age 50. However, once he stopped using cocaine, he became progressively more depressed, lost all interest in being with friends, and stopped going out to dinners. He plunged into an anhedonic abyss, from which the Cymbalta was not lifting him.

Knowing that the chronic use of cocaine can deplete the concentration of dopamine in the brain's reward centers, I started him on L-phenylalanine (precursor of dopamine) to enable the neurons to synthesize more dopamine (and subsequently, norepinephrine). We started at 500 mg just once per day, being careful not to ignite any tendency to mania that might have been present.

He tolerated the L-phenylalanine well, and so we increased it to three times per day. We added the herbal *Rhodiola rosea* (100 mg/d) to further enhance mood and energy. The Cymbalta was continued without change, at 60 mg/d. Within 2 weeks of being on this regimen, he started going out to dinner with friends, and reported a greatly increased sense of well-being. He told me that his brain no longer felt like "mush."

Within a year, he had married his girlfriend of several years, and he stood by her when she had to undergo cardiac surgery for valve defects.

This case illustrates the ability of nutritional and herbal supplements to serve as complementary agents, greatly augmenting the efficacy of prescription medications when the latter are not performing adequately (which is quite often the case).

D,L-PHENYLALANINE FOR DRUG ABUSE AND DEPRESSION
Richard M. Carlton, MD
Psychiatry
New York, New York

PATRICIA: 15 YEARS OF NEARLY CONTINUOUS ABUSE OF COCAINE AND HEROIN, WITH COMORBID DEPRESSION

Patricia, a 32-year-old single woman, was a computer programmer who had been seriously abusing cocaine and heroin for 15 years, frequently shooting them up intravenously. She was referred to me by the private outpatient drug treatment facility that had been treating her for several years, to little avail. She was still abusing, despite all the modalities she had tried over the years, which included 12-step programs, individual counseling, psychiatric medications, auricular acupuncture, and more.

Knowing that chronic abuse of cocaine and/or opiates can leave the brain chronically depleted of endogenous opiates (and can also chronically decrease dopamine levels in the reward centers), I started Patricia on D,L-phenylalanine (DLPA) at a dose of 500 mg, 1 capsule b.i.d.

- The L-isomer of phenylalanine improves mood
  - By increasing synthesis of the neuromodulator phenylethylamine
  - By being converted to tyrosine (which in turn increases the synthesis of dopamine and/or norepinephrine)
- The D-isomer inhibits enkephalinase, the enzyme that inactivates enkephalin. By inhibiting the breakdown of enkephalin, the D-isomer increases the net availability of endogenous enkephalins, so that more of the opiate receptors are bound to ligand, more of the time. That alleviates the cravings, while decreasing perceived pain (psychological as well as physical).

It can take about a week's time for D-phenylalanine to produce clinically meaningful inhibition of enkephalinase. Therefore, I urged Patricia to not expect much change for a week or so. When she returned to the office 2 weeks after the first appointment, she told me a remarkable story:

About 8 days after starting the DLPA, Patricia completely stopped using cocaine and heroin. She had lost all cravings for them. But her boyfriend, still an active junkie, was angry at these improvements in her behavior, and around day 10 he left her, taking with him her keys, her credit cards, and her ATM card.

Patricia told me, "In the past I would have shot up. I would know that wouldn't do me any good, but it never stopped me. Instead, this time around, I called the police to have him arrested. I called the bank and credit card companies to get new cards. And I called a locksmith to get the lock changed."

That was it. After 15 years of snorting and shooting these drugs, despite numerous social and psychopharmacological modalities, this over-the-counter pill had turned off all of her cravings.

Two years later Patricia happened to call me to ask a question. She was continuing to take the DLPA and had been "clean" the entire time, without any relapses whatsoever. She was enjoying her life and was doing well in her career as a computer programmer.

This case illustrates a phenomenon I have observed repeatedly for the 40 years I have been using this nutritional approach: When we offer the brain the nutrients it needs to increase its synthesis of the neurotransmitters that regulate mood, hungers, and drives, it responds to that "offer" with a sharp reduction in drives that are abnormal and destructive. Those negative drives seem to be soothed and sated.

GLUTAMINE TO INCREASE GABA IN ALCOHOLISM
Richard M. Carlton, MD
Psychiatry
New York, New York

A 52-Year-Old Alcoholic Housewife

In 1985, the *American Journal of Psychiatry* published an article documenting that chronic alcoholics tend to have chronically low brain CSF (cerebrospinal fluid) and serum levels of GABA (gamma-aminobutyric acid). Given that it was already known to science that supplements of L-glutamine (the precursor amino acid for GABA) will enhance the rate of synthesis of this important inhibitory and calming neurotransmitter, I predicted that glutamine supplements would help chronic alcoholics stop drinking. I looked forward to the opportunity to try it out.

A few months later a new patient told me that his 52-year-old wife was drinking seven martinis after dinner, on a nightly basis. He said that this got her "sloshed" every night, to the point that she had become dysfunctional and difficult. She denied having a problem with alcohol, stating that her drinking was just her way of coping with "stress." She refused to go to Alcoholics Anonymous (AA) meetings.

I told my patient that glutamine supplements, 500 mg twice a day, might be helpful to his wife, and that he could tell her that this supplement would help her with her "stress." She agreed to take it, and within a week or so, her consumption of alcohol decreased from seven martinis per day to just one per day. He would ask her if she would like a second martini, and she would say, "No thanks, I don't need it."

About 4 months later, she decided to decrease her dose of glutamine from 2 capsules per day to 1 per day, and within a week or so, the number of martinis she drank increased to three to four per day. This was nevertheless a great deal better than the baseline seven martinis per day. A few things struck me at the time:

- We had a dose–response curve here: The higher the dose, the less was the drinking. This was anecdotal, of course, with an "*n*" of 1. But it encouraged me to keep using this approach.

- This approach had worked even in the absence of any "inner reckoning." Over the years I have referred many patients to AA, hoping they would get the inner reckoning, and I consider myself a "physician friend of AA." But it can take some people many *years* of 12-step meetings until they get "sick and tired of being sick and tired" and maintain sobriety.
- This nutrient approach is therefore very humane, in that it can help even those who cannot or will not turn to a higher source for help. And it can bring great relief to those who have turned to a higher source but continue to suffer.

In the years since that first case, I have helped an estimated 50 alcoholics gain control of their drinking with the help of glutamine and a few additional nutrients (particularly B complex vitamins, and magnesium). In addition, this approach has saved about a dozen marriages, where the patients I was treating were at the end of their rope with alcoholic spouses and were thinking of filing for divorce. I would urge these patients to offer glutamine supplements to their spouses; in each case, the spouses agreed to take it; and in each case, the spouses stopped drinking, completely.

In one case, after 6 months of abstinence, the husband of one of my patients was looking forward to a visit from an old high school drinking buddy, and as he wanted to go drinking with this buddy, he stopped taking the glutamine. For several days he got drunk with the "friend," kept on drinking even after the friend left town, and would not resume taking the glutamine. Two months later his wife, my patient, filed for divorce. People with this condition need to keep taking the glutamine, to keep GABA levels up to a "safe" level.

These cases illustrate that while there are certainly personality problems and spiritual issues underlying the addictions, coexisting with that there are a host of problems with brain chemistry. In many cases, these problems with brain chemistry can be corrected by supplementing with pharmacological dosages of nutrients. While the primary nutrient I have focused on is L-glutamine, other investigators have published controlled studies showing that nutrients such as magnesium, zinc, D,L-phenylalanine, B vitamins (especially vitamin B1), *N*-acetylcysteine (NAC), and vitamin C are helpful in controlling alcohol addiction/abuse.

TRANSDERMAL ESTRADIOL FOR PREMENSTRUAL SYNDROME MOOD AND COGNITIVE DYSFUNCTION

Ann Hathaway, MD
Integrative Functional Medicine and Bioidentical Hormones
San Rafael, California

42-YEAR-OLD WOMAN WITH DEBILITATING PMS, MOOD, AND COGNITIVE SYMPTOMS

This woman had a height of 5 foot, 9 inches, and weight of 130 pounds. Following are additional details:

- High-functioning mother of three, chief executive officer (CEO) of her own company, and a triathlete.
- She had never noticed significant premenstrual syndrome (PMS) symptoms until the previous 8 months, when she noted marked dysphoria and irritability. She found herself snapping at her children and fighting with her husband over inconsequential things.
- She recalled that she had suffered from unexplained sadness for the first few months after each child was born, but was able to struggle through it with the help of her very supportive husband.
- At the time of my evaluation, she was very compromised premenstrually and could not do any productive work for a week prior to her menses each month.

- She also noted that her breasts, which were always on the small side, had gotten smaller.
- She experienced some hot flashes and feelings of warmth at night during her severe PMS.

Labs during the PMS phase were as follows:

Estradiol 17 pg/mL (very low)
Estrone 11 pg/mL (low)
Progesterone 4.7 ng/dL (adequate)
Testosterone 24 ng/dL (adequate)

Treatment

- A compounded topical cream of 0.4 mg of estradiol applied to the inner arm once daily was prescribed for the last 10 to 12 days of her cycle, and this yielded beneficial results within the first month, though she still was not yet back to normal.
- The estradiol dose was increased to 0.6 mg/d.
- Her mood and cognition returned to normal by the next cycle, and she and her husband were very pleased with the results.
- Her estradiol level increased to 36 pg/mL (therapeutic) on this regimen.

HORMONAL TREATMENT OF POSTPARTUM DEPRESSION
Ann Hathaway, MD
Integrative Functional Medicine and Bioidentical Hormones
San Rafael, California

32-YEAR-OLD FIRST-TIME MOTHER, 6 WEEKS POSTPARTUM, WITH SYMPTOMS OF DEPRESSION

- This woman was happily married, and her pregnancy was planned.
- She had an uncomplicated pregnancy with a forceps-assisted vaginal delivery after 11 hours of labor.
- The infant was healthy, nursing well, and gaining weight appropriately.
- The patient stated there were no major problems in her life, yet she was experiencing continuous sadness and tearfulness, feelings of imminent doom, lack of self-worth, anxiety about minor decisions, and fear that she is not taking good care of her baby.
- In detailed discussion with her, it was clear that the patient was taking good care of her child, and there was no risk of her harming her child.
- She was not suicidal.

Previous History

- She had a history of mild depression, lasting 6 months in her mid 20s due to a relationship breakup.
- She had also experienced PMS in the past, with mild to moderate mood and anxiety symptoms during the last 5 days before her period.

Labs 6 Weeks Postnatal

- Estradiol 16 pg/mL (low)
- Progesterone 1.2 ng/dL (expected postpartum level)

Treatment

- She began a 0.1-mg estradiol transdermal patch, twice weekly application, and noted her depression improved significantly in 3 days.
- She felt she was back to her normal self, she felt calmer and much more confident.

- She had an improved sense of pleasure in mothering her child.
- After 20 days on the estradiol patch, oral micronized progesterone 200 mg was added for 10 days each month, and it was well tolerated.

Follow-Up Labs
- Estradiol was 79 pg/mL.
- Several months later, estradiol was 87 pg/mL.
- Progesterone after 10 days of P4 was 5.3 ng/dL.
  - This progesterone level provides adequate protection for uterine endometrial lining given her current estradiol level.

Course of Treatment
- She stayed on this treatment for 8 months and then transitioned off.
- She continued to do well, although she did not begin menstrual cycles for an additional 4 months.
- She was able to nurse successfully until her child was 19 months old.

TESTOSTERONE AND POSTMENOPAUSAL SEXUAL FUNCTIONING
Ann Hathaway, MD
Integrative Functional Medicine and Bioidentical Hormones
San Rafael, California

60-YEAR-OLD WOMAN, 9 YEARS POSTMENOPAUSAL
- On topical estradiol 0.4 mg and topical progesterone 35 mg/d for 17 days per month for 8 years.
- She feels well on this regime, with good mental clarity, positive mood, sound sleep, and excellent physical energy.
- However, she noted a gradual decline in her sexual interest, much slower arousal, and decreased ability to climax.
- She notes mild vaginal dryness and some discomfort with intercourse.
- She does not experience any difference when on or off progesterone.

Labs
- Estradiol 28 pg/mL
- Estrone 34 pg/mL
- Sex hormone binding globulin (SHBG) 95
- Testosterone 9 ng/dL
- Progesterone 2.3 ng/dL on day 17 of her progesterone use
  - Her total testosterone is quite low.
  - With her high SHBG level, the free testosterone is very low since what little testosterone she has is bound to the SHBG and is not bioavailable.
  - I do not generally measure the free testosterone in women because the concentration is very low, so the sensitivity of the laboratory measurement is unreliable in women.

Treatment
- Estriol 1 mg/g with testosterone 1.5 mg/g cream was compounded for this patient.
- She used 0.5 g applied to the genital area and the vaginal area daily for 4 weeks.
- She called the office to say she noted marked benefit in the vaginal dryness but only a small increase in her sexual function.

- She was advised to continue daily use for another 3 weeks, at which time she reported a marked improvement in her libido and sexual pleasure, and vaginal moisture was much improved.
- The dosing was then changed to use the testosterone and estriol mixture only two to three times per week. The patient was cautioned that excess testosterone applied to the genitals over a long period of time may result in clitoromegaly.

DIETARY CHANGES AND HIGH-DOSE PROGESTERONE FOR PREMENSTRUAL SYNDROME
Ann Hathaway, MD
Integrative Functional Medicine and Bioidentical Hormones
San Rafael, California

A 45-year-old woman with anxiety, insomnia, and food cravings in the 10 days before menses was seen. She had a height of 5 feet, 4 inches; her weight was 162, and BMI was 28.

- A comprehensive gastrointestinal (GI) evaluation with stool testing for dysbiosis and adequacy of digestion was performed, and multiple beneficial interventions were made.
- Dietary changes, including an elimination diet trial and a fermentable oligo-di-monosaccharides and polyols (FODMAPs) diet were initiated, and yielded significant benefits in decreasing anxiety.
- Food cravings were improved, but persisted.
- Her weight decreased to 151.

MIDLUTEAL LABS

- Estradiol 459 pg/mL (high)
- Estrone 302 pg/mL (high)
- Progesterone 5.1 ng/dL (low for midluteal, suggesting suboptimal ovulation, excess estrogen/progesterone [E/P] ratio)
- Testosterone 38 ng/dL (adequate)

TREATMENT

- She was prescribed compounded vaginal suppositories with 400 mg of progesterone twice daily, for a total dose of 800 mg per day, during the last 12 days of her cycle.
- She noted a significant improvement in sleep, less anxiety and less food cravings, and noted no deleterious effects from the treatment.

MENOPAUSAL DEPRESSION AND DYSPHORIA WITH PROGESTERONE
Ann Hathaway, MD
Integrative Functional Medicine and Bioidentical Hormones
San Rafael, California

A 54-year-old woman who is 4 years postmenopausal was treated as follows:

- Her climacteric symptoms were initially treated with oral conjugated equine estrogen (CEE) daily and cyclic medroxyprogesterone (MPA) 2.5 mg 12 days per month by her gynecologist.
- She noted improved mood on CEE, but worsening mood on MPA days, so she discontinued the MPA.

- She tried discontinuing the CEE, but experienced diminished mood when she went off.
- Her gynecologist advised her to go off CEE and take an SSRI for depression.
- She tried several SSRIs without benefit. She felt more fearful, less willing to try new things, more sensitive to criticism, and cried for no reason. She stated that low-level dysphoria was continually present in spite of the SSRI treatment.
- She came in to my office for an evaluation, off all hormones, with the following new labs:
    - Estradiol 8 pg/mL (low)
    - Estrone 39 pg/mL (expected)
    - Testosterone 9 ng/dL (low)
    - DHEA-S 41 mcg/dL (low)

TREATMENT

- A low-dose estradiol 0.0375 mg transdermal patch was initiated.
- In the second month, we added transdermal progesterone cream 30 mg per day for 15 days a month. There was no benefit.
- A repeat estradiol blood level was 22 pg/mL.
- The estradiol patch dose was increased to 0.05 mg, and in 2 days, she noted a dramatic improvement in mood and her sense of well-being.

FOLLOW-UP LAB

- Estradiol 36 pg/mL (good level)

COURSE OF TREATMENT

- She began compounded transdermal progesterone cream the following month at 30 mg/d, 20 days per month, and felt dysphoric within 5 days of starting.
- Various progesterone doses were tried topically, and then various doses of oral micronized progesterone, from 50 to 100 mg for 20 days per month, and 250 mg/d for 10 days every 2 or 3 months.
- She remained very intolerant of the progesterone, as it caused depression, anxiety, and irritability.
- The decision was made to continue her on unopposed transdermal estradiol (no progesterone) with regular pelvic sonograms to evaluate the endometrial thickness, alternating with endometrial biopsies every 6 months.
- She had one study every 6 months for the first 3 years.
- After 3 years, her screening frequency was decreased to once a year, with pelvic sonograms alternating with endometrial biopsies.
- No endometrial hyperplasia has developed.

COMMENTS

- The goal in using estradiol for mood symptoms generally requires achieving an estradiol level of 25 to 40 pg/mL, but this varies from woman to woman.
- Early in menopause, there may be a need for higher estradiol levels, and it is generally safe to go higher in women if they can tolerate higher progesterone dosing, which would allow keeping the estrogen:progesterone ratio in balance.

- There is interesting Swedish research on using very high-dose progesterone (800 mg/d) in vaginal suppositories, which surprisingly yielded very good results in women who did not tolerate 400 mg.
- This was not tried with this patient.
- See the progesterone section of Chapter 11 for more information.

PSYCHOTHERAPY AUGMENTED WITH NUTRIENTS AND MIND-BODY APPROACHES

Amelia Villagomez, MD
Child and Adolescent Psychiatry
University of Arizona
Tucson, Arizona

A 12-year-old Caucasian female was brought into the emergency department (ED) with worsening suicide ideation (SI) and a plan to hang herself.

- Further evaluation revealed worsening symptoms of *tearfulness, insomnia, depressed mood, anhedonia, anxiety, irritability, difficulty concentrating,* and *poor appetite* over the past 1 to 2 years.
- Of note, she also had a history of *poor body image, restrictive eating,* and since she was 5 years old, she was *reported to wear her bathing suit in the shower.*
- She also reported *nightmares* at least four nights a week. Mom states patient was *afraid of the dark* and would regularly join mom and dad in bed.
- She was the daughter of a well-to-do investment banker father, and her mom was a CEO at a health-care company.
- Mom had history of anorexia nervosa and alcoholism and posttraumatic stress disorder (PTSD) from physical, sexual, and emotional abuse by the patient's uncle.
- The parents were separated for a year but had not officially filed for divorce at the time of admission.
- In the course of the psychiatric evaluation, the patient became tearful when asked about any history of trauma, and reported she was *sexually molested by her uncle starting at age 5,* and had never told anyone about this out of fear. She stated she felt responsible and guilty for her parents' separation.

Her labs were significant for *25-OH vitamin D level of 15.*

Child protective services were involved, and the parents were informed of the patient's report of past trauma. The parents were very supportive, though shocked by the news, and proceeded to get legal support. The patient worked closely with the clinical team to form a safety plan prior to discharge.

TREATMENT PLAN

- She was started on omega-3 fatty acids 2.4 g each day (EPA: 1400 mg; DHA: 960 mg); 2000: IU/day.
- Melatonin 3 mg qhs (at bedtime) was given as necessary for insomnia.
- Upon admission to the psychiatric unit, the patient was initially very guarded and unable to feel safe, but within a few individual sessions with the provider, she was able to let her guard down a bit and participate in treatment.
- She was open to using meditation (focused attention, diaphragmatic breathing), guided imagery (PTSD CD by Belleruth Naparstek), creative arts, music, journaling (writing out

her feelings of anger, frustration, sadness, disappointment toward her family), and body-mind approaches such as yoga and shaking meditation.

- She expressed her dream of one day healing to the point that she would be able to create an institute for the rehabilitation and care of abused animals.

OUTCOME

The patient achieved significant improvement of her depressive symptoms, sleep, appetite, and anxiety over the 3-week hospitalization. Her outpatient therapist continued to support her over the next 6 months despite very challenging dynamics with the family.

HPAT AXIS DYSFUNCTION MASQUERADING AS DYSTHYMIA, FATIGUE, AND BRAIN FOG

Sara Gottfried, MD
Gottfried Institute for Functional Medicine
Berkeley, California

The patient is Sara, age 56. Her plea for help was, "I'm flat and dull—this is not the dynamic fifty-something I expected to be."

Sara is an alluring 56-year-old woman who first came to see me in 2008. At the time, she had just entered menopause and felt foggy, flat, and doughy—not the qualities she wanted to bring to the second half of her life. She wanted to be certain that I understood the depth of her fatigue, because other doctors were dismissive. I listened carefully, and fortunately, we were able to turn her symptoms around within several weeks.

Originally from Houston, Sara is an acclaimed artist who lives and works in San Francisco. I could hear a slight Texan drawl to her voice as she asked me at her first visit, "Who is this bone-tired person? I don't recognize her. Why do I opt out of social invitations when earlier in the week they seems like a good idea?" To deal with her fatigue, she would try to boost her energy by grazing carbs, especially crackers with cheese.

At the time, I did not yet have answers to her questions, but I had a hunch her ennui was hormonal, and from the constellation of symptoms, a combination of thyroid and adrenal problems. Sara felt too young to feel so old, and it was affecting her painting and the logistics of mothering. She was newly divorced, and her 10-year-old daughter was the light of her life. Her work in the studio was often cut short because she needed a nap or simply did not feel motivated to create.

In her first questionnaire, Sara added that she felt low in energy and slowed down most of the time, and even worse, blamed herself for it. Her lowest energy was 1 to 4 p.m., but mornings were difficult too: she slept well but did not wake up in the morning feeling restored. She worked hard (harder than she felt she should) with a trainer three times per week to keep her body around 138 pounds on her 5-foot, 5-inch frame.

Sara had been diagnosed with hypothyroidism in 1989. Her doctor put her on the leading thyroid medication, and initially it helped her sluggish energy, foggy memory, and moodiness, and despite exercise, her 20-pound weight gain. However, with time, her low thyroid symptoms crept back into her daily experience. She stayed at approximately the same dose for 19 years—her doctor checked her thyroid function with standard labs (thyroid stimulating hormone [TSH], and free-T4) every 6 or so months and would adjust her dose slightly up or down, but it did not seem to resolve her symptoms. She received her care at a prestigious medical center.

We began by testing her hormones. I suspected that Sara's adrenal function, stress hormones, and thyroid were the primary culprits behind her lack of energy and vitality. I also believed that the reason she felt initially good on the thyroid medication in 1989, and then crashed, was that her adrenal function and cortisol levels were not in the happy medium range that we all need and deserve.

RESULTS

I tested Sara's free-T4 and free-T3 levels, because both are vital to healthy thyroid function. Free-T3 is the active thyroid hormone—the T4 that her doctor had been checking was a storage hormone that I find does not correlate as well with vitality.

I mention this not to blame her primary care doctor; testing TSH and T4 is the standard protocol in mainstream medicine, because we all learn in medical school that if T4 is working properly, it will convert into T3. This often is not the case. I have learned after taking care of women for more than 20 years that many women do not convert T4 into T3 as planned. The most commonly prescribed thyroid medications are T4, and T4 can be measured in the blood as therapeutic, yet the T3 level in the blood may be low. Low T3 levels can result in extreme fatigue and poor mood. Besides, mainstream medicine also tells women that it is normal to feel tired and cranky as you age, and I do not believe that either.

When the labs arrived at my office, I found the following.

Low Free T3

Sara's thyroid function was within the so-called "normal" range as estimated merely by her TSH and free T4 level, but her free T3 level was low, suggesting she was not converting her T4 into T3 as planned.

Her level was 2.5 pg/mL. (I recommend that practitioners aim for the top half of the reference range at their lab, and for Sara's lab, that optimal range is 3.3 to 4.2 pg/mL.)

High Thyroid-Stimulating Hormone (TSH)

This test confuses a lot of people: TSH rises when your thyroid is too slow.
I believe the healthy range is 0.3 to 2.5 mIU/L, and Sara's result was 6.65 mIU/L.

Autoimmune Thyroiditis

The root cause of her slow thyroid was that her immune system was attacking her thyroid.
Her thyroid peroxidase antibodies were 70 IU/mL, and normal is <35.

Low Vitamin D

Sara's vitamin D level was 35 ng/mL.
While most conventional doctors would be fine with this level, I wanted Sara's level to be approximately 50 to 70.
Vitamin D serves many purposes in the body and brain—in Sara's case, it could be helpful for her thyroid function and to boost metabolism, as well as to potentially improve her brain fog.

High Cortisol and Low DHEA-S

Sara's morning blood cortisol level was elevated at 23 mcg/dL, and I advise my patients to aim for 10 to 15 mcg/dL.
Her DHEA-S was 173 ng/dL, and while this hormone varies according to age, her level was low for her age.
Overall, her cortisol and DHEA-S suggested Sara was under long-standing stress and her body could not keep up with the demand.

Borderline High Triglycerides

Sara had triglycerides of 150.

TREATMENT PROTOCOL

We discovered that Sara's T3 was subpar and addressed it with The Gottfried Protocol for the combination of thyroid and adrenal issues. Here is the protocol we used for Sara:

- Step 1. Targeted lifestyle changes and nutraceuticals
  - Sara began a high-potency multivitamin that filled nutritional gaps needed for her thyroid and adrenals, including copper, zinc, selenium, and iodine. She also started vitamin D, 2000 IU/d.
  - For diet, I suggested a gluten-free, sugar-free food plan, as I suspected that the gluten could be aggravating her autoimmune thyroiditis and that sugar was raising her triglycerides. I asked her to experiment with a mostly vegan diet as we next tested her for leaky gut syndrome and food allergies.
  - For contemplative practice, Sara already had a hodgepodge of spiritual practices—I asked that she become consistent about meditation 30 minutes each day.
- Step 2. Herbal Therapies
  - For her high cortisol, I recommended *Rhodiola*, 200 mg twice/day.
- Step 3. Bioidentical Thyroid and Adrenal Hormones
  - For her low T3 and high TSH, I prescribed 16.25 mg of Nature-Throid® (later, this was replaced by Westhroid-P®, which contains medium-chain triglycerides and no fillers, but that was not available at the time). She took her Nature-Throid first thing in the morning, on an empty stomach, with nothing else to eat or drink for 60 minutes. Sara stayed on her T4 medication (Synthroid®) until a year later when she noted hair loss, a common side effect of Synthroid, and we switched her to the equivalent dose of Tirosint®.
  - DHEA 5 mg/day for additional adrenal support since her levels were low for her age.

FOLLOW-UP

- Since her thyroid medication was managed by her primary care physician at one of the leading Bay Area Medical Centers, I called Sara's doctor to touch base about my recommendations. Sadly, her doc was not open to my ideas, and treated me as unworthy of serious consideration. She listened to me describe the TSH and free T3, and cut me off midsentence with a curt reply: "I don't believe in topping off thyroid medication to help a patient get skinny." I was stunned. I held my ground, kindly informed the doctor what I would prescribe, and called it in to Sara's local pharmacy.
- After 6 weeks on her protocol, Sara felt like a new person. She realized the "self blame" was actually hormonal in origin. She retested her labs, and we found that her thyroid was now normal, her thyroid antibodies were undetectable, and her triglycerides dropped to the optimal range.
- Sara returned for her follow-up appointment and her verve was undeniable. She had turned a pivotal corner and she was glowing. Her weight dropped without changing her exercise, her general malaise lifted, and she could remember where she left the car keys. "I didn't know that the reason I felt so off was my hormones. I thought it was a psychological or emotional failing. Now I'm back in my studio and fully present. Energy is flowing through me and feeding my passion, my creativity, and my work. Overall, my vitality has gone way up, and I've lost weight without trying. My chronic need to take a nap has subsided. Ever since I could remember, as an adult, I've had bouts of walking around in a daze, wondering when the fog would lift. Well, those days are gone. The shift is subtle, yet quite profound to my experience of myself and of life. I feel better. I look better. I love what's happening!"

10-DAY DETOX FOR SEVERE DEPRESSION WITH SUICIDE IDEATION

Myrto A. Ashe, MD
Functional Medicine
San Rafael, California

M is a 32-year-old man who presented with persistent major depression and a history of substance abuse:

- Was on Wellbutrin® 300 mg QD, Lexapro® 40 mg QD, and was about to start Abilify®
- Had severe anhedonia on a daily basis
- Had stopped working since being hospitalized 3 months before the visit due to having a suicidal plan
- Attended a day treatment psychiatric program

M comes from a large Catholic family. He reports serious health-related stress due to his mother's cancer diagnosis before his birth. He says he felt like "an afterthought" in his family. It was busy, cluttered, and financially on a worsening trajectory, though he enjoyed having many siblings to spend time with.

M was a healthy baby, though he had minor surgery as an infant. As a toddler and school-aged child, he had asthma and was frequently ill, repeatedly receiving antibiotics and missing school. He also remembers feeling sad a lot as a child.

M did very well in high school and college but also partied a lot and got into financial difficulty while not completing his degree. His mother passed away from cancer when he was 22, shortly before college graduation. M moved back in with his father and resented having to contribute financially. These were very difficult years. M began overusing alcohol. He became more reckless and suicidal. He met his present wife. They married 7 years ago. They just had their first baby a few months ago.

After his wedding, M turned to Alcoholics Anonymous, Prozac®, and therapy all at the same time. He felt better for a while but then returned to feeling depressed. Venlafaxine® was tried, but he had an adverse reaction (hot flashes). His medications were changed to the present combination. He believes he is having more anxiety on this combination.

M has also tried psychotherapy: cognitive-behavioral therapy (CBT) and dialectical behavior therapy (DBT).

M reported trying the Master Cleanse a few times and noticing that he felt a lot better while on it. The Master Cleanse is a juice fast that consists of consuming only tea and lemonade with maple syrup. While on this regimen, M felt brighter, his brain clear, and he had more energy. Unfortunately, this is not a sustainable diet, so after completing a few days on it, M resumed a conventional diet and began to feel unwell again.

When asked what is meaningful to him at this time, he mentions helping others, animal rescue, and sharing experiences. He did not mention his wife (sitting next to him) or his baby daughter.

FAMILY HISTORY

M does not have a family history of mental illness.

His brother Dave, who now has multiple sclerosis, had a brief episode with a striking personality change in high school. His doctor now believes it was an early manifestation of MS.

His mother died in her 70s. She lived in Slovakia during WWII. She was overweight and survived breast cancer in her 40s. In 2002, she was diagnosed with bone cancer and died. His father is in his 70s, has colon cancer, had skin cancer, and does not take good care of himself.

INTERVENTION

M and his wife explained that they were financially very limited, and were fearful that a Functional Medicine approach would be expensive and ineffective. I recommended that instead of repeated visits with me to explain a complicated plan of action, M follow a predesigned plan detailed in the book *The 10-Day Detox Diet* by Hyman. This entails a very low glycemic index diet based on natural foods only, daily meditation, sweating, daily exercise, and basic supplements. Supplements included a high-quality multivitamin, essential fatty acids, vitamin D, and probiotics. Blood tests were performed and excluded frank deficiencies in B12, iron, other B vitamins, and vitamin D.

After 10 days on this plan, the patient wrote the following e-mail:

"My depression is greatly reduced, all puffiness and inflammation are gone, my cravings are reduced, my brain fog is gone and I haven't felt this mentally sharp since I was 16."

As he had also just started on Abilify and his wife felt that this could be a positive effect of this new medication, he did "a little experiment yesterday and had my usual fill of sugar, dairy, and gluten, and started to feel terrible."

M explained his transformation to his colleagues at the day treatment and several of them purchased the book and embarked on this plan.

At this time (1 month later), he is actively engaged in his life, spending time learning new computer programs relevant to his work, looking for a job, cooking dinner along with his wife, being more engaged with his daughter, looking forward to the future, and looking for a psychiatrist who will help him gradually reduce his medications.

MEDITATION AND MINDFULNESS FOR DEPRESSION AND ANXIETY

Healy Smith, MD, ABIHM
New York Presbyterian Hospital/Weill Cornell Medical College
New York, New York

Fiona is a lovely married woman in her early 30s who presented with a long history of depression and anxiety, on one to two antidepressants and a benzodiazepine as needed for the previous 12 years. She was interested in lowering her medications pre-pregnancy. She had a history of panic disorder for a few years, since resolved, and described her anxiety now as mainly physical symptoms, particularly dizziness as well as nausea, and a feeling of urgency, not clearly related to thoughts or worry or identifiable triggers. She also reported an extensive family history of anxiety.

She described waves of depression lasting a couple weeks or more, with anhedonia, tearfulness, fatigue, low appetite, low motivation, irritability, and emotional reactivity. She reported a few episodes of suicidal thoughts amid her depressions, and before entering treatment superficially scratched her wrist with a sharp knife while drinking; she did not bleed but was very frightened. She was unable to identify triggers to these depressive episodes that would occur every few months.

Medical history was relevant for childhood asthma, a history of stomach ulcers understood to be due to stress and anxiety, and intervertebral disk inflammation. She has a strong social network, was successful in her high-stress, creative job, had a healthy diet, enjoyed exercise, the arts, time with friends and family, and, as an introvert, alone time.

We started weekly therapy and medication management, with her stated goals of minimizing medication, better managing stress, and improving and stabilizing mood. Early on, I introduced meditation to her as a means of supporting her health while we started to adjust her medications. We started with relaxing breathing techniques, first practicing during our session. She described initially feeling relaxed, but then dizzy. I observed that her breathing was quick and shallow, and introduced her to slower belly breathing. She committed to 5 min/d practicing slower belly breathing, breathing in to a count of four, and out to a count of five. We also agreed to start each of our sessions with 7 minutes of meditation.

She attended to her breathing in moments during the day, which she found more difficult to do when anxious. When anxious, she noticed that she would either breathe quickly or hold her breath, and felt unable to think clearly. We discussed the anxiety-producing effects of hyperventilation, and started practicing Vipassana meditation, focused on following the breath, mindful of the flow of thoughts and sensations.

She generally meditated two to five times per week, for 7 min/session, and also regularly checked in with her breathing throughout the day. Within 6 weeks of treatment, she described feeling calmer, happier, and more resilient. She was more able to recognize upsetting thoughts and feelings in the moment, and to take a step back before reacting, which then made her feel better about herself. She found that the alone time she spent in meditation recharged her, and began to place higher priority on making time for herself, and recognizing and enjoying the moments of alone time she did have, such as while brushing her teeth.

After a couple of months, she described this being the longest stretch she'd had with minimal anxiety, and also noted improvements in her back pain. When she would feel the physical symptoms of anxiety creep in, she would bring her attention to her breathing, which would tend to be shallow. She would slow and deepen her breath, which would reduce her anxiety. She said that starting our sessions with meditation helped clear her mind, and helped her to be more present for our session.

She described that often in the last 1 to 2 minutes of her home meditation sessions, she would start to feel nervous and antsy, sometimes stopping early. We discussed an alternative reaction to these feelings, a mindful approach—bringing an interested attention to them, breathing them in, and exploring their texture.

We successfully tapered her off medications during the fourth through seventh months of treatment. She noted increased irritability off of medication.

As she continued practicing mindfulness meditation, she became increasingly aware of its effects—on the days she meditated, she felt more patient and clear, and less irritable. She became more aware of a cycle in which she would overextend herself, then become irritable, which would rouse feelings of guilt, and then poor self-esteem. In an effort to bring more balance to her stressful life, we explored incorporating more self-care. She had long been highly driven to be productive, including in her leisure time, but after experiencing the effects of meditation on increasing her effectiveness at work (through increased patience and clarity, and less irritability and reactivity, engendering more effective teamwork and leaving her feeling better about herself), as well as her overall happiness, she longed for more restorative down-time. She began to make room for quiet time by herself during her weeks, and noticed a corresponding decrease in irritability when she took this time.

She described her irritability as quick shifts into a sense of time speeding up, feeling overwhelmed and out of control, getting frustrated and angry, always followed by regret, guilt, and feelings of depression. She started to bring mindful attention to these moments, just noticing the thoughts and feelings, without having to change them. Primarily in the interest of addressing her tendency to be harsh with herself, and increasing her capacity for nonjudgmental presence, I taught her loving-kindness meditation, silently repeating the phrases, "May I be safe, May I be happy, May I be healthy, May I live with ease."

I asked her to initially focus on sending these wishes to herself, which she found most difficult, and then extending them out to widening circles. She soon described being able to engage her difficult feelings differently, with more acceptance versus resistance or resignation, and with more ease versus feeling drained. She described feeling more grounded, connected, and kind to herself, as well as feeling calmer, and more forgiving of herself when she did not meet her expectations.

For example, when tired and grumpy one weekend day, she allowed herself a rare nap, and woke feeling much better. She began to discover a correlation between being very tough on herself and getting more irritable; and between being kinder to herself and feeling more emotional stability. She described increasing ability to step back in an emotional moment, versus her old pattern of getting sucked into the emotion, with tunnel vision. She developed a technique for moments when she would start to feel the pull of strong emotion. She would visualize a stop sign, introduce a pause.

Always goal-oriented, she began to take more interest in the process versus just in the outcome, letting herself enjoy and appreciate moments along the path. For example, during a day with much housework to be done, she described really enjoying the process and result of painting a room, while in the past she would have quickly moved onto the next task, not feeling satisfied until all her goals were accomplished.

Upon reflecting on mindfulness meditation versus metta (loving-kindness) meditation, she described generally feeling clearer and more refreshed after mindfulness meditation, and feeling kinder to herself after loving-kindness meditation.

While she continues to have times when she gets pulled into floods of emotion, she describes a different way of relating to them—instead of feeling hopeless and stuck, she recognizes their temporary nature, and indeed, they tend to pass more quickly. She has described feeling more resilient and stronger, and is now expecting her first child.

MEDITATION/MINDFULNESS: AN UNEXPECTED OBSTACLE

Healy Smith, MD, ABIHM
New York Presbyterian Hospital/Weill Cornell Medical College
New York, New York

Dana is a married woman in her late 30s with a long history of dysthymia, depression, and poor self-esteem. She suffered from postpartum depression after the births of both her children, but had been doing well for about a year on an SSRI. She was slowly tapered off, and continued to do well for many months, before relapsing into another episode, characterized by insomnia, near-anhedonia, rumination, fatigue, low motivation, and low appetite, with difficulty fulfilling her roles as a stay-at-home mother.

In addition to restarting medication, I introduced the supplemental use of meditation, beginning with a couple minutes of following her breath. She reported that during this quiet time, her undistracted mind would fill with ruminative depressive thoughts, making her feel worse. We tried tools for a couple weeks to increase her capacity for observing her thoughts versus being drawn into them, but without success.

I then suggested trying loving-kindness meditation, repeating a series of kind wishes toward herself, thus not leaving space for rumination, and recommended for background Sharon Salzberg's book *Lovingkindness*, which describes the Buddhist path and practices toward cultivating loving-kindness and other life-enhancing qualities. This is a book several of my patients have enjoyed and found useful.

The next week, however, Dana expressed discomfort in doing a practice rooted in a spiritual/religious philosophy, a concern that I had not previously encountered, and that caught me off guard. We let go of meditation, and focused on other approaches toward wellness.

In her case, amid an acute depression, her depressive ruminations appeared too strong to distance from. It is possible that a group intervention, such as Mindfulness-Based Stress Reduction (MBSR) or possibly Mindfulness-Based Cognitive Therapy (MBCT) would have been more supportive and effective, but her skepticism of these practices would have likely overcome the motivation and commitment needed.

While more and more people are interested in meditation and mindfulness, it is important to keep in mind and respect the discomfort that some people will have toward techniques born from spiritual and religious practice. Perhaps a better approach with her would have been to introduce mindfulness practices more distanced from religion, as taught in Acceptance and Commitment Therapy (ACT).

After several months of euthymia and significant progress in psychotherapy—including increased awareness of the high cost to her happiness and relationships of her tendency to retreat into her thoughts instead of expressing and asserting her opinions, ideas, and needs—Dana brought up on her own initiative that she was interested in revisiting practices to become more present. She continued to articulate what she disliked about her associations with meditation, including the language often used, with its potential for spiritual or New Age associations.

We discussed her concerns, and, utilizing more of an ACT approach, have been creatively developing practices that have helped to cultivate her observing self, to gain distance from unhelpful but routinized thought patterns, to ground herself in her body, and to increase her self-confidence and assertiveness in the moment.

MINDFULNESS MEDITATION FOR LONG-STANDING DISABLING DEPRESSION
Susan Evans, PhD
Weill Cornell Medical College
New York, New York

Henry is a middle-aged married male who has suffered for years from bouts of Major Depression. Past episodes of depression have included suicide attempts requiring hospitalization. Following one hospitalization several years ago, the patient went on disability and has remained unemployed. Henry, who is highly intelligent, well read, and with a cynical sense of humor, had never received a course of cognitive behavioral therapy (CBT) and was referred by his psychopharmacologist for a course of standard CBT. Initially, the patient expressed skepticism that CBT would be helpful to him and perceived himself as a "hopeless case."

Despite a rather pessimistic attitude, Henry was willing to collaborate with the treatment plan and began learning the cognitive model. He assiduously completed his homework assignments, including the dysfunctional thought record (DTR). His automatic thoughts often related to negative self-schemas including the belief he was a "loser," "fraud," and "worthless." He often described himself in session in scathing and self-condemning terms, and while critical examination of his thoughts led him to identify significant distortions in his thinking, he continued to hold on to his core belief of worthlessness. He would often respond by saying, "I still feel like a lazy, useless, worthless excuse for a human being."

After several sessions of gaining little traction with cognitive restructuring, I asked the patient, with a bit of trepidation (half expecting a cynical response), if he would be interested in learning mindfulness. In fact, Henry seemed quite interested and went on a quest to learn as much about it as he could. I started by introducing Henry to the body scan as well as other mindfulness strategies (i.e., sitting meditation), and he began to practice regularly.

Over a relatively short period of time, both Henry and I noted a remarkable shift in his attitude toward himself. Rather than his habitual self-loathing stance, he began to respond to himself with an attitude of self-compassion. In the past, Henry would take any small opportunity to beat himself up. Now, after practicing mindfulness for a few weeks, he began to "talk back" to himself in positive and encouraging terms. He gave an example in one session of attending a neighborhood party and rather than his usual behavior of falling into rumination afterward about how socially inept he is, Henry remarked that he was aware of these thoughts but "let them go."

Within a few weeks of beginning a daily meditation practice, Henry's depression remitted, and he began to experience himself and the world in a new way. He commented to me that he felt the mindfulness practice was helping him to step back and look at things from a distance and not take things so personally. He also felt he had developed a sense of compassion toward himself that he had never felt before.

Over time, Henry titrated down from therapy sessions but continued his mindfulness practice. At one point, he suffered a serious stroke and was incapacitated for several months and required extensive rehabilitation. When I saw him for a follow-up visit several months later, Henry told me that the meditation practice got him through the recovery period.

MINDFULNESS-BASED STRESS REDUCTION FOR ANXIETY
Barbara Wingate, MD
Rittenhouse Healing Collaborative
Philadelphia, Pennsylvania

For many patients, the reliable, predictable tried-and-true schedule and teaching of Mindfulness-Based Stress Reduction (MBSR) is reassuring. They benefit from the group setting and hearing of others' struggles and successes in the important tasks to:

- Still and quiet the mind
- Take note of their bodies and emotions
- Tolerate their unpredictable feelings, thoughts, and sensations

They get support on how to bring the morning (or evening) practice into their day.

They hear how others struggle to find time, skip sessions, practice daily, yet still move imperfectly forward and derive benefits.

Over the last 15 to 20 years, I have referred well over 100 patients for such an experience, and been with them through the process. The fact that I have taken the MBSR courses (and indeed taken the teaching apprenticeship and have practiced teaching MBSR) promotes trust in this fairly arduous 8-week process.

Meditation is not instant bliss and relaxation, but most often is quite challenging at first, and it continues to be so for many of us. But the daily benefits are worth the efforts.

Patients are on occasion too depressed to tolerate the thoughts that feel like painful rumination. I have faced the tough decision to advise at least 10 of my referrals to drop out and try again later, or perhaps try a different form of meditation, and advised them to have medication management and/or other forms of therapy instead.

In my experience, patients with mild to moderate depression and anxious features do best with mindfulness meditation. My most recent referral fit this category exactly:

A gentleman in his mid-50s with chronic anxiety and somatic fears about dying early was encouraged to try the 8-week MBSR course.

His symptoms had worsened after he was diagnosed (ultimately incorrectly) with mild emphysema. He had earlier responded to an SSRI and clonazepam, as well as marital counseling to minimize stress at home, and he was demoralized by the return of symptoms. I had at some point added Buspar®, which allowed for less benzodiazepine use, an important goal for all, but especially those who are older with the increased risk of Alzheimer's disease. We both were aiming for adding a more natural self-healing tool.

His pleasure in the course was palpable, and he was pleased and surprised to find a former therapist of his in his class. The democracy of the playing field—the notion that we all get anxious and have troublesome thoughts—was very reassuring to him.

He practiced diligently and felt his symptoms reduce by about week 4.

To quote Anne Lamott, "My mind is a bad neighborhood that I try not to go into alone."[1]

MINDFULNESS-BASED COGNITIVE THERAPY PROGRAM FOR DEPRESSION IN AN ELDERLY WOMAN
Susan Evans, PhD
Weill Cornell Medical College
New York, New York

Martha is an elderly frail woman who signed up for the Mindfulness-Based Cognitive Therapy (MBCT) program because she wanted to learn meditation in an effort to find some peace in her life.

She had lost her beloved husband to cancer in recent years, and had been struggling with loneliness and depression since his death.

Martha had rejected the idea of medication or therapy for her depression but was open to meditation training. Throughout the program Martha appeared quiet, reserved, and at times sad and withdrawn. She seemed reluctant to engage in any of the group discussions, but listened with a tone of interest and respect. Although Martha did not speak in class, she always arrived early and reported that she was regularly practicing the meditation as well as the awareness and cognitive exercises.

Martha completed the 8-week course and relayed that she had found a greater sense of inner peace. She noted that she had been struggling with early morning awakening since her husband had died, and since starting the program she began to practice the body scan she learned during these early hours.

Martha acknowledged a growing sense of control and calm as she integrated meditation into her daily routine.

Toward the end of the class, Martha approached the group leader and said she was ready to consider getting help for her depression. It appeared that the course allowed her to confront her sadness, and provided a gateway for further treatment.

MULTIMODAL GRIEF THERAPY: DIET, NUTRIENTS, EXERCISE, ART, AND FAMILY THERAPY

Lewis Mehl-Madrona, MD, PhD
Coyote Institute
Orono, Maine

CASE STUDIES IN GERIATRIC DEPRESSION

Ms. TN was an 80-year-old female whose husband had recently died from an acute coronary event. She had been grieving and was brought in by her daughter, who believed that the grief was taking too long. Hearing this, her mother was indignant, saying that she would grieve as long as she wished. Her daughter had read extensively on the stages of grief and felt that her mother had entered into what could have been called "pathological bereavement," a concept to which her mother objected greatly.

Assessment revealed that Ms. TN met the DSM-V criteria for major depressive disorder. However, her feeling was that she was just grieving and should be left alone to do that. We agreed to continue to meet with her and the daughter.

The first step in the treatment was to convince the patient that she should taper and stop the alprazolam and oxycodone that her primary care physician had prescribed for her grief and for her knee osteoarthritis. We explained to her that Alprazolam tended to make sadness worse, and that she would do better without it. We also explained that Oxycodone was not indicated for nonlethal conditions, because it actually made pain worse over time. The best treatment for osteoarthritis of the knee was to keep moving.

We continued weekly meetings to give Ms. TN an opportunity to express her grief about her husband and to pay tribute to his life and to their marriage, as this was quite important to her. The primary care physician had proposed starting her on Sertraline®, to which we responded that it was reasonable if she wanted, or she could continue to work with some nondrug means to determine what was necessary. We have learned that the first response of primary care physicians is usually medication, since they do not have access to nonpharmacological means of working with depression. They tend to rely solely on drugs.

Meanwhile, we were exploring Ms. TN's diet. She was largely eating pasta and bread, quick to fix items that were not necessarily nutritious. We focused on what she could do quickly to improve her diet and found that she was willing to cook fish, since it was quick. We encouraged her to replace pasta with fish and to eat less desserts and breads.

She began to take that recommendation to heart and to make those changes in her diet, which were associated with slow improvement in her mood. When she began to have trouble eating enough fish, we proposed fish oil supplements, to which she agreed. Then we were able to upgrade her vitamins to EMPowerplus®, which is a brand we recommend because it is pharmaceutical grade and broadly comprehensive. She began taking EMPowerplus and fish oil supplements in adequate doses.

During each meeting, which lasted between 40 minutes and one hour, we continued to do a combination of family therapy with her and her children, and to encourage her to express her grief, both verbally and artistically.

She was eating less carbohydrates and more protein, taking broad-spectrum micronutrients and fish oil, so our next move was to increase her activity. We began to explore her objections to walking, and we suggested that to walk was definitely cool. Over the next 4 weeks, she started walking between 2 and 3 km per day.

Over the course of 4 months, she finished her grieving, completed several art projects dedicated to her deceased husband, moved her diet in the direction of more protein and vegetables, reduced her intake of simple carbohydrates (pasta, bread, and desserts), started walking 2 to 3 km/d, added a multiple vitamin of high quality, and added fish oil.

The family therapy sessions were interpreted as resolving some of the difficulties (long-term) between mother and daughter.

I find the key in cases like this is often to keep meeting, regardless of other considerations, with the idea that frequent meetings will dislodge logjams and move the patient toward progress.

HEALING THROUGH STORYTELLING, EMPOWERMENT, CONTINUITY, AND RADICAL ACCEPTANCE
Lewis Mehl-Madrona, MD, PhD
Coyote Institute
Orono, Maine

Ms. NN was a 65-year-old woman, mother of three, and grandmother of nine children. When she first came to consult Lewis Mehl-Madrona (LMM) and Barbara J. Mainguy (BJM), she was a 20-year veteran of the psychiatric system. She had been hospitalized over 300 times in the past 20 years and had attempted suicide almost 100 times. She immediately challenged LMM with how he was going to fix her, to which he replied that he did not know and invited her to come again.

NN had a number of therapists, who, to LMM's perspective, seemed to encourage her passivity and to mitigate against recovery. She appeared to terrify them with her suicide threats so as to mobilize them to attempt to rescue her.

NN continued to come, and LMM continued to reflect that he did not know how to help her, but he could tell her stories. This patient was part Native American, so he began to tell her Native American stories aimed at promoting self-agency and casting NN as heroic in her journeys through life. During this time, NN proposed a variety of medication changes, none of which were unreasonable, and all of which LMM agreed to do. None of these changes appeared to make any difference.

NN continued to come for weekly appointments and chose to join an ongoing group that LMM and BJN ran, which was called "Complicated Minds." She began coming every week. She also joined their "Pain Group," which was required of her since she had come on an Oxycodone dose for chronic musculoskeletal pain. Our policy was to manage patients who came on opiate therapy in group medical visits, which they were required to attend twice monthly in order to continue to receive their opiates. (We never started opiates for nonterminal, chronic conditions.) Eventually, NN joined our third group, which we called "Fragile Minds," and which was mostly art therapy for people who were, in fact, quite fragile.

Over this time, little appeared to change, but with one year of contact, NN had no hospitalizations and no suicide attempts, which had not happened for her in over 20 years. We believed it was our relationship with her in which we were radically accepting and nonjudgmental that was making the difference.

In her second year of coming to us, she suddenly decided to eat differently. This was after 18 months of hearing about the anti-inflammatory diet and the importance of avoiding carbohydrates and sugars. She had previously been eating mostly sugar and simple carbohydrates. Without explanation, she decided to eat a vegetarian diet with complete organic ingredients and no simple carbohydrates or sugars. She began to produce her own Kombucha, a fermented drink of high vitamins and minerals. She began to lose weight (she had previously been of high body mass index [BMI]) and her mood improved. She slowly began to leave her house and walk. She found ways to get vitamins for low-income people and began to take a comprehensive vitamin supplement. She began to practice her wiccan spirituality again.

By 3 years into the treatment, NN had still not had any further hospitalizations or suicide attempts. She was off opiates and benzodiazepines and, in fact, all medications. Her blood pressures had normalized. She was no longer borderline diabetic. She had normalized her BMI. She was attending regular spiritual gatherings, socializing with others, interacting with her grandchildren, eating organically, exercising, doing yoga, and attending groups. Through her ongoing relationships, she continued to improve, off all medications.

We believe that the key ingredients again consisted of radical acceptance and nonjudgment coupled with frequent meetings. LMM uses hypnotic principles in most of his sessions and gave her many suggestions to be the hero of her own life and to gain self-agency. These were embedded in the stories he told her, some of which he recorded for her to hear at home.

NARRATIVE THERAPY FOR DEPRESSION
Antolin C. Trinidad, MD, PhD
Department of Psychiatry, Norwalk Hospital
Norwalk, Connecticut
Yale University School of Medicine
New Haven, Connecticut

At the time of his presentation to therapy, Doug was a 19 year-old male college student who initially presented for treatment in the emergency room of the university hospital of the university where he matriculated as a sophomore undergraduate student in anthropology. He presented to treatment because of depression and suicidal ideation. He did not present with a plan to kill himself; rather, on many days, he thought that he would rather not be alive.

Despite being very lonely, Doug could not get himself to think about dating because he could not define his sexual orientation. He had fallen behind in his classes, and because he was on full scholarship, he believed that his stay at the university was endangered. The thought of having to go back to his family in Pennsylvania was so difficult to accept that he wished he would "just die."

He talked to his roommate about his thoughts, and his roommate facilitated bringing him in to the emergency room (ER) for evaluation. After being seen in the ER, Doug was discharged with an appointment to see a therapist the following day.

In therapy, it came to light that Doug has always felt the odd child out. Introspective and introverted, he did not think anyone in his family understood him. His father was a mail carrier in their small town, his mother worked at the local school cafeteria, and his younger siblings (a brother and a sister) seemed to be interested in the "normal" things like soccer and the cheerleading team at the local high school.

Doug remembered that he has always dressed differently. Though tall and attractive, he wore nonprescription eyeglasses that he picked out at local thrift stores along with colorful, unconventional clothes and accessories, with the result that often other students drew away from him because of this unusual style. He said that because he was different, he was bullied both in grade and high school, where he felt like he did not have friends.

Doug received an academic scholarship and felt relief that he could finally get out of his small town to a bigger, more diverse city and university. But soon, the familiar feeling of not fitting in returned. He felt sexually attracted to both men and women. Although the university provided an accepting environment to different sexual orientations, Doug felt restricted by the pressure to define himself as either straight or gay, because not doing so confused the small circle of acquaintances he had.

During Christmas breaks and holidays, he would go back to Pennsylvania and would feel compelled to wear conventional clothing, such as plaid flannel shirts, jeans and high-top shoes so he would not stand out as much during family gatherings. However, he still loved scouring thrift shops and picking out unusual outfits such as different hats, scarves, and coats. Though he did not cross dress, he occasionally picked accessories such as scarves and sunglasses in the women's section of stores. He liked a different hairstyle and wore his hair longer than most students.

In narrative therapy, the first discussion revolved around the idea of the dominant narrative and how it influenced Doug's own self-narrative. In his small town, few people went to college. Indeed, he was the first one in his family to go to college. Most people stayed in town, few people left, and it was his perception that his parents expected that of him as well. It had always been assumed that Doug would get married, have children, and be part of his extended family. After college, Doug's parents believed that he would get a teaching job at the local community college, and even if he did not settle exactly within the same town, he would live close by. None of these elements were ever articulated, but Doug interpreted many conversations through the years with his parents as having those themes of leading a life similar to the rest of his family.

Doug's role models did not live lives that comported with Doug's own sense of who he was as a person, and so the dominant narrative formed in his mind by observation alone. Doug assumed that because he never planned on living that life expected of him, he would be somewhat of a pariah in his family, especially given his own perception of his different sexual orientation. In therapy, he often mused that he wished he were just more conventional and not so different, that it would have been "much easier."

Regarding his unconventional clothing style, Doug said that he regarded his body as his own artistic experimentation. He experienced much enjoyment in color and in unusual combinations of clothing elements. His mood lifted when he found the right combination of clothes. When the therapist expressed interest in the meaning of his sartorial experiments for the day, Doug would light up, saying he wanted his clothing choices to be an academic, scholarly interest in the future. He had many ideas about the interplay of meanings and how it affected moods, how his clothes reflected elements of the past since they were mostly vintage clothing from thrift shops, and how the past can be brought back artistically into the present. The therapist explored how such unconventional clothing style became one reason why he was bullied in his younger years.

A long conversation ensued, leading to the conclusion that in fact there are forces in society that discourage novelty and self-expression, and that a self-narrative such as Doug's can often meet with adversities. Doug concluded that there is a price, but to be able to be true to one's self, one must be brave enough to stand up to these oppositions.

This conversation also led to his sexual orientation. Like a different narrative expressed in clothing and style, sexuality can also be expressed and identified in more than one way. Doug observed that at the university, he noticed that certain students dressed much more conservatively—students majoring in business and finance, for example, whom Doug sometimes ridiculed because he said they all seemed like clones. The therapist noted this and asked Doug what that meant. Doug said he guessed he was starting to see how his personal choices, and his self-narrative, were beginning to make sense to him because he found them superior in the sense that it was a refreshing change from being a cliché. Not only were they more authentic and courageous, but they also provided much-needed diversity.

The idea of courage also sparked the therapist's interest. Doug was encouraged to reflect on that issue some more and how it related to his depression. Doug took the challenge and came up with the conclusion that if one was not true to one's own story, then depression is more likely. Courage is what it takes to get your story heard because other people may not understand it, or they may actually dislike your story. But the story is yours and yours alone.

This is the point of departure which the therapist noted—that we are here on earth not to follow the stories or rules others have followed for generations, but to bravely chart our own courses. There is something heroic about this process. Doug's and the therapist's conclusion during the ending of his therapy was that the world would be very boring if everyone wanted to be the same person as everybody else.

What Doug did, with the help of the therapist, was to recognize that he was the author of his own story and that he had always been courageous in owning up to it, despite the bullying and the feeling of being alone. In considering the effects of this new, re-authored story to the alleviation of his depression, they concluded that depression is a state of helplessness, whereas the re-authored story was definitely not helplessness, but agency—a state whose appropriate accompanying affect is definitely not depression.

In other words, a narrative of persecution and isolation was re-authored into a narrative akin with heroism, recognizing the value of diversity and the importance of artistic expression.

A FUNCTIONAL APPROACH TO ANXIOUS DEPRESSION
Dean Raffelock, DC, Dipl. Ac., DAAIM
Raffelock and Associates, Inc.
Ashland, Oregon

Anne W., a 37-year-old Caucasian female with two young children, presented with

- Anxious depression—moderate to severe
- Severe fatigue in the mid to late afternoon
- Trouble falling back to sleep after 3 hours of sleep
- Orthostatic blood pressure changes
- Chronic digestive disturbances
- Multiple food sensitivities
- Chronic knee, lower back, and neck pain
- Family history of breast cancer

Anne had been to four physicians, and the only treatment offered for her depression and anxiety were selective serotonin reuptake inhibitors (SSRIs) and benzodiazepines. A neighbor had committed suicide shortly after going on an SSRI, and another had gained over 40 pounds on one, so Anne was unwilling to try the pharmaceutical route for these symptoms.

Her lifestyle was stressful. Her occupation required travel to remote areas with questionable sanitation. She was afraid that her poor health and moods would make her "an overall failure in life" along with being "an inadequate absentee mother and wife." She had little energy for her family when she returned from her travels each month.

Exercise was sporadic. She had no meditation or stress reduction practice. She ate a vegetarian diet, but her diet did not include many *green vegetables* or adequate protein.

Anne stated that her health began to fail 4 years prior, shortly after the birth of her second child. At that time a friend had given her a copy of my book, *A Natural Guide to Pregnancy and Postpartum Health*[2] which discusses the concept that a mother's hormones, neurotransmitters, and overall nutrient reserves can become drained by donating all the nutrients to form her baby's body, the placenta, and milk for breastfeeding. Anne had also lost a lot of blood during her delivery.

These notions made sense to her, and she had tried to get her hometown primary care provider (PCP) to run some of the tests recommended in my book, to no avail. After 4 years of her symptoms getting progressively worse, Anne decided to fly in to have a consultation with me.

After examining her and taking her history, I recommended the following tests in the order I thought most important:

- A 24-hour comprehensive adrenal and reproductive steroid test with metabolites and added free T3 and free T4
- A comprehensive urine neurotransmitter excretion test including 5-hydroxyindoleacetate, vanilmandelate, and homovanillate
- A comprehensive digestive stool analysis with an additional intestinal permeability (leaky gut) test
- A comprehensive, customized blood chemistry panel that included vitamin D, HbA1c, homocysteine, full thyroid panel including TSH, fT3, fT4, and thyroid antibodies, as well as iron panel with ferritin
- An individualized optimal nutrition (ION) panel including fatty acids, amino acids, intracellular minerals, organic acids, and antioxidants

Individual tests were run at the rate of one to two per month as finances were tight. Nonetheless, Anne was committed to "go for it," so we proceeded with testing at the rate she could afford.

The first tests we received back were the 24-hour comprehensive urine hormone test and the comprehensive neurotransmitter excretion test. Based on these tests, we started with the following strategy:

- Progesterone metabolites were extremely low. This was expected due to Anne's anxiety, as progesterone is necessary to sensitize GABA receptors.
- Total estrogens, E1, E2, and E3, and all estrogen metabolites were very low.
- Although low, her 2-OH estrone:16-OH estrone ratio was not ideal.
- Adequate estrogen is required to sensitize serotonin receptors.
- DHEA-S was borderline low, and the DHEA metabolites were also borderline low.
- Total cortisol was borderline low, but its metabolites were extremely low.
- Free T3 was slightly elevated.
- 5-HIAA was low, GABA low, catecholamine metabolites were in the upper normal range.

I first recommended 100 mg of bio-identical progesterone cream (a relatively modest dosage) taken from day 12 to the first menstrual bleed of her menstrual cycle.

I also recommended a 200-mg dose of a sublingual pharmaGABA nutritional supplement, taken at least once per day but more often if she was particularly anxious.

Within 10 days her anxiety had improved 85% to 90%, along with some lessening of fatigue, possibly since progesterone is a precursor steroid for cortisol production.

Anne was very encouraged and motivated to continue with care.

The next intervention was to start a very low dosage (0.25 mg) of bio-identical Biest® cream (estradiol + estriol), along with 50 mg of 5-HTP (an amino acid that is a precursor to serotonin) TID to enhance the production of serotonin and the sensitization of the serotonin receptors.

Taking extra precaution because of the family history of breast cancer, I prescribed

- DIM (Di-indolymethane, a phytonutrient found in cruciferous vegetables and known to support estrogen metabolism)
- Calcium-D-glucarate (supports glucuronidation of estrogen in phase 2 detox)
- A combination methyl donor product (P-5-P, methylcobalamin, 5-MTHF, betaine and R-5-P)

These three additions helped to support liver phase II detoxification of estrogens (especially the potentially carcinogenic 16-OH estrone) via sulfation, glucuronidation, and methylation.

This small addition of estrogens, 5-HTP, and the estrogen detoxifying agents made another big improvement in Anne's care. She now felt that a dark cloud had lifted, and she began to enjoy life again. Her anxious depression was virtually gone.

I chose to not prescribe any DHEA because it can be antagonistic to GABA, plus I was hoping that her low DHEA levels would improve with better sleep.

A 3-week experiment with very low-dose cortisol (2 mg in the morning and 2 mg at noon) improved her energy greatly, and Anne began to sleep through the night. This confirmed my suspicion that she was waking after a few hours of sleep because she did not have enough glucocorticoid activity to sustain her blood sugar throughout the night, thus epinephrine levels would elevate due to hypoglycemia and wake her up.

I then switched the low-dose cortisol to my favorite adaptogenic herb for women, *Eleutherococcus senticosus* (Siberian ginseng), and this allowed her body to produce adequate cortisol on its own. Her sleep issues were now resolved.

Now Anne said she was "back" and very happy with her results. I recommended we retest her hormones in another month and suggested she have someone in her own city take over her care. I felt it was not worthwhile to spend the money on the ION panel since she was doing so well. I recommended a concentrated fish oil supplement and high-quality multivitamin along with continued improvements in her diet.

Ann said that she had already done her blood tests and her comprehensive digestive stool analysis (CDSA) with intestinal permeability (IP), and would like to fly in one more time to go over these.

Her CDSA revealed significant dysbiosis including a high concentration of a rare paramecium, lowered amounts of beneficial probiotics, and a moderate *Candida* yeast overgrowth. I decided to temporarily prescribe low-dose DHEA to help upregulate her intestinal immunity while I gave her an herbal formula to kill off the unfriendly microbes; plus, I recommended natural sauerkraut instead of probiotics. Within 5 weeks her joint pain was gone.

Her blood results showed low iron and borderline low ferritin, so we discussed her vegetarian diet and how to obtain adequate iron via her diet. This helped to resolve her postural hypotension which I theorized was caused by low cortisol and low blood volume.

Anne decided to spend 8 summer weeks in Boulder, Colorado, where I practiced at that time, and follow-up testing allowed us to continue with appropriate nutrient dosages and to track our progress.

We achieved great success with this treatment strategy. It was gratifying that her most distressing symptom, the anxious depression, resolved quite quickly with low-dose progesterone, very low-dose estrogen, and the two neurotransmitter-related nutrients.

RESOLUTION OF GAD, POSTPARTUM-ONSET OCD, AND COMORBID ALOPECIA WITH NUTRIGENOMIC INTERVENTIONS

Kelly Brogan, MD, ABHIM
Integrative Psychiatry
New York, New York

The patient is a 36-year-old married female, employed as a librarian, with a history of generalized anxiety, nightmares, nail biting, and self-medication of social anxiety with cocaine and alcohol. She presented for consultation around alternatives to medication.

She described the above symptoms as chronic, along with repeated intrusive catastrophic images (e.g., after her dog went in an elevator, of his being mangled by the leash getting caught), and vivid, violent nightmares beginning postpartum (4 years prior). She noted alopecia (areata) just prior to presentation, which made her concerned about more systemic imbalances.

She endorsed anhedonia secondary to anxiety around task completion and socializing, and described feelings of hopelessness related to living her "entire life in this state" and "never being present." She denied any significant stressors, and described her anxiety as self-generated.

She endorsed persistent hunger, with irritability if more than 2 hours lapse without eating. There were no other complaints around appetite or sleep (besides the nightmares). Her energy was described as medium to low. There was no history of panic, compulsions, or eating disordered behaviors.

She experienced complete resolution of her psychiatric and physical symptoms within 6 months of dietary change, relaxation response, and targeted nutraceuticals.

PREVIOUS PSYCHIATRIC HISTORY

The patient described the onset of violent nightmares, as well as chronic nail biting, at age 4 to 5. Tearfulness and poor adjustment in college yielded a prescription for Adderall®, which she took for 2 months. She discontinued the Adderall because of black-outs when drinking alcohol.

She describes long-standing social anxiety and difficulty "looking people in the eye," with associated binge drinking and cocaine use.

She had been treated previously with psychotherapy, acupuncture, self-administered Valerian root (with good effect), and Wellbutrin for smoking cessation.

There is no clear history of depression, mania, panic, obsessive-compulsive disorder (OCD), psychosis, or self-injury. There is no suicidal ideation or planning. And there is no eating-disordered behavior.

SUBSTANCE ABUSE HISTORY

The patient reports nightly alcohol (one glass of wine) since college. She uses cocaine approximately one time per month. She smokes approximately three cigarettes on the weekends.

MEDICAL HISTORY

Height 5 foot, 6 inches; weight 145 lbs
Menarche at age 12; regular cycles
G2 P1, termination at age 19, daughter born October 7, epidural, breastfed 3 months
Mirena IUD recently placed
She complains of significant PMS, including irritability, moodiness, and leg aching
Alopecia areata
Anemia
Headaches, occasional
Bunion surgery

DIET AND EXERCISE

Diet: Her typical diet includes coffee, beans, avocado wrap, yogurt with granola, sandwiches, and tomato soup.

She eats meat, eggs, fish, baked goods, and dark chocolate.
She uses olive oil to cook.

Allergies: Pitted fruits and raw nuts
No complaints on review of systems. Has a daily bowel movement.
Exercise: recently competed in a triathalon, does Yoga once/month.

MEDICATIONS/SUPPLEMENTS

She was generally inconsistent with the following:

Multivitamin
Omega-3 fatty acids
Iron
Vitamin D3

FAMILY HISTORY

Father: depression, anxiety, history of hallucinogen use
Maternal: ETOH abuse on mother's side of the family

SOCIAL HISTORY

The patient was born and raised in New Jersey—the second child after an infant death. Her mother was 22 when she conceived the patient. There were no notable pregnancy or milestone issues.

The patient is the eldest of six siblings. Her mother attended nursing school, and her father held "many jobs" in addition to the couple running a drop-in center, in the house, for troubled teens up until the patient was 4 years old. She describes her parents as "very much in love," but the household as chaotic, stating that she was largely responsible for care of her siblings beginning at age 9. The family often gave refuge to wayward individuals, and the patient feels that this impacted the quality of her family life.

She attended college in Maine for 2 years prior to leaving and traveling (Wisconsin; Massachusetts) when funds ran low. She completed college in New Jersey and worked for 6 years in a magazine layout department before achieving a master's degree in library science. She now works at the New York Public Library as a librarian.

She met her husband in college, and they have been married for 10 years. She was ambivalent about having children but states that she "worships" her daughter, and the couple are satisfied with their current family structure. She states that her husband is very private, and that he "doesn't deal with his issues directly." He travels most days of the week.

They have two dogs.

MENTAL STATUS EXAM

The patient was dressed in casual attire with shoulder-length, dark hair, glasses, earrings, no makeup. She was cooperative and friendly throughout the session, and was initially soft spoken. Speech was normal. Mood was "overwhelmed." Affect was reactive, stable, and appropriate. Thought process was logical and linear. Thought content—no suicidal ideation (SI)/homicidal ideation (HI)/paranoid ideation (PI)/auditory hallucinations (AH)/visual hallucinations (VH), she was focused on chronic symptoms. Insight and judgment were good. She was alert and oriented ×3.

IMPRESSION

Axis I: GAD, OCD, r/o substance-induced anxiety/mood disorder, r/o alcohol abuse/dependence, r/o cocaine abuse, r/o nicotine abuse
Axis II: deferred
Axis III: alopecia, anemia, PMS, headaches
Axis IV: husband's travel schedule, chronic symptoms
Axis V: 70

TREATMENT

I recommended a modified Paleo diet (grain free, diary free, whole foods) for 30 days, to include organic/pastured meat, wild fish, pastured eggs, low glycemic fruit, nuts, and seeds, and organic vegetables, excluding starch.

We incorporated starchy root vegetables and potatoes after one month.

I also recommended:

Total amino solution—two before meals
L-theanine—one twice daily
Magnesium threonate—one to three at night
PharmaGABA 200 mg prn anxiety
Chromium 600 mcg daily
Selenium 200 mcg daily
Zinc glycinate 30 mg daily
N-acetylcysteine 900 mg bid
Methylated B complex

ONE-MONTH FOLLOW-UP

Her 24-hour salivary cortisol testing revealed normal levels upon awakening and mid-day, but elevated cortisol by 6 p.m., and significantly elevated cortisol at bedtime.
I added:
Cortisol manager—three before dinner and three before bed

TWO-MONTH FOLLOW-UP

Comprehensive stool testing revealed:

Chymotrypsin (digestive enzyme) 0.6 (0.9–26.8 U/g)
Rare meat fibers
2+ Lactobacillus (should be 3–4+)
4+ Citrobacter, 4+ Bacillus (these are potential pathogens at this level)

I added:

MicroDefense (probiotics) for 2 weeks before starting VSL-3 capsules (probiotics)—
    one before breakfast and dinner for a month, then one a day with food thereafter.
GlutAleoMin (for gut healing)—one scoop twice a day for a month, then once a day for a month
Panxyme (digestive enzyme)—with each meal

She enrolled in a mindfulness-based stress reduction meditation course 2 months after presentation.

OUTCOME AND FOLLOW-UP

Two months later, the patient experienced resolution of anxiety and irritability and had increased stress resilience.
    She had mild obsessive ruminations, and less frequent intrusive images.
    She had notable resolution of food cravings and her occasional headaches.
    Her stool test recommendations were implemented, along with replacement of the Mirena IUD (that had synthetic hormones) with a copper IUD.
    She presented 6 weeks later stating that her alopecia had resolved in its entirety, as had her presenting anxiety symptoms.
    She reported feeling calm, stable, and without physical complaints.

Discussion

This patient exemplifies the role of the gut-brain axis in chronic disease, and the nature of psychiatric symptoms such as depression and anxiety in a greater physiologic context of imbalance. There is a precedent for considering the microbiota as central to behavioral symptoms, including discussion of OCD as a result of dysbiosis.

This patient was minimally breastfed, exposed to toxicants, stress, and a nutrient-poor diet. The origins of her dysbiosis are likely the cumulative impact of these evolutionary mismatches.

A review by Dinan et al.[3] encompasses the clinical basis for the use of probiotics in mental health, with reference to animal studies in which behavioral changes resulted from exposure to bacterial strains such as *Bifidobacterium* and *Lactobacillus*. In placebo-controlled trials in humans, measures of anxiety, chronic fatigue, and depression and anxiety associated with irritable bowel syndrome have shown positive outcomes with probiotic administration.

The role of gut microbiota in epigenetic expression encompasses a myriad of physiologic tasks, including the following (Selhub et al.[4]):

- Direct protection of the intestinal barrier
- Influence on local and systemic antioxidant status, reduction in lipid peroxidation
- Direct, microbial-produced neurochemical production, for example, gamma-aminobutyric acid (GABA)
- Indirect influence on neurotransmitter or neuropeptide production
- Prevention of stress-induced alterations to overall intestinal microbiota
- Direct activation of neural pathways between gut and brain
- Limitation of inflammatory cytokine production
- Modulation of neurotrophic chemicals, including brain-derived neurotrophic factor (BDNF)
- Limitation of carbohydrate malabsorption
- Improvement of nutritional status, for example, omega-3 fatty acids, minerals, dietary phytochemicals
- Limitation of small intestinal bacterial overgrowth
- Reduction of amine or uremic toxin burden
- Limitation of gastric or intestinal pathogens
- Analgesic properties

Given widespread fermentation practices in traditional cultures, it appears that this dietary wisdom may serve to ameliorate gut-based inflammation and promote optimal nutrient assimilation as described in Dinan et al.[3]: "Traditional dietary practices have completely divergent effects of blood LPS (lipopolysaccharides or endotoxins in the outer membrane of Gram-negative bacteria); significant reductions (38%) have been noted after a one-month adherence to a prudent (traditional) diet, while the Western diet provokes LPS elevations."

In addition to increasing bioavailability and production of minerals, and neurochemicals, fermented foods actually produce methylfolate, an activated form of folate required for methylation, fatty acid and brain chemical synthesis, detox, and gene expression.

Because of the complex co-evolution of bacterial strains, cultivated through our food supply, and complementary to our inner microbiomes, we have an opportunity to use therapeutic foods to re-educate an immune system that has been drawn off course. Additionally, psychobiotics (probiotics) have the potential to modulate multiple different relevant factors at once:

"This could manifest, behaviorally, via magnified antioxidant and anti-inflammatory activity, reduction of intestinal permeability and the detrimental effects of LPS, improved glycemic control, positive influence on nutritional status (and therefore neurotransmission and neuropeptide production), direct production of GABA, and other bioactive chemicals, as well as a direct role in gut-to-brain communication via a beneficial shift in the intestinal microbiota itself."[4]

It is therefore compelling to consider the power of reconnecting to the natural world through our food; communicating through our guts to our brains, that nutrients are plentiful, our bodies are safe, and that our inflammatory systems can be put at ease. It is under these circumstances that the infinite complexity of the endocrine, immune, and gastrointestinal systems can play out, unhindered in support of mental health and wellness.

Labs:

Prediabetes - HbA1c 5.8
Hashimoto thyroiditis – thyroglobulin Ab 40.73
ANA + 1:80
hsCRP 8.16 (quite inflamed)

These were all normalized 6 months later.

		9/12	3/13
Glucose	70–99 mg/dL	92	84
Total cholesterol	<200 mg/dL	134	148
HgA1c	<5.7%	5.8	5.1
Free T3	1.7–3.7 pg/mL	3.63	2.96
TSH	0.35–4.94 uIU/mL	1.8	1.8
Thyroglobulin Ab	<4.11 IU/mL	40.73	9.62
Free T4	0.70–2.48 ng/dL	0.91	0.93
MTHFR	Compound heterozygote		
Vitamin D	30–100 ng/mL	28.2	32.4
ANA	<1:80	1:80, homogenous	Negative
Hs-CRP <3 mg/dL	<1.0	8.16	1.07

A FUNCTIONAL APPROACH AND TESTOSTERONE REPLACEMENT FOR DEPRESSION IN A 75-YEAR-OLD MAN

Kat Toups, MD, DFAPA
Functional Medicine Psychiatry
Walnut Creek, California

Mr. A is a 75-year-old successful businessman, retired from two previous careers, who was still actively working when he developed his first ever case of major depression in 2011.

He was profoundly depressed, suicidal, uninterested in eating, had major insomnia, and was not interested in any social contact.

At that time, he was treated successfully with Wellbutrin and Remeron, and returned to his baseline after 9 months. He also returned back to work.

Mr. A remained well for almost 2 years, and had continued Wellbutrin, but stopped Remeron during that time. After two nights of not being able to sleep in February 2014, he plunged back into another episode of depression, with symptoms similar to the first episode, although he did not experience suicidal ideation with the second episode.

Remeron was restarted for his insomnia with good results with regard to sleep. For the continued depression, Mr. A was tried on Effexor, which made him sweat excessively, and then tried on multiple antidepressants and Abilify in addition to the Wellbutrin and Remeron, without any benefit.

The patient and his wife came to see me to explore a functional medicine approach since he was not improving. At that time, he was taking Remeron, Wellbutrin, and Pristiq®.

The patient's presenting symptoms were

- No desire to interact with others—he preferred to watch TV all day and was previously very gregarious socially and occupationally
- Loss of appetite—severe, with undesired weight loss
- Lack of energy
- Poor concentration
- Lack of confidence
- Excessive preoccupation and worry about his need to regain weight he had lost from depression

Mr. A's medical history included a long history of ulcerative colitis, hypothyroidism, type 2 diabetes, and hyperlipidemia. He was on medications for several of these conditions, including treatment with a Statin medication and no CoQ10 replacement. (Note: Statins are known to completely block CoQ10 absorption, so it is advisable to augment with CoQ10 to prevent myopathies and other sequelae of blocking this important antioxidant.)

It is interesting to note that with this "depression," this patient had no feelings of sadness. When I see depression in an elderly patient with no prior history, it often can portend the development of Alzheimer's disease, but this patient was extremely intact cognitively, with a sharp intellect and quick sense of humor.

It definitely seemed advisable to initiate a functional medicine evaluation, as I suspected inflammation to be a potential culprit in his symptomatology. As Mr. A had a history of ulcerative colitis and limited food intake with his depression, it was important to evaluate nutritional factors, as well as to optimize his nutrition, glucose control, lipids, hormones, and exercise.

As Mr. A had many chronic illnesses that were inflammatory in nature, I had him start by eating a diet of whole foods (no processed foods), and also to eliminate gluten, which is known to be inflammatory even if one is not allergic. I asked him to minimize other grains as well, since carbs = sugar, and his glycemic control was poor. I advised incorporating more vegetables in place of the carbs, to consider juicing vegetables to increase his phytonutrients and antioxidants, and to strive for eating "all the colors of the rainbow" every day. (Note: Juicing is a good way to maximize servings of vegetables, and juiced foods can be more easily absorbed by people with impaired gut functioning.)

I also asked Mr. A to eat lots of healthy fats at every meal: coconut oil and coconut milk, avocados, olive oil, free range meat and chicken, wild-caught fish, nuts, and seeds. The statin treatment had improved his lipids at the expense of his brain. As the brain is 65% fat, when the lipid levels get too low, the brain can suffer. (Statins now carry a U.S. Food and Drug Administration [FDA] warning about memory loss with use.)

As for exercise, I asked Mr. A to endeavor to at least take a walk every day. This can be good for energy, brain, and depression, as well as blood pressure and glucose control.

Screening labs revealed poor glucose control (this is also a side effect of statin medications), low vitamin D (27), low CoQ10, and a TSH of 1.9 with free T4 and free T3 at the bottom of the range, while reverse T3 was normal. (This is "subclinical hypothyroidism" with an impaired brain axis since the TSH was not elevated, as it should be with low free thyroid hormone levels.)

The other striking finding was that Mr. A's testosterone level was quite low: 4.1 (6.6–18.1), as was his DHEA-S level. His hs-estradiol was not elevated, so he was not aromatizing toward estrogen. LH was also quite elevated.

His comprehensive stool analysis revealed very low levels of healthy probiotic bacteria, with subsequent overgrowth of multiple commensal strains of bacteria. He also had poor levels of his pancreatic elastase digestive enzymes and impaired fat digestion, as well as a slightly increased lactoferrin and red blood cells consistent with his latent ulcerative colitis.

In addition to the dietary changes already instituted, we added digestive enzymes to further aid in food breakdown and nutrient absorption, as well as VSL-3, a very high-potency probiotic.

He was also started on vitamin D 10,000 IU per day, fish oil with an EPA:DHA ratio of 3:2–1.5 g BID, and high-potency B vitamins. All three of these nutrients are vitally important for production of neurotransmitters, methylation (he had no MTHFR mutations, but still needed methylation cofactors), and brain function. CoQ-10, a potent anti-oxidant and the rate-limiting step for mitochondrial production of ATP for energy, was also added at 120 mg BID.

Cytomel 5 mcg BID was started for additional thyroid support, given his low energy and depression.

We added turmeric (curcumin) 500 mg BID, both for his depression as well as its anti-inflammatory and healing properties for his GI disease. (There is a randomized study showing turmeric worked as well as Prozac for depression, and other research showing turmeric is as effective as mesalamine for colitis.)

Pristiq was slowly weaned, as it had not been effective and was possibly contributing to the flatness and apathy that Mr. A was experiencing.

Four weeks later, Mr. A reported he was feeling better. He was more engaging with people, doing more social things and exercising again. He had altered his diet, but had not fully eliminated gluten.

I had Mr A consult with his urologist about starting testosterone, since he had a past history of an elevated PSA (a possible contraindication for testosterone therapy), though it was normal when I evaluated him. The brain has testosterone receptors, and I felt that replacing the deficient testosterone might have a beneficial effect for his brain functioning. The urologist re-tested and confirmed the low testosterone levels, and agreed with a trial of testosterone.

At our next follow-up, Mr. A said that as soon as he started using Androgel®, he felt completely fine in 10 days. Previously forcing himself to eat, his appetite had returned to normal. His sleep was good, and he began tapering his Remeron. He woke up feeling rested.

Mr. A immediately returned back to work and resumed his successful real estate practice.

He reported that his energy was good, and he was exercising regularly. He felt enthusiastic about life again. This was quite a change, after spending almost a year sitting in a chair in front of the TV.

REFERENCES

1. Lamott, A. 1993. *Operating Instructions: A Journal of My Son's First Year.* New York, NY: Pantheon.
2. Raffelock, D., *A Natural Guide to Pregnancy and Postpartum Health*, 2002, New York: Avery.
3. Dinan, T.G., Stanton, C., and Cryan, J.F. 2013. Psychobiotics: A novel class of psychotropic. *Biol Psychiatry* 74(10): 720–726. doi:10.1016/j.biopsych.2013.05.001. Epub 2013 Jun 10. Review. [PubMed PMID: 23759244].
4. Selhub, E.M., Logan, A.C., and Bested, A.C. 2014. Fermented foods, microbiota, and mental health: Ancient practice meets nutritional psychiatry. *J Physiol Anthropol* 33: 2. doi:10.1186/1880-6805-33-2. Review. [PubMed PMID: 24422720]. [PubMed Central PMCID: PMC3904694].

Index

Printed in the United States
by Baker & Taylor Publisher Services

Printed in the United States
by Baker & Taylor Publisher Services